ATHEROSCLEROSIS AND AUTOIMMUNITY

ATHEROSCLEROSIS AND AUTOIMMUNITY

Editors:

Yehuda Shoenfeld
Department of Medicine 'B'
The Research Center of Autoimmune Diseases
Sheba Medical Center, Tel-Hashomer
Sackler Faculty of Medicine, Tel-Aviv University
Israel

Dror Harats
The Institute of Lipid and Atherosclerosis Research
Sheba Medical Center, Tel-Hashomer
Israel

Georg Wick
The Institute of Biomedical Aging Research
Austrian Academy of Science
Institute for General and Experimental Pathology
University of Innsbruck
Medical School, Innsbruck
Austria

Section V – Anti-Endothelial Cell Antibodies and Atherosclerosis
Edited by Pierre Youinou, *Brest, France* and
Pier-Luigi Meroni, *Milano, Italy*

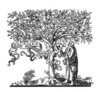

2001
ELSEVIER
Amsterdam – Lausanne – New York – Oxford – Shannon – Singapore – Tokyo

ELSEVIER SCIENCE B.V.
Sara Burgerhartstraat 25
P.O. Box 211, 1000 AE Amsterdam, The Netherlands

Library of Congress Cataloging in Publication Data
A catalog record from the Library of Congress has been applied for.

ISBN: 0-444-50669-1

⊗ The paper used in this publication meets the requirements of ANSI/NISO Z39.48-1992 (Permanence of Paper).
Printed in The Netherlands.

Dedication

We dedicate this book to our wives:
Irit, Rika, and Traudi

Thanks

We are indebted to Ms. Rachel Guri and Ms. Sara Tessler
for their secretarial assistance.

PREFACE

Atherosclerosis is a prolonged process that starts in the second decade of life, progresses slowly and the clinical manifestations appear in the 4–5th decade onwards. The early lesions, i.e., fatty streaks, may be seen already during fetal development and regress soon after birth [1], but reappear in early adolescence and may progress into more complex lesions, that take many years to regress [2]. Evidence based on large studies provided proof that hypercholesterolemia is a leading risk factor for atherogenesis [3]. In addition, other risk factors, such as hypertension, smoking, diabetes, low HDL, homocysteinemia were identified.

Within the last two decades it was recognized that risk factors interact to promote development of coronary artery disease (CAD) [3]. Thus, smoking as a single risk factor, manifests clinically as a respiratory disease, but in conjunction with high LDL cholesterol levels enhances CAD very markedly [4]. The same is true for hypertension and diabetes, that in presence of hypercholesterolemia will increase the risk for CAD several-fold. It has been generally accepted that the known risk factors account for only 50% of patients with CAD [5]. One plausible explanation for underestimation of the contribution of known risk factors to mortality and morbidity of CAD could be that the definition of "normality" requires more rigorous re-evaluation. Three decades ago, 300 mg/dL of plasma cholesterol, 180 mg/dL of LDL cholesterol, blood pressure of 160/95 mm Hg, were considered to be within *upper normal* limits. Information from large-scale intervention studies for secondary prevention of CAD permitted to redefine these limits. Thus the upper normal limit for LDL cholesterol has been continuously decreasing to <100 mg/dL, and recently even <80 mg/dL is considered as a therapeutic goal. The latter values start to approach those found in free living non-human primates, who also develop atherosclerosis when exposed to "western type" diets.

Since the formulation by R.Ross of the "response to injury hypothesis of atherosclerosis" [6–9], it became accepted that this process is an outcome of a chronic inflammatory reaction in the artery. This book deals with knowledge accrued in the past decade concerning the role of immunity in the initiation and perpetuation of atherosclerosis [10–13]. The participation of monocyte derived macrophages and lymphocytes, the latter mostly activated T-cells [14] pointed to the involvement of the immune system in this inflammatory reaction. There is convincing evidence that LDL, once modified by macrophages within the arterial wall, can be responsible for T-cell activation [15]. Circulating antibodies to oxidized LDL have been demonstrated in animals and humans [15]. Immune activation was invoked also for other antigens, such as heat shock proteins [16, 17]. The above mentioned antigens were found to be present in atherosclerotic lesions [15, 18]. In IL-4 knockout mice fewer atherosclerotic lesions after heat shock protein injection were seen, indicating an important role of this cytokine in the response to heat shock protein [19]. Involvement of CD40 and CD40 ligand in atherogenesis (mediators of immune responses) is supported by their expression in most cellular elements of the atheroma [20]. In LDL receptor deficient mice, injection of anti-CD40L antibodies reduced atherosclerosis markedly [20]. In addition, various infections of microbial (chlamydia pneumoniae) or viral (adenoviruses and herpesviridae) origin [21, 22] have been proposed as candidates for vascular injury which may culminate in atherogenesis. Among them herpesviruses were shown to activate the coagulation system and accelerate progression of atherosclerosis [23].

The immune approach to atherosclerosis led also to the use of immunization against oxidized LDL. Thus injection of homologous malonyl dialdehyde modified LDL (MDA-LDL) to WHHL rabbits resulted in reduction of atherosclerosis [24]. Similar results were obtained also in apoE deficient mice hyperimmunized with homologous MDA-LDL [25].

On the other hand, immunization to heat shock proteins of mice fed an atherogenic diet resulted in enhancement of fatty streak formation [26]. In analogy, when LDL receptor deficient [27] and apoE deficient mice were immunized to β-2-glycoprotein I (a target of autoimmune anticardiolipin antibodies) they responded with an accelerated development of atherosclerosis [28]. This antigen was found also in human atherosclerotic lesions co-localizing with CD4-lymphocytes [29]. When primed lymphocytes from β2GPI immunized mice were injected into LDL-receptor deficient mice, atherosclerotic lesions were enhanced [30].

Future research that will be designed to test the relative importance of the immune hypothesis in atherogenesis will determine the approach to be taken in CAD prevention and treatment. In the meantime, introduction of a primary prevention program that encompasses all known risk factors for CAD, throughout the school curriculum, seems to us a logical approach, and with the escalating costs of clinical care of CAD becomes an inescapable conclusion.

Olga Stein and Yechezkiel Stein
Jerusalem, 16th July 2000

REFERENCES

1. Napoli C, D'Artmiento FP, Mancini FP, Postiglione A, Witztum JL, Palumbo G, Palinski W. Fatty streak formation occurs in human fetal aortas and is greatly enhanced by maternal hypercholesterolemia. Intimal accumulation of low density lipoprotein and its oxidation precede monocyte recruitment into early atherosclerotic lesions. J Clin Invest 1997;100:2680–2690.
2. Stein Y, Stein O. Does therapeutic intervention achieve slowing of progression or bona fide regression of atherosclerotic lesions? Arterioscler Thromb Vasc Biol 2000; In press .
3. Prevention of Coronary Heart Disease: Scientific Background and New Clinical Guidelines. Recommendations of the European Atherosclerosis Society prepared by the International Task Force for Prevention of Coronary Heart Disease. Nutr Metab Cardiovasc Dis 1992;2:113–156.
4. Stein Y, Harats D, Stein O. Why is smoking a major risk factor for coronary heart disease in hyperlipidemic subjects? Annals N Y Acad Sci 1992;686:66–71.
5. Oliver MF. Prevention of coronary heart disease – propaganda, promises, problems, and prospects. Circulation 1986;73:1–9.
6. Ross R, Glomset JA. The pathogenesis of atherosclerosis. N Engl J Med 1976;295:369–377; 420–425.
7. Ross R. The pathogenesis of atherosclerosis – an update. N Engl J Med 1986;314:488–500.
8. Ross R. The pathogenesis of atherosclerosis: a perspective for the 1990s. Nature 1993;362:801–809.
9. Ross R. Atherosclerosis – an inflammatory disease. N Engl J Med 1999;340:115–126.
10. Witztum JL, Palinski W. Editorial. Are immunological mechanisms relevant for the development of atherosclerosis? Clin Immunol 1999;90:153–156.
11. Wick G, Perschinka H, Xu Q. Autoimmunity and atherosclerosis. Am Heart J 1999;138:5444–5449.
12. Palinski W, Witztum JL. Immune responses to oxidative neoepitopes on LDL and phospholipids modulate the development of atherosclerosis. J Int Med 2000;247:371–380.
13. Nicoletti A, Caligiuri G, Hansson GK. Immunomodulation of atherosclerosis: myth and reality. J Int Med 2000;247:397–405.
14. Hansson GK. Cell-mediated immunity in atherosclerosis. Curr Opin Lipidol 1997;8:301–311.
15. Steinberg D, Witztum JL. Lipoproteins, lipoprotein oxidation, and atherogenesis. In "Molecular Basis of Cardiovascular Disease" (KR Chien, Ed.), Saunders, Philadelphia, 1999:458–475.
16. Xu W, Dietrich H, Steiner HJ, Gown AM, Mikuz G, Kaufmann SHE, Wick G. Induction of arteriosclerosis in normocholesterolemic rabbits by immunization with heat shock protein 65. Arterioscler Thromb 1992;12:789–799.
17. Kol A, Lichtman AH, Finberg RW, Libby P, Kurt-Jones EA. Cutting edge: heat shock protein (HSP) 60 activates the innate immune response: CD14 is an essential receptor for HSP60 activation of mononuclear cells. J Immunol 2000;1644;13–17.
18. Berberian PA, Myers W, Tytell M, Challa V, Bond MG. Immuno- histochemical localization of heat shock protein-70 in normal-appearing and atherosclerotic specimens of human arteries. Am J Pathol 1990;136:71–80.
19. George J, Shoenfeld Y, Gilburd B, Afek A, Shaish A, Harats D. Requisite role for interleukin-4 in the acceleration of fatty streaks induced by heat shock protein 65 or *Mycobacterium tuberculosis*. Circ Res 2000;86: 1203–1210.
20. Mach F, Schonbeck U, Sukhova GK, Atkinson E, Libby P. Reduction of atherosclerosis in mice by inhibition of CD40 signalling. Nature 1998;394:200–203.
21. Danesh J, Collins R, Peto R. Chronic infections and coronary heart disease: is there a link? Lancet

1997;350:430–436.

22. Nieto FJ. Infections and atherosclerosis: new clues from an old hypothesis? Am J Epidemiol 1998;148:937–948.

23. Nicholson AC, Hajjar DP. Herpesviruses and thrombosis: activation of coagulation on the endothelium. Clin Chim Acta 1999;286:23–29.

24. Palinski W, Miller E, Witztum JL. Immunization of LDL receptor-deficient rabbits with homologous malondialdehyde-modified LDL reduced atherogenesis. Proc Natl Acad Sci USA 1995;92:821–825.

25. George J, Afek A, Gilburd B, Levkovitz H, Shaish A, Goldberg I, Kopolovic Y, Wick G, Shoenfeld Y, Harats D. Hyperimmunization of apo-E-deficient mice with homologous malondialdehyde low-density lipoprotein suppresses early atherogenesis. Atherosclerosis 1998;138:147–152.

26. George J, Shoenfeld Y, Afek A, Gilburd B, Keren P, Shaish A, Kopolovic J, Wick G, Harats D. Enhanced fatty streak formation in C57BL/6J mice by immunization with heat shock protein-65. Arterioscler Thromb Vasc Biol 1999;19:505–510.

27. George J, Afek A, Gilburd B, Blank M, Levy Y, Aron-Maor A, Levkovitz H, Shaish A, Goldberg I, Kopolovic J, Shoenfeld Y. Induction of early atherosclerosis in LDL receptor deficient mice immunized with β2GPI. Circulation 1998;15:1108–1105.

28. Afek A, George J, Shoenfeld Y, Gilburd B, Levy Y, Shaish A, Keren P, Janackovic Z, Goldberg I, Kopolovic J, Harats D. Enhancement of atherosclerosis in beta-2-glycoprotein I-immunized apolipoprotein E-deficient mice. Pathobiology 1999;67:19–25.

29. George J, Harats D, Gilburd B, Afek A, Levy Y, Schneiderman J, Barshack I, Kopolovic J, Shoenfeld Y. Immunolocalization of β_2-glycoprotein I (apolipoprotein H) to human atherosclerotic plaques. Potential implications for lesion progression. Circulation 1999;99:2227–2230.

30. George J, Gilburd B, Afek A, Levy Y, Kopolovic J, Harats D, Shoenfeld Y. Adoptive transfer of β2 glycoprotein I (β2GPI)-reactive lymphocytes enhances atherosclerosis in LDL receptor deficient mice. Circulation 2000;102:1822–1827.

List of Contributors

Olga Amengual
Lupus Research Institute
The Rayne Institute
St. Thomas' Hospital
London
United Kingdom

Tatsuya Atsumi
Department of Medicine II
Hokkaido University
School of Medicine
Sapporo
Japan

Paul A. Bacon
Department of Rheumatology
University of Birmingham
Birmingham
United Kingdom

Khalil Bdeir
Department of Pathology
Laboratory Medicine
University of Pennsylvania
Philadelphia, PA 19104
USA

II. Michael Belmont
Hospital for Joint Diseases
NYU Medical Center
New York
USA

A. Biasiolo
Department of Clinical and Experimental Medicine
Thrombosis Center
University of Padova
Via Gattamelata 64
I-35128 Padova
Italy

Miri Blank
Department of Medicine B and the
Research Center of Autoimmune Diseases
Sheba Medical Center
Tel Hashomer
Israel

Anne Bodron
Laboratory of Immunology
Institut de Synergie des Sciences
et de la Santé
Brest University Medical School
Brest
France

Dan Buskila
Rheumatic Disease Unit and Epidermiology Department
Soroka Medical Center
Faculty of Health Sciences
Ben Gurion University of the Negev
Beer Sheva
Israel

Richard Cervera
Systemic Autoimmune Diseases Unit
Hospital clinic
Barcelona, Catalonia
Spain

Jacques Chevalier
INSERM U430
Hôpital Broussais
Paris
France

Douglas B. Cines
Department of Pathology
Laboratory Medicine
University of Pennsylvania
Philadelphia, PA 19104
USA

T. Del Ros
Department of Medical and Surgical Sciences
University of Padova
Via Gattamelata 64
I-35128 Padova
Italy

Mordechai Deutsch
The Jerome Schottenstein Cellscan Center
Department of Physics
Bar-lan University
Ramat Gan
Israel

B. Devulder
Internal Medicine Department
University Hospital of Lille
59035 Lille Cedex
France

Maryvonne Dueymes
Laboratory of Immunology
Institut de Synergie des Sciences
et de la Santé
Brest University Medical School
Brest
France

Jean-Paul Duong Van Huyen
Laboratoire d'Anatomie Pathologique
Hôpital Européen Georges Pompidou
France

P. Duriez
Research Laboratory on Lipids and Atherosclerosis
INSERM U325
Pasteur Institute of Lille
Lille
France

Stephen E. Epstein
Cardiovascular Research Institute
Washington Hospital Center
110 Irving Street
Washington, DC 20010
USA

Mario Febbraio
Center of Vascular Biology
Cornell University Medical College
1300 York Avenue
New York, NY 10021
USA

Josep Font
Systemic Autoimmune Diseases Unit
Hospital clinic
Barcelona, Catalonia
Spain

J. Frostegard
Department of Medicine and CMM
Karolinska Hospital
Karolinska Institutet
17176 Stockholm
Sweden

J-C. Fruchart
Research Laboratory on Lipids and Atherosclerosis
INSERM U325
Pasteur Institute of Lille
Lille
France

J. Bruce German
Department of Food Science & Technology
University of California at Davis
Davis, CA 95616
USA

Jacob George
Department of Medicine B and the
Research Center of Autoimmune Diseases
Sheba Medical Center
Tel Hashomer
Israel

M.E. Gershwin
Department of Rheumatology/Allergy and
Clinical Immunology
University of California at Davis
Davis, CA 95616
USA

Tzipora Goldkorn
Signal Transduction
UC Davis School of Medicine
TB149, Davis Campus
Davis, CA 95616
USA

Antonio M. Gotto, Jr
Center of Vascular Biology
Cornell University Medical College
1300 York Avenue
New York, NY 10021
USA

Sandeep Gupta
Department of Cardiology
Whipps Cross Hospital
Leytonstone
London E11 1 NR
United Kingdom

E. Hachulla
Internal Medicine Department
University Hospital of Lille
59035 Lille Cedex
France

David P. Hajjar
Weill Medical College of Cornell University
Department of Pathology, A-626
1300 York Avenue
New York, NY 10021
USA

Jihong Han
Center of Vascular Biology
Cornell University Medical College
1300 York Avenue
New York, NY 10021
USA

Göran K. Hansson
Center for Molecular Medicine L8:03
Karolinska Hospital
S-17176 Stockholm
Sweden

Dror Harats
Institute of Lipid and Atherosclerosis Research
Shcba Medical Center
Tel Hashomer, Sackler faculty of Medicine
Tel-Aviv University
Tel-Aviv
Israel

Abd Al-Roof Higazi
Department of Clinical Biochemistry
Hebrew University – Hadassah Medical Center
Jerusalem
IL-91120 Israel

Graham R.V. Hughes
Lupus Research Institute
The Rayne Institute
St. Thomas' Hospital
London
United Kingdom

Norman T. Ilowite
Schneider Children's Hospital
Long Island Jewish Medical Center
Albert Einstein College of Medicine
New Hyde Park, NY 11040
New York
USA

Miguel Ingelmo
Systemic Autoimmune Diseases Unit
Hospital clinic
Barcelona, Catalonia
Spain

Luigi Iuliano
Institute of Clinical Medcine I
University La Sapienza
Via del Policlinico 155
00185 Rome
Italy

Sònia Jiménez
Systemic Autoimmune Diseases Unit
Hospital clinic
Barcelona, Catalonia
Spain

Katsunori Jinnouchi
Second Department of Pathology
Kumamoto University
School of Medicine
Kumamoto 860-0811
Japan

Keiko Kaihara
Department of Cell Chemistry
Institute of Cellular and Molecular Biology
Okayama University Medical School
Okayama
Japan

Junko Kasahara
Department of Cell Chemistry
Institute of Cellular and Molecular Biology
Okayama University Medical School
Okayama
Japan

Srinivas V. Kaveri
INSERM U430
Hôpital Broussais
Paris
France

Michel D. Kazatchkine
INSERM U430
Hôpital Broussais
Paris
France

Munther A. Khamashta
Lupus Research Institute
The Rayne Institute
St. Thomas' Hospital
London
United Kingdom

G.D. Kitas
Department of Rheumatology
University of Birmingham
Birmingham
United Kingdom

Kazuko Kobayashi
Department of Cell Chemistry
Institute of Cellular and Molecular Biology
Okayama University Medical School
Okayama
Japan

Takao Koike
Department of Medicine II
Hokkaido University School of Medicine
Sapporo
Japan

Nitza Lahat
Lady Davis Carmel Medical Center
Bruce Rappaport Faculty of Medicine
7 Michal Street
Haifa, 34632
Israel

Marc Lambert
Internal Medicine Department
University Hospital of Lille
59035 Lille Cedex
France

Pnina Langevitz
The Heller Institute of Medical Research
Sheba Medical Center
Tel Hashomer and Sackler Faculty of Medicine
Tel Aviv University
Tel Aviv
Israel

Eduardo C. Lau
Specialty Laboratories, Inc.
Research Laboratory
2211 Michigan Avenue
Santa Monica, CA 90404
USA

S.N. Lavrentiadou
Signal Transduction
UC Davis School of Medicine
TB149, Davis Campus
Davis, CA 95616
USA

Yair Levi
Department of Medicine B and the
Research Center of Autoimmune Diseases
Sheba Medical Center
Tel Hashomer
Israel

Avi Livneh
The Heller Institute of Medical Research
Sheba Medical Center
Tel Hashomer and Sackler Faculty of Medicine
Tel Aviv University
Tel Aviv
Israel

Jukka Luoma
A.I. Virtanen Institute of Molecular Sciences
University of Kuopio
P.O. Box 1627
70211 Kuopio
Finland

Galina S. Marder
Long Island Jewish Medical Center
New York
USA

Eiji Matsuura
Department of Cell Chemistry
Institute of Cellular and Molecular Biology
Okayama University Medical School
Okayama
Japan

Werner-J. Mayet
First Medical Department
University of Mainz
Langenbeckstrasse 1
55101 Mainz
Germany

Pier Luigi Meroni
Allergy & Clinical Immunology Unit
Department of Internal Medicine
University of Milan
IRCCS Istituto Auxologico Italiano
Milan
Italy

Fausta Micheletta
Institute of Clinical Medcine I
University La Sapienza
Via del Policlinico 155
00185 Rome
Italy

U. Michon-Pasturel
Internal Medicine Department
University Hospital of Lille
59035 Lille Cedex
France

Gunda Millonig
Institute for Biomedical Aging Research
Austrian Academy of Sciences
Rennweg 10
A-6020 Innsbruck
Austria

Diana Milojevic
Schneider Children's Hospital
Long Island Jewish Medical Center
Albert Einstein College of Medicine
New Hyde Park, NY 11040
New York
USA

Outi Närvänen
A.I. Virtanen Institute of Molecular Sciences
University of Kuopio
P.O. Box 1627
70211 Kuopio
Finland

Lily Neumann
Rheumatic Disease Unit and Epidermiology
Department
Soroka Medical Center
Faculty of Health Sciences
Ben Gurion University of the Negev
Beer Sheva
Israel

Andrew C. Nicholson
Center of Vascular Biology
Cornell University Medical College
1300 York Ave
New York, NY
USA

Antonino Nicoletti
INSERM U430
Hôpital Broussais
Paris
France

Gerlinde Obermoser
Department of Dermatology
University of Innsbruck
Innsbruck
Austria

S. Frieda A. Pearce
Center of Vascular Biology
Cornell University Medical College
1300 York Avenue
New York, NY 10021
USA

Vittorio Pengo
Department of Clinical and Experimental Medicine
Thrombosis Center
University of Padova
Via Gattamelata 64
I-35128 Padova
Italy

Michelle Petri
Johns Hopkins University School of Medicine
Division of Rheumatology
1830E Monument street
Baltimore, MD 21205
USA

Sonja Praprotnik
Department of Rheumatology
University Medical Center
Ljubljana
Slovenia

Mordechai Pras
The Heller Institute of Medical Research
Sheba Medical Center
Tel Hashomer and Sackler Faculty of Medicine
Tel Aviv University
Tel Aviv
Israel

Manuel Ramos-Casals
Systemic Autoimmune Diseases Unit
Hospital clinic
Barcelona, Catalonia
Spain

Elena Raschi
Allergy & Clinical Immunology Unit
Department of Internal Medicine
University of Milan
IRCCS Istituto Auxologico Italiano
Milan
Italy

Lubica Rauová
Research Institute of Rheumatic Diseases
Piest'any
Slovak Republic

T. Ravid
Signal Transduction
UC Davis School of Medicine
TB149, Davis Campus
Davis, CA 95616
USA

Ronan Révélen
Laboratory of Immunology
Institut de Synergie des Sciences
et de la Santé
Brest University Medical School
Brest
France

Monica Riboni
Allergy & Clinical Immunology Unit
Department of Internal Medicine
University of Milan
IRCCS Istituto Auxologico Italiano
Milan
Italy

Giovanni Ricevuti
Section of Internal Medicine and Nephrology
Department of Internal Medicine and Therapeutics
University of Pavia
Piazzale Golgi 4
I-27100 Pavia
Italy

Jozef Rovenský
Research Institute of Rheumatic Diseases
Nábr. I. Krasku 4
92101 Piest'any
Slovak Republic

A. Ruffati
Department of Medical and Surgical Sciences
University of Padova
Via Gattamelata 64
I-35128 Padova
Italy

Naomi Sakashita
Second Department of Pathology
Kumamoto University
School of Medicine
Kumamoto 860-0811
Japan

Andreas Schwarting
First Medical Department
University of Mainz
Langenbeckstrasse 1
55101 Mainz
Germany

R. Scognamiglio
Department of Clinical and Experimental Medicine
Thrombosis Center
University of Padova
Via Gattamelata 64
I-35128 Padova
Italy

Norbert Sepp
Department of Dermatology
University of Innsbruck
Innsbruck
Austria

Amarjit S. Sethi
Department of Experimental Therapeutics
The William Harvey Research Institute
London
United Kingdom

Yana Shafran
The Jerome Schottenstein Cellscan Center
Department of Physics
Bar-lan University
Ramat Gan
Israel

Aviv Shaish
Institute of Lipid and Atherosclerosis Research
Sheba Medical Center
Tel Hashomer
Israel

S. Shapiro
Lady Davis Carmel Medical Center
Bruce Rappaport Faculty of Medicine
7 Michal Street
Haifa, 34632
Israel

Yaniv Sherer
Department of Medicine B and the
Research Center of Autoimmune Diseases
Sheba Medical Center
Tel Hashomer
Israel

Joshua Shemer
The Heller Institute of Medical Research
Sheba Medical Center
Tel Hashomer and Sackler Faculty of Medicine
Tel Aviv University
Tel Aviv
Israel

Yehuda Shoenfeld
Department of Medicine 'B' and the
Research Center of Autoimmune Diseases
Sheba Medical Center
Tel Hashoner
Israel

Yechezkiel Stein
Department of Medicine
Haddassa Hospital Ein Kerem
Jerusalem
Israel

Viera Stvrtinová
Mecial Faculty
Comenius University
Bratislava
Slovak Republik

Kiyoshi Takahashi
Second Department of Pathology
Kumamoto University
School of Medicine
Kumamoto 860-0811
Japan

Motohiro Takeya
Second Department of Pathology
Kumamoto University
School of Medicine
Kumamoto 860-0811
Japan

Cinzia Testoni
Allergy & Clinical Immunology Unit
Department of Internal Medicine
University of Milan
IRCCS Istituto Auxologico Italiano
Milan
Italy

Ella Trubiankov
Department of Medicine B and the
Research Center of Autoimmune Diseases
Sheba Medical Center
Tel Hashomer
Israel

A. Tsaba
Signal Transduction
UC Davis School of Medicine
TB149, Davis Campus
Davis, CA 95616
USA

Alena Tuchynová
Research Institute of Rheumatic Diseases
Piest'any
Slovak Republic

O. Vaarala
Department of Immunobiology
National Public Health Institute
Helsinki
Finland

Francesco Violi
Institute of Clinical Medcine I
University La Sapienza
Via del Policlinico 155
00185 Rome
Italy

Steven M. Watkins
FAME Analytics, Inc.
2545 Boatman Avenue
West Sacramento, CA 95691
USA

Georg Wick
Institute for Biomedical Aging Research
Austrian Academy of Sciences
Rennweg 10
A-6020 Innsbruck
Austria

Christian J. Wiedermann
Department of Internal Medicine
University of Innsbruck
Anichstrasse 35
A-6020 Innsbruck
Austria

Ruihua Wu
Specialty Laboratories, Inc.
221 Michigan Avenue
Santa Monica, CA 90404
USA

Qingbo Xu
Institute for Biomedical Aging Research
Austrian Academy of Sciences
Rennweg 10
A-6020 Innsbruck
Austria

Seppo Ylä-Herttuala
A.I. Virtanen Institute of Molecular Sciences
University of Kuopio
P.O. Box 1627
70211 Kuopio
Finland

Mika Yoshimatsu
Second Department of Pathology
Kumamoto University
School of Medicine
Kumamoto 860-0811
Japan

Pierre Youinou
Laboratory of Immunology
Brest University Medical School Hospital
BP 824
F 29 609 Brest Cedex
France

Yi Fu Zhou
Cardiovascular Research Institute
Washington Hospital Center
110 Irving Street
Washington, DC 20010
USA

Jianhui Zhu
Cardiovascular Research Institute
Washington Hospital Center
110 Irving Street
Washington, DC 20010
USA

Naomi Zurgil
The Jerome Schottenstein Cellscan Center
Department of Physics
Bar-lan University
Ramat Gan
Israel

CONTENTS

Atherosclerosis and Autoimmunity
Y. Shoenfeld, D. Harats and G. Wick, editors

Introduction: Autoimmunity as an Additional 'Risk Factor' for Atherosclerosis

Yehuda Shoenfeld[1], Dror Harats[2] and Georg Wick[3]

[1]Department of Medicine 'B' and the Research center of Autoimmune Diseases, Sheba Medical Center, Tel Hashomer, Israel; [2]Institute of Lipid and Atherosclerosis Research, Sheba Medical Center, Tel-Hashomer, Sackler faculty of Medicine, Tel-Aviv University, Tel-Aviv, Israel; [3]Institute for Biomedical Aging Research, Austrian Academy of Sciences and Inst. for General and Experimental Pathology, University of Innsbruck, Innsbruck, Austria

This book deals with autoimmune aspects of atherosclerosis.

Atherosclerosis is the most prevalent disease responsible for death from myocardial infarction, cerebrovascular events and renal failure. Hardening of the arteries and narrowing of their lumen results from the deposition of macrophages laden with lipids, mainly oxidized LDL and formation of the atherosclerotic plaque. For years the traditional risk factors such as high cholesterol levels hypertension, diabetes mellitus, smoking, family history and others were believed to be the major factors playing in the pathogenicity of atherosclerosis. In the last decade it has been realized that atherosclerosis, an inflammatory process may have infectious and *autoimmune components*. Correlation between many inflammatory markers such as CRP, adhesion molecules, cytokines and others with the incidence and severity of the disease were reported. Bacteria, such as Chlamidya, and viruses, such as EBV and CMV, were implicated in the pathogenesis of the disease and several reports have shown beneficial effects of an antibiotic treatments. Last but not least, autoantigens and autoantibodies seem to be involved in the induction of atherosclerosis. This main autoantigens being heat shock proteins, oxLDL and B2GPI. The later findings were also followed by successful trials to immunomodulate the disease.

Atherosclerosis is a process that involves lipid accumulation in the walls of arteries leading to a compromised flow to nearly any target organ. The final common pathways of advanced atherosclerosis is ischemia of the heart (myocardial infarction), brain (cerebrovascular events) and to the legs (claudication and necrosis).

The modern view of atherosclerosis is that of a chronic inflammatory disorder. It is based on the realization that immune-competent cells are abundant in the vicinity of the plaque starting from its initial stages (i.e. fatty streak formation). Thus, activated T lymphocytes macrophages (the major components of the evolving plaque) and major histocompatibility complex (MHC) bearing cells (i.e. endothelial and smooth muscle cells) constitute, invariable relations in the atherosclerotic plaque.

A recent 'extension' of the inflammatory view of atherosclerosis has been provided in recent years by several laboratories including ours. Thus, it has been speculated that autoimmunity to various autoantigens can act to influence the fate of the advancing lesion.

To demonstrate that a disease has an autoimmune component, we have to show that upon immunization of a naive animal with the implicated autoantigen, the disease can be modified. Specifically, it was shown that autoimmunity to heat shock protein 60 plays an initiatory role in the development of atherosclerosis in experimental animals and in humans. Similar results were achieved following immunization with another compound called ß2GPI. The later is also the autoantigen in SLE patients and in subjects having the antiphospholipid syndrome.

1

The third candidate autoantigen the oxidized LDL known to be the noxious agent in atherosclerosis was found to be protective in the disease upon active immunization.

The induced disease, like the natural one was characterized by many autoimmune features such as deposition of autoantigens, autoantibodies and involvement of the immune cells the lymphocytes.

The ultimate evidence that indeed atherosclerosis has an autoimmune component is based on our ability to transfer the disease from an induced mice to a naive mice just by transferring the lymphocytes.

It is not surprising that if atherosclerosis has an autoimmune component, that it can be treated by immunomodulation. Indeed, favorable results were achieved with high dose intravenous immunoglobulin (IVIG) which is employed also in other autoimmune diseases such as SLE, polydermatomyositis and by depletion of lymphocytes. Anti CD40/Ligand antibodies treatment and other molecules were also been used successfully by immunomodulating the disease.

Thus atherosclerosis is an additional disease found to have an autoimmune pathogenesis and treatment.

In this book world known experts gathered following a meeting that took place on March 2001 in Geneva, Switzerland. It summarized the diverse aspects of the interrelationship between the immune system and atherosclerosis.

AUTOIMMUNITY AND ATHEROSCLEROSIS

Atherosclerosis and Autoimmunity
Y. Shoenfeld, D. Harats and G. Wick, editors

The Autoimmune Pathogenesis of Atherosclerosis – An Evolutionary-Darwinian Concept

Georg Wick[1,2], Gunda Millonig[1,2] and Qingbo Xu[1]

[1]Institute for Biomedical Aging Research, Austrian Academy of Sciences, Innsbruck, Austria; [2]Institute for General and Experimental Pathology, University of Innsbruck, Medical School, Innsbruck, Austria

1. INTRODUCTION

During the last decade, the main classical theories of atherogenesis, i.e. the "response-to-injury" and the "altered lipoprotein" hypotheses and their modifications have been supplemented by the concept that immunologic-inflammatory processes play a major role at various stages of this disease. Interestingly, these ideas about the formation of atherosclerotic lesions have already been discussed since the 19th century. For a long time it has, however, not been clear if the observed inflammatory phenomena in the arterial wall were of a primary or secondary nature. The indications for a participation of immuno-inflammatory processes in the development of atherosclerotic lesions included the deposition of immunoglobulins and co-distributed complement components in the arterial wall, the participation of lymphoid cells in addition to macrophages in the intimal mononuclear infiltrate, and the occurrence of pro-inflammatory cytokines, chemokines and growth factors and their receptors. In addition, serum markers of inflammation, such as acute phase proteins and indicators for activation of the immune system, e.g. neopterin, were found to be correlated with the occurrence of atherosclerotic lesions. Most importantly, infections have been discussed as possible atherosclerosis-associated or even causally relevant phenomena. In this respect, viral and bacterial infections were discussed, the former including herpes viruses and cytomegaloviruses (CMV), the latter including *Chlamydiae, Helicobacter pylori* and others. Finally, *bona fide* autoimmune reactions against biochemically altered autoantigens, e.g. oxidized low density lipoproteins (oxLDL), have also been considered as possible causes for or phenomena connected with the development of atherosclerosis.

Based on these data and on our own long standing interest in experimentally induced and spontaneously occurring animal models for autoimmune diseases and their respective human counterparts as well as our previous work on the role of the lipid metabolism for lymphocyte reactivity with special emphasis on age-related changes of the immune response, we decided more than a decade ago to investigate the question if humoral and/or cellular immune reactions play an *initiating* role in the development of atherosclerosis. In case that these endeavours were successful, we, of course, finally aimed at identifying the antigen(s) that is/are possibly involved in this process. Our work, that has in the meantime been supported by data from many other laboratories, has shown that the antigen in question is a certain stress protein, heat shock protein 60 (HSP 60). As will be detailed below, HSP 60 is expressed by vascular endothelial cells upon being subjected to various forms of stress, mainly including those that are already known as classical risk factors for atherogenesis.

In this contribution, we will take atherosclerosis as a paradigmatic age-related disease that can be taken as a price that we pay later in life for genetic traits that are of benefit in younger years, i.e. up to the time of reproduction. As we will see, in the case of atherosclerosis we pay for our potential to raise protective immunity against microbial (viral, bacterial, parasitic) HSP 60 that allows for survival until the time of reproduction, but that may be detrimental later on under circumstances that have not been subject to evolutionary pressure since reaching an old age and living beyond the fertility period of an indivudual was obviously not "forseen" by nature.

2. EXPERIMENTAL AND CLINICAL DATA THAT FORMED THE BASIS FOR THE AUTOIMMUNE HYPOTHESIS OF ATHEROGENESIS

2.1. Classical Concepts for the Development of Atherosclerosis

In developed countries, cardiovascular diseases are notorious as the main cause of mortality, and atherosclerosis plays an important role in this context. It is, therefore, one of the diseases that has been most extensively studied from various viewpoints in numerous laboratories around the world.

Atherosclerosis is a multi-factorial disease based on the action of various risk factors that become effective on an appropriate genetic background. The disease is characterized by the appearance of mononuclear cells in the vessel wall at certain predelection sites, such as arterial branching points, which are known to be subject to altered haemodynamic stress. With progression of lesions, smooth muscle cells (SMC) from the media immigrate into the intima, where they proliferate and lead to the deposition of extracellular matrix (ECM) proteins, notably collagen fibers. This sequence of events leads to thickening and hardening of arteries (*arteriosclerosis*). *Atherosclerosis* is characterized by the additional formation of foam cells, i.e. macrophages and SMC that have taken up chemically modified, e.g. oxidized low density lipoproteins (oxLDL) via non-saturable scavenger receptors, leading to overloading of these cells with lipids and the eventual deposition of extracellular cholesterol crystals. According to a conventional classical view of atherogenesis, whitish cushion-like lesions, so-called fatty streaks, with a predominance of foam cells constitute the precursors of more severe, rupture-prone, often exulcerated and even calcified lesions, i.e. atherosclerotic plaques.

The classical concepts of atherogenesis do not ascribe a major significance to inflammatory-immunologic processes as possible primary pathogenetic factors. The *"response to injury"* hypothesis [1] originally postulated an alteration of the endothelium (mechanical injury, toxins, free radicals, etc.) as the initiating event leading to endothelial cell (EC) dysfunction, followed by increased permeability, expression of adhesion molecules and release of growth factors and chemotactic factors. As a consequence, platelet aggregation and monocyte adhesion and activation take place, the latter being attracted into the subendothelial space of the intima where they meet with SMC immigrating from the media, followed by foam cell formation, as mentioned above. As the lesion progresses, a fibrotic "cap" and a rupture-prone "shoulder" region characterized by ECM deposition are formed.

Recently, the "response to injury" hypothesis has been complemented and extended by the so called *"athero-ELAM"* hypothesis (endothelial-dependent mechanisms of leukocyte recruitment in atherogenesis) [2, 3]. This hypothesis focuses on endothelial dysfunction as the main initiating factor of atherogenesis. Non-adaptive changes of endothelial structure or function caused by pathophysiological stimuli may lead to localized acute or chronic alterations in the interaction of ECs with cellular and humoral circulating blood components and other layers of the vascular wall. These changes include increased permeability and subsequent oxidative modification of plasma proteins, a hyper-tendency for adhesion of blood leukocytes and a functional imbalance of pro- and antithrombotic factors, growth- and inhibitory factors as well as dilatory and constrictive vasoactive substances.

The *"altered-lipoprotein"* hypothesis [4] postulates an initiating role of chemically-altered lipoproteins, notably oxLDL, that lead to the primary formation of foam cells in the intima. This hypothesis has recently been modified, since it has been shown that only native rather than oxLDL is found in the circulation, and that native LDL transported into the intima through the endothelium is modified (oxidized) and retained there, where it acts as a chemoattractant for monocytes and SMC and is later taken up by these cells, resulting in foam cell formation (*"retention of modified LDL"* hypothesis) [5].

A third classical concept, less significantly supported by experimental and clinical data, is the *"monoclonal SMC proliferation"* hypothesis [6] which suggests initiation of the disease by clonally-proliferating SMC.

3. PREVIOUS OBSERVATIONS THAT SUPPORT THE ROLE OF INFLAMMATORY-IMMUNE PROCESSES IN THE DEVELOPMENT OF ATHEROSCLEROSIS

An association between inflammatory processes and atherogenesis has been postulated by many authors in the past, but, surprisingly, were ignored for a long time by groups engaged in "classical" atherosclerosis research or considered to be only a secondary phenomenon [7, 8]. Such changes include, the occurrence of granular deposits of immunoglobulins and co-distributed complement components, increased expression of C3b receptors (CR1) and C3b1 receptors (CR3) on macrophages within atherosclerotic lesions, but not in unaltered vessels [9, 10]. However, B cells are only found in very low numbers in various stages of atherosclerotic lesions, and the site of production for these immunoglobulins must, therefore, be sought elsewhere [11]. Various candidates against which these antibodies could be directed have been discussed, among them oxLDL [12] and, as shown by ourselves, certain stress proteins [13].

Other than these humoral immune phenomena, it is now clear that T cells are among the first cells infiltrating the intima of arteries during the earliest stages of atherosclerosis, most probably before monocytes [14]. In an immunohistological study of vascular arterial specimens of young (<35 years) and old (>65 years) patients who died from non-atherosclerosis-associated diseases, we were able to show that the earliest mononuclear cells infiltrating the intima at sites of the development of atherosclerotic lesions were T cells, in contrast to current dogma, rather than macrophages, the latter dominating at later stages together with SMC immigrating from the intima. A majority of these early T cells are CD4+, HLA-DR+ and interleukin-2 receptor+ (IL-2R+), i.e. activated [11, 15]. Other authors were able to show that T cells in late atherosclerotic plaques express the low molecular variant of the "leukocyte common antigen" (CD45RO) and the integrin "very late activation antigen-1" (VLA-1)

[16]. Hansson et al. [17, 18], analyzing the rearrangement of T cell receptor (TCR) genes in these latter cells derived from advanced lesions, showed that they represent a polyclonal population rather than displaying restricted T-cell receptor TCR usage. Mosorin et al. [19] have recently confirmed our data in rabbits [20] by showing HSP60 to be the main antigenic candidate against which T cell clones derived from human atherosclerotic plaques are reacting.

Regardless of which antigen these lymphocytes may recognize, it seems unprobable that ECs that aberrantly express major histocompatibility complex (MHC) class II antigens act as primary antigen-presenting cells for T cell sensitization. In our own experiments, we were only able to show MHC class II expression by EC at sites where T cell accumulations, and thus production of gamma-interferon (IFNγ), where present in the intima directly beneath these areas [11]. Therefore, we and others concluded that the expression of MHC class II molecules by EC represents a secondary rather than a primary phenomenon [21, 22]. We originally reasoned that sensitization of T cells takes place at other sites, e.g. the draining lymph nodes. This concept was indirectly supported by the demonstration of increased serum levels of neopterin in patients with atherosclerosis, speaking for a systematic activation of macrophages by IFNγ [23, 24]. However, as will be detailed below, we have recently made the surprising discovery that a whole network of dendritic cells (DC) resembling Langerhans cells in the skin is present in the arterial intima [25], an observation that has completely changed our ideas with respect to the possible in situ T cell sensitization in the vascular system.

The large majority of CD3+ in the mononuclear infiltrate in atherosclerotic lesions expresses the TCRα/ß, but an unexpectedly high proportion also expresses the TCRγ/δ [15]. While the latter type of cells only constitutes approximately 1% in peripheral blood, enrichment to 10% and more within early atherosclerotic lesions can be observed. The majority of these latter cells express the TCRγ2 chain, i.e. resembles the TCRγ/δ+ population found in the intestinal mucosa. On the other hand, TCR Vγ9δ2+ cells characteristic of circulating TCRγ/δ+ cells are not proportionally increased in the intima. Furthermore, we were able to demonstrate considerable accumulations of T cells at various sites of the *normal* arterial intima of adults and even children and babies, i.e. without concommitant occurrence of atherosclerotic lesions [26]. Together with the above-mentioned accumulations of TCRγ/δ+ cells, notoriously present in the so-called mucosa-associated lymphoid tissue (MALT) compared to other lymphatic organs, e.g. the spleen, this observation prompted us to put forward the hypothesis of the existence of a "vascular-associated lymphoid tissue" (VALT). We hypothesized that the VALT may fulfill a task similar to MALT, i.e. monitoring exogenous or autologous antigenic material that comes into contact with bodily surfaces, in this case that of the vascular system [27]. It later turned out that the observation of an enrichment of TCRγ/δ+ cells may have special importance, since they are known to preferentially react with certain stress proteins (heat shock proteins – HSP) [28], a phenomenon that will be detailed below.

Finally, it was possible to demonstrate on the protein- and mRNA-level that EC as well as leukocytes occurring in atherosclerotic lesions are able to produce a variety of immunological-inflammatory mediators. Among others, these include interleukin-1 (IL-1: EC, SMC, macrophages), tumor necrosis factor α (TNFα: SMC, T cells, macrophages), lymphotoxin (LT: T cells), IL-2 (T cells), IL-6 (EC, SMC, macrophages), IL-8 (EC, macrophages), monocyte-chemotactic peptide-1 (MCP-1: EC, SMC, macrophages) and IFNγ (T cells) [1, 7, 8]. Together, these molecules can modulate the local cellular immune response within emerging atherosclerotic lesions [2]. In addition, growth factors, such as platelet-derived growth factor (PDGF), exert a mitogenic effect on mesenchymal cells and stimulate leukocyte migration. Thus, they play an important role in the maintenance of the immunologic-inflammatory reaction. Normal vascular tissues do not display a high content of PDGF-ß receptors, but in the case of arterial diseases associated with an activation of macrophages and T cells, a considerable expression of such receptors can be observed. The immune reaction within the arterial wall, therefore, seems to entail an increased responsivity to PDGF-ß [1, 2].

Based on these data, we performed a large series of studies in experimental animals and humans that are summarized in the next paragraph, and that

finally led to the formulation of our new *"autoimmune" hypothesis* for the development of atherosclerosis.

4. SUMMARY OF THE AUTOIMMUNE HYPOTHESIS OF ATHEROGENESIS

Our initial experiments attempted to identify the antigen(s) that may incite the cellular and/or humoral immune response at the beginning of the development of atherosclerotic lesions. Among the many candidate antigens, microbial constituents, e.g. confronting the immune system in the course of various infections, and oxLDL emerged as the most prominent. Our experimental and clinical data suggest that the earliest stage of atherogenesis consists of an autoimmune reaction against a stress protein, *viz.* HSP60 [13, 29, 30].

HSPs are expressed by prokaryontic and eukaryontic cells constitutively and/or under stress conditions [31, 32]. Physiologically, they fulfill important functions in conjunction with the folding and intracellular transport of proteins. Under stress (e.g. mild heat — hence the name toxins, oxygen radicals, infection, mechanical stress, etc.), some HSPs exert a chaperone function, i.e. associate with other cellular proteins and protect them from denaturation. HSPs are classified into several families according to their molecular mass (Table 1). The main groups are the 100 kD, 70 kD, 60 kD, 40 kD and low molecular weight families. HSPs are phylogenetically highly conserved. Thus, HSP 60 of mycobacteria (mHSP65), *Chlamydiae* (cHSP60), and *E.coli* (GroEL) show over 95% homology on the DNA and protein level. In fact, human HSP60 (hHSP60) and mHSP65 are still approximately 55% homologous [33]. Since HSP60 quantitatively and qualitatively constitute very important antigenic components of bacteria, parasites and even viruses (often contained in the envelope of the latter [34], nearly all humans show humoral and cellular immune reactivity against them. Due to the high degree of sequence homology, this protective immune reactivity (including that derived from vaccinations) may have to be "paid for" by the danger of cross-reactivity with autologous animal or human HSP60 [35].

Our evidence that such an (auto)immune reaction against HSP60 may be instrumental in initiat-

Table 1. The HSP superfamily: Physiological role and possible relation to the immune response of major HSPs

Family	Major members	Important physiological function	Possible role in the immune response
HSP90	HSP90, HSP83	Prevention of steroid receptor binding to DNA; tyrosine kinase phosphorylation	Tumor resistance; autoimmunity
HSP70	HSP70, BiP hsc70, grp78 dnak	Protein folding and unfolding; protein translocation; assembly of multimeric complexes	Immunoglobulin assembly; class II antigen processing; antigen of many pathogens; autoimmunity
HSP60	HSP65, groEL	Protein folding and unfolding; assembly of multimeric complexes	Antigen of many pathogens; autoimmunity
Ubiquitin	Ubiquitin	Protein degradation	Class I – antigen processing; lymphocyte homing; autoimmunity

ing atherosclerosis can be summarized as follows:

- Immunization of normocholesterolemic rabbits with heat-killed mycobacteria or recombinant mHSP led to the emergence of arteriosclerotic lesions, i.e. intimal infiltration by MNC with a preponderance of activated CD4+ T cells, but no foam cells, at sites of the arterial tree known to be predisposed to disease development [36].

- Rats, rabbits and humans express HSP60 in EC at these sites, providing a prerequisite for inter-action of specific T cells and antibodies elicited previously by infection or vaccination [15, 19, 26, 37].

- *In vitro*, the same stressors lead to the *simultaneous* expression of HSP60 and adhesion molecules (intercellular adhesion molecule-1 – ICAM-1; endothelial leukocyte adhesion molecule-1 – ELAM-1; vascular cell adhesion molecule-1 – VCAM-1) by EC at the mRNA and protein levels [38]. However, arterial EC seem to be more sus-ceptible than venous EC to the action of various stressors (notably oxLDL), probably based on a lower threshold for the latter due to the pre-stressing effect of life-long exposure to the higher arterial blood pressure. It is known that venous bypasses of occluded arteries often undergo severe restenosis and "venosclerosis" subsequent to being subjected to the higher arterial blood pressure conditions. We have recently developed a mouse model [39] for carotid bypasses that allows for an indepth study of this issue using appropriate donor (e.g. cytokine or adhesion mol-ecule knock out mice) and recipient combina-tions, as well as various therapeutic (drugs, anti-sense oligonucleotide, etc.) interventions [40, 41].

There is ample evidence that infections may be involved in atherogenesis. Thus, Marek dis-ease virus (MDV), an avian herpes virus leading to neurolymphomatosis in chickens [42], also induces atherosclerosis and CMV [43, 44], herpes virus [45] and *Chlamydia pneumoniae* [46, 47, 48] have been discussed as being associated with the development of human atherosclerotic lesions.

Our own studies of this problem were based on our long-standing experience with experimen-tally-induced and spontaneously occurring organ-specific autoimmune diseases in humans and var-ious animal models [49, 50] and our interest in a possible role of an altered lipid metabolism in the decrease of immune reactivity in older age [51].

- The first, presumably autoimmune, step of athero-sclerosis that can be induced by three immu-nizations of rabbits at five week intervals with mHSP65 is still reversible, i.e. subsides after an interval of 32 weeks, while the more severe atherosclerotic lesions induced by feeding a cho-lesterol-rich diet only or following immunization plus feeding a cholesterol-rich diet do not regress during this period of time [52]. Immunosup-pression of rabbits by treatment with an anti-rabbit pan T cell mouse monoclonal antibody in combination with prednisolone (to prevent the formation of anti-mouse Ig antibodies) inhibits the development of atherosclerosis induced by immunization with mHSP65 [53].

- The mild atherosclerotic aortic lesions that develop in C57BL/6J mice upon feeding a cholesterol-rich diet are aggravated by immunization with mHSP65 [54, 55]. Interestingly, immunization of such mice with chemically-modified LDL prevents the emergence of atherosclerosis. The results of these experiments, which are even more significant when ApoE-/- mice are used [56], proved that (a) immunity to HSP is pathogenic, and (b) an immune reaction to oxLDL may be beneficial, probably by removing oxLDL via immune complex formation.

- As expected, the peripheral blood as well as the arterial lesions induced in rabbits by immunization with mHSP65 are enriched for HSP65-reactive T cells compared to unimmunized controls. It was, however, notable that T cell lines derived from atherosclerotic lesions of unimmunized rabbits fed a cholesterol-rich diet also showed a significantly increased proportion of HSP65 specificity compared to T cell lines derived from the peripheral blood of the same animals [19], pointing to a preferential activation of such cells in the lesions.

- *In vitro* data obtained from examination of arterial and venous cells, including human umbilical vein EC (HUVECs) as well as macrophages of animals and man, showed that HSP60 can be induced in the cytoplasma of these cells by various types of stress factors, e.g. TNFα, H_2O_2, LPS, elevated temperature, or chemical stress [37, 57]. Furthermore, HSP60 is expressed on the surface of stressed cells, thus providing the basis for lysis of these, but not unstressed cells, by human and animal anti-mHSP65 antibodies via complement-mediated cytotoxicity or antibody-dependent cellular cytotoxicity (ADCC) [57, 58]. *In vitro* and *in vivo* experiments in rats involving mechanical stressing of EC have provided evidence for a significant upregulation of HSP60 and adhesion molecule expression under these circumstances [59].

- Studies on the effect of an immunosuppressive treatment performed in *in vitro* experiments showed that treatment with aspirin leads to the induction of HSP60 by ECs, but is also able to suppress the TNFα-induced expression of adhesion molecules (ICAM-1, VCAM-1, ELAM-1), thus potentially inhibiting the interaction of HSP60-specific T cells with their targets [60].

- In a large study of sera from a clinically-healthy group of human volunteers, aged 40–90 years (the so-called "Bruneck Study" [61, 62]), we showed a correlation of anti-mHSP65 antibody titers with the presence of sonographically-demonstrable atherosclerotic lesions in the *A.carotis* [63]. Statistical analyses revealed that these antibodies reflected a risk factor independent of classical risk factors for atherogenesis, except age. Furthermore, it was shown that these antibodies not only react with mHSP65, but show strong cross-reactivity with HSP60 of *Chlamydia pneumoniae* (cHSP60), mHSP65, GroEL and, most importantly, hHSP60 [64]. As mentioned, it was then shown that human affinity chromatography-purified anti-cHSP60 or anti-GroEL antibodies were also able to lyse stressed human EC [58] or macrophages [57] in a complement-dependent fashion or via ADCC. That the mitochondrial protein HSP60 is transported to the cell surface [65] has, in the meantime, been unequivocally corroborated by our collaborators Soltys and Gupta [66], although the possible functional role at that location is still elusive.

- In a recent follow-up study to our work on anti-HSP65/60 antibodies in the sera of the "Bruneck Study", we were able to show that this parameter is very robust, and thus a good indicator of morbidity, but it is also an indicator of mortality, since patients who died during the period from 1990 to 1995 had significantly elevated antibody titers [67].

- Initial attempts to identify mHSP65/HSP60 cross-reactive epitopes recognized by human antibodies using overlapping peptides spanning the whole mHSP65 molecule, revealed three linear epitopes, i.e. at the N-terminus AA 91-105, the C-terminus AA 501-515, and a less well defined AA 171-185 stretch in between [68]. Since antibodies, in contrast to T cells, generally recognize conformational rather than linear epitopes, it is of interest that computer modelling of hHSP60 based on the known structure of GroEL showed that the N- and C-terminal linear epitopes seemed to associate to form a conformational epitope in the native hHSP60 molecule [35].

- The association of high titers of anti-HSP60/65 antibodies with cardiovascular disease is not only valid for carotid, but also for coronary atherosclerosis [69–72]. Interestingly, myocardial infarction entails decreased titers of these antibodies presumably due to complex formation of endogenously released HSP60 with pre-existing antibodies and removal of immune complexes via the reticular EC system. Cardiac ischemia which leads to the release of endogenous antigenic HSP60, has recently been demonstrated in a perfused rat heart model [73].

- We were able to show that the ability to develop atherosclerosis increases with the "infectious load" to which an individual has been subjected. The incidence of atherosclerosis is not only associated with the presence of serum antibodies against *Chlamydia* and high levels of the acute-phase C reactive protein (CRP), but is further significantly augmented if respiratory infections are simultaneously present [74]. These observations show that infectious agents in general can stimulate immune responses to HSP60/65, and we have demonstrated a several-fold increase of anti-mHSP65 antibody titers during the course of an infection with Gram-negative bacteria [75]. In addition to *chlamydial* infections, anti-mHSP65 antibodies were found to closely correlate with immune reactions to endotoxin in the general population. Interestingly, bacterial cell wall LPS can concomitantly induce hHSP60 and adhesion molecules on EC, a prerequisite for the cellular immune response to hHSP60 [37].

- Furthermore, we have recently demonstrated that levels of soluble HSP60 (sHSP60) are elevated in subjects with atherosclerosis in the general population [76].
- We have begun to approach the question of how signal transduction in mechanically stressed EC is achieved, and if this process is altered during *in vitro* aging. Based on previous results, these experiments concentrated on the mitogen-activated protein kinase (MAP-kinase) pathway. MAP-kinases include a family of tyrosine/threonine-kinases, especially stress-activated protein kinase (SAPK) or c-Jun NH2-terminal kinases (JNK), extracellular signal-regulated kinase (ERK) and p38/MAP-kinase [77].

Our quest to identify the "sensors" for mechanical stress has been successful in the SMC system. Interestingly, mechanical (tension) stress on SMC directly entails the phosphorylation of the PDGF-receptor α chain, and thus receptor activation [78]. When GRB2, an adaptor protein, is isolated from thus stressed SMC and analyzed in Western blots with anti-phosphotyrosine, anti-PDGF-Rα and anti-GRB2-antibodies, a positive reaction for phosphotyrosine emerged at the PDGF-Rα band. These results prove the activation of PDGF-Rα by mechanical stress. The cell culture supernatant of stressed SMC did not lead to the phosphorylation of the PDGF-Rα, nor was the stress-induced activation of PDGF-Rα inhibited by antibodies against PDGF. Therefore, mechanical stress seems to directly influence the cell surface or alter the receptor conformation, thus triggering a signal pathway that is normally employed by growth factors. These observations may substantially add to our understanding of how a physical stimulus can be translated into a physiologic signal cascade normally used by growth factors. We plan to apply this methodological know-how to the study of mechanically-stressed EC.

Finally, it should be mentioned that immunization of rabbits with recombinant mHSP65 results in development of atherosclerosis, but not arthritis [29], while the reverse is true for rats [79, 80]. This phenomenon seems to be due to the recognition of different HSP60 epitopes by the immune system of these two species. Detailed analyses aimed at the identification of the epitopes responsible for sensitizing HSP65/60-reactive T cells found in atherosclerotic lesions of rabbits compared to those known to play a role in the induction of arthritis in rats (peptide AA 180-188 of the 573 AA long HSP65) [81] as well as in human rheumatoid arthritis are still lacking.

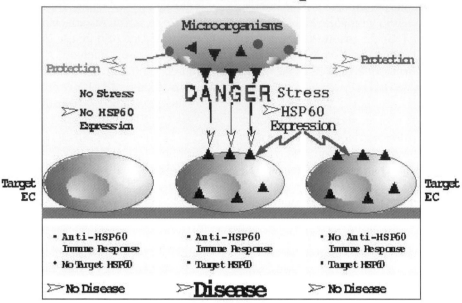

Figure 1. Cellular and humoral immune response to HSP60.

4.1. The Autoimmune Hypothesis of Atherogenesis

The "immunologic" hypothesis obviously may encompass the "response-to-injury" as well as the "altered lipoprotein" hypotheses. The reaction of EC to stress is a primary response that entails an inflammatory reaction mediated by HSP65/60-reactive T cells and HSP60/65-specific antibodies, finally resulting in the development of the classical atherosclerotic lesions when additional risk factors come into play. Biochemically altered lipoproteins, such as oxLDL, may first act as stressors on EC and only later lead to the transformation into foam cells of blood-born macrophages and SMC immigrating from the media into the intima. Moreover, it is not yet clear where the sensitization of HSP60-reactive lymphocytes occurs, and whether we are dealing with a cross-reaction between microbial HSP60 and hHSP60 triggered by an exogenous antigen only, e.g. during infection, or are witnessing a *bona fide* autoimmune reaction against chemically altered autologous hHSP6o. However, we have solid data that *all* individuals studied so far in our laboratory (aged one month to 80 years) show inflammatory foci in the arterial intima at areas subjected to major haemodynamic stress.

Figure 1 summarizes our concept of the autoimmune pathogenesis of atherosclerosis. This concept is based on the fact that most individuals possess antibodies and T cells recognizing HSP60 epitopes that may result in cross-reactivity between microbial (bacterial, parasitic-viral) antigens and hHSP60. In addition, non-HSP microbial epitopes are, of course, also recognized by the human immune system. Together, these immune mechanisms confer protection to the individual, who "pays" for this protective immunity when arterial EC are maltreated by atherogenic risk factors, e.g. hypertension, smoking, oxygen radicals, infections, etc. In this case, the anti-microbial HSP60 response will recognize autologous HSP60 and lead to the first inflammatory stage of atherosclerosis, which may be followed by the development of more severe lesions, i.e. plaques, including the formation of foam cells, ECM and extracellular lipid depositon, exulceration and even calcification. The specificity of the immune response for cross-reactive atherogenic HSP60 epitopes depends on the individual T and B cell repertoire and the association of the relevant peptides with appropiate MHC class II and class I molecules. Occasionally, protection against infections may rely only on immunity against non-HSP60 epitopes or HSP60 epitopes that are not cross-reactive with the eukaryontic homologues, and these individuals will, therefore, not run into the danger of cross-reaction with autologous HSP60 expressed on stressed arterial EC.

Thus far, we do not know whether cellular or humoral effector mechanisms are the first to mediate vascular damage. From immunohistological data in humans and early observations in mice, we presently favour the concept that atherosclerosis is initiated by CD4+/TH1 cells, and that humoral antibodies play an accelerating and aggravating role. Parallel studies in mice and humans to clarify this crucial issue are now being performed.

5. OUTLOOK

It is obvious that our novel autoimmune hypothesis for atherogenesis opens new and exciting perspectives for diagnosis, prevention and therapy of this disease. Diagnostic approaches include the determination of humoral antibodies against pro- and eukaryontic HSP 60 with special emphasis on the relevant conformational epitopes, as well as similar approaches, however focussing on linear epitopes, for T cell reactivity. Special attention is, of course, given to the identification of cross-reactive microbial and human HSP 60 epitopes. However, reactivity with altered autologous HSP 60 in the sense of a *bona fide* autoimmune reaction should also be considered. This approach will not only allow for diagnosis of already established disease, but also provide the means for identification of persons at risk and initiation of appropriate preventive measures.

Finally, the already applied anti-inflammatory strategies for prevention and treatment of atherosclerosis, e.g. via non-steroidal drugs such as aspirin, may in the future be complemented and made more specific and efficient by administration of appropriate native, modified or fragmented HSP 60 peptides via different routes and in different galenic combinations.

ACKNOWLEDGEMENT

Our work is supported by grants of the Austrian Science Fund (project no. 12213) and the State of Vorarlberg.

REFERENCES

1. Ross R. The pathogenesis of atherosclerosis: a perspective for the 1990s. Nature 1993; 362;801–809.
2. Ross R. Atherosclerosis-an inflammatory disease. N Engl J Med 1999;340:115–126.
3. Gimbrone MA. Vascular endothelium: an integration of pathophysiologic stimuli in atherosclerosis. Am J Cardiol 1995;75:67B-70B.
4. Steinberg D. Modified forms of low-density lipoprotein and atherosclerosis. J Intern Med 1993;233:227–232 .
5. Witztum JL, Steinberg D. Role of oxidized low density lipoprotein in atherogenesis. J Clin Invest 1991;88:1785–1792.
6. Schwartz SM, Murry CE. Proliferation and the monoclonal origins of atherosclerotic lesions. Annu Rev Med 1998;49:437–460.
7. Hansson GK, Jonasson L, Seifert PS, Stemme S. Immune mechanisms in atherosclerosis. Arteriosclerosis 1989;9:567–578.
8. Libby P, Hansson GK. Involvement of the immune system in human atherogenesis: current knowledge and unanswered questions. Lab Invest 1991;64:5–15.
9. Niculescu F, Rus H. Complement activation and atherosclerosis. Mol Immunol 1999;36:949–955.
10. Seifert PS, Hugo F, Hansson GK, Bhakdi S. Prelesional complement activation in experimental atherosclerosis. Terminal C5b-9 complement deposition coincides with cholesterol accumulation in the aortic intima of hypercholesterolemic rabbits. Lab Invest 1998;60:747–754.
11. Xu Q, Oberhuber G, Gruschwitz M, Wick G. Immunology of atherosclerosis: cellular composition and major histocompatibility complex class II antigen expression in aortic intima, fatty streaks, and atherosclerotic plaques in young and aged human specimens. Clin Immunol Immunopathol 1990;56:344–359.
12. Yla-Herttuala S, Palinski W, Butler SW, Picard S, Steinberg D, Witztum JL. Rabbit and human atherosclerotic lesions contain IgG that recognizes epitopes of oxidized LDL. Arterioscler Thromb 1994;14:32–40
13. Wick G, Kleindienst R, Dietrich H, Xu Q. Is atherosclerosis an autoimmune disease? Trends Food Sci Technol 1992;3:114–119.
14. Emeson EE, Robertson AL. T lymphocytes in aortic and coronary intimas. Their potential role in atherogen-

esis. Am J Pathol 1988;130:369–376.

15. Kleindienst R, Xu Q, Willeit J, Waldenberger FR, Weimann S, Wick G. Immunology of atherosclerosis: demonstration of heat shock protein 60 expression and T lymphocytes bearing alpha/beta or gamma/delta receptor in human atherosclerosic lesions. Am J Pathol 1993;142:1927–1937.

16. Stemme S, Holm J, Hansson GK. T lymphocytes in human atherosclerotic plaques are memory cells expressing CD45RO and the integrin VLA-1. Arterioscler Thromb 1992;12:206–211.

17. Stemme S, Rymo L, Hansson GK. Polyclonal origin of T lymphocytes in human atherosclerotic plaques. Lab Invest 1991;65:654–660.

18. Paulsson G, Zhou X, Tornquist E, Hansson GK. Oligoclonal T cell expansions in atherosclerotic lesions of apolipoprotein E-deficient mice. Arterioscler Thromb Vasc Biol 2000;20:10–17.

19. Mosorin M, Surcel HM, Laurila A, Lehtinen M, Karttunen R, Juvonen J, Paavonen J, Morrison RP, Saikku P, Juvonen T. Detection of Chlamydia pneumoniae–Reactive T Lymphocytes in Human Atherosclerotic Plaques of Carotid Artery. Arterioscler Thromb Vasc Biol 2000;20:1061–1067.

20. Xu Q, Kleindienst R, Waitz W, Dietrich H, Wick G. Increased expression of heat shock protein 60 coincides with a population of infiltrating T lymphocytes in atherosclerotic lesions of rabbits specifically responding to heat shock protein 65. J Clin Invest 1993;91:2693–2702.

21. Hansson GK, Jonasson L, Holm J, Clowes MK, Clowes A. Gamma interferon regulates vascular smooth muscle proliferation and la expression in vivo and in vitro. Circ Res 1988;63:712–719.

22. Van der Wal AC. Atherosclerotic lesions in human. In situ immunophenotypic analysis suggesting an immune mediated response. Lab Invest 1989;61:166–170.

23. Tatzber R, Rable H, Korsika K, Erhart U, Puhl H, Waeg G, Krebs A, Esterbauer H. Elevated serum neopterin levels in atherosclerosis. Atherosclerosis 1991;89:203–208.

24. Xu Q, Wick G, Wacher H, Reibnegger G. Relationship among serum hsp 65 antibodies, neopterin, autoantibodies and atherosclerosis. Pteridines 1994;5;139–141.

25. Millonig G, Hochleitner BW, Rabl W, Niederegger H, Romani N, Wick G. Vascular-associated dendritic cells. (submitted for publication).

26. Waltner-Romen M, Falkensammer G, Rabl W, Wick G. A previously unrecognized site of local accumulation of mononuclear cells. The vascular-associated lymphoid tissue. J Histochem Cytochem 1998;46:1347–1350.

27. Wick G, Romen M, Amberger A, Metzler B, Mayr M, Falkensammer G, Xu Q. Atherosclerosis, autoimmunity, and vascular-associated lymphoid tissue. FASEB J 1997;11:1199–1207.

28. Young RA, Elliot TJ. Stress proteins, infection and immune surveillance. Cell 1989;59:5–8.

29. Wick G, Schett G, Amberger A, Kleindienst R, Xu Q. Is atherosclerosis an immunologically mediated disease? Immunol Today 1995;16:27–33.

30. Xu Q, Wick G. The role of heat shock proteins in protection and pathophysiology of the arterial wall. Mol Med Today 1996;2:372–379.

31. Young D, Roman E, Moreno C, O'Brien R, Born W. Molecular chaperones and the immune response. Philos Trans R Soc Lond B Biol Sci 1993;339:363–367.

32. Morimoto RI. Regulation of the heat shock transcriptional response: cross talk between a family of heat shock factors, molecular chaperones, and negative regulators. Genes Dev 1998;12:3788–3796.

33. Jones DB, Coulson AF, Duff GW. Sequence homologies between hsp60 and autoantigens. Immunol Today 1993;14:115–118.

34. Bartz SR, Pauza CD, Ivanyi J, Jindal S, Welch WJ, Malkovsky M. An Hsp60 related protein is associated with purified HIV and SIV. J Med Primatol 1994;23:151–154.

35. Wick G, Perschinka H, Xu Q. Autoimmunity and atherosclerosis. Am Heart J 1999;138:444–449.

36. Xu Q, Dietrich H, Steiner HJ, Gown AM, Schoel B, Mikuz G, Kaufmann SH, Wick G. Induction of arteriosclerosis in normocholesterolemic rabbits by immunization with heat shock protein 65. Arterioscler Thromb 1992;12:789–799.

37. Seitz CS, Kleindienst R, Xu Q, Wick G. Coexpression of heat shock protein 60 and intercellular-adhesion molecule-1 is related to increased adhesion of monocytes and T cells to aortic endothelium of rats in response to endotoxin. Lab Invest 1996;74:242.

38. Amberger A, Maczek C, Jürgens G, Michaelis D, Schett G, Trieb K, Eberl T, Jindal S, Xu Q, Wick G. Co-expression of ICAM-1, VCAM-1, ELAM-1 and Hsp60 in human arterial and venous endothelial cells in response to cytokines and oxidized low-density lipoproteins. Cell Stress Chaperones 1997;2:94–103.

39. Zou Y, Dietrich H, Hu Y, Metzler B, Wick G, Xu Q. Mouse model of venous bypass graft arteriosclerosis. Am J Pathol 1998;153:1301–1310.

40. Hu Y, Zou Y, Dietrich H, Wick G, Xu Q. Inhibition of neointima hyperplasia of mouse vein grafts by locally applied suramin. Circulation 1999;100:861–868.

41. Zou Y, Hu Y, Mayr M, Dietrich H, Wick G, Xu Q. Reduced neointima hyperplasia of vein bypass grafts in intercellular adhesion molecule-1-deficient mice. Circ Res 2000;86:434–440.

42. Hajjar DP. Viral pathogenesis of atherosclerosis: Impact

of molecular mimicry and viral genes. Am J Pathol 1991;139:1195–1211.

43. Adam E, Probtsfield JL, Burek J, McCollum CH, Melnick JL, Petrie BL, Bailey KR, Debakey ME. High levels of cytomegalovirus antibody in patients requiring vascular surgery for atherosclerosis. Lancet 1987;8:291–293.

44. Zhou YF, Shou M, Guetta E, Guzman R, Unger EF, Yu ZX, Zhang J, Finkel T, Epstein SE. Cytomegalovirus infection of rats increases the neointimal response to vascular injury without consistent evidence of direct infection of the vascular wall. Circulation 1999;100:1569–1575.

45. Yamashiroya HM, Ghosh L, Yang R, Robertson Al jr. Herpesviridae in the coronary arteries and aorta of young trauma victims. Am J Pathol 1988;130:71–79.

46. Saikku P, Leinonen M, Mattila K, Ekman MR, Nieminen MS, Makela PH, Huttunen JK, Valtonen V. Serological evidence of an association of a novel Chlamydia, TWAR, with chronic coronary heart disease and acute myocardial infarction. Lancet 1988;2:983–986.

47. Thom DH, Grayston JT, Siscovick DS, Wang SP, Weiss NS, Daling JR. Association of prior infection with Chlamydia pneumoniae and angiographically demonstrated coronary artery disease. JAMA 1992;268:68–72.

48. Shor A, Phillips JI. Chlamydia pneumoniae and atherosclerosis. JAMA 1999;282:2071–2073.

49. Wick G, Brezinschek HP, Hála K, Dietrich H, Wolf H, Krömer G. The obese strain of chickens: an animal model with spontaneous autoimmune thyroiditis. Adv Immunol 1989;47:433–500.

50. Wick G, Sgonc R, Kroemer G. Autoimmune disease, spontaneous animal models; In: Encyclopedia of Immunology, 2nd Edition – PJ Delves, IM Roitt (eds.) Academic Press 1998;280–287.

51. Wick G, Huber LA, Xu QB, Jarosch E, Schönitzer D, Jürgens G. The decline of the immune response during aging: the role of an altered lipid metabolism. Ann N Y Acad Sci 1991;621:277–290.

52. Xu Q, Kleindienst R, Schett G, Waitz W, Jindal S, Gupta RS, Dietrich H, Wick G. Regression of arteriosclerotic lesions induced by immunization with heat shock protein 65-containing material in normocholesterolemic, but not hypercholesterolemic, rabbits. Atherosclerosis 1996;123:145–155.

53. Metzler B, Mayr M, Dietrich H, Singh M, Wiebe E, Xu Q, Wick G. Inhibition of arteriosclerosis by T-cell depletion in normocholesterolemic rabbits immunized with heat shock protein 65. Arterioscler Thromb Vasc Biol 1999;8:1905–1911.

54. George J, Shoenfeld Y, Afek A, Gilburd B, Keren P, Shaish A, Kopolovic J, Wick G, Harats D. Enhanced fatty streak formation in C57BL/6J mice by immuniza-

tion with heat shock protein-65. Arterioscler Thromb Vasc Biol 1999;3;505–510.

55. George J, Shoenfeld Y, Gilburd B, Afek A, Shaish A, Harats D. Requisite role for interleukin-4 in the acceleration of fatty streaks induced by heat shock protein 65 or mycobacterium tuberculosis. Circ Res 2000;86:1203–1210.

56. George J, Afek A, Gilburd B, Levkovitz H, Shaish A, Goldberg I, Kopolovic Y, Wick G, Shoenfeld Y, Harats D. Hyperimmunization of apo-E-deficient mice with homologous malondialdehyde low-density lipoprotein suppresses early atherogenesis. Atherosclerosis 1998;138:147–152.

57. Schett G, Metzler B, Mayr M, Amberger A, Niederwieser D, Gupta RS, Mizzen L, Xu Q, Wick G. Macrophage-lysis mediated by autoantibodies to heat shock protein 65/60. Atherosclerosis 1997;128:27–38.

58. Schett G, Xu Q, Amberger A, Van der Zee R, Recheis H, Willeit J, Wick G. Autoantibodies against heat shock protein 60 mediate endothelial cytotoxicity. J Clin Invest 1995;96:2569–2577.

59. Hochleitner BW, Hochleitner EO, Obrist P, Eberl T, Amberger A, Xu Q, Margreiter R, Wick G. Fluid shear stress induces heat shock protein 60 expression in endothelial cells in vitro and in vivo. Arterioscl Throm Vasc Biol 2000;20:617–623.

60. Amberger A, Hala M, Saurwein-Teissl M, Metzler B, Grubeck-Loebenstein B, Xu Q, Wick G. Suppressive effects of anti-inflammatory agents on human endothelial cell activation and induction of heat shock proteins. Mol Med 1999;5:117–128.

61. Kiechl S, Willeit J, Egger G, Poewe W, Oberhollenzer F. Body iron stores and the risk of carotid atherosclerosis: prospective results from the Bruneck study. Circulation 1997;96:3300–3307.

62. Kiechl S, Aichner F, Gerstenbrand F, Egger G, Mair A, Rungger G, Spogler F, Jarosch E, Oberhollenzer F, Willeit J. Body iron stores and presence of carotid atherosclerosis. Results from the Bruneck Study. Arterioscler Thromb 1994;14:1625–1630.

63. Xu Q, Willeit J, Marosi M, Kleindienst R, Oberhollenzer F, Kiechl S, Stulnig T, Luef G, Wick G. Association of serum antibodies to heat-shock protein 65 with carotid atherosclerosis. Lancet 1993;341:255–259.

64. Mayr M, Metzler B, Kiechl S, Willeit J, Schett G, Xu Q, Wick G. Endothelial cytotoxicity mediated by serum antibodies to heat shock proteins of Escherichia coli and Chlamydia pneumoniae: immune reactions to heat shock proteins as a possible link between infection and atherosclerosis. Circulation 1999;99:1560–1566.

65. Xu Q, Schett G, Seitz CS, Hu Y, Gupta RS, Wick G. Surface staining and cytotoxic activity of heat-shock protein 60 antibody in stressed aortic endothelial cells.

Circ Res 1994;75:1078–1085.

66. Soltys BJ, Gupta RS. Immunoelectron microscopic localization of the 60-kDa heat shock chaperonin protein (Hsp60) in mammalian cells. Exp Cell Res 1996;222:16–27.

67. Xu Q, Kiechl S, Mayr M, Metzler B, Egger G, Oberhollenzer F, Willeit J, Wick G. Association of serum antibodies to heat-shock protein 65 with carotid atherosclerosis: clinical significance determined in a follow-up study. Circulation 1999;100:1169–1174.

68. Metzler B, Schett G, Kleindienst R, van der Zee R, Ottenhoff T, Hajeer A, Bernstein R, Xu Q, Wick G. Epitope specificity of anti-heat shock protein 65/60 serum antibodies in atherosclerosis. Arterioscler Thromb Vasc Biol 1997;17:536–541.

69. Mukherjee M, De Benedictis C, Jewitt D, Kakkar VV. Association of antibodies to heat-shock protein-65 with percutaneous transluminal coronary angioplasty and subsequent restenosis. Thromb Haemost 1996;75:258–260.

70. Hoppichler F, Lechleitner M, Traweger C, Schett G, Dzien A, Sturm W, Xu Q. Changes of serum antibodies to heat-shock protein 65 in coronary heart disease and acute myocardial infarction. Atherosclerosis 1996;126:333–338.

71. Birnie DH, Holme ER, McKay IC, Hood S, McColl KE, Hillis WS. Association between antibodies to heat shock protein 65 and coronary atherosclerosis. Possible mechanism of action of Helicobacter pylori and other bacterial infections in increasing cardiovascular risk. Eur Heart J 1998;19:387–394.

72. Gruber R, Lederer S, Bechtel U, Lob S, Riethmüller G, Feucht HE. Increased antibody titers against mycobacterial heat-shock protein 65 in patients with vasculitis and arteriosclerosis. Int Arch Allergy Immunol 1996;110:95–98.

73. Schett G, Metzler B, Kleindienst R, Amberger A, Recheis H, Xu Q, Wick G. Myocardial injury leads to a release of heat shock protein (hsp) 60 and a suppression of the anti-hsp65 immune response. Cardiovasc Res 1999;42:685–695.

74. Mayr M, Kiechl S, Willeit J, Wick G, Xu Q. Infections, immunity and atherosclerosis: Association of antibodies to *C. Pneumoniae*, *H. Pylori* and cytomegalovirus with immune reactions to heat shock proteins 60 and carotid or femoral atherosclerosis. Circulation 2000;102:833–839.

75. Mayr M, Xu Q, Wick G. Atherogenic effects of chronic infections: The role of heat shock protein 60 in autoimmunity. Israel Med Assoc J 1999;1:272–277.

76. Xu Q, Schett G, Perschinka H, Mayr M, Willeit J, Kiechl S, and Wick G. Serum soluble heat shock protein 60 is elevated in subjects with atherosclerosis in a general population. Circulation 2000;102:14–20.

77. Zou Y, Hu Y, Metzler B, Xu Q. Signal transduction in arteriosclerosis: mechanical stress-activated MAP kinases in vascular smooth muscle cells (review). Int J Mol Med 1998;1:827–834.

78. Hu Y, Bock G, Wick G, Xu Q. Activation of PDGF receptor alpha in vascular smooth muscle cells by mechanical stress. FASEB J 1998;12;1135–1142.

79. Anderton SM, Van Eden W. T-lymphocyte recognition of hsp 60 in experimental arthritis. In: Stress Proteins in Medicine 1996; W Van Eden, DB Young (eds.) Marcel Dekker, Inc., New York.

80. Van Eden W, Thole JER, Van der Zee R, Noordzij A, Van Embden JDA, Hensen EJ, Cohen IR. Cloning the mycobacterial epitope recognized by T lymphocytes in adjuvant arthritis. Nature 1988;331:171.

81. Hogervorst EJM, Wagenaar JPA, Boog CJP, Van der Zee R, Van Embden JDA, Van Eden W. Adjuvant arthritis and immunity to the mycobacterial 65kD heat shock protein. Intern Immunol 1992;4:719.

Atherosclerosis and Autoimmunity
Y. Shoenfeld, D. Harats and G. Wick, editors

Autoimmune Aspects of Atherosclerosis

Göran K. Hansson[1] and Antonino Nicoletti[2]

[1]Center for Molecular Medicine, Karolinska Institute, Stockholm, Sweden; [2]INSERM U430, Hôpital Broussais, Paris, France

1. INTRODUCTION

Atherosclerosis remains the principal cause of death in the world [1]. Its etiologic and pathogenic mechanisms have not been completely elucidated [2, 3] although epidemiological studies have identified a number of risk factors associated with cardiovascular disease. These include family history, smoking, hypertension, and elevated serum cholesterol levels. However, such "risk factors" are associated with only about 50% of cases of cardiovascular disease [4, 5] and consequently, all the efforts to control them have led to a rather modest decrease in the clinical manifestations of the disease.

The sequence of events in plaque formation and analysis of its components can shed light on the mechanisms involved in the pathogenesis of atherosclerosis. At an early stage, monocytes adhere to morphologically intact endothelium, then traverse the endothelium, accumulate as a subendothelial layer and start to accumulate lipid, forming so-called foam cells [6–9]. The lesion is further expanded by an invasion of smooth muscle cells, presumably deriving from the media, and which will produce extracellular matrix, forming a cap that surrounds the "core" containing foam cells and extracellular cholesterol. This sequence of events has been well described in experimental hypercholesterolemic animals [10–15]. As the disease progresses, the plaque may be complicated by calcification and eventually may rupture to the lumen. Indeed, clinical symptoms such as ischemic heart disease develop as a consequence of plaque complication [16].

Thus, the non cellular components of the plaque are mainly extracellular matrix components and LDL while the cellular compartment is represented by macrophages and migrated smooth muscle cells. About 15 years ago, it was demonstrated that 20% of the infiltrating inflammatory cells in the atheromas are T lymphocytes [17], which are in an activated state [18, 19]. This led to the proposal of a completely new pathogenetic mechanism. Nowadays, it is suggested by many authors that a specific immune response could initiate and/or perpetuate the atherosclerotic process. However, establishing a harmful or protective role of the immune response in any pathologic process is not trivial and many different aspects need to be characterized by experimental studies. In the present review, some studies that have evaluated the involvement of the immune system during atherogenesis will be discussed and these findings will be confronted to concepts of fundamental immunology. Finally, the validation of these concepts by experimental immunomodulation will be considered.

2. DESCRIPTIVE STUDIES IN HUMANS

The idea of atherosclerosis as an inflammatory disorder was proposed already in the nineteenth century [20], but more firm evidence for this view was presented through light microscopic studies in the 1960s, when lymphocyte-like cells were demonstrated in the adventitia surrounding the atheromatous arteries [21]. The development of immunohistochemical techniques provided definitive evidence for the presence of T lymphocytes in the plaque [17] and quantitative analysis revealed that up to 20% of the cells in some regions of the plaque were T cells [22]. These studies were thereafter confirmed by many other studies [18, 23-25]. The presence of T cells in the plaque has been the basis for theories of the local immune response in atherogenesis postulating that T cells may affect the surrounding tissues [26, 27]. The characterization of the T cells in the human plaque has been pursued in great detail and it is now known that these T cells are polyclonal [28] memory T cells, mainly of the CD4+ TCRαβ+ type [19]. The demonstration that T cells isolated from the human plaque were reactive against oxidized LDL (oxLDL) [29] identified a major target of the cellular immune response in the plaque.

The association of elevated levels of circulating antibodies to oxidized LDL in patients with advanced atherosclerosis [30] suggests a possible involvement also of a B cell-mediated response in the pathogenesis of ischemic heart disease [31]. Immune complexes with the modified LDL would favour the uptake of oxidized LDL contributing to foam cell formation [32, 33] and eventually activate the complement cascade [34–36] leading to amplification of the inflammatory component in the plaque.

The limitation of epidemiological and pathologic studies consists in their focusing on the most readily available explanations, such as the chronic atherosclerotic background, thrombosis and plaque fissure, as plausible triggers of ischemic events. Thus experimental studies are necessary to understand the role of the single pathogenic component in the initiation and perpetuation of atherosclerotic disease. Here we will focus on the immune components of atherogenesis.

3. DESCRIPTIVE STUDIES IN EXPERIMENTAL MODELS

For those interested in the involvement of the immune system in atherosclerosis, good experimental animal models have become available during recent years. A good animal model in this field could be postulated as presenting lesions similar in structure and composition to those found in humans, developing lesions in a relatively short time, with an immune system well characterized, easy to manipulate, and maintained preferably at a reasonable cost. While the rabbit fullfills some of these requirements, the mouse models are the ones best suited for

this kind of studies.

The pioneering studies performed in the mouse were aimed at finding the strain of mice most susceptible to atherosclerosis. Paigen et al established that wild-type mice are relatively resistant to the disease and develop fatty streak lesions but not fibrofatty atherosclerotic plaques [37, 38]. The most susceptible strain was found to be the C57Bl/6 strain and thus it was used for the development of transgenic strains more sensitive to atherosclerosis than the wild-type mice (see [39] for review). The most used atherosclerotic mouse is the apoE knockout mouse [40] which is deficient in apolipoprotein E, a important ligand for lipoprotein clearance. As a consequence of this deficiency, these mice develop severe hypercholesterolemia and fibrofatty atherosclerotic plaques resembling those observed in humans [41, 42]. These lesions are exacerbated when the mice are fed a high-cholesterol, high-fat, Western-type diet. The similarity with the human lesions goes beyond the morphology. Indeed, as humans, apoE knockout mice show modified LDL in the aortic lesions and elevated serum levels of antibodies against modified LDL [43]. B cell hybridomas producing monoclonal autoantibodies to epitopes of oxidized lipoproteins were cloned from apoE KO mice [44], demonstrating that spontaneous oxidation of lipoproteins in vivo can be the source of the specific epitopes of these antibodies. A cell-mediated response has also been shown in the plaques of apoE KO mice. Zhou et al [45] have shown that the aortic lesions of apoE mice contains CD4+ and CD8+ T cells and that hypercholesterolemia can effectively affect the T helper (Th) 1/Th2 switch in the atherosclerosis- related immune response [46]. T cells of early atherosclerotic lesions in the the apoE KO mouse show restricted heterogeneity with regard to T cell receptor (TCR) gene rearrangement patterns [47]. This implies that oligoclonal expansions of specific T cells take place during atherogenesis.

4. THE TARGETS

The non-cellular components of the plaque are mainly extracellular matrix and LDL. The composition of LDL renders it sensitive to modification by oxidative reactions. The presence of oxLDL in the plaque is thought to be able to trigger the infiltration of macrophages and the deposition of specific autoantibodies. Macrophages reduce the extracellular accumulation of LDL modified by oxidative reactions by uptake via scavenger receptors [48, 49]. This pathway has no negative feed-back and thus the macrophage continues to take up oxLDL until cholesterol ester accumulation results in the characteristic foam cell. We have shown that scavenger receptors A can mediate uptake of modified antigens such as oxLDL for presentation to antigen-specific T cells [50]. T cells specific for oxLDL are present in the human plaques [29] and can be isolated from the lymphoid organs of apoE KO mice [51, 52]. These data place oxLDL as a strong candidate antigen.

The discovery that human plaque contains heat shock proteins [53] and that immunization of rabbit with bacterial HSP-65 could induce arteriosclerosis despite a normocholesterolemic diet [54] has shed light on HSPs as potential targets of the immune response in atherosclerosis [55]. This theory is founded in basic concepts of immunology since there is evidence for an antigenicity of HSPs [56, 57]. However, the priming element is not yet well defined and could either be the microbial HSP or the self HSP. On the other hand, the lesions induced in these immunization protocols are not mature atherosclerotic lesions and could represent an inflammatory vascular lesion that may or may not progress into atherosclerosis depending on other factors such as lipids and hemodynamics. Thus, HSP may play an aggravating rather than a causative role.

A possible role for infectious agents is suggested by the presence of viral genomes in human atheromas such as Herpesvirus [58] or cytomegalovirus [59–61] and experimental murine infection with cytomegalovirus is associated with an inflammatory response in the aortic lumen [62]. *Chlamydia pneumoniae* (*Cp*), a human respiratory pathogen that causes acute respiratory disease and approximately 10% of community-acquired pneumonia, has been associated with coronary artery disease [63–68] suggesting that *Cp* may be involved in the atherosclerotic process. Nevertheless, this association is not confirmed by other studies [69]. We shall consider that *Cp* infection is geographically widespread. Seroepidemiological studies have shown that virtually everyone is infected with the *Cp* organ-

isms at some time and that reinfection is common. Other bacterial organisms have also been proposed, although results are contradictory. For instance, *Helicobacter pylori* strains were associated with ischemic heart disease in one study [70] while other studies did not find such an association [71]. One should keep in mind that none of these studies could provide evidence of active pathogenic activity of the microorganisms in situ.

New concepts in this field of research are emerging, and particularly the notion of "multiple infections". The presence serological responses towards more than one pathogen seems to be associated with an increased prevalence of coronary artery disease. Since many different common pathogens may be associated with clinical manifestations of coronary artery disease, one might speculate that the complexity of the specific immune responses directed against each pathogen could yield to a balanced Th1/Th2 environment. In this view, prevalent infections occurring spontaneously as well as provoked by strategies aiming at eradicating or suppressing one or a few pathogens could break this equilibrium.

Before postulating a cause-effect relationship between infections and atherosclerosis [72, 73], it should be kept in mind that atherosclerosis could actually be the causal element and the infection an opportunistic event. Indeed, the lesions could be considered as wounds where opportunistic infectious agents could home. This point of view does not preclude a modulating role for the infectious agents that could either be protective (for instance promoting a Th2 immune response and thus an anti-inflammatory environment) or deleterious (directly due to the cytotoxicity of the microorganism or indirectly through a boosting of a proinflammatory Th1 immune response). Experimental studies should be specifically designed to investigate the role of the antimicrobial cell-mediated and humoral immune responses in atherosclerosis.

Given the growing interest of microbial infections in atherosclerosis, animal models have been established, including mouse models [74]. One warning in that domain of research is that most pathogens involved so far are not natural pathogens of the animal models. Thus the effect observed with these microorganisms might not represent the effects they exert in humans. This is illustrated by the fact that

Helicobacter pylori does not provoke ulcers in mice, clearly indicating that the targets of these bacteria in the mouse are distinct from the human ones.

5. IMMUNE DEFECTS, IMMUNOMODULATION AND ATHEROSCLEROSIS

To study the role of the immune system in atherosclerosis, several immunocompromised models have been developed. This has been achieved either by selective or total immunosuppression and produced by genetic engineering or immunomodulation induced by drugs or antibodies.

6. GENETIC IMMUNODEFICIENCY

Studies on C57Bl/6 mice may give clues on the role of the immune system in fatty streak formation although the early stage and variable extent of fatty streaks in these animals reduce the power of the analysis. Results obtained in genetically immunodeficient C57Bl/6 mice are not so clear in interpretation and present several contradictions. Given that TNF-α promotes numerous inflammatory reactions associated with atherosclerosis, the absence of the TNF receptor (p55) in mice was expected to protect against atherosclerosis. Surprisingly, p55 KO mice (C57Bl/6 strain) show aortic sinus lesion sizes >2 fold larger than C57BL/6 wild type mice when fed an atherogenic diet despite equivalent lipid levels between strains [75]. Moreover, class I MHC deficient mice, and to a lesser extent severe combined immune deficiency (SCID), have increased lesions compared to wildtype C57BL/6J mice despite similar lipoprotein profiles [76], suggesting a major role for the T cytotoxic response in fatty streak formation.

Defective recruitment mechanisms for mononuclear leukocytes result in significant reduction of atherosclerosis in murine models. Thus, LDL receptor deficient mice that carry targeted deletions of the gene for monocyte chemoattractant protein-1 (MCP-1) or its receptor CCR2 exhibit significantly less atherosclerosis than LDL receptor-knockouts with intact MCP-1 signaling [77, 78]. Similarly,

apoE deficient mice that are also deficient in P-selectin or intercellular adhesion molecule-1 (ICAM-1) are protected against atherosclerosis [79]. Macrophage colony-stimulating factor deficient mice show decreased counts of total leukocytes and lymphocytes as well as blood monocytes and peritoneal macrophages [80]. Smith et al [81] have shown that apoE KO mice lacking the macrophage colony-stimulating factor develop 70% less lesions than single apoE KO mice despite very high cholesterol levels (1300 mg/dL). This strongly suggests that macrophages and/or lymphocytes are pro-atherogenic.

ApoE KO crossed with interferon-γ receptor KO mice substantiate the interpretation that lymphocytes are proatherogenic since they exhibit 60% less lesions than apoE KO mice [82] suggesting that interferon-γ and thus T cells (the source of interferon-γ is exclusively the T and NK cells) promote atherosclerosis. These results were not confirmed in Rag2-apoE double KO (lacking mature T and B cells) [83]. However, in this study, the levels of total serum cholesterol were extremely elevated (>2000 mg/dL) and such a non-physiologic concentration of cholesterol would surely mask the effective role of the immune system in atherosclerosis. This is substantiated by the work of Dansky et al [84] who showed that on chow diet (cholesterol levels ~400 mg/dL), Rag1-apoE double KO mice exhibit almost 50% less lesions than apoE single-KO mice. The group of mice put on Western diet, which developed very high cholesterol levels (~1000 mg/dL), showed only minor effects on lesions. Taken together, these results suggest that the cellular immune response is deleterious rather than protective in physiologic conditions.

This conclusion is confirmed in our recent study of SCID/apoE mice, which lack T and B cells [85]. They have a 70% reduction in lesions, however, reconstitution with CD4+ T cells returns lesion size almost to the level of immunocompetent apoE KO mice.

7. OTHER TYPES OF IMMUNOMODULATIONS

7.1. Immunosuppression

Emeson et al [86] showed that cyclosporin A treatment moderately accelerated atherosclerosis in hyperlipidemic C57BL/6 mice which supports the hypothesis of a protective role of the cell-mediated response at the fatty streak stage. However, a different study from the same group [87] showed that CD4+ and CD8+ T cell depletion reduced fatty streak formation in C57BL/6 hyperlipidemic mice indicating that T cells would actually aggravate fatty streak formation. It is possible that the results of cyclosporin treatment are due to effects on vascular as well as immune cells, since this drug can inhibit growth factor-induced smooth muscle proliferation [88, 89].

The cytokines interleukin 1 (IL-1) and tumor necrosis factor (TNF) are secreted by the different cell populations of the vascular wall and have been suggested to promote atherosclerosis. Their respective roles in atherogenesis were investigated in apoE KO mice by use of IL-1 receptor antagonist and TNF binding protein [90]. Blocking TNF or IL-1 was protecting apoE KO mice from atherosclerosis, demonstrating that these inflammatory cytokines play a deleterious role in lesion formation.

Recently, new reports have been published on more fine tuning of the immune response in atherosclerosis providing interesting insight into the mechanisms involved in atherogenesis. Cells in human atherosclerotic lesions express the immune mediator CD40 and its ligand CD40L [91]. The interaction of CD40 with CD40L is important in both humoral and cell-mediated immune responses and treatment with antibody against mouse CD40L limited atherosclerosis in mice lacking the receptor for low-density lipoprotein which had been fed a high-cholesterol diet for 12 weeks [92]. This study indicates a role for CD40 signaling in atherogenesis and suggests that the immune response may be pro-atherogenic.

We evaluated whether immune modulation in apoE KO mice could affects disease development by using intravenous immunoglobulins (ivIg) which is a therapeutic tool for autoimmune and systemic inflammatory diseases [93, 94]. The immunomodulating action of ivIg is still unclear and may involve both Fc- and V region-dependent mechanisms (see ref. [95] for review). The Fc portion of ivIg may block Fc receptors on phagocytic cells of the reticuloendothelial system, inhibiting antibody synthesis by B cells, modulating suppressor and helper functions of T cells, affecting the production of cytokines by monocytes/macrophages, and interfering with complement-mediated tissue damage. V region-dependent mechanisms, on the other hand, include specific antibodies that bind antigens in the recipient.

Injections of apoE KO mice with ivIg reduced by 35% fatty streak formation and by 50% mature fibrofatty lesions [96]. In this study, we also found that ivIg treatment reduced IgM antibodies to oxidized LDL and led to inactivation of spleen and lymph node T cells. These data indicate that ivIg inhibits atherosclerosis both during the fatty streak and mature lesion phases, and that this protection could be explained by the modulation of T cell activity and/or antibody production. Of note, ivIg preparations also contain anti-CD40 and anti-CD40L antibodies (Kaveri S., personal communication).

7.2. Passive and Active Immunization

Several authors have demonstrated that anticardiolipin antibodies (aCL) can activate platelets and endothelial cells as well as increase oxidized low density lipoprotein (LDL) uptake by macrophages and immunization with aCL [97, 98] resulted in accelerated fatty streak formation. Similarly, immunization to HSPs is proatherogenic [55, 99]. In contrast, immunization with modified LDL epitopes leads to reduced atherosclerotic lesions [100-103] as well as reduced neointimal formation after balloon injury [104]. Of note, most of these studies employed hyperimmunization strategies with incomplete Freund's adjuvant. Such strategies promote a humoral immune response but are rather poor activators of cell-mediated immunity. Therefore, such studies suggest that the humoral immune response to oxLDL is likely protective. Alternatively to the hyperimmunization strategies, tolerance strategies have also to be considered. We are currently exploring this possibility.

21

8. CONCLUSION

Taken together, all the experimental studies in immunomodulated atherosclerotic mice show that the immune response protect from atherogenesis in the early stages of the disease but results in accelerated atherosclerotic progression at the later stages. However, results in hypercholesterolemic atherosclerotic mice models have to be taken with caution, since it is now clear that hypercholesterolemia can substantially affect the T helper response in these mice [46]. Furthermore, different epitopes may exert diverse kind of immune response, resulting either in protection or worsening of atherosclerosis. The reactivity to some antigens may well be more complex than thought with dichotomic effects, an effect mediated by the humoral immune response and an effect mediated by the cell-mediated immune response.

A fine modulation of the immune response, aimed at targeting the right epitopes, by immunization or tolerization, and controlling the T cell phenotype, may become a powerful tool in prevention and treatment of atherosclerosis in humans.

REFERENCES

1. Murray CJ, Lopez AD. Global mortality, disability, and the contribution of risk factors: Global Burden of Disease Study. Lancet 1997;349:1436–42.
2. James TN. Presidential address. AHA 53rd scientific sessions, Miami Beach, Florida, November 1980. Sure cures, quick fixes and easy answers. A cautionary tale about coronary disease. Circulation 1981;63:1199A–202A.
3. Ross R. The pathogenesis of atherosclerosis: a perspective for the 1990s. Nature 1993;362:801–9.
4. Braunwald E. Shattuck lecture-cardiovascular medicine at the turn of the millennium: triumphs, concerns, and opportunities. N Engl J Med 1997;337:1360–9.
5. Oliver MF. Prevention of coronary heart disease-propaganda, promises, problems, and prospects. Circulation 1986;73:1–9.
6. Stary HC. The intimal macrophage in atherosclerosis. Artery 1980;8:205–7.
7. Stary HC. Evolution and progression of atherosclerotic lesions in coronary arteries of children and young adults. Arteriosclerosis 1989;9:I19-32.
8. Stary HC. The sequence of cell and matrix changes in atherosclerotic lesions of coronary arteries in the first forty years of life. Eur Heart J 1990;11:3–19.
9. Stary HC. Composition and classification of human atherosclerotic lesions. Virchows Arch A 1992;421:277–90.
10. Rosenfeld ME, Tsukada T, Gown AM, Ross R. Fatty streak initiation in Watanabe Heritable Hyperlipemic and comparably hypercholesterolemic fat-fed rabbits. Arteriosclerosis 1987;7:9–23.
11. Rosenfeld ME, Tsukada T, Chait A, Bierman EL, Gown AM, Ross R. Fatty streak expansion and maturation in Watanabe Heritable Hyperlipemic and comparably hypercholesterolemic fat-fed rabbits. Arteriosclerosis 1987;7:24–34.
12. Gerrity RG. The role of the monocyte in atherogenesis: I. Transition of blood-borne monocytes into foam cells in fatty lesions. Am J Pathol 1981;103:181–90.
13. Gerrity RG. The role of the monocyte in atherogenesis: II. Migration of foam cells from atherosclerotic lesions. Am J Pathol 1981;103:191–200.
14. Faggiotto A, Ross R. Studies of hypercholesterolemia in the nonhuman primate. II. Fatty streak conversion to fibrous plaque. Arteriosclerosis 1984;4:341–56.
15. Faggiotto A, Ross R, Harker L. Studies of hypercholesterolemia in the nonhuman primate. I. Changes that lead to fatty streak formation. Arteriosclerosis 1984;4:323–40.
16. Libby P. Molecular bases of the acute coronary syndromes. Circulation 1995;91:2844–50.
17. Jonasson L, Holm J, Skalli O, Gabbiani G, Hansson GK. Expression of class II transplantation antigen on vascular smooth muscle cells in human atherosclerosis. J Clin Invest 1985;76:125–31.
18. Hansson GK, Holm J, Jonasson L. Detection of activated T lymphocytes in the human atherosclerotic plaque. Am J Pathol 1989;135:169–75.
19. Stemme S, Holm J, Hansson GK. T lymphocytes in human atherosclerotic plaques are memory cells expressing CD45RO and the integrin VLA-1. Arterioscler Thromb 1992;12:206–11.
20. Virchow R. Der atheromatose Prozess der Arterien. Wien Med Wochenschr 1856;6:825-8.
21. Schwartz CJ, Mitchell JRA. Cellular infiltration of the human arterial adventitia associated with atheromatous plaque. Circulation 1962;26:73–8.
22. Jonasson L, Holm J, Skalli O, Bondjers G, Hansson GK. Regional accumulations of T cells, macrophages, and smooth muscle cells in the human atherosclerotic plaque. Arteriosclerosis 1986;6:131–8.
23. Munro JM, van der Walt JD, Munro CS, Chalmers JA, Cox EL. An immunohistochemical analysis of human aortic fatty streaks. Hum Pathol 1987;18:375–80.
24. Emeson EE, Robertson AL, Jr. T lymphocytes in aortic

and coronary intimas. Their potential role in atherogenesis. Am J Pathol 1988;130:369–76.

25. van der Wal AC, Das PK, Bentz van de Berg D, van der Loos CM, Becker AE. Atherosclerotic lesions in humans. In situ immunophenotypic analysis suggesting an immune mediated response. Lab Invest 1989;61:166–70.

26. Hansson GK, Jonasson L, Seifert PS, Stemme S. Immune mechanisms in atherosclerosis. Arteriosclerosis 1989;9:567–78.

27. Libby P, Hansson GK. Involvement of the immune system in human atherogenesis: current knowledge and unanswered questions. Lab Invest 1991;64:5–15.

28. Stemme S, Rymo L, Hansson GK. Polyclonal origin of T lymphocytes in human atherosclerotic plaques. Lab Invest 1991;65:651–60.

29. Stemme S, Faber B, Holm J, Wiklund O, Witzum JL, Hansson GK. T lymphocytes from human atherosclerotic plaques recognize oxidized low density lipoprotein. Proc Natl Acad Sci USA 1995;92:3893–7.

30. Parums DV, Brown DL, Mitchinson MJ. Serum antibodies to oxidized low-density lipoprotein and ceroid in chronic periaortitis. Arch Pathol Lab Med 1990;114:383–7.

31. Salonen JT, Yla-Herttuala S, Yamamoto R, Butler S, Korpela H, Salonen R, et al. Autoantibody against oxidised LDL and progression of carotid atherosclerosis. Lancet 1992;339:883–7.

32. Griffith RL, Virella GT, Stevenson HC, Lopes-Virella MF. Low density lipoprotein metabolism by human macrophages activated with low density lipoprotein immune complexes. A possible mechanism of foam cell formation. J Exp Med 1988;168:1041–59.

33. Palinski W, Rosenfeld ME, Yla-Herttuala S, Gurtner GC, Socher SS, Butler SW, et al. Low density lipoprotein undergoes oxidative modification in vivo. Proc Natl Acad Sci USA 1989;86:1372–6.

34. Seifert PS, Hansson GK. Decay-accelerating factor is expressed on vascular smooth muscle cells in human atherosclerotic lesions. J Clin Invest 1989;84:597–601.

35. Seifert PS, Hugo F, Hansson GK, Bhakdi S. Prelesional complement activation in experimental atherosclerosis : terminal C5b-9 complement deposition coincides with cholesterol accumulation in the aortic intima of hypercholesterolemic rabbits. Lab Invest 1989;60:747–54.

36. Seifert PS, Hansson GK. Complement receptors and regulatory proteins in human atherosclerotic lesions. Arteriosclerosis 1989;9:802–11.

37. Paigen B, Morrow A, Brandon C, Mitchell D, Holmes P. Variation in susceptibility to atherosclerosis among inbred strains of mice. Atherosclerosis 1985;57:65–73.

38. Paigen B, Ishida BY, Verstuyft J, Winters RB, Albee D. Atherosclerosis susceptibility differences among progenitors of recombinant inbred strains of mice. Arteriosclerosis 1990;10:316–23.

39. Breslow JL. Mouse models of atherosclerosis. Science 1996;272:685–8.

40. Plump AS, Smith JD, Hayek T, Aalto-Setala K, Walsh A, Verstuyft JG, et al. Severe hypercholesterolemia and atherosclerosis in apolipoprotein E-deficient mice created by homologous recombination in ES cells. Cell 1992;71:343–53.

41. Palinski W, Ord VA, Plump AS, Breslow JL, Steinberg D, Witztum JL. ApoE-deficient mice are a model of lipoprotein oxidation in atherogenesis. Demonstration of oxidation-specific epitopes in lesions and high titers of autoantibodies to malondialdehyde-lysine in serum. Arterioscler Thromb 1994;14:605–16.

42. Nakashima Y, Plump AS, Raines EW, Breslow JL, Ross R. ApoE-deficient mice develop lesions of all phases of atherosclerosis throughout the arterial tree. Arterioscler Thromb 1994;14:133–40.

43. Palinski W, Ylä-Herttuala S, Rosenfeld ME, Butler SW, Socher SA, Parthasarathy S, et al. Antisera and monoclonal antibodies specific for epitopes generated during oxidative modification of low density lipoprotein. Arteriosclerosis 1990;10:325–35.

44. Palinski W, Horkko S, Miller E, Steinbrecher UP, Powell HC, Curtiss LK, et al. Cloning of monoclonal autoantibodies to epitopes of oxidized lipoproteins from apolipoprotein E-deficient mice. Demonstration of epitopes of oxidized low density lipoprotein in human plasma. J Clin Invest 1996;98:800–14.

45. Zhou X, Stemme S, Hansson GK. Evidence for a local immune response in atherosclerosis. CD4+ T cells infiltrate lesions of apolipoprotein-E-deficient mice. Am J Pathol 1996;149:359–66.

46. Zhou X, Paulsson G, Stemme S, Hansson GK. Hypercholesterolemia is associated with a T helper (Th) 1/Th2 switch of the autoimmune response in atherosclerotic apo E-knockout mice. J Clin Invest 1998;101:1717–25.

47. Paulsson G, Zhou, X., Törnquist, E., Hansson, G. K. Oligoclonal T cell expansions in atherosclerotic lesions of apolipoprotein E-deficient mice. Arterioscl Thromb Vasc Biol 2000;20:10-7.

48. Brown MS, Goldstein JL. Lipoprotein metabolism in the macrophage: Implifications for cholesterol deposition in atherosclerosis. Annu Rev Biochem 1983;52:223–61.

49. Steinberg D, Parthasarathy S, Carew TE, Khoo JC, Witztum JL. Beyond cholesterol: modifications of low-density lipoprotein that increase its atherogenicity. N Engl J Med 1989;320:915–24.

50. Nicoletti A, Caligiuri G, Tornberg I, Kodama T, Stemme S, Hansson GK. The macrophage scavenger receptor type A directs modified proteins to antigen presentation. Eur J Immunol 1998;28:1–10.

51. Nicoletti A, Paulsson G, Hansson E, Törnberg I, Hansson GK. T helper lymphocytes specific for modified LDL in apoB transgenic and apoE knockout mice. (Submitted).

52. Caligiuri G, Nicoletti, A., Törnberg, I., Hansson, G. K. Effects of sex and age on atherosclerosis and autoimmunity in apoE-deficient mice. Atherosclerosis 1999;145:301–8.

53. Berberian PA, Myers W, Tytell M, Challa V, Bond MG. Immunohistochemical localization of heat shock protein-70 in normal-appearing and atherosclerotic specimens of human arteries. Am J Pathol 1990;136:71–80.

54. Xu Q, Dietrich H, Steiner HJ, Gown AM, Schoel B, Mikuz G, et al. Induction of arteriosclerosis in normocholesterolemic rabbits by immunization with heat shock protein 65. Arterioscler Thromb 1992;12:789–99.

55. Wick G, Schett G, Amberger A, Kleindienst R, Xu Q. Is atherosclerosis an immunologically mediated disease? Immunol Today 1995;16:27–33.

56. Feige U, van EW. Infection, autoimmunity and autoimmune disease. Exs 1996;77:359–73.

57. Kaufmann SH. Heat shock proteins and the immune response. Immunol Today 1990;11:129–36.

58. Benditt EP, Barrett T, McDougall JK. Viruses in the etiology of atherosclerosis. Proc Natl Acad Sci USA 1983;80:6386–9.

59. Nieto FJ, Adam E, Sorlie P, Farzadegan H, Melnick JL, Comstock GW, et al. Cohort study of cytomegalovirus infection as a risk factor for carotid intimal-medial thickening, a measure of subclinical atherosclerosis. Circulation 1996;94:922–7.

60. Melnick JL, Hu C, Burek J, Adam E, DeBakey ME. Cytomegalovirus DNA in arterial walls of patients with atherosclerosis. J Med Virol 1994;42:170–4.

61. Chen S, Li W, Yang Y. Detection of human cytomegalovirus DNA in vascular plaques of atherosclerosis by in situ hybridization:. Chung Hua I Hsueh Tsa Chih; 1995;75:592-3,638.

62. Berencsi K, Endresz V, Klurfeld D, Kari L, Kritchevsky D, Gonczol E. Early atherosclerotic plaques in the aorta following cytomegalovirus infection of mice. Cell Adhes Commun 1998;5:39–47.

63. Halme S, Syrjala H, Bloigu A, Saikku P, Leinonen M, Airaksinen J, et al. Lymphocyte responses to Chlamydia antigens in patients with coronary heart disease. Eur Heart J 1997;18:1095–101.

64. Kuo CC, Shor A, Campbell LA, Fukushi H, Patton DL, Grayston JT. Demonstration of Chlamydia pneumoniae in atherosclerotic lesions of coronary arteries. J Infect Dis 1993;167:841–9.

65. Maass M, Gieffers J. Cardiovascular disease risk from prior Chlamydia pneumoniae infection can be related to certain antigens recognized in the immunoblot profile. J Infect 1997;35:171–6.

66. Maass M, Bartels C, Engel PM, Mamat U, Sievers HH. Endovascular presence of viable Chlamydia pneumoniae is a common phenomenon in coronary artery disease. J Am Coll Cardiol 1998;31:827–32.

67. Molestina RE, Dean D, Miller RD, Ramirez JA, Summersgill JT. Characterization of a strain of Chlamydia pneumoniae isolated from a coronary atheroma by analysis of the omp1 gene and biological activity in human endothelial cells. Infect Immun 1998;66:1370–6.

68. Puolakkainen M, Kuo CC, Shor A, Wang SP, Grayston JT, Campbell LA. Serological response to Chlamydia pneumoniae in adults with coronary arterial fatty streaks and fibrolipid plaques. Eur Heart J 1993;14:12–6.

69. Weiss SM, Roblin PM, Gaydos CA, Cummings P, Patton DL, Schulhoff N, et al. Failure to detect Chlamydia pneumoniae in coronary atheromas of patients undergoing atherectomy. J Infect Dis 1996;173:957–62.

70. Pasceri V, Cammarota G, Patti G, Cuoco L, Gasbarrini A, Grillo RL, et al. Association of virulent Helicobacter pylori strains with ischemic heart disease. Circulation 1998;97:1675–9.

71. Regnstrom J, Jovinge S, Bavenholm P, Ericsson CG, De FU, Hamsten A, et al. Helicobacter pylori seropositivity is not associated with inflammatory parameters, lipid concentrations and degree of coronary artery disease. J Intern Med 1998;243:109–13.

72. Nieminen MS, Mattila K, Valtonen V. Infection and inflammation as risk factors for myocardial infarction. Eur Heart J 1995;273:375–6.

73. Mehta JL, Saldeen TG, Rand K. Interactive role of infection, inflammation and traditional risk factors in atherosclerosis and coronary artery disease. J Am Coll Cardiol 1998;31:1217–25.

74. Moazed TC, Kuo C, Grayston JT, Campbell LA. Murine models of Chlamydia pneumoniae infection and atherosclerosis. J Infect Dis 1997;175:883–90.

75. Schreyer SA, Peschon JJ, LeBoeuf RC. Accelerated atherosclerosis in mice lacking tumor necrosis factor receptor p55. J Biol Chem 1996;271:26174–8.

76. Fyfe AI, Qiao JH, Lusis AJ. Immune-deficient mice develop typical atherosclerotic fatty streaks when fed an atherogenic diet. J Clin Invest 1994;94:2516–20.

77. Boring L, Gosling, J., Cleary, M., Charo, I. F. Decreased lesion formation in CCR2-/- mice reveals a role for chemokines in the initiation of atherosclerosis. Nature 1998;394:894–7.

78. Gosling J, Slaymaker, S., Gu, L., Tseng, S., Zlot, C. H., Young, S. G., Rollins, B. J., Charo, I. F. MCP-1 deficiency reduces susceptibility to atherosclerosis in mice that overexpress human apolipoprotein B. Journal of Clinical Investigation 1999;103:773–8.

79. Collins RG, Velji R, Guevara NV, Hicks MJ, Chan L,

Beaudet AL. P-Selectin or intercellular adhesion molecule (ICAM)-1 deficiency substantially protects against atherosclerosis in apolipoprotein E- deficient mice. J Exp Med 2000;191:189-94.

80. Wiktor-Jedrzejczak WW, Ahmed A, Szczylik C, Skelly RR. Hematological characterization of congenital osteopetrosis in op/op mouse. Possible mechanism for abnormal macrophage differentiation. J Exp Med 1982;156:1516–27.

81. Smith JD, Trogan E, Ginsberg M, Grigaux C, Tian J, Miyata M. Decreased atherosclerosis in mice deficient in both macrophage colony- stimulating factor (op) and apolipoprotein E. Proc Natl Acad Sci USA 1995;92:8264–8.

82. Gupta S, Pablo AM, Jiang XC, Wang N, Schindler C. IFNg potentiates atherosclerosis in apoE knock-out mice. J Clin Invest 1997;99:2752–561.

83. Daugherty A, Pure E, Delfel-Butteiger D, Chen S, Leferovich J, Roselaar SE, et al. The effects of total lymphocyte deficiency on the extent of atherosclerosis in apolipoprotein E-/- mice. J Clin Invest 1997;100:1575–80.

84. Dansky HM, Charlton SA, Harper MM, Smith JD. T and B lymphocytes play a minor role in atherosclerosis plaque formation in the apoliprotein E-deficient mouse. Proc Natl Acad Sci USA 1997;94:4642–6.

85. Zhou X, Nicoletti A, Elhage R, Hansson GK. Transfer of CD4+ T cells aggravates atheroclerosis in immunodeficient apoE knockout mice. Circulation 2000; in press.

86. Emeson EE, Shen ML. Accelerated atherosclerosis in hyperlipidemic C57BL/6 mice treated with cyclosporin A. Am J Pathol 1993;142:1906–15.

87. Emeson EE, Shen ML, Bell CG, Qureshi A. Inhibition of atherosclerosis in CD4 T-cell-ablated and nude (nu/nu) C57BL/6 hyperlipidemic mice. Am J Pathol 1996;149:675–85.

88. Jonasson L, Holm J, Hansson GK. Cyclosporin A inhibits smooth muscle proliferation in the vascular response to injury. Proc Natl Acad Sci USA 1988;85:2303–6.

89. Thyberg J, Hansson GK. Cyclosporine A inhibits induction of DNA synthesis by PDGF and other peptide mitogens in cultured rat aortic smooth muscle cells and dermal fibroblasts. Growth Factors 1991;4:209–19.

90. Elhage R, Maret A, Pieraggi MT, Thiers JC, Arnal JF, Bayard F. Differential effects of interleukin-1 receptor antagonist and tumor necrosis factor binding protein on fatty-streak formation in apolipoprotein E-deficient mice. Circulation 1998;97:242–4.

91. Mach F, Schonbeck U, Sukhova GK, Bourcier T, Bonnefoy JY, Pober JS, et al. Functional CD40 ligand is expressed on human vascular endothelial cells, smooth muscle cells, and macrophages: implications for CD40-CD40 ligand signaling in atherosclerosis. Proc Natl Acad Sci USA 1997;94:1931–6.

92. Mach F, Schonbeck U, Sukhova GK, Atkinson E, Libby P. Reduction of atherosclerosis in mice by inhibition of CD40 signalling. Nature 1998;394:200–3.

93. Dwyer JM. Manipulating the immune systel with immune globulin. N Engl J Med 1992;326:107–16.

94. Kaveri SV, Dietrich G, Hurez V, Kazatchkine MD. Intravenous immunoglobulins (IVIg) in the treatment of autimmune diseases. Clin Exp Immunol 1991;86:192–8.

95. Kazatchkine MD, Dietrich G, Hurez V, Ronda N, Bellon B, Rossi F, et al. V region-mediated selection of autoreactive repertoires by intravenous immunoglobulin (i.v.Ig) Immunol Rev 1994;139:79–107.

96. Nicoletti A, Kaveri S, Caligiuri G, Bariety J, Hansson GK. Immunoglobulin treatment reduces atherosclerosis in apo E knockout mice. J Clin Invest 1998;102:910–8.

97. George J, Afek A, Gilburd B, Levy Y, Blank M, Kopolovic J, et al. Atherosclerosis in LDL-receptor knockout mice is accelerated by immunization with anticardiolipin antibodies. Lupus 1997;6:723–9.

98. George J, Afek A, Gilburd B, Blank M, Levy Y, Aron MA, et al. Induction of early atherosclerosis in LDL-receptor-deficient mice immunized with beta2-glycoprotein I. Circulation 1998;98:1108–15.

99. Roma P, Catapano AL. Stress proteins and atherosclerosis. Atherosclerosis 1996;127:147–54.

100. Ameli S, Hultgardh-Nilsson A, Regnstrom J, Calara F, Yano J, Cercek B, et al. Effect of immunization with homologous LDL and oxidized LDL on early atherosclerosis in hypercholesterolemic rabbits. Arterioscl Thromb 1996;16:1074–9.

101. Palinski W, Miller E, Witztum JL. Immunization of low density lipoprotein (LDL) receptor-deficient rabbits with homologous malondialdehyde-modified LDL reduces atherogenesis. Proc Natl Acad Sci USA 1995;92:821–5.

102. George J, Afek A, Gilburd B, Levkovitz H, Shaish A, Goldberg I, et al. Hyperimmunization of apo-E-deficient mice with homologous malondialdehyde low-density lipoprotein suppresses early atherogenesis. Atherosclerosis 1998;138:147–52.

103. Freigang S, Horkko S, Miller E, Witztum JL, Palinski W. Immunization of LDL receptor-deficient mice with homologous malondialdehyde-modified and native LDL reduces progression of atherosclerosis by mechanisms other than induction of high titers of antibodies to oxidative neoepitopes. Arterioscler Thromb Vasc Biol 1998;18:1972–82.

104. Nilsson J, Calara F, Regnstrom J, Hultgardh-Nilsson A, Ameli S, Cercek B, et al. Immunization with homologous oxidized low density lipoprotein reduces neointi-

mal formation after balloon injury in hypercholesterolemic rabbits. J Am Coll Cardiol 1997;30:1886–91.

PATHOGENETIC IMMUNE MECHANISM OF ATHEROSCLEROSIS

Atherosclerosis and Autoimmunity
Y. Shoenfeld, D. Harats and G. Wick, editors

The Role of Macrophage Scavenger Receptors in Atherogenesis

Kiyoshi Takahashi, Motohiro Takeya, Naomi Sakashita, Mika Yoshimatsu and Katsunori Jinnouchi

Second Department of Pathology, Kumamoto University School of Medicine, Kumamoto 860–0811, Japan

1. INTRODUCTION

The development of atherosclerosis is induced by deposition of low density lipoproteins (LDL) in the arterial walls and followed by migration of monocytes from peripheral blood into the arterial walls, uptake of oxidized LDL (OxLDL) by macrophages, accumulation of cholesterol ester in macrophages, their transformation into foam cells, and numerical increment of foam cells in the atherosclerotic lesions [1]. The atherosclerotic lesions are classified into the diffuse intimal thickening, fatty streak lesions, atherosclerotic plaques, and complicated lesions [1–3]. In the diffuse intimal thickening, monocytes start to invade into the arterial intima and differentiate into macrophages [1–3]. Macrophages ingest modified LDL (mLDL), including OxLDL, and transform into foam cells. In the fatty streak lesions, the number of macrophage-derived foam cells increases in the arterial intima and a part of macrophage-derived foam cells proliferate *in loco* [1, 4, 5]. During the processes of foam cell transformation, OxLDL is actively ingested by macrophages, is digested and degraded into amino acids and free cholesterol within lysosomes [6]. Free cholesterol is released from the lysosomes into the cytosol, excess of cholesterol ester is accumulated in membrane-free lipid droplets by catalyzing with acyl coenzyme A:cholesterol acyltransferase-1 (ACAT-1), and intracellular accumulation of lipid droplets changes macrophages into foam cells [6, 7]. In the atherosclerotic plaques, the number of macrophage-derived foam cells increases more than in the fatty streak lesions, and besides the macrophage-derived foam cells, smooth muscle cells migrate from the subintimal layer and media of arteries, accumulate lipid droplets in the cytoplasm, and transform into foam cells. In the center of the plaques, necrotic lipid cores are formed. In the complicated lesions, the central lipid cores become enlarged with increased numbers of foam cells of both macrophage and smooth muscle cell origins, accompanied by arterial surface ulceration, thrombosis, and calcification.

About 20 years ago, Brown and Goldstein [8] proposed on macrophages the presence of specific receptors which participate in uptake of mLDL, including acetyl-LDL (AcLDL) and OxLDL, and called the receptors as scavenger receptors (SRs). In 1988, Kodama *et al.* [9] purified a 220 kDa trimeric membrane glycoprotein having the ability of macrophages to bind to AcLDL, and subsequently two bovine cDNAs encoding class A type I and type II macrophage SR (MSR-AI,II) were cloned [10, 11]. Further, cloning of cDNA for MSR-AI,II was reported in humans [12], mice [13, 14], and rabbits [14]. Since 1990, the present authors have performed collaboration studies on MSR-AI,II with Prof. T. Kodama, University of Tokyo, in human and experimental animal research fields. On the basis of the results obtained in our studies and from those of other groups of investigators, the authors review the role of MSR-AI,II and their relationship to monocyte chemoattractant protein-1 (MCP-1) and macrophage colony-stimulating factor (M-CSF) in atherogenesis.

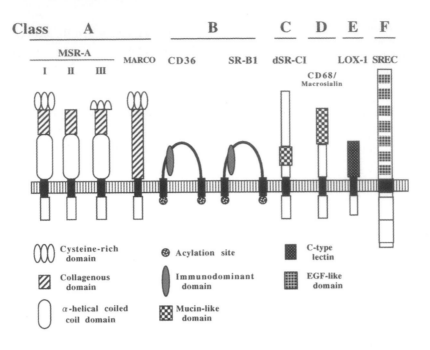

Figure 1. Classification and molecular structures of SRs.

2. CLASSIFICATION OF SRS

SRs are defined to be receptors binding to OxLDL, are heterogeneous in molecular structure, and include various types of receptors. Recently, they are classified into class A, B, C, D, E and F, and different types of receptors are included in each class (Fig. 1). In the class A, type I, type II, type III MSR, and MARCO (macrophage receptor with collagenous structure) are included, because these receptors possess a collagenous domain. All of the receptors are expressed on macrophages and are called MSR-A [15, 16]. CD36 and SR-BI (scavenger receptor type BI) belong to the class B. CD36 is an 88-kDa glycoprotein expressed on monocyte/macrophages, platelets, and endothelial cells; it serves as a receptor for both the adhesive glycoprotein thrombospondin and collagen [17, 18]. SR-BI is a CD36-related receptor and is regarded as a high density lipoprotein (HDL) receptor [19]. In the class C receptor, dSR-CI (Drosophila scavenger receptor) is included; it is expressed on macrophages in fetal stage [20]. CD68/macrosialin, classified in the class D, is a member of LAMP (lysosomal associated membrane protein) family and is expressed in the endolysosomal compartments and partly on the cell surface of macrophages [21–23]. Although Fcγ RII-B2 is a Fc receptor of IgG, is expressed on macrophages, and binds to OxLDL in mice [24], its function as MSR has not been proven in humans [25]. Besides these receptors, certain receptors such as LOX-1 (lectin-like LDL receptor) or SREC (scavenger receptor expressed by endothelial cells) can bind to OxLDL, are known to be expressed on vascular endothelial cells, and are classified as class E or class F scavenger receptor, respectively [26–28]. However, LOX-1 is also expressed on macrophages in humans and mice [27].

3. MOLECULAR STRUCTURE AND FUNCTION OF MSR-A

MSR-AI, II, and III are generated from the alternative splicing of a single gene located at the chromosomal region 8p22 in humans. These three types of the MSR consist of six domains: I, N-terminal cytoplasmic (residues 1–50), II, transmembranous (51–76), III, spacer (77–109), IV, α-helical coiled coil (110–272), V, collagen-like (273–341), VI, C-terminal type-specific (342–451 and 342–358 for type I and type II, respectively) (Fig. 2). MSR-AI,

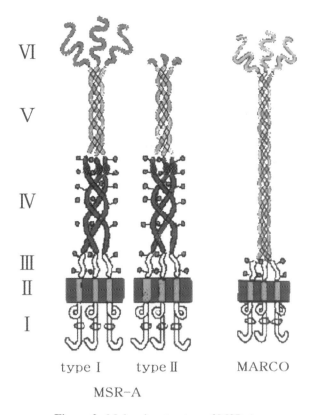

VI

V

IV

III

II

I

type I   type II   MARCO

MSR–A

Figure 2. Molecular structure of MSR-A.

II are expressed on the cell membrane of macrophages ubiquitously distributed in tissues of humans [29, 30], bovines [31], and mice [32]. Among these domains, the C-terminal 22 amino acids of the collagen-like domain are highly conserved among bovine, human, rabbit, and murine MSR-A molecules, and deletion mutation experiments indicated that these amino acids mediate ligand binding [14]. This region can bind to a diverse array of negatively charged macromolecules such as OxLDL, AcLDL, apoB-100, advanced glycation end products (AGE), polyanions such as polyguanyl or polyinosinic acids, lipoteichoic acid of Gram-positive bacteria, lipopolysaccharide (LPS) of Gram-negative bacteria, negatively charged collagens, crocidolite asbestos, or apoptotic cells. In this region, lysine residues are positively charged and responsible for binding to the negatively charged ligands [14]. The α-helical coiled coil domain mediates the assembly of functional trimeric receptors; its N-terminus is responsible for the formation of a stable trimer and its C-terminus exhibits pH-dependent conformational

changes which induce ligand dissociation [33, 34]. On the contrary, a study with anti-murine monoclonal antibody for MSR-AI,II, 2F8, demonstrated that the antibody inhibits cation-independent macrophage adhesion, suggesting that the α-helical coiled coil domain is involved in an adhesion function [35]. Although the C-terminal type-specific domain is called "cysteine-rich" domain, its function has not been known yet. MSR-AIII is localized in cytoplasmic vesicles and is not expressed on the cell surface. Thus, this receptor is unable to bind to any ligands existing extracellularly [36].

MARCO is a 210 kDa membrane glycoprotein consisting of a similar trimeric molecular structure to MSR-A, I,II, and III [37]. However, this receptor has an extremely long collagenous domain and a short α-helical coiled coil domain, suggesting that it lacks functions as adhesion molecule and dissociation from ligands within endosomes [37]. Thus, ligands bound to MARCO seem to be directly transported into lysosomes without dissociation. In unstimulated normal mice, MARCO receptor is expressed on marginal zone macrophages of spleen, macrophages in the marginal sinuses and medulla of lymph nodes, some peritoneal and pulmonary alveolar macrophages, and Kupffer cells in the liver [37–39]. MARCO selectively binds to bacterial antigens and neutral polysaccharides [37] and stimulation with LPS to mice induces enhanced expression of the receptor on Kupffer cells, pulmonary alveolar macrophages, and macrophages in other organs of the animals [39], suggesting that it is involved in host defense against bacterial infection. We have confirmed that a similar MARCO expression is induced by high cholesterol feeding to mice (data, not published).

4. TISSUE DISTRIBUTION, SUBCELLULAR LOCALIZATION, AND ENDOCYTIC PATHWAY OF MSR-AI,II IN MACROPHAGES DURING ENDOCYTOSIS

In humans, bovines, and mice, immunohistochemical studies using monoclonal antibodies against human, bovine, and murine MSR-AI,II clearly demonstrated the distribution and localization of the receptors on macrophages ubiquitously distributed

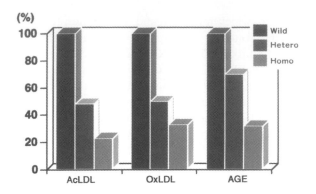

Figure 3. Percentages of uptake and degradation of AcLDL, OxLDL, and AGE by thioglycolate-elicited peritoneal macrophages in homozygous, heterozygous MSR-A-deficient mice relative to wild-type mice.

in tissues [29–32]. Our immunoelectron microscopic studies disclosed the localization of MSR-AI,II on the cell surface membrane of human and bovine macrophages [29, 31, 40, 41]. However, it is not expressed in monocytes and their precursor cells.

Our biochemical studies [42, 43] demonstrated that, when bovine macrophages were incubated with I^{125}-labeled AcLDL, OxLDL, and AGE, the association and degradation of the ligands by macrophages are increased in a dose-dependent manner at saturated conditions, the association of OxLDL is two times higher than that of AcLDL, and the degradation of OxLDL is one third of AcLDL. Based on these *in vitro* data, it seems that macrophages show more resistant proteolysis for OxLDL than for AcLDL [42]. To examine this notion *in vivo*, mice deficient in MSR-AI,II were generated by disrupting exon 4 which encodes α-helical coiled coil domain, an essential domain for the assembly of the functional trimeric structure [42, 43]. In the MSR-A-deficient mice, the degradation of I^{125}-labeled AcLDL, OxLDL, and AGE by thioglycolate-elicited peritoneal macrophages was reduced to one third of the wild-type mice (Fig. 3). These data show that MSR-AI,II is important for the uptake of these ligands by macrophages *in vivo* [42]. However, the reason why the ligands are taken up by MSR-AI,II-deficient macrophages seems to be explained by the involvement of MSRs other than MSR-AI,II.

Our previous *in vitro* studies on the endocytic processes of gold-labeled OxLDL, AcLDL, and AGE in bovine alveolar macrophages [40, 41] dem-

onstrated that on one hour incubation of the macrophages with these ligands at 4 °C, MSR-AI,II bind to the ligands but remain not internalized (Fig. 4A). On shift of temperature from 4 °C to 37 °C, the ligands bound to MSR-AI,II are concentrated in coated pits and are internalized into coated vesicles within a few minutes (Fig. 4B). With the lapse of time, the ligand-MSR-AI,II complexes are found on the membrane of vesicles and are transferred into early endosomes (Fig. 4C). Ten minutes later, the dissociation of the ligands from the receptors occurs within the endosomes and the ligands are found in their center of late endosomes and are transferred into lysosomes (Fig. 4D). In the lysosomes, immunoreactivity of the ligands disappears about 30 minutes later and gold particles remain for long time. These findings imply that the ligands are degraded within the lysosomes into cholesterol and amino acids. In our previous study on the endocytosis of the ligands in CHO cells transfected with a mutant receptor in which valine was changed into histidine at amino acid 168 from the C-terminus of α-helical coiled coil domain, we found that the ligands were not dissociated from MSR-AI,II within endosomes and that the ligand-receptor complexes remained for long time within endosomes, and were finally transported into lysosomes and degraded therein [33]. These data showed that the α-helical coiled coil domain is involved in ligand-receptor dissociation. About 15 to 20 minutes after incubation at 37 °C, transport vesicles containing MSR-AI,II appear around Golgi complexes and are transported into a trans-Golgi system (Fig. 4E). In the trans-Golgi system, MSR-AI,II are packed into secretory vesicles. The vesicles are transported into the cell periphery of macrophages (Fig. 4F), recycling MSR-AI,II to the cell membrane for reutilization [40, 41].

5. EXPRESSION OF MSR-AI,II DURING ATHOGENEIS IN HUMANS

In humans, the expression of MSR-AI,II in atherosclerotic lesions of human aortas was demonstrated immunohistochemically using a polyclonal antibody for synthetic peptides of human MSR-AI,II or monoclonal antibodies for human MSR-AI molecules [12, 29, 30]. In the diffuse intimal thickening, macrophages are scattered in the thickened intima and

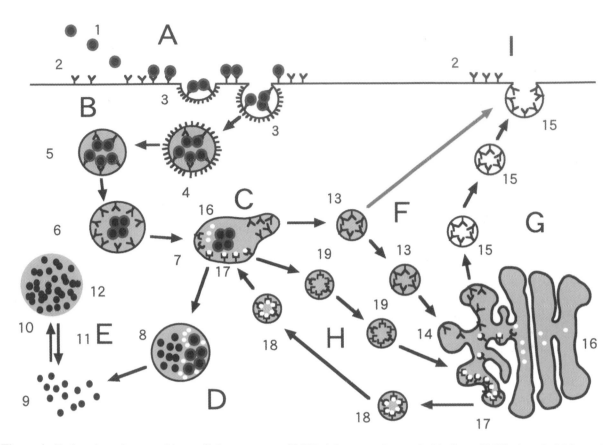

Figure 4. Endocytic pathway and intracellular transport of MSR-A in macrophages. A: binding of MSR-A to OxLDL on the cell surface, B: internalization, C: ligand-receptor dissociation in endosomes, D: lysosomal degradation, E: cholesterol ester cycle, F: transport of MSR-A to trans-Golgi system, G: transport of MSR-A by secretory vesicles to the cell membrane, H: transport of lysosomal hydrorases from Golgi complexes to endosomes, I: receptor recycling, 1: OxLDL, 2: MRS-A, 3: coated pit, 4: coated vesicle, 5, 6, 7: endosomes, 8: lysosomes, 9: free cholesterol, 10: esterification, 11: de-esterification, 12: lipid droplet, 13: trasport vesicles containing MSR-A, 14: trans-Golgi system, 15: secretory vesicles, 16: Golgi stacks, 17, 18: transport vesicles carrying lysosomal hydrolases, 19: transport vesicles returning from endosomes to trans-Golgi system.

arc intensely immunoreactive for these antibodies. In the fatty streak lesions, macrophages and macrophage-derived foam cells infiltrate in cluster or densely and are also immunoreactive. Compared with the foam cells, the immunoreactivity of the macrophages is more intense for the MSR-A antibodies. In the atherosclerotic plaques or complicated lesions, the numbers of MSR-A-positive cells are varied: however, the immunoreactivity for MSR-A is decreased in advanced lesions. Foam cells are occasionally negative for the antibodies and these MSR-A-negative foam cells are mostly of smooth muscle cell origin.

Immunohistochemical studies using a murine monoclonal antibody for human OxLDL, FOH1a/DLH3, which recognizes oxidized phosphatidylcholine of OxLDL, demonstrated intracellular accumulation of OxLDL in macrophages and macrophage-derived foam cells in the atherosclerotic lesions [44, 45]. In addition, OxLDL was also deposited in the other structures, including swollen collagen fibers, cellular debris in necrotic cores, and endothelial cells. Double staining with anti-human MSR-A antibodies and FOH1a/DLH3 revealed double positive reactions in macrophages and macrophage-derived foam cells, suggesting that extracellularly produced OxLDL is ingested by macrophages via MSR AI,II [44].

In order to examine immunohistochemical distribution and localization of AGEs in the atherosclerotic lesions, we used three distinct AGE-specific monoclonal antibodies, 6D12, 1F6, and 2A2: 6D12 recognizes N^ε-(carboxymethyl)lysine (CML), a nonfluororescent and noncrosslinked AGE structure, 1F6 recognizes fluorolink, a fluorescent and crosslinked AGE structure, and the epitope of 2A2 is unknown but is different from that of CML, fluorolink or other known AGE structures such as pyrrline, pentosidine, and crosslines. These AGE-specific molecular structures were demonstrated intra- or extracellularly in the atherosclerotic lesions of various stages. AGEs were localized in macrophages, macrophage-derived foam cells, smooth muscle cells, and endothelial cells, while they were also deposited in the extracellular spaces of the intima, media, and adventitia, as well as in collagen fibers [46, 47]. Double immunostainings with anti-human MSR-A antibodies and one of three AGE-specific monoclonal antibodies disclosed double positive reactions in macrophages and macrophage-derived foam cells [45, 46]. Immunoelectron microscopic studies revealed intralysosomal localization of AGEs in macrophage-derived foam cells, often associated with ceroid granules [46]. These findings suggested that the extracellularly produced AGEs were taken up by macrophages at least via MSR-AI,II receptors and were accumulated in lysosomes, although the other receptors such as RAGE (receptor for AGE), Galectin-3, and lyzozyme may be involved in the uptake of AGEs by macrophages [47].

Although MCP-1, MCP-2, MCP-3, MCP-4, macrophage inflammatory protein-1, tumor necrosis factor-α, transforming growth factor-β, M-CSF, granulocyte/macrophage colony-stimulating factor, and RANTES (regulated on activation, normal T expressed and secreted) are known to be factors inducing monocyte chemotaxis and migration, MCP-1 is the most intense monocyte chemotactic factor [48]. This protein was first cloned by Yoshimura *et al.* in 1989 [49]. Since 1991, we have performed collaboration studies with Dr. Yoshimura and generated murine anti-human and anti-rat MCP-1 monoclonal antibodies [50, 51]. Our immunohistochemical study using a mouse anti-human MCP-1 monoclonal antibody showed the expression of MCP-1 in vascular endothelial cells, macrophages, smooth muscle cells, foam cells, and infiltrated lymphocytes in the atherosclerotic lesions of various stages of aorta obtained from autopsy cases [52]. However, no expression of MCP-1 was demonstrated in normal-looking aorta and mild diffuse intimal thickening without cellular infiltration.

M-CSF is a growth factor which induces the development of monocytic cells in bone marrow, differentiation of monocytes into macrophages in tissues, proliferation and survival of tissue macrophages [53]. In the human atherosclerotic lesions, immunohistochemical expression of M-CSF or colony-stimulating factor-1 (CSF-1) were found in vascular endothelial cells, macrophages, foam cells, medial smooth muscle cells, and adventitial cells [54], in agreement with the results obtained from our previous study of cholesterol-fed rabbits [5] and from studies of other investigators in humans and animals [54, 55]. In the processes of monocyte migration into atherosclerotic lesions, their differentiation into macrophages, and foam cell transformation, MCP-1 and M-CSF are considered to be important for the expression of MSR-AI,II on macrophages and formation of foam cells in the lesions.

6. FUNCTIONAL ROLES OF MSR-AI,II DURING ATHEROGENESIS IN MICE

In order to clarify the role of MSR-AI,II in atherogenesis, we used two strains of atherogenic model mice, apolipoprotein E (apoE)-deficient mice and LDLR-deficient mice and mated them with MSR-A-deficient mice to generate apoE/MSR-A- or LDLR/MSR-A-double deficient mice [42, 43, 56]. In apoE-deficient mice, atherosclerosis spontaneously develops at several months after birth [57], whereas LDLR-deficient mice must be fed a high cholesterol diet to induce atherosclerosis [58]. Total serum cholesterol levels of apoE/MSR-A-double deficient mice were slightly higher than that of apoE-single deficient mice [42, 43]. However, the average size of atherosclerotic lesions in the double deficient mice was reduced to nearly 60% of the single deficient mice. LDLR-single deficient mice and LDLR/MSR-A-double deficient mice started to be fed a 1.25% high cholesterol diet at 3 months of age to induce atherosclerosis [56]. At 4 and 12 weeks after high cholesterol feeding, the lesion size in the double

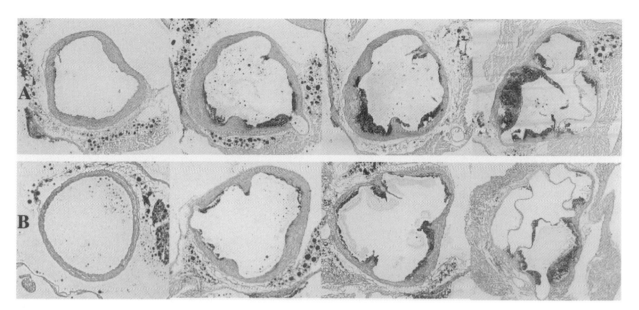

Figure 5. Light-microscopic observation of atherosclerotic lesions in the aortic arch of LDLR-single deficient mouse (A) and LDLR/MSR-A-double deficient mouse (B) after 12 weeks of a high cholesterol diet. Original magnifications: A, B, × 20.

deficient mice (Fig. 5B) was reduced to about 20% of the LDLR-single deficient mice (Fig. 5A). These size reductions in both models of the double deficient mice obviously imply that MSR-A is important for the development of atherosclerosis. Total plasma cholesterol levels of LDLR-single deficient mice fed a high cholesterol diet for 4 weeks were significantly higher than those of double deficient mice [56]. However, there was no statistical correlation between plasma cholesterol levels and atherosclerotic lesions between the single deficient mice and double deficient mice, suggesting the importance of local factors in atherogenesis [56]. In the remaining atherosclerotic lesions of apoE/MSR-A-double deficient mice and LDLR/MSR-A-double deficient mice, SRs other than MSR-AI,II, such as MARCO, CD36, and macrosialin/CD68, were clearly demonstrated by immunohistochemistry or by reverse transcriptase-polymerase chain reaction, suggesting that these SRs other than MSR-AI,II are involved in the uptake of OxLDL and in foam cell transformation during atherogenesis [56].

In apoE-deficient and MCP-1-transgenic mice, the expression of MCP-1 by macrophages is enhanced and the progression of atherosclerosis is accelerated by increasing both macrophage numbers and OxLDL accumulation in the atherosclerotic lesions [59], whereas MCP-1 deficiency reduces the development of atherosclerosis in MCP-1-deficient apoB-transgenic mice [60] or high cholesterol diet-induced MCP-1/LDLR-double deficient mice [61]. The selective absence of CCR2, the receptor for MCP-1, which is mainly expressed on monocytes, decreases the formation of early atherosclerotic lesions in CCR2/apoE-double deficient mice, compared with apoE-deficient mice [62]. These data reveal a role for MCP-1 in the development of early atherosclerotic lesions *in vivo*. Our recent study revealed that the expression of MCP-1 messenger RNA in response to inflammatory stimuli was delayed in MSR-A-deficient mice, compared with the wild-type mice [63], suggesting that MSR-AI,II play a signaling receptor and are related to MCP-1 production.

Ten years ago, Nishikawa and associates first found the complete absence of M-CSF in osteopetrotic (*op*) mice, which was caused by an osteopetrosis (*op*) mutation, resulting in a failure in the coding region of M-CSF gene [64, 65]. In collaboration studies of *op/op* mice with Prof. Nishikawa and his group, we reported a complete or nearly complete absence of monocytes in peripheral blood, a developmental failure of monocytic cells in bone marrow, and marked deficiencies of tissue macro-

Figure 6. Transmission electron microscopic observation of monocytes (A), their differentiation into macrophages (B), and their transformation into foam cells (C) in a 2-coculture system with rabbit aortic endothelial cells (AECs), aortic smooth muscle cells (ASMCs), and a mixture of matrix proteins with OxLDL and/or MCP-1 on polyethylene filters in chemotaxis chambers. A: At 2 hours of coculture with a mixture of MCP-1 into collagen gel layer, monocytes (mono) adhere to AECs covering collagen gel layer. B: At 4 days after coculture, transmignant monocytes differentiate into macrophages (Mφ). C: On day 7 after coculture with a mixture of OxLDL into a collagen gel layer, macrophages transform into foam cells by accumulating lipid droplets (Mφ). Original magnifications: A, × 3,000; B, × 3,500; C, × 1,500.

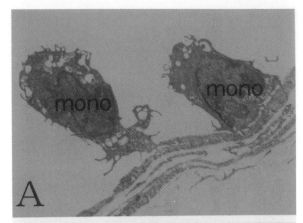
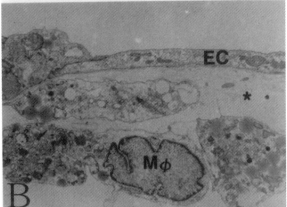
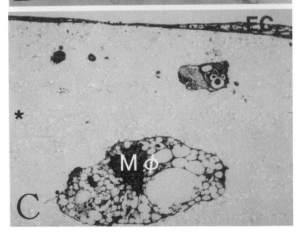

phages in various organs and tissues [65–68]. In *op/op* mice, monocyte migration into inflammatory foci is severely impaired [66]. In mice deficient in both M-CSF (*op*) and apoE, the frequency of atherosclerosis development is severely reduced, demonstrating that M-CSF is important for atherogenesis [69–71]. In apoE-deficient *op/op* mice, MSR-A expression is reduced in proportion to decreases in macrophage number [71]. It is known that M-CSF markedly and selectively increases MSR-AI,II synthesis in murine macrophages: posttranslationally, the receptors appear more stable and shift to a predominantly surface distribution, and functionally, M-CSF enhances OxLDL uptake for macrophages [63].

7. REAPPEARANCE EXPERIMENT OF MONOCYTE TRANSMIGRATION AND FOAM CELL FORMATION IN AN IN VITRO COCULTURE MODEL SYSTEM

In the early stage of atherosclerosis, blood monocytes migrate into the subendothelial space, differentiate into macrophages in the intima, and transform into foam cells by the uptake of OxLDL *in vivo*. To reappear these phenomena *in vitro*, we developed a 2-coculture system with rabbit aortic endothelial cells, aortic smooth muscle cells, and a mixture of matrix proteins on polyethylene filters in chemotaxis chambers [72]. Rabbit aortic endothelial cells were seeded on a mixture of type I and type IV collagen with or without various types of serum lipoproteins or on matrix proteins secreted by smooth muscle cells. In these coculture systems,

the aortic endothelial cells can maintain a well-preserved monolayer for up to 2 weeks. When human CD14-positive monocytes were added in the upper medium of the systems with MCP-1 treatment, monocytes adhered to the endothelial cells covering the collagen gel layer (Fig. 6A), approximately 60% of the monocytes transmigrated into the subendothelial space within 24 hours and were retained for up to 7 days, whereas without MCP-1 treatment, less than 30% of monocytes transmigrated [72]. On day 1, transmigrant monocytes were negative for immunostaining with anti-human MSR-AI,II monoclonal antibodies; however, on day 3, they differentiated into macrophages (Fig. 6B) and became positive for MSR-AI,II. When OxLDL was added to the matrix layer of type I and type IV collagen, on day 4, MSR-A-positive macrophages became enlarged, accumulating lipid droplets, and by day 7, they had the appearance of typical foam cells (Fig. 6C). This coculture system seems to be useful for dissecting the cellular and molecular events in the early stage of atherogenesis.

ACKNOWLEDGEMENT

We thank Prof. Tatsuhiko Kodama, Department of Molecular Biology and Medicine, Research Center for Advanced Science and Technology, University of Tokyo, Prof. Takefumi Doi, Faculty of Pharmaceutical Sciences, Osaka University, Prof. Makoto Naito, Second Department of Pathology, Niigata University School of Medicine, Prof. Seikoh Horiuchi, Second Department of Biochemistry, Kumamoto University School of Medicine, Dr. Teizo Yoshimura, Immunopathology section, Laboratory of Immunobiology, National Cancer Institute, Frederick Cancer Research and Development Center, and Dr. Leonard D. Shultz, Jackson Laboratory, USA, for their collaboration studies with us.

REFERENCES

1. Ross R. The pathogenesis of atherosclerosis: a perspective for the 1990's. Nature 1993;326:801–809.

2. Haust MD. The natural history of human atherosclerotic lesions. In: Vascular Injury and Atherosclerosis, Moore S, editor, Marcel Dekker, Inc., New York, 1981; 1–23.

3. Mclyill HC, Geer JC, Stron JP. Natural history of human atherosclerotic lesions. In: Atherosclerosis and Its Origin, Sander M, Bourne GH, editors, Academic Press, New York, 1963;39–65.

4. Rosenfeld ME, Ross R. Macrophage and smooth muscle cell proliferation in atheroscleroticlesion of WHHL and comparably hypercholesterolemic fat-fed rabbits. Arteriosclerosis 1990;10:680–687.

5. Ruan Y, Takahashi K, Naito M. Immunohistochemical detection of macrophage-derived foam cells and macrophage colony-stimulating factor in pulmonary atherogenesis of cholesterol-fed rabbits. Pathol Int 1995;45:195–195.

6. Brown MS, Goldstein JL. Lipoprotein metabolism in the macrphage: Implications for choleterol deposition in atherosclerosis. Annu Rev Biochem 1983;52:223–261.

7. Sakashita N, Miyazaki A, Takeya M, Horiuchi S, Chang CCY, Chang T-Y, Takahashi K. Localization of human acyl-coenzyme A: cholesterol acyltransferase-1 (ACAT-1) in macrophages and in various tissues. Am J Pathol 2000;156:227–236.

8. Goldstein JL, Ho YK, Basu SK, Brown MS. Binding site on macrophages that mediates uptake and degradation of acetylated low density lipoprotein, producing massive cholesterol deposition. Proc Natl Acad Sci USA 1979;76:333–337.

9. Kodama T, Reddy P, Kishimito C, Krieger M. Purification and characterization of a bovine acetyl low density lipoprtein receptor. Proc Natl Acad Sci USA 1988;85:9238–9242.

10. Kodama T, Freeman M, Rohrer L, Zabrecky M, Matsudaira P, Krieger M. Type I macrophage scavenger receptor contains alpha-helical and collagen-like coiled coils. Nature 1990;343:531–535.

11. Rohrer L, Freeman M, Kodama T, Penman M, Krieger M. Coiled coil fibrous domains mediate ligand binding by macrophage scavenger receptor type II. Nature 1990;343:570–572.

12. Matsumoto A, Naito M, Itakura H, Ikemoto S, Asaoka H, Hayakawa I, Kanamori H, Aburatani H, Takaku F, Suzuki H, Kobari Y, Miyai T, Takahashi K, Cohen EH, Wydro R, Housman DE, Kodama T. Human macrophage scavenger receptors: Primary structure, expression, and localization in atherosclerotic lesions. Proc Natl Acad Sci USA 1990;87:9133–9137.

13. Freeman M, Ashkenas J, Rees DJ, Kingsley DM, Copeland NG, Jenkins NA, Krieger M. An ancient, highly conserved family of cystein-rich protein domians revealed by cloning type I and type II murine macropohage scavenger receptors. Proc Natl Acad Sci USA 1990;87:8810–8814.

14. Doi T, Higashino K, Kurihara Y, Wada Y, Miyazaki T, Nakamuta H, Uesugi S, Imanishi T, Kawabe Y, Itakura H, Yazaki Y, Matsumoto A, Kodama T. Charged collagen structure mediates the recognition of negatively charged macromolecules by macrophage scavenger receptors. J Biol Chem 1993;268:2126–2133.

15. Krieger M, Herz J. Structure and functions of mul-

tiligand lipoprotein receptors: macrophage scavenger receptors and LDL receptor-related protein(LRP). Annu Rev Biochem 1994;63:601–637.

16. Kodama T, Doi T, Suzuki H, Takahashi K, Wada Y, Gordon S. Collagenous macrophage scavenger receptors. Curr Opin Lipidol 1996;7:287–291.

17. Huh HY, Pearce SF, Yesner LM, Shindler JL, Silverstein RL. Regulated expression of CD36 during monocyte-to-macrophage differentiation. Potential role of CD36 in foam cell formation. Blood 1996;87:2020–2028.

18. Han J, Hajjar DP, Febbraio M, Nicolson AC. Native and modified low density lipoproteins increase in functional expression of the macrophage class B scavenger receptor, CD36. J Biol Chem 1997;272:21654–21659.

19. Acton S, Rigotte A, Landschulz KT, Xu S, Hobbs HH, Krieger M. Identification of scavenger receptor SR-BI as a high density lipoprotein receptor. Science 1996;271:518–52.

20. Pearson A, Lux A, Krieger M. Expression cloning of dSR-CI, a class C macrophage-specific scavenger receptor from Drosophila melanogaster. Proc Natl Acad Sci USA 1995;92:4056–4060.

21. Ramprasad MP, Fischer W, Witztum JL, Sambrano GR, Quehenberger O, Steinberg D. The 94- to 97-kDa mouse macrophage membrane protein that recognizes oxidized low density lipoprotein and phosphatidyl-serine-rich liposomes is identical to macrosialin, the mouse homologue of CD68. Proc Natl Acad Sci USA 1995;92:9580–9584.

22. Ramprasad MP, Terpstra V, Kondratenko N, Quehenberger O, Steinberg D. Cell surface expression of mouse macrosialin and human CD68 and their role as macrophage receptors for oxidized low density lipoprotein. Proc Natl Acad Sci USA 1996;93:14833–14838.

23. Holness CL, da Silva RP, Fawcett J, Gordon S, Simmons DL. Macrosialin, a mouse macrophage-restricted glycoprotein, is a member of the lamp/lgp family. J Biol Chem 1993;268:9661–9666.

24. Stanton LW, White RT, Bryant CM, Protter AA, Endemann G. A macrophage Fc receptor for IgG is also a receptor for oxidized low-density lipooprotein. J Biol Chem 1992;267:22446–22451.

25. Morganelli PM, Groveman DS, Pfeifer JR. Evidence that human Fc gamma receptor IIA (CD32) subtypes are not receptors for oxidized LDL. Arterioscler Thromb Vasc Biol 1997;17:3248–3254.

26. Sawamura T, Kume N, Aoyama T, Moriwaki H, Hoshikawa H, Aiba Y, Tanaka T, Miwa S, Katsura Y, Kita T, Masaki T. An endothelial receptor for oxidized low-density lipoprotein. Nature 1997;386:73–77.

27. Moriwaki H, Kume N, Kataoka H, Murase T, Nishi E, Sawamura T, Masaki T, Kita T: Expression of lec-tin-like oxidized low density lipoprotein receptor-1 in human and murine macrophages: upregulated expression by TNF-α. FEBS Lett. 1998;440:29–32.

28. Adachi H, Tsujimoto M, Arai H, Inoue K. Expression cloning of a novel scavenger receptor from human endothelial cells. J Biol Chem 1997;272:31217–31220.

29. Naito M, Suzuki H, Mori T, Matsumoto A, Kodama T, Takahashi K. Coexpression of type I and type II human macrophage scavenger receptors in macrophages of various organs and foam cells in atherosclerotic lesions. Am J Pathol 1992;141:591–599.

30. Takeya M, Tomokiyo R-I, Jinnouchi K, Sakaguchi H, Hagiwara S-I, Honda M, Wada Y, Suzuki H, Kodama T, Takahashi K. Macrophage scavenger receptors: Structure, function, and tissue distribution. Acta Histochem Cytochem 1999;32:47–51.

31. Naito M, Kodama T, Matsumoto A, Doi T, Takahashi K. Tissue distribution, intracellular localization, and in vitro expression of bovine macrophage scavenger receptors. Am J Pathol 1991;139:1411–1423.

32. Huges DA, Fraser IP, Gordon S. Murine macrophage scavenger receptor: in vivo expression and function as receptor for macrophage adhesion in lymphoid and non-lymphoid organs. Eur J Immunol 1995;25:466–473.

33. Doi T, Kurasawa M, Higashino Y, Wada Y, Matsumoto A, Kodama T. The histidine interruption of an alpha-helical coiled coil allosterically mediates a pH-dependent ligand dissociation from macrophage scavenger receptors. J Biol Chem 1994;269:25598–25604.

34. Suzuki K, Doi T, Imanishi T, Kodama T, Tanaka T. The conformation of the α-helical coiled coil domain of macrophage scavenger receptor is pH dependent. Biochemistry 1997;36:15140–15146.

35. Fraser I, Hughes D, Gordon S. Divalent cation-independent macrophage adhesion inhibited by monoclonal antibody to murine scavenger receptor. Nature 1993;364:343–346.

36. Gough PJ, Greaves DR, Gordon S. A naturally occurring isoform of the human macrophage scavenger receptor (SR-A) gene generated by alternative splicing blocks modified LDL uptake. J Lipid Res 1998;39:531–543.

37. Elomaa O, Kangas M, Sahlberg C, Tuukkanen J, Sormunen R, Liakka A, Thesleff I, Kraal G, Tryggvason K. Cloning of a novel bacteria-binding receptor structurally related to scavenger receptors and expressed in a subset of macrophages. Cell 1995;80:603–609.

38. Van Der Laan LJW., Kangas M, Döpp EA, Brouge-Holub E, Elomaa O, Tryggvason K, Kraal G. Macrophage scavenger receptor MARCO: In vito and in vivo regulation and involvement in the anti-bacterial host defense. Immunol Lett 1997;57:203–208.

39. Ito S, Naito M, Kobayashi Y, Takatsuka H, Jiang S,

Umezu H, Hasegawa G, Arakawa M, Shultz LD, Elomaa O, Tryggvason K. Roles of a macrophage receptor with collagenous structure (MARCO) in host defense and heterogeneity of splenic marginal zone macrophages. Arch Histol Cystol 1999;62:83–95.

40. Mori T, Takahashi K, Naito M, Kodama T, Hakamata H, Saki M, Miyazaki A, Horiuchi S, Ando M. Endocytic pathway of scavenger receptors via trans-Golgi system in bovine alveolar macrophages. Lab Invest 1994;71:409–416.

41. Mori T, Takahashi K, Higashi T, Takeya M, Kume S, Kawabe Y, Kodama T, Horiuchi S. Localization of advanced glycation end products of Maillard reaction in bovine tissues and their endocytosis by macrophage scavenger receptors. Exp Molec Pathol 1995;63:135152.

42. Suzuki H, Kurihara Y, Takeya M, Kamada N, Kataoka M, Jishage K, Ueda O, Sakaguchi H, Higashi T, Suzuki T, Takashima Y, Kawabe Y, Cybshi O, Wada Y, Honda M, Kurihara H, Aburatani H, Doi T, Matsumoto A, Azuma S, Noda T, Toyoda Y, Itakura H, Yazaki Y, Horiuchi S, Takahashi K, Kruijt JK, Berkel TJC, Steinberger UP, Ishibashi S, Maeda N, Gordon S, Kodama T. A role for macrophage scavenger receptors in atherosclerosis and susceptibility to infection. Nature 1997;386:292–296.

43. Suzuki H, Kurihara Y, Takeya M, Kamada N, Kataoka M, Jishage K, Sakaguchi H, Kruijt JK, Higashi T, Suzuki T, Berkel TJC, Horiuchi S, Takahashi K, Yazaki Y, Kodama T. The multiple roles of macrophage scavenger receptors (MSR) in vivo: Resistance to atherosclerosis and susceptiblity to infection in MSR-knockout mice. J Atheroscler Thromb 1997;4:1–11.

44. Itabe H, Takeshima E, Iwasaki H, Kimura J, Yoshida Y, Imanaka T, Takano T. A monoclonal antibody against oxidized lipoprotein recognizes foam cells in atherosclerotic lesions. J. Biol. Chem. 1994;27:15274–15279.

45. Itabe H, Yamamoto H, Imanaka T, Shimamura K, Uchiyama H, Kimura J, Sanaka T, Hata Y, Takano T. Sensitive detection of oxidatively modified low density lipoprotein using a monoclonal antibody. J Lipid Res 1996;37:45–53.

46. Kume S, Takeya M, Mori T, Araki N, Suzuki H, Horiuchi S, Kodama T, Miyauchi Y, Takahashi K. Immunohistochemical and ultrastructural detection of advanced glycation end products in atherosclerotic lesions of human aorta with a novel specific monoclonal antibody. Am J Pathol 1995;147:654–667.

47. Ling X, Sakashita N, Takeya M, Nagai R, Horiuchi S, Takahashi K. Immunohistochemical distribution and subcellular localization of three distinct specific molecular structures of advanced glycation end products in

human tissues. Lab Invest 1998;78:1591–1606.

48. Ogata H, Takeya M, Yoshimura T, Takagi K, Takahashi K. The role of monocyte chemoattractant protien-1 (MCP-1) in the pathogenesis of collagen-induced artheritis in rats. J Pathol 1997;182:106–114.

49. Yoshimura T, Robinson EA, Tanaka S, Appella E, Leonard EJ. Purification and amino acid analysis of two human monocyte chemoattractants produced by phytohemagglutinin-stimulated human blood mononuclear leukocytes. J Immunol 1989;142:1956–1962.

50. Yoshimura T, Takeya M, Takahashi K, Kuratsu J, Leonard EJ. Production and characterization of mouse monoclonal antibodies against human monocyte chemiattractant protein-1. J Immunol 1991;147:2229–2233.

51. Sakanashi Y, Takeya M, Yoshimura T, Feng L, Morioka T, Takahashi K. Kinetics of macrophage subpopulations and expression of monocyte chemoattractant protein-1 (MCP-1) in bleomycin-induced lung injury of rats studied by a novel monoclonal antibody against rat MCP-1. J Leukoc Biol 1994;56:741–750.

52. Takeya M, Yoshimura T, Leonard EJ, Takahashi K. Detection of monocyte chemoattractant protein-1 in human atherosclerotic lesions by an anti-monocyte chemoattractant protein-1 monoclonal antibody. Hum Pathol 1993;24:534–539.

53. Kawasaki ES, Lander MB. Molecular biology of macrophage colony-stimulating factor. In: Colony-Stimulating Factors, Molecular and Cellular Biology, In: Dexter, TM, Garland JM, Testa NG, editors, Marcel Dekker Inc., New York-Basel, (Immunol Ser) 1990;49:155–176.

54. Rosenfeld ME, Yla-Herttuala, Lipton BA, Ord VA, Witztum JL, Steinberg D. Macrophage colony-stimulating factor mRNA and protein in atherosclerotic lesions of rabbits and humans. Am J Pathol 1992;140:291–300.

55. Clinton SK, Underwood R, Hayes L, Sherman ML, Kufe DW, Libby P. Macrophage colony-stimulating factor gene expression in vascular cells and in experimental and human atherosclerosis. Am J Pathol 1992;140:301–316.

56. Sakaguchi H, Takeya M, Suzuki H, Hakamata H, Kodama T, Horiuchi S, Gordon S, Van Der Laan LJ, Kraal G, Ishibashi S, Kitamura N, Takahashi K. Role of macrophage scavenger receptors in diet-induced atherosclerosis in mice. Lab Invest 1998;78:423–434.

57. Zhang SH, Reddick RL, Piedrahita JA, Maeda N. Spontaneous hypercholesterolemia and arterial lesions in mice lacking apolipoprotein E. Science 1992;258:468–471.

58. Ishibashi S, Goldstein JL, Brown MS, Herz J, Burns DK. Massive xanthomatosis and atherosclerosis in cholesterol-fed low density lipoprotein recptor-negative mice. J Clin Invest 1994;93:1885–1893.

59. Aiello RJ, Bourassa P-AK, Lindsey S, Weng W,

Natoli E, Rollins BJ, Milos PM. Monocyte chemoattractant protein-1 accelerates atherosclerosis in apolipoprotein E-deficient mice. Arterioscler Thromb Vasc Biol 1999;19:1518–1525.

60. Gosling J, Slaymaker S, Gu L, Tseng S, Zlot CH, Young SG, Rollins BJ, Charo IF MCP-1 deficiency reduces susceptibility to atherosclerosis in mice that overexpress human apolipoprotein B. J Clin Invest 1999;103:773–778.

61. Gu L, Okada Y, Clinton SK, Gerard C, Sukhova GK, Libby P, Rollins BJ. Absence of monocyte chemosttroctant protein-1 reduces atherosclerosis in low density lipoprotein receptor-deficient mice. Mol Cell 1998;2:275–281.

62. Boring L, Gosling J, Cleary M, Charo IF. Decreased lesion formation in CCR2$^{-/-}$ mice reveals a role for chemokines in the initiation of atherosclerosis. Nature 1998;394:894–897.

63. De Villiers WJS, Fraser IP, Hughes DA, Doyle AG, Gordon S. Macrophage colony-stimulating factor selectively enhances macrophage scavenger receptor expression and function. J Exp Med 1994;180:705–709.

64. Yoshida H, Hayashi S-I, Kunisada T, Ogawa M, Nishikawa S, Okamura H, Shultz LD. The murine mutation "osteopetrosis" (op) is a mutation in the coding region of the macrophage colony-stimulating factor (Csfm) gene. Nature 1990;345:442–444.

65. Nishikawa S-I, Hayashi S-I, Yoshida H, Naito M, Takahashi K, Shultz LD. A model mouse defective in M-CSF production: Molecular biology and pathology of osteopetrosis mouse (*op/op*). In: Dendritic Cells in Lymphoid Tissues, Imai Y, Tew JG, Hoefsmit ECM, editors, Excerpta Medica, Amsterdam, 1991;225–231.

66. Naito M, Hayashi S, Yoshida H, Nishikawa S-I, Shutuz LD, Takahashi K. Abnormal differentiation of tissue macrophage populations in "osteopetrosis" (op) mice

defective in the production of macrophage colony-stimulating factor. Am J Pathol 1991;139:657–667.

67. Takahashi K, Naito M, Umeda S, Shultz LD. The role of macrophage colony-stimulating factor in hepatic glucan-induced granuloma formation in the osteopetrosis mutant mouse defective in the production of macrophage colony-stimulating factor. Am J Pathol 1994;144:1381–1392.

68. Umeda S, Takahashi K, Shultz LD, Naito M, Takagi K. Effects of macrophage colony-stimulating factor on macrophages and their related cell populations in the osteopetrosis (*op*) mouse defective in the production of functional macrophage colony-stimulating factor protein. Am J Pathol 1996;149:559–574.

69. Smith JD, Trogan E, Ginsberg M, Grigaux C, Tian J, Miyata M. Decreased atherosclerosis in mice deficient in both macrophage colony-stimulating factor (*op*) and apolipoprotein E. Proc Natl Acad Sci USA 1995;92:8264–8268.

70. Qiao JH, Tripathi J, Mishra NK, Tripathi S, Wang XP, Imes S, Fishbein MC, Clinton SK, Libby P, Lusis AJ, Rajavashisth TB. Role of macrophage colony-stimulating factor in atherosclerosis. Am J Pathol 1997;150:1687–1699.

71. De Villiers WJ, Smith JD, Miyata M, Dansky HM, Darley E, Gordon S. Macrophage phenotype in mice deficient in both macrophage-colony-stimulating factor (op) and apolipoprotein E. Arterioscler Thromb Vasc Biol 1998;18:631–640.

72. Takaku M, Wada Y, Jinnouchi K, Takeya M, Takahashi K, Usuda H, Naito M, Kurihara H, Yazaki Y, Kumazawa Y, Okimoto Y, Umetani M, Noguchi N, Niki, E, Hamamoto T, Kodama T. An *in vitro* coculture model of transmigrant monocytes and foam cell formation. Arterioscler Thromb Vasc Biol 1999;19:2330–2339.

Atherosclerosis and Autoimmunity
Y. Shoenfeld, D. Harats and G. Wick, editors

CD36, the Macrophage Class B Scavenger Receptor: Regulation and Role in Atherosclerosis

Andrew C. Nicholson, Jihong Han, Maria Febbraio, S. Frieda A. Pearce, Antonio M. Gotto, Jr. and David P. Hajjar

Center of Vascular Biology, Cornell University Medical College, 1300 York Ave., New York, NY, USA

Oxidation of low density lipoproteins is a critical early event in the pathogenesis of atherosclerosis. OxLDL is present in human atheroma [1] and is the proximal source of lipid that accumulates within cells of the atherosclerotic lesion [2]. Furthermore, platelets, monocytes, and endothelial cells exposed to OxLDL are converted to a pro-thrombotic, pro-inflammatory, pro-atherogenic phenotype. Considerable experimental work has illuminated pathways of LDL oxidation in the vessel wall, and preventative strategies in animal models and in humans based on anti-oxidant therapy are ongoing and show promise. Several cellular receptors involved in binding and internalizing modified LDL particles (including OxLDL) have been identified and are termed "scavenger receptors". Although their physiological roles are unclear, they presumably have a significant role in atherosclerotic foam cell development [2–5].

A receptor for acetylated LDL (now referred to as the type A scavenger receptor) was the first macrophage scavenger receptor identified, isolated, and cloned [6, 7]. Two alternatively spliced mRNAs, types I and II, have been identified, both encoding homotrimeric membrane proteins that differ only at the C terminus [8–10]. These receptors are expressed on macrophages (but not freshly isolated peripheral blood monocytes) and exhibit broad ligand binding specificity, recognizing modified forms of LDL, four-stranded nucleic acids, polysaccharides, and endotoxin [11].

Modification of LDL by acetylation, acetoacetylation or malondialdehyde treatment [12] abolishes the positive charge on lysine residues of LDL and prevents recognition by the LDL receptor, while facilitating scavenger receptor binding [13]. Since these modifications do not occur under physiological conditions, the natural ligand for this receptor was unclear until Steinberg et al demonstrated by that OxLDL competes for the binding of acetylated LDL (AcLDL) to macrophages [14]. LDL particles are presumably subjected to oxidative modification in the vessel wall by reactive oxygen metabolites produced by monocytes, neutrophils, and other cells in the developing lesion [15]. The competitive inhibition of AcLDL binding by OxLDL, however, was only partial. Subsequent binding and cross competition studies with both OxLDL and AcLDL in macrophages and numerous transfected and normal cell lines has clearly demonstrated the existence of multiple scavenger receptor functional classes [16–18]; receptor(s) for AcLDL, receptor(s) for OxLDL, and receptor(s) that recognize both. Since the type I and II receptors exhibit identical binding specificity it does not appear that differences at the C terminus account for differences in ligand recognition [18]. Steinberg and his colleagues have recently shown that oxidatively damaged erythrocytes bind to macrophages, and that OxLDL, but not AcLDL or native LDL, blocks this binding [19], providing further evidence for a receptor other than the cloned type I/II receptor for oxidized lipid on the macrophage surface. They have subsequently shown that this receptor is identical to macrosialin, the mouse homologue of CD68 [20].

In addition to that of macrophages, scavenger receptor activity has also been detected on hepatic endothelial cells (EC), Kupffer cells, and, on parenchymal cells of the liver [21, 22]. *In vivo* and *in vitro* studies suggest that scavenger receptor function on EC and Kupffer cells is probably not mediated by type A scavenger receptor. Rabbit and bovine EC bind and degrade AcLDL, but do not express mRNA for type A receptors [23]. Intravenously injected [125I]AcLDL in rats is taken up primarily by liver ECs [21], while [125I]OxLDL is cleared predominantly by Kupffer cells [24]. When Kupffer cell membranes were analyzed by ligand blotting, two sites of [125I]OxLDL binding were identified; a major binding site at 95kD and a minor site at 220kD, representing the type I/II receptor [25]. These data suggest that the smaller protein may function as a specific OxLDL receptor in the liver.

Because of the importance of OxLDL in the pathogenesis of atherosclerosis and the data suggesting that the Type I/II receptor cannot account for most OxLDL binding to macrophages and vascular cells, considerable efforts have been taken to identify other scavenger receptors. Endemann and her colleagues used an expression cloning strategy to identify murine macrophage receptors that recognized OxLDL but not AcLDL. The initial clone identified by this method encoded FcγRII, a receptor for the Fc portion of IgG [26]. While transfection of this cDNA into a cell line conferred on these cells the capacity to internalize and degrade OxLDL, inhibition of FcγRII on macrophages by antibodies or by immune complexes did not influence OxLDL binding or uptake, suggesting strongly that FcγRII is not a bona fide macrophage scavenger receptor [26]. The second clone identified by this strategy encoded the murine homologue of CD36 (platelet gpIV) [27], an 88kD transmembrane glycoprotein.

CD36 is now referred to as a type B scavenger receptor. It is a member of family of receptors which also includes SR-B1/CLA-1, an HDL receptor [28–30]. CD36 is expressed by monocyte/macrophages [31], platelets [32], microvascular endothelial cells [33], and adipose tissue [34]. Like the type A scavenger receptors [35], CD36 recognizes a broad variety of ligands including OxLDL [27, 36], anionic phospholipids [37], apoptotic cells [38], thrombospondin (TSP) [39], collagen [40], *Plasmodium falciparum*-infected erythrocytes [41], and long-chain fatty acids [34]. Unlike the class

A receptors, which recognize the oxidized apoprotein portion of the lipoprotein particle [13], CD36 binds to the lipid moiety of OxLDL [36]. Binding of OxLDL to CD36-transfected cells is inhibited by anionic phospholipid vesicles [37]. CD36 also binds HDL [42], however SR-BI mediates uptake of HDL CE with much greater efficiency than CD36 [43]. Recently, CD-36 was also identified as the major receptor for LDL modified by monocyte-generated reactive nitrogen species [44].

The cDNAs for human, murine, and rat CD36 have been cloned and sequenced [34, 45] and are highly homologous. The carboxy terminus includes a stretch of 27 hydrophobic residues consistent with a classic transmembrane domain, followed by a short 6 to 9 amino acid intracellular domain. At the N-terminus, the predicted initiator methionine is followed by another long hydrophobic region suggesting a secretory signal sequence. Since there is no obvious signal peptidase cleavage site and since the amino acid sequence of purified platelet CD36 begins at the residue immediately after the initiator methionine, it is probable that this signal sequence remains part of the mature molecule. A CD36 truncation mutant lacking the carboxy terminal transmembrane domain is secreted by transfected cells, suggesting that the N-terminal hydrophobic domain is extracellular (exofacial), and not a second transmembrane domain [46]. We have utilized a series of recombinant bacterial glutathione S-transferase/CD36 fusion proteins that span nearly the entire CD36 molecule to characterize the structural domain on CD36 that recognizes Ox-LDL [47]. The Ox-LDL-binding domain is different from the thrombospondin-1-binding domain located at amino acids 93–120. A fusion protein containing the region extending from amino acids 5 to 143 formed specific, saturable, and reversible complexes with Ox-LDL. As with intact CD36, binding was blocked by excess unlabeled Ox-LDL and antibodies to CD36. The stoichiometry and affinity of the fusion protein for Ox-LDL were similar to those of the intact protein [47]. This fusion protein competitively inhibited binding of Ox-LDL to purified platelet CD36 and to CD36 expressed on peripheral blood monocytes and CD36 cDNA-transfected melanoma cells [47]. The use of smaller peptides and fusion proteins including those spanning amino acids 28–93 and 5–93 has further narrowed the binding site to a region from amino acids 28 to 93, although participation of a sequence in the noncontiguous region 120–155 cannot be excluded [47].

CD36-transfected cells bind OxLDL in a saturable manner. Binding, internalization, and degradation of OxLDL is increased 4-fold in CD36 transfected cells relative to cells transfected with vector alone [36]. More than half of the binding of OxLDL by human monocyte-derived macrophages is inhibited by anti-CD36 antibodies [36]. In our experiments, LDL and acetylated LDL (AcLDL) bind equivalenty to control and CD36-transfected cells [36]. However, others have reported that CD36 will bind native LDL [42]. Expression of CD36 in monocyte/macrophages is dependent both on the differentiation state as well as exposure to soluble mediators [48, 49]. We studied the effect of lipoproteins, native LDL and modified LDL (AcLDL and OxLDL) on the expression of CD36 in J774 cells, a murine macrophage cell line [50]. Exposure to lipoproteins resulted in a marked induction of CD36 mRNA expression (4–8 fold). Maximum induction was observed 2 hr. after treatment with AcLDL and at 4 hr. with LDL and OxLDL. Expression of CD36 mRNA persisted through 24 hr. with each treatment group. Induction of CD36 mRNA expression was paralleled by an increase in CD36 protein as determined by Western blot, with the greatest induction by OxLDL (4-fold). In the presence of actinomycin D, treatment of macrophages with LDL, AcLDL or OxLDL did not affect CD36 mRNA stability, implying that CD36 mRNA was transcriptionally regulated by lipoproteins [50]. Incubation of macrophages with cholesterol acceptor proteins (BSA or HDL) reduced expression of CD36 mRNA in a dose-dependent manner [50]. The effects of lipoproteins on CD36 expression were mimicked by alterations in macrophage cellular cholesterol content [51]. Depletion of cellular cholesterol by treatment with cyclodextrins significantly decreased the expression of both CD36 mRNA and ^{125}I-OxLDL binding. In contrast, macrophages that are cholesterol-loaded with cyclodextrin:cholesterol complexes increased both CD36 mRNA expression and ^{125}I-OxLDL binding [51]. Results of these experiments demonstrate that, unlike the LDL receptor, which is down-regulated by cellular cholesterol, expression of CD36 is enhanced by cholesterol and down-regulated by cholesterol efflux.

The effect of OxLDL on CD36 is due, in part, to its ability to activate the transcription factor, PPARγ (peroxisome proliferator activated receptor-γ) [52, 53]. PPAR-γ is a member of a nuclear hormone superfamily that can heterodimerize with the retinoid X receptor (RXR) and act as a transcriptional regulator of genes encoding proteins involved in adipogenesis and lipid metabolism [54]. Other PPARγ ligands (15-deoxyΔ^{12,14} prostaglandin J2 (15d-PGJ2) and the thiazolidinedione class of antidiabetic drugs) also increase CD36 expression [52, 53]. These results further imply that macrophage expression of CD36 and foam cell formation in atherosclerotic lesions may be perpetuated by a cycle in which lipids continue to drive expression of a lipoprotein receptor in a self-regulatory manner.

We evaluated signaling pathways involved in the induction of CD36 mRNA. Treatment of RAW264.7 cells (a murine macrophage cell line) with protein kinase C (PKC) activators (diacylglycerol (DAG) and ingenol) up-regulated CD36 mRNA expression. Specific inhibitors of PKC reduced CD36 expression in a time-dependent manner. In contrast, protein kinase A (PKA) and cyclic AMP agonists had no effect on CD36 mRNA expression. PKC inhibitors reduced basal expression of CD36 and blocked induction of CD36 mRNA by 15d-PGJ2 and OxLDL. In addition, PKC inhibitors decreased both PPARγ mRNA and protein expression. Treatment of human monocytes with OxLDL, but not 15d-PGJ2, resulted in increased expression of PKC-α as well as its translocation from the cytosol to the plasma membrane. Finally, PKC inhibitors blocked induction of CD36 protein surface expression by OxLDL and 15d-PGJ2 in human monocytes, as determined by FACS. These results demonstrate that activation of CD36 gene expression by OxLDL involves initial activation and translocation of PKC with subsequent PPARγ activation.

Phorbol esters (PMA), M-CSF and IL-4 have also been shown to increase monocyte/macrophage expression of CD36 [49], while expression of CD36 is down-regulated in response to cholesterol efflux [51], LPS [49], dexamethasone [49], and interferon-γ [55]. With the exception of OxLDL, which activates PPAR-γ leading to CD36 gene transcription, the mechanism(s) by which this diverse collection of factors modulates CD36 expression remains undefined. Transforming growth factor-β1 (TGF-β1) and

TGF-β2 are multifunctional mediators that regulate cellular growth, migration, adhesion, extracellular matrix formation, and apoptosis [56]. We investigated the effect of transforming growth factor-β1 (TGF-β1) and TGF-β2 on the expression of CD36 in macrophages. Treatment of phorbol ester-differentiated THP-1 macrophages with TGF-β1 or TGF-β2 significantly decreased expression of CD36 mRNA and surface protein. TGF-β1/TGF-β2 also inhibited CD36 mRNA expression induced by OxLDL and 15-deoxyΔ^{12,14} prostaglandin J$_2$ (15d-PGJ$_2$), a PPAR-γ ligand, suggesting that the TGF-β1/TGF-β2 down-regulated CD36 expression by inactivating PPAR-γ mediated signaling. TGF-β1/TGF-β2 increased phosphorylation of both MAP kinase and PPAR-γ while MAP kinase inhibitors reversed suppression of CD36 and inhibited PPAR-γ phosphorylation induced by TGF-β1/TGF-β2. Finally, MAP kinase inhibitors alone increased expression of CD36 mRNA and surface protein but had no effect on PPAR-γ protein levels. Our data demonstrate that TGF-β1 and TGF-β2 decrease expression of CD36 by a mechanism involving phosphorylation of MAP kinase, subsequent MAP kinase phosphorylation of PPAR-γ, and a decrease in CD36 gene transcription by phosphorylated PPAR-γ.

Generation of null and transgenic mice, in which specific genes are targeted, has led to an important leap forward in our ability to understand the pathogenesis of this atherosclerosis. Before the invention of these techniques, mice were all but resistant to atherosclerosis and therefore not useful. Mouse models are valuable because mice can be studied in large numbers, the genetics of many strains is well documented, inbred strains provide virtual clones in which to do experiments, environmental factors can be altered, and crossbreeding and now, genetic techniques, allow manipulation of genetic factors. To date, there are several important murine models, including Apo E and low density lipoprotein receptor nulls, which have been created specifically to mimic human atherosclerosis.

The role of type A scavenger receptor in atherosclerosis has been evaluated in several murine models. On an apoE-deficient background, type A scavenger receptor-deficient mice showed a 60% reduction in atherosclerotic lesion development, suggesting a strong pro-atherogenic role for the SR-A [57]. However, on an LDLR-deficient background, absence of the type A scavenger receptor resulted in only a 20% reduction in atherosclerosis [58] and no decrease in atherosclerosis was observed when SR-A-deficient mice are crossed with APOE3-Leiden mice [59]. Thus, the genetic background of these mice has important effects on extent of atherosclerosis seen when crossed with type A scavenger receptor knockout mice. Interestingly, when uptake of oxidized LDL is examined in macrophages from mice in which the type A scavenger receptor gene had been disrupted, it was reduced by only 30% [60]. This indicates that about 70% of the uptake of oxidized LDL in macrophages is attributable to oxidized LDL receptor(s) other than the type A receptor.

We hypothesized that knocking out CD36 would also alter the course of atherosclerosis by delaying or preventing foam cell and fatty streak formation. To test this hypothesis, we created a mouse null in CD36 [61]. These mice produced no detectable CD36 protein, were viable, and bred normally. A significant decrease in binding and uptake of OxLDL lipoprotein was observed in peritoneal macrophages of null mice as compared with those from control mice [61]. This reduced binding and uptake of OxLDL was expected based on previous data in human macrophages. A genetic polymorphism in the CD36 gene has been identified in an Asian population [62] and shown to result in deficient expression of CD36 (NAK^a-phenotype). Monocyte-derived macrophages isolated from these patients bound 40% less Ox-LDL and accumulated 40% less cholesterol ester than cells derived from normal controls , further implicating CD36 as a physiological OxLDL receptor [63].

CD36 null animals had a significant increase in fasting levels of cholesterol, non-esterified free fatty acids, and triacylglycerol [61]. The increase in cholesterol was mainly within the high density lipoprotein (HDL) fraction, while the increase in triacylglycerol was within the very low density lipoprotein fraction [61]. Null animals had lower fasting serum glucose levels when compared with wild type controls. Uptake of ^{3}H-labeled oleate was significantly reduced in adipocytes from null mice [61]. However, the decrease was limited to the low ratios of fatty acid:bovine serum albumin, suggesting that CD36 was necessary for the high affinity component of the uptake process [61].

To assess the role of the class B scavenger receptor CD36 in atherogenesis, we crossed a CD36-null strain with the atherogenic apo E–null strain and quantified lesion development [64]. There was a 76.5% decrease in aortic tree lesion area (Western diet) and a 45% decrease in aortic sinus lesion area (normal chow) in the CD36-apo E double-null mice when compared with controls, despite alterations in lipoprotein profiles that often correlate with increased atherogenicity [64]. Macrophages derived from CD36-apo E double-null mice bound and internalized 60% less copper-oxidized LDL and LDL modified by monocyte-generated reactive nitrogen species [64]. A similar inhibition of in vitro lipid accumulation and foam cell formation after exposure to these ligands was seen. These results support a major role for CD36 in atherosclerotic lesion development in vivo and suggest that blockade of CD36 can be protective even in more extreme proatherogenic circumstances [64].

In summary, research *in vitro* and in murine models of atherosclerosis supports the hypothesis that CD36 is a major receptor for pro-atherogenic lipids. However, the specific role that CD36 plays in the development of the human atheroma remains to be determined. In support of a role for CD36 in human vascular disease, lipid-laden macrophages in human atherosclerotic lesions exhibit strong immunoreactivity to CD36, but a low or moderate level of immunoreactivity to the type A scavenger receptor [65]. This high level of expression of CD36 in lipid-laden macrophages may reflect increased expression in response to OxLDL-derived PPAR-γ ligands, which, in turn, activate CD36 gene transcription. Thus, CD36 and PPAR-γ are both potential targets for therapeutic intervention to block macrophage foam cell development during atherosclerosis.

REFERENCES

1. Haberland M, Fong D, Cheng L. Malondialdehyde-altered protein occurs in atheroma of Watanabe heritable hyperlipidemic rabbits. Science 1988;241:215–218.
2. Steinberg D, Parthasarathy S, Carew T, Khoo J, Witztum J. Beyond cholesterol. Modifications of low-density lipoprotein which increase its atherogenicity. N Engl J Med 1989;320:915–919.
3. Steinberg D. Lipoproteins and the pathogenesis of atherosclerosis. Circ 1987;76:508–514.
4. Gown A, Tsukada T, Ross R. Human atherosclerosis. II. Immunocytochemical analysis of the cellular composition of human atherosclerotic lesions. Amer J Pathol 1986;125:191–207.
5. Fogelman A, Van Lenten B, Warden C, Haberland M, Edwards P. Macrophage lipoprotein receptors. J Cell Sci 1988;Suppl.9:135–149.
6. Kodama T, Reddy P, Kishamoto C, Krieger M. Purification and characterization of a bovine acetyl low density lipoprotein receptor. Proc Natl Acad Sci USA 1988;85:9238–9242.
7. Via D, Dresel H, Cheng S-L, Gotto A. Murine macrophage tumors are a source of a 260,000-dalton acetyl- low density lipoprotein receptor. J Biol Chem 1985;260:7379–7386.
8. Kodama T, Freeman M, Rohrer L, Zabrecky J, Matsudaira P, Krieger M. Type I macrophage scavenger receptor contains alpha-helial and collagen-like coiled coils. Nature 1990;343:531–535.
9. Rohrer L, Freeman M, Kodama T, Penman M, Krieger M. Coiled-coil fibrous domains mediate ligand binding by macrophage scavenger receptor type II. Nature 1990;343:570–572.
10. Matsumoto A, Naito M, Itakura H, et al. Human macrophage scavenger receptors: Primary structure, expression, and localization in atherosclerotic lesions. Proc Natl Acad Sci USA 1990;87:9133–9137.
11. Hampton R, Golenbock D, Penman M, Krieger M, Raetz C. Recognition and plasma clearance of endotoxin by scavenger receptors. Nature 1991;352:342–344.
12. Haberland M, Fogelman A, Edwards P. Specificity of receptor-mediated recognition of malondialdehyde-modified low density lipoproteins. Proc Natl Acad Sci USA 1982;79:1712–1716.
13. Parthasarathy S, Fong L, Otero D, Steinberg D. Recognition of solubilized apoproteins from delipidated, oxidized low density lipoprotein (LDL) by the acetyl-LDL receptor. Proc Natl Acad Sci USA 1987;84:537–540.
14. Parthasarathy S, Printz D, Boyd D, Joy L, Steinberg D. Macrophage oxidation of low density lipoprotein generates a modified form recognized by the scavenger receptor. Arteriosclerosis 1986;6:505–510.
15. Palinski W, Rosenfeld M, Yla-Herttuala S, et al. Low density lipoprotein undergoes oxidative modification in vivo. Proc Natl Acad Sci USA 1989;86:1372–1376.
16. Sparrow C, Parthasarathy S, Steinberg D. A macrophage receptor that recognizes oxidized low density lipoprotein but not acetylated low density lipoprotein. J Biol Chem 1989;264:2599–2604.
17. Arai H, Kita T, Yokode M, Narumiya S, Kawai C. Multiple receptors for modified low density lipoproteins in mouse peritoneal macrophages: differently

uptake mechanisms for acetylated and oxidized low density lipoproteins. Biochem Biophys Res Comm 1989;159:1375–1382.

18. Freeman M, Ekkel Y, Rohrer L, et al. Expression of type I and type II bovine scavenger receptors in Chinese hamster ovary cells: lipid droplet accumulation and nonreciprocal cross competition by acetylated and oxidized low density lipoprotein. Proc Natl Acad Sci USA 1991;88:4931–4935.

19. Sambrano G, Parthasarathy S, Steinberg D. Recognition of oxidatively damaged erythrocytes by a maraphage receptor with specificity for oxidized low density lipoprotein. Proc Natl Acad Sci USA 1994;91:3265–3269.

20. Ramprasad M, Fischer W, Witztum J, Sambrano G, Quehenberger O, Steinberg D. The 94- to 97-kDa mouse macrophage membrane protein that recognizes oxidized low density lipoprotein and phosphatidyl-serine-rich liposomes is identical to macrosialin, the mouse homologue of CD68. Proc Natl Acad Sci USA 1995;92:9580–9584.

21. Nagelkerke J, Barto K, Van Berkel T. In vivo and in vitro uptake and degradation of acetylated low density lipoprotein by rat liver endothelial, Kupffer, and parenchymal cells. J Biol Chem 1983;258:12221–12227.

22. Kamps J, Kruijt J, Kuipur J, Van Berkel T. Characterization of the interaction of acetylated LDL and oxidatively modified LDL with human liver parynchymal and Kupffer cells in culture. Arterio and Thromb 1992;12:1079–1087.

23. Bickel P, Freeman M. Rabbit aortic smooth muscle cells express inducible macrophage scavenger receptor messenger RNA that is absent from endothelial cells. J Clin Invest 1992;90:1450–1457.

24. Van Berkel T, De Rijke Y, Kruijt J. Different fate in vivo of oxidatively modified low density lipoprotein and acetylated low density lipoprotein in rats. J Biol Chem 1991;266:2282–2289.

25. De Rijke Y, Van Berkel T. Rat liver Kupffer cells and endothelial cells express different binding proteins for modified low density lipoprotein. J Biol Chem 1994;269:824–827.

26. Stanton L, White R, Bryant C, Protter A, Endemann G. A macrophage Fc receptor for IgG is also a receptor for oxidized low density lipoprotein. J Biol Chem 1992;267:22446–22451.

27. Endemann G, Stanton L, Madden K, Bryant K, White RT, Protter A. CD36 is a receptor for oxidized low density lipoprotein. J Biol Chem 1993;268:11811–11816.

28. Acton S, Attilio R, Landschultz K, Xu S, Hobbs H, Krieger M. Identification of scavenger receptor SR-B1 as a high density lipoprotein receptor. Science 1996;271:518–520.

29. Acton S, Scherer P, Lodish H, Krieger M. Expression cloning of SR-BI, a CD36-related class B scavenger receptor. J Biol Chem 1994;269:21003–21009.

30. Calvo D, Vega MA. Identification, primary structure, and distribution of CLA-1, a novel member of the CD36/LIMPII gene family. . J Biol Chem 1993;268:18929–18935.

31. Talle M, Rao P, Westberg E, et al. Patterns of antigenic expression on human monocytes as defined by monoclonal antibodies. Cell Immunol 1983;78:83–99.

32. Li YS, Shyy YJ, Wright JG, Valente AJ, Cornhill JF, Kolattukudy PE. The expression of monocyte chemotactic protein (MCP-1) in human vascular endothelium in vitro and in vivo. Mol Cell Biochem 1993;126:61–68.

33. Greenwalt D, Lipsky R, Ockenhouse C, Ikeda H, Tandon N, Jamieson G. Membrane glycoprotein CD36: A review if its roles in adherence, signal transduction, and transfusion medicine. Blood 1992;80:1105–1115.

34. Abumrad N, El-Maghrabi MR, Amri E, Lopez E, Grimaldi P. Cloning of a rat adipocyte membrane protein implicated in binding or transport of long-chain fatty acids that is induced during preadipocyte differentiation. J Biol Chem 1993;268:17665–17668.

35. Krieger M, Acton S, Ashkenas J, Pearson A, Penman M, Resnick D. Molecular flypaper, host defense, and atherosclerosis. J Biol Chem 1993;268:4569–4572.

36. Nicholson A, Pearce SFA, Silverstein R. Oxidized LDL binds to CD36 on human monocyte-derived macrophages and transfected cell lines. Evidence implicating the lipid moiety of the lipoprotein as the binding site . Arterio and Thromb 1995;15:269–275.

37. Rigotti A, Acton S, Krieger M. The class B scavenger receptors SR-B1 and CD36 are receptors for anionic phospholipids. J Biol Chem 1995;270:16221–16224.

38. Ren Y, Silverstein R, Allen J, Savill J. CD36 gene transfer confers capacity for phagocytosis of cells undergoing apoptosis. J Exp Med 1995;181:1857–1862.

39. Asch A, Barnwell J, Silverstein R, Nachman R. Isolation of the thrombospondin membrane receptor. J Clin Invest 1987;79:1054–1061.

40. Tandon N, Kralisz U, Jamieson G. Identification of GPIV (CD36) as a primary receptor for platelet-collagen adhesion. J Biol Chem 1989;264:7576–7583.

41. Barnwell J, Ockenhouse C, Knowles D. Monoclonal antibody OKM5 inhibits the in vitro binding of *Plasmoium falciparum* infected erythrocytes to monocytes, endothelial, and C32 melanoma cells. J Immunol 1985;135:3494–3497.

42. Calvo D, Gomez-Coronado D, Suarez Y, Lasuncion M, Vega MA. Human CD36 is a high affinity receptor for the native lipoproteins HDL, LDL, and VLDL. J Lipid Res 1998;39:777–788.

43. Connelly MA, Klein S, Azhar S, Abumrad N, Williams DL. Comparison of Class B Scavenger Receptors,

CD36 and Scavenger Receptor BI (SR-BI), Shows That Both Receptors Mediate High Density Lipoprotein-Cholesteryl Ester Selective Uptake but SR-BI Exhibits a Unique Enhancement of Cholesteryl Ester Uptake. J Biol Chem 1999;274:41–47.

44. Podrez EA, Febbraio M, Sheibani N, et al. Macrophage scavenger receptor CD36 is the major receptor for LDL modified by monocyte-generated reactive nitrogen species. J Clin Invest 2000;105:1095–1108.

45. Oquendo P, Hundt E, Lawler J, Seed B. CD36 directly mediates cytoadherence of plasmodium falciparum parasitized erythrocytes. Cell 1994;58:95–101.

46. Pearce SFA, Wu J, Silverstein R. A carboxy terminal truncation mutant of CD36 is secreted and binds to thrombospondin. Blood 1994;84:384–389.

47. Pearce SFA, Roy P, Nicholson AC, Hajjar DP, Febbraio M, Silverstein R. Recombinant glutathione S-Transferase/CD36 fusion proteins define an oxidized low density lipoprotein-binding domain. J Biol Chem 1998;273:34875–34881.

48. Huh H-Y, Pearce SFA, Yesner L, Silverstein RL. Regulated expression of CD36 during monocyte-to-macrophage differentiation: Potential role of CD36 in foam cell formation. Blood 1996;87:2020–2028.

49. Yesner L, Huh H, Pearce SFA, Silverstein R. Regulation of monocyte CD36 and thrombospondin-1 expression by soluble mediators. Arterio and Thromb 1996;16:1019–1025.

50. Han J, Hajjar DP, Febbraio M, Nicholson AC. Native and modified low density lipoproteins increase the functional expression of the macrophage class B scavenger receptor, CD36. J Biol Chem 1997;272:21654–21659.

51. Han J, Hajjar DP, Tauras JM, Nicholson AC. Cellular cholesterol regulates expression of the macrophage type B scavenger receptor, CD36. J Lipid Res 1999;40:830–838.

52. Tontonoz P, Nagy L, Alvarez J, Thomazy V, Evans R. PPAR_ promotes monocyte/macrophage differentiation and uptake of oxidized LDL. Cell 1998;93:241–252.

53. Nagy L, Tontonoz P, Alvarez J, Chen H, Evans R. Oxidized LDL regulates macrophage gene expression through ligand activation of PPAR_. Cell 1998;93:229–240.

54. Tontonoz P, Hu E, Spiegelman B. Regulation of adipocyte gene expression and differentiation by peroxisome proliferator activated receptor gamma. Curr Opin Genet Dev 1995;5:571–576.

55. Nakagawa T, Nozaki S, Nishida M, et al. Oxidized LDL increases and interferon-gamma decreases expression of CD36 in human monocyte-derived macrophages. Arterioscler Thromb Vasc Biol 1998;18:1350–1357.

56. Sporn M, Roberts A, Wakefield L, Crombrugghe B. Some recent advances in the chemistry and biology of transforming growth factor-beta. J Cell Biol 1987;105:1039–1045.

57. Suzuki H, Kurihara Y, Takeya M, et al. A role for macrophage scavenger receptors in atherosclerosis and susceptability to infection. Nature 1997;386:292–296.

58. Hisashi S, Takeya M, Sozuki H, et al. Role of macrophage scavenger receptors in diet-induced atherosclerosis in mice. Lab Invest 1998;78:423–433.

59. de Winther MP, Gijbels MJ, van Dijk KW, et al. Scavenger receptor deficiency leads to more complex atherosclerotic lesions in APOE3Leiden transgenic mice. Athero 1999;144:315–321.

60. Lougheed M, Lum C, Ling W, Suzuki H, Kodama T, Steinbrecher U. High affinity saturable uptake of oxidized low density lipoprotein by macrophages from mice lacking the scavenger receptor class A type I/II. J Biol Chem 1997;272:12938–12944.

61. Febbraio M, Abumrad NA, Hajjar DP, et al. A null mutation in murine CD36 reveals an important role in fatty acid and lipoprotein metabolism. J Biol Chem 1999;274:19055–19062.

62. Kashiwagi H, Tomiyama Y, Kosugi Y, et al. Identfication of the molecular defects in a subject with type I CD36 deficiency. Blood 1994;83:3545–3552.

63. Nozaki S, Kashiwagi H, Yamashita S, et al. Reduced uptake of oxidized low density lipoproteins in monocyte-derived macrophages from CD36-deficient subjects. J Clin Invest 1995;96:1859–1865.

64. Febbraio M, Podrez EA, Smith JD, et al. Targeted disruption of the class B scavenger receptor CD36 protects against atherosclerotic lesion development in mice. J Clin Invest 2000;105:1049–1056.

65. Nakata A, Nakagawa Y, Nishida M, et al. CD36, a novel receptor for oxidized low-density lipoproteins, is highly expressed on lipid-laden macrophages in human atherosclerotic aorta. Arterioscler Thromb Vasc Biol 1999;19:1333–1339.

Atherosclerosis and Autoimmunity
Y. Shoenfeld, D. Harats and G. Wick, editors

Atherosclerosis, Matrix-Metalloproteinases (MMPs) and Ischemia/Hypoxia

N. Lahat and S. Shapiro

Immunology Research Unit, Lady Davis Carmel Medical Center, and Bruce Rappaport Faculty of Medicine, Technion – Israel Institute of Technology, Haifa, Israel

1. ATHEROSCLEROSIS AS AN INFLAMMATORY DISEASE – POSSIBLE INVOLVEMENT OF ISCHEMIA

Atherosclerosis is a complex and multifactorial process, and yet there is no single theory that explains all its varied aspects. Inflammatory phenomena at sites of atherosclerotic plaques are increasingly thought to be major determinants of the progression and clinical outcome of disease [1]. The atherosclerotic lesions, which occur principally in large and medium sized elastic and muscular arteries, can lead to ischemia of the heart, brain or extremities, resulting in infarction. Primary manifestations of atherosclerosis, the so-called "fatty streaks", which appear already in arteries of the developing fetus [2], are composed of lipids accumulating in inflammatory cells - monocyte derived macrophages and T lymphocytes [3]. While ischemia is clearly the abrupt clinical detrimental end of the atherosclerotic process, it can also be implicated in the induction of disease. The prevailing theory explaining mechanisms leading to the formation of atherosclerotic plaques is the "response to injury". According to this theory, the initial damage may be caused by a variety of insults including elevated oxidized low density lipoproteins (OX-LDL), hypertension, infectious microorganisms, diabetes, genetic alternations, and ischemia/reperfusion episodes with or without clinical significance [4, 5]. Alternative theories suggest that arterial hypoxia, whether resulting from ischemic or non-ischemic processes, involving or not involving inflammatory patholo-

gies, is the primary mechanism leading to atherosclerosis, or at least is a very early occurrence in the atherosclerotic process [6–9]. Reperfusion of ischemic tissues or reoxygenation of hypoxic cells is critical for salvage and repair of cell injury. Paradoxically they may also, at least temporarily, aggravate the damage [10].

The key event in the "response to injury" hypothesis is endothelial dysfunction, leading to adherence of activated platelets, monocytes and T cells, the subsequent migration of the inflammatory mononuclear cells into the intima and local secretion of hydrolytic enzymes, cytokines, chemokines and growth factors [1]. The injury induces the endothelium, to increase its permeability, to exhibit procoagulation properties and to secrete factors similar to those produced by activated immune cells such as: vasoactive molecules, cytokines, chemokines and growth factors [11]. The inflammatory environment causes migration of smooth muscle cells (SMC), residing in the media of the injured artery, into the intima, and their local proliferation. These SMC generate the fibrous cap of the nascent atherosclerotic plaque [12].

During the ongoing inflammation, enlargement and restructuring of the atherosclerotic plaque is compensated for by dilation of the artery wall, termed "remodelling". Cycles of ischemia/reperfusion (I/R) including hypoxia/reoxygenation (H/R) may be part of the dynamic process, at any stage, of atherosclerosis, without causing an immediate destructive effect. However, at some point the complicated lesion may rupture, resulting in hemorrhage in the plaque, a pro-thrombotic response and rapid total occlusion of the artery.

2. MMPS AND THEIR PATHOGENIC ROLE IN ATHEROSCLEROSIS

The interactions among endothelial cells, immune cells and SMC, the three main cell types participating in the formation, remodelling and growth of the atherosclerotic-plaque, require continuous cell traffic into and inside the vessel. Extracellular matrix (ECM) degradation is essential for these movements. The matrix-metalloproteinases (MMPs), a family of enzymes, 24 of which have been identified to-date, degrade all types of ECM. These enzymes which are associated with both physiological and pathological conditions [13, 14] were suggested to have an important role in the development of atherosclerosis and plaque rupture. MMPs share structural and functional features that include a variation on a five-domain modular structure, dependence on a Zn^{++} ion in their catalytic site, and secretion from cells as inactive zymogens, except for membrane type (MT)-MMPs which are anchored in the cell membranes. The inactive zymogens, require activation through proteolysis, which is performed mainly by serine proteases. Unlike the other MMPs, the activation of Collagen IV degrading MMP2 occurs principally through proteolysis, involving MT1-MMP, while thrombin and integrin $\alpha V\beta3$ may also independently lead to its activation. The MMPs are divided into sub-families according to substrate specificities though a considerable degree of overlap exists: the Collagenases (MMP1, MMP8, MMP13) degrade collagen type I, the Gelatinases (MMP2 and MMP9) degrade gelatin and collagen type IV and the Stromelysins (MMP3, MMP10, MMP11) degrade stromal-proteoglycans.

Regulation of the MMP's activity occurs at different levels including gene transcription, zymogen activation and binding to specific endogenous tissue inhibitors of metalloproteinases (TIMPs), four of which (TIMP1–4) have been reported to date. Similar to the MMPs themselves, TIMPS are produced by different cell types, including those participating in inflammatory responses. Although TIMP2, in low concentrations, has been implicated in activation, rather than inhibition of MMP2, the ratio between MMPs/TIMPs appears to determine the net activity of MMPs. TIMP1 inhibits the activity of all MMPs while having a higher affinity for MMP1, MMP2, MMP3 and MMP9, and TIMP2 specifically inhibits MMP2. Excessive degradation of cell basement membranes and matrix tissue in pathological conditions is related to high concentrations of MMPs, or elevated MMP/TIMP ratios. Inflammatory cytokines, chemokines and growth factors, secreted from T lymphocytes, monocytes/ macrophages, epithelial cells, mesencymal cells, SMC and endothelium induce this elevated expression.

An important role of MMPs in the formation and outcome of atherosclerosis was assessed by in-vitro experiments and in-vivo observations and experiments. Already in 1991 stromelysin mRNA was shown in areas enriched with macrophages in human atherosclerotic plaques [15]. In 1994/5 immunoreactive MMP1, MMP2 and MMP3 were co-localized to lesional lipid-containing macrophages [16], and freshly isolated rabbit plaque macrophages were found to exhibit MMP1, MMP3 and MMP9 activity [17]. More recent studies revealed that MT1-MMP, the main activator of the gelatinase MMP2 (which is principally involved in the degradation of cellular basement membranes) was expressed in SMC and macrophages in human atherosclerotic plaques. Furthermore the proinflammatory molecules, tumor necrosis factorα (TNFα), interleukin1 (IL-1) and OX-LDL were found to lead to an elevation in MT1-MMP expression in these cells in-vitro. OX-LDL was also shown to enhance the expression of the second gelatinase, MMP9, in these cells, while reducing the level of its natural inhibitor TIMP1 [18]. Immunohistochemical analysis of human atherosclerotic plaques revealed the expression of TIMP1 in only a minority of macrophage- and IL-8-rich areas. Moreover, *in-vitro* studies performed with cholesterol-loaded human derived macrophages demonstrated that IL-8, a potent pro-inflammatory chemokine, induced effective inhibition of TIMP1 expression [19]. Gene therapy, using an adenoviral vector containing the human TIMP-1 gene, was attempted in apolipoprotein-E deficient mice, which spontaneously develop human-like atherosclerosis. In-vivo transfection of diseased mice resulted in overexpression of TIMP-1, which was accompanied by increased matrix formation and elevated concentrations of smooth muscle components in the plaques. These findings point to TIMP-1 mediated inhibition of disease progression, or facilitation of lesion regression [20].

Several recent studies classified plaques as those prone to rupture (vulnerable, atheromatous plaques) or those less frequently associated with acute thrombic manifestations (stable, fibrous plaques). A thin fibrous cap and accumulation of lipid containing macrophages ("foam cells") characterized vulnerable plaques. Enhanced local release of MMPs, mainly MMP1 and MMP13 (interstitial collagenases) from resident macrophages, was demonstrated in these plaques, as well as a high content of inflammatory cytokines, such as IL-1β, TNFα, and interferon γ (IFNγ) [21]. Thus a potential role for macrophage derived MMPs in the fragility and rupture of plaques was suggested [22].

3. EFFECTS OF ISCHEMIA/REPERFUSION AND HYPOXIA/REOXYGENATION ON MMPS IN ATHEROSCLEROTIC PLAQUES

Ischemia/reperfusion (I/R) and the resulting hypoxia/reoxygenation (H/R) may be associated with atherosclerosis, as suggested earlier in this review. However, their influence on the progression of disease, particularly their modulation of MMPs in relation to disease progression has not been elucidated. Extensive literature exists, concerning the separate effects of I/R and H/R on each of the three cell types involved in the atherosclerotic lesion: monocytes/macrophages, endothelium and SMC. It was shown that H/R lead to death of SMC both by apoptosis and necrosis [23]. The surviving SMC, resistant to H/R, exhibited major alternations in the amount and composition of matrix synthesis, and in their ability to bind LDL [24]. These cells were also found to produce elevated level of CO, a vasodilator with properties similar to those of NO, whose inhibition in endothelial cells denotes their dysfunction [25]. Interactions may thus be formed between SMC, endothelial cells and other cells in the vicinity. Though OX-LDL, the matrix itself, and NO are known as modulators of MMPs, and secretion of MMPs from SMC was also demonstrated, no studies were reported as to the effects mediated by H/R and I/R on the expression of MMPs in these cells.

Monocytes/macrophages accumulate in hypoxic areas of atherosclerotic plaques [26, 27]. Local H/R or I/R may lead to their apoptotic or necrotic death [28], thus providing a possible explanation for the disintegrated areas observed within atherosclerotic lesions. A 150 kDa oxygen-regulated protein, expressed in atherosclerotic residing macrophages was hypothesized to protect them from cell death during H/R [29]. The resistant macrophage subpopulations, which survived repeated H/R cycles [30], exhibited marked changes in their secretory activity. They produced enhanced levels of inflammatory cytokines [31] and proangiogenic substances such as vascular endothelial growth factor (VEGF), fibroblast growth factor (FGF) and platelet derived growth factor (PDGF), which through their affect on endothelial cells, may enhance the formation of new blood vessels [32].

It has been suggested that hypoxia, via its suppression of local chemoattractants [33], inhibits the migratory activity of monocytes/macrophages by immobilizing them in hypoxic areas. Using the Mono Mac-6 human monocytic cell line, we have recently found that hypoxia reduced and reoxygenation gradually elevated the secretion of active MMP9, while not affecting MMP2. (N. Lahat, B. Marom, H. Bitterman, M. Rahat, unpublished results.) These results offer an additional possible explanation for the monocytes/macrophages retention in hypoxic tissues, amongst them atherosclerotic lesions.

Proangiogenic and inflammatory molecules secreted from hypoxic macrophages induce activation of endothelial cells which, on the one hand, may acerbate "endothelial dysfunction", and on the other hand may enhance neovascularization [34]. The endothelium is one of the most hypoxia–tolerant mammalian cell types. Induction of resistance in these cells involves upregulation of proteins, whose identity and exact protective roles are not entirely understood [35]. Production of MMPs, as a part of endothelial survival characteristics, can be induced in endothelial cells indirectly as described, but also directly as a result of low oxygen tension. We evaluated the effects of H/R on the modulation of MMP2, its main activator MT1-MMP, and its endogenous inhibitor TIMP2, in human endothelial cells [36]. Hypoxia was found to enhance the transcription of the MMP2 gene and the secretion of its zymogen form, though it inhibited both MT1-MMP and TIMP2 gene transcription. Reoxygenation enhanced both MMP2 and MT1-MMP gene expression and elevated MMP2 activity, suggesting that both hypoxia and reoxygenation were necessary for active angiogenesis. Protective "preconditioning" of endothelial cells by repeated I/R or H/R cycles has also been reported, however its mechanisms are not yet clear [34, 37]. The effects of this preconditioning on MMPs expression by endothelial cells has not been reported.

4. POSSIBLE DUAL ROLE FOR ISCHEMIA/REPERFUSION OR HYPOXIA/REOXYGENATION IN ATHEROSCLEROSIS: DO MMPS PLAY A BENEFICIAL ROLE?

The role of I/R and H/R in the pathogenesis and progress of atherosclerosis is equivocal. They may evoke or aggravate the vicious cycle of inflammatory cascades described, involving endothelium, monocytes/macrophages and SMC. However, intermittent I/R were found to exert anti-atherogenic effects on experimental atherosclerosis in rabbits [38] and preconditioning by H/R cycles was shown to have protective effects against primary induced endothelial damage [34, 37]. The coronary artery collateral circulation is frequently associated with atherosclerosis, and there now remains little doubt that it may be beneficial in limiting myocardial infarction in the face of coronary artery stenosis and active coronary occlusion [39]. It is evident that collaterals are the result of neoangiogenesis, of which I/R and H/R are major stimulators [40]. A pathogenic role for MMPs in atherosclerosis formation, plaque growth and sensitivity to rupture was strongly suggested in *in-vitro* studies, *in-vivo* observations, and the efficient therapeutic intervention implementing MMPs inhibitors. However, these studies did not take into consideration possible positive effects of MMP secretion, which may be triggered during non-occlusive short I/R or H/R episodes in atherosclerotic plaques, promoting beneficial angiogenesis. As with other potent biological factors, induction of destructive versus advantageous effects may be timing, local concentration and types of additional, interacting-molecules. To date

the regulation of MMPs during I/R and H/R accompanying atherosclerosis, and their active role in disease progression or therapy awaits further research.

REFERENCES

1. Ross A. Ateroslerosis – An inflammatory disease. N Engl J Med 1999;340:115–126.
2. Napoli C, D'Armiento FP, Mancini FP, Postiglione A., Witztum JL, Palumbo G, Palinski W. Fatty streak formation occurs in human fetal aortas and is greatly enhanced by maternal hypercholesterolemia: intimal accumulation of low density lipoprotein and its oxidation precede monocyte recruitment into early atherosclerotic lesions. J Clin Invest 1997;100:2680–2690.
3. Stary HC, Chandler AB, Glagov S, Guyton W Jr, Rosenfeld ME, Schaffer SA, Schwartz CJ, Wagner WD, Wissler RW. A definition of initial, fatty streak, and intermediate lesion of atherosclerosis: a report from the committee on vascular lesions of the council on arteriosclerosis. American Heart Association. Circulation 1994;89:2462–2478.
4. Yang ZH, Richard V, von-Segesser L, Bauer E, Stultz P, Turina M, Luscher TF. Threshold concentrations of endothelin-1 potentiate contractions to norepinephrine and serotonin in human arteries. A new mechanism of vasospasm? Circulation 1990; 82:188–195.
5. Fischer S, Claus M, Wiesnet M, Renz D, Schaper W, Karliczek GF. Hypoxia induced permeability in brain microvessel endothelial cells via VEGF and NO. Am J Physiol 1999;276:C812–C820.
6. Simanonok JP. Non ischemic hypoxia of the arterial wall is the primary cause of atherosclerosis. Med Hypotheses 1996;46:155–161.
7. Mohri M, Takeshita A. Coronary microvascular disease in humans. Jpn Heart J 1999; 40:97–108.
8. Sinisalo J, Syrjala M, Mattila KJ, Kerman T, Nieminen MS. Endothelial release of tissue type plasminogen activator and ischemia-induced vasodilatation are linked in patients with coronary heart disease. Blood Coagul Fibrinolysis 1999;10:181–187.
9. Lowe GD. Etiopathogenesis of cardiovascular disease: hemostatis, thrombosis and vascular medicine. Ann Periodontal 1998;3:121–126.
10. Zimmerman BJ, and Granger DN. Reperfusion injury. Surg Clin N Am 1992;72:65–83.
11. Pohlman TH, Harlan M. Adaptive responses of the endothelium to stress. J Surg Res 2000;89:85–119.
12. Libby P, Ross R. Cytokines and growth regulatory molecules. In: Fuster V, Ross R, Topol EJ, editors. Atherosclerosis and coronary artery diseases. Vol I. Philadel-

phia, Lippincott-Raven, 1996;585–594.

13. Cawston T. MMPs and TIMP properties and implications for the rheumatic disease. Mol Med Today 1998;3:130–137.

14. Borden P, Heller RA. Transcriptional control of MMPs and TIMPs. Crit Rev in Eucaryotic Gene Expression 1997;7:159–178.

15. Henney AM, Wakeley PR, Davies MI, Foster K, Hembry R, Murphy G, Hemphries S. Localization of stromolysin gene expression in atherosclerotic plaques by in situ hybridization. Proc Natl Acad Sci USA 1991;88:8154–8158.

16. Galis ZS, Sukhova G, Lark M, Libby P. Increased expression of MMPs and matrix degrading activity in vulnerable regions of human atherosclerotic plaques. J Clin Invest 1994;94:2493–2503.

17. Galis, ZS Sukhova G, Kranzhefer R, Clark S, Libby P. Macrophage foam cells from experimental atheroma constitutively produce matrix degrading proteinase. Proc Natl Acad Sci USA 1995;92:402–406.

18. Rajavshisth TB, Xiao-Ping X, Jovinge S, Meisels, Xiao-Ou X, Ning Ning C, Fishbein MC, Kaul S, Cercek B, Sharipi B, Shah PK. Membrane-Type1 MMP expression in human atherosclerotic plaques. Circulation 1999;99:3103–3109.

19. Moreau M, Brocheriou I, Petit L, Ninio E, Chapman J, Rauis M. IL-8 mediates downregulation of TIMP1 expression in cholesterol loaded human macrophages. Circulation 1999;99:420–426.

20. Rovis M, Adamy C, Duverger N, Lesnik P, Horellou P, Moreau M, Emmanuel F, Caillaud JM, Lapland PM, Dachet C, Chapman MJ. Adenovirus mediated over-cxpression of TIMP1 reduces atherosclerotic lesions in apolipoprotein E deficiency mice. Circulation 1999;100:533–540.

21. Libby P, Sukhova L, Lee RT, Galis ZS. Cytokines regulate vascular functions related to stability of atherosclerotic plaque. J Cardiovasc Pharmacol 1995;25:S9–S12.

22. Sukhova GK, Schonbeck V, Rabkin E, Shoen FJ, Poole R, Billingshurst RC, Libby P. Evidence for increased collagenolysis by interstitial collagenase 1 and 3 in vulnerable human atheromatous plaques. Circulation 1999;99:2503–2509.

23. Saikumar P, Dong Z, Weinberg JM, Venkatachalan MA. Mechanism of cell death in hypoxia/reoxygenation injury. Oncogene 1998;17:3341–3349.

24. Figueroa JE, Tao Z, Sarphie TG, Smart FW, Glancy DL, Vijayagapal P. Effect of hypoxia and hypoxia/reoxygenation on proteoglycan metabolism by vascular smooth muscle cells. Atherosclerosis 1999;143:135–144.

25. Kounembanas S, Morita T, Liu Y, Christou H. Mechanisms by which oxygen regulates gene expression and cell interaction in the vasculature. Kidney Int 1997;51:438–443.

26. Bjornheden T, Levin M, Evaldsson M, Wiklung O. Evidence of hypoxic areas within the arterial wall in vivo. Arterioscler Thromb Vasc Biol 1999;19:870–876.

27. Knierriem HJ, Jurukova Z. Proteolytic enzyme release by macrophages in the destabilization process of atherosclerotic plaques. Atherosclerosis 1997;134:233.

28. Rymsa B, Becker HD, Lauchart W. De Groot H. Hypoxia/reoxygenation in liver injury: Kupfer cells are more vulnerable to reoxygenation than to hypoxia. Res Commun Chem Pathol Pharmacol 1990;68:264–266.

29. Tsukamoto Y, Kuwabara K, Hirota S, Ikeda J, Sterm P, Yanai H, Matsumoto M, Ogawa S, Kitamura Y. 150 kDa oxygen regulated protein is expressed in human atherosclerotic plaques and allows mononuclear phagocytes to withstand cellular stress on exposure to hypoxia and modified LDL. J Clin Invest 1996;98:1930–1941.

30. Yun IK, Mc Cormick TS, Villabona C, Judware RR, Espinosa MB, Lapentina EG. Inflammatory mediators are perpetuated in macrophages resistant to apoptosis induced by hypoxia. Proc Natl Acad Sci USA 1997;94:13903–13908.

31. Rahat M, Lahat N, Smollar J, Brod V, Kinarty A and Bitterman H. Divergent effects of ischemia – reperfusion and NO donor on TNFα mRNA accumulation in rat organs. Shock 2000 (in press).

32. Lewis JS, Lee JA, Underwood JCE, Harris AL, Lewis CE. Macrophage response to hypoxia: relevance to disease mechanisms. J Leuk Biol 1999;66:889–900.

33. Negos RP, Turner L, Burk F, Balkwill FR. Hypoxia down regulates MCP-1 expression: implications for macrophage distribution in tumors. J Leuk Biol 1998;64:758–765.

34. Pohlman TH and Harlan JM. Adaptive responses of the endothelium on stress. J Surg Res 2000;89:85–119.

35. Graven K and Farber HW. Endothelial cell hypoxic stress proteins. J Lab Clin Med 1998;132:456–63.

36. Ben-Bassat Y, Miller A, Shapiro S, Bitterman H, Lahat N. Effects of hypoxia and reoxygenation on expression of MMP2 and its regulatory molecules in endothelial cells. (abst.) 2nd Internat Conf on Tumor Microenvironment, Progression, Therapy and Prevention 2000.

37. Beauchamp P, Richard V, Tamion F, Lallemand F, Leberton JP, Vaudry h, Daueau M, Thuillez C. Protective effects of preconditioning in cultured rat endothelial cells. Circulation 1999;100:541–546.

38. Kitaev MI, Aitbaev K, Liamtsev VT. Effect of hypoxic hypoxia on development of atherosclerosis in rabbits. Aviakosm Ekaolog Med 1999;33:54–57.

39. Schultz A, Lavie L, Hochberg I, Begar R, Tsachi S, Shorecki K, Lavie P, Rouin A, Levi AP. Interindividual heterogeneity in the hypoxic regulation of VEGF. Cir-

culation 1999;100:547–552.

40. Isner JM. Manipulating angiogenesis against vascular disease. Hospital Practice 1999; 34:79–80.

Atherosclerosis and Autoimmunity
Y. Shoenfeld, D. Harats and G. Wick, editors

Ceramide Pathway and Apoptosis in Autoimmunity and Atherosclerosis

T. Goldkorn, J. George, S.N. Lavrentiadou, T. Ravid, A. Tsaba,Y. Shoenfeld and D. Harats

Signal Transduction, UC Davis School of Medicine, TB149, Davis Campus, Davis CA 95616, USA

Abbreviations: *ApoE:* apolipoprotein E, *aPLs:* antiphospholipid antibodies, *aSMase:* acidic sphingomyelinase β*2GPI:* β2-glycoprotein I, *BSO:* DL-buthionine-[S,R]-sulfoximine, *CF:* cystic fibrosis, *Cyt C:* cytochrome C, *DAG:* diacylglycerol, *DD:* death domain, *DISC:* death-inducing signal complex, *HSP:* heat shock protein, *IFN:* interferon, *FADD:* Fas-associated death domain protein, *FAN:* factor associated with nSMase activation, *IL1:* interleukin 1, *LDL:* low-density lipoprotein, *MAPK:* mitogen-activated protein kinase, *NSD:* neutral SMase domain, *PI3K:* phosphatidyl 3-kinase, *PKC:* protein kinase C, *OxLDL:* oxidized LDL, *RA:* rheumatoid arthritis, *ROS:* reactive oxygen species, *S-1-P:* sphingosine-1-phosphate, *SLE:* systemic lupus erythematosus, *SM:* sphingomyelin, *nSMase:* neutral sphingomyelinase, *NGF:* nerve growth factor, *TRADD:* TNFR1 associated death domain protein, *TNF:* tumor necrosis factor, *TNFR:* tumor necrosis factor receptor, *TR55:* tumor necrosis factor receptor-55.

1. INTRODUCTION

Multicellular animals are facing daily death at the cellular level. Cells usually die by apoptosis, a death process that is controlled by built-in cellular mechanisms. However, in cases of severe injury, cells may alternatively undergo necrosis, which is a non-programmed death resulting in cellular lysis.

Apoptotic cell death was originally distinguished from necrosis based on morphological differences and on the tendency of necrotic, but not apoptotic, cells to induce an inflammatory response. Although it is still not clear how necrotic cells trigger inflammation, this capacity may be critical in relating tissue damage to the generation of an immune response.

Apoptotic cell death, which concludes in the execution, packaging, and removal of the dying cells, has emerged as a physiological response to developmental and environmental signals. The pathways suggested for this significant process may vary between different types of cells. Two main classes of lipids participate in signaling pathways in immune cells. One includes glycerol-based lipids with diacylglycerol (DAG) as its most studied member that mediates the activation of protein kinase C (PKC) molecules. The second group depends on the sphingolipids, with the most-studied agents being sphingosine, sphingosine-1-phosphate, and ceramide. It is presently clear that sphingolipids are ubiquitously distributed in all eukaryotic cells, especially in cellular membranes, where they were previously thought to maintain only a structural role. However, in recent years ceramide has especially received substantial interest for its modulatory role in the path of apoptosis. These studies have led to new understanding of some of the underlying pathology of several diseases with imbalances in the sphingolipid metabolism leading to undesired cell activation, imbalance in apoptosis and inflammatory processes.

2. CERAMIDE PATHWAY AND APOPTOSIS

The morphologic features of apoptosis are typical and well conserved in diverse cell types. This suggests a possible convergence of multiple sign-

55

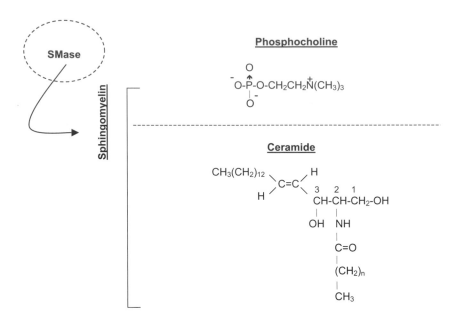

Figure 1. Sphingomyelin (SM) hydrolysis by sphingomyelinase (SMase) generated ceramide.

aling pathways, which ultimately culminate in one common route towards apoptosis. The ceramide/ sphingomyelin (SM) pathway may constitute that common step. Our studies have begun to identify a receptor-activated pathway of signal transduction involving the sphingolipid SM and its hydrolysis product ceramide [1].

Agonists of the ceramide pathway include cytokines such as Tumor Necrosis Factorα (TNFα) [2–5], interleukin1β((IL1β)) [6, 7], interferonγ(IFN γ) [8], vitamin D3 [9], nerve growth factor (NGF) [10], as well as anti-CD28 [11, 12], anti-CD40 [13] and anti-CD95 antibodies [14, 15], and various other stress agents including oxidized LDL [16, 17]. The observation that membrane-permeant synthetic ceramides could mimic the biological effects of most ceramide pathway agonists has provided significant weight to the role of ceramide in signal transduction and apoptosis [18].

In the past, sphingolipids were mainly considered as major structural cell membrane lipid compounds. The studies of Hannun et al [19] showed for the first time a role of one of these sphingolipids, sphingosine, as an effective signaling molecule. This led to the discovery of the sphingomyelin pathway that is a ubiquitous, evolutionarily conserved signaling system analogous to the cAMP and phosphoinositide pathways [9]. Sphingomyelin (N-acylsphingosin-1-phosphocholine) is a sphingolipid preferentially concentrated in the plasma membrane of mammalian cells. Sphingomyelin catabolism occurs via the action of sphingomyelin-specific forms of phospholipase C, termed sphingomyelinases (SMases), which hydrolyze the phosphodiester bond of sphingomyelin [2, 5, 14, 20], yielding ceramide and phosphorylcholine (Figure 1).

To date, several types of SMases have been identified. The main forms of SMases are distinguished by their pH optima [5, 11]. Human and murine acid sphingomyelinase (aSMase; pH optimum 4.5–5.0) have been cloned and determined to be the products of a conserved gene, whereas Mg^{2+}-dependent or -independent neutral SMases (nSMase; pH optimum 7.4) have yet to be molecularly characterized. Interestingly, neutral (membrane) nSMase does not gain access to the signaling events activated by the acidic (lysosomal) aSMase and vice versa, indicating that ceramide action may be determined by the subcellular site of its production [21–23].

Ceramide has been shown to act as an intracellular second messenger [7, 24]. In addition to demonstrating cell growth inhibitory effects and reacting to stress with apoptosis [14, 15, 24–34] it mediates various cellular responses, such as those control-

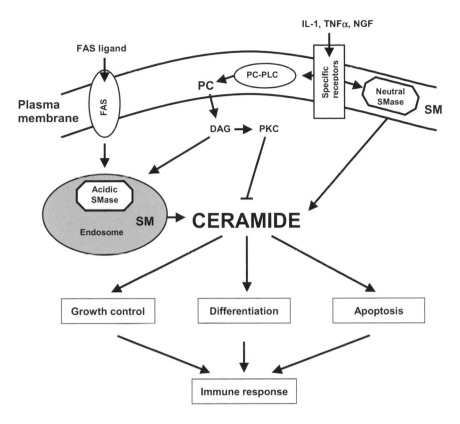

Figure 2. Ceramide-mediated signal transduction. Ceramide is generated via the receptor-mediated activation of discrete acid and neutral SMases, located in distinct subcellular compartments. Different mechanisms are involved in the activation of each SMase (see Figure 3). Ceramide then transduces downstream signals through the modulation of the activities of a variety of target enzymes/transcriptional activators.

ling cell proliferation [11, 12, 35, 36] and differentiation [8, 9, 37] (Figure 2). The molecular signals which mediate these events may be transduced by a variety of putative proteins such as members of the mitogen-activated protein kinase (MAPK) family, protein kinase C (PKC) isoenzymes, raf and small GTPases, ceramide-activated protein phosphatase, the kinase suppressor of ras, a proline-directed protein- kinase, and transcription factors [25–31]. In addition, phosphatidyl 3-kinase (PI3K), which is a critical signaling molecule involved in regulating cell survival and proliferation pathways, was shown recently to cross-talk with ceramide generation within cells, and to provide a mechanism for regulation of cell survival/death decisions [35]. Taken together, the variety of mediators and molecular targets involved in ceramide signaling has led to the notion that ceramide is an important lipid mediator of cellular responses in organisms from

yeast to humans [27, 36, 37].

More general reviews on the signaling functions of sphingolipids are available [25, 27, 28, 31, 38–41]. The general role of sphingomyelin metabolites in vascular cell signaling and atherogenesis [42] and the role of glycosphingolipids in vascular biology has been also recently reviewed [43]. Therefore, the goal of this chapter is to focus on ceramide pathway in vascular cell signaling mainly in conjunction with apoptosis in autoimmunity and atherosclerosis.

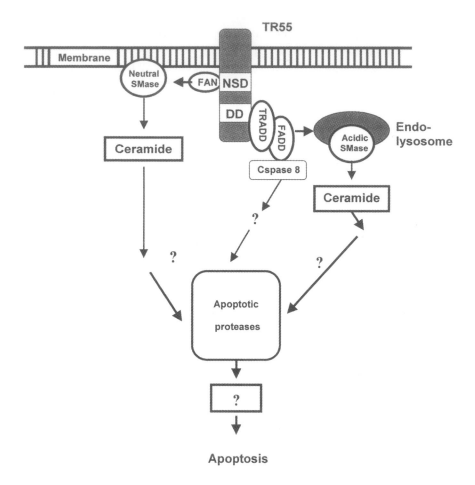

Figure 3. Proposed model for the activation mechanism of nSMase and aSMase through TNF-R55 (TR55 or TNFR-1). TR55 initiates the nSMase pathway via interaction between its NSD domain and FAN, whereas the aSMase is activated via the recruitment of the TRADD/ FADD complex to the death domain (DD) of TR55.

3. REGULATORS OF APOPTOSIS AND CERAMIDE

3.1. Death Receptors

Death receptors are a subset of the TNF Receptor family, including the 55-kDa receptor for TNF (TNFR1, or TNF-R55 (TR55)), Fas/CD95, and the TRAIL receptors, among others. The death receptors are a family of trans plasma membrane proteins sharing a homologous cytoplasmic domain, the death domain (DD) (Figure 3). This domain is responsible for the recruitment of adapter proteins and the initiation of the apoptotic signaling cascade [44]. Activation of death receptors triggers the assembly of DISC (death-inducing signal com-

plex), composed of multiple cytosolic proteins with different functional roles [44]. Of these cytosolic proteins, TRADD (TNFR1 associated death domain protein), which is recruited by some receptors (e.g., TNFR1 and death receptor 3), serves as an adapter to the binding of FADD (Fas-associated death domain protein) and other transductional proteins [44]. Once associated, FADD binds a specific pro-protease, pro-caspase 8, whose proteolytic activation at the receptor level triggers the evolvement of the cascade of apoptotic-signaling events leading to cell death [45, 46] (Figure 3).

Kronke and colleagues developed a model, in which distinct cytoplasmic domains of TNF-R55 signal the activation of an aSMase and nSMase [5, 47–50]. The death domain (DD) uses the two pro-apoptotic adapter proteins, TRADD and FADD, for the activation of aSMase (Figure 3). Notably, FADD involvement was also suggested in the Fas activation of aSMase [51]. A second signaling domain, which was termed the neutral SMase domain (NSD) is located upstream of the death domain (DD) and directly links the TNF-R55 to the activation of the nSMase. A novel adapter protein, FAN (factor associated with nSMase activation), has been identified that specifically binds to the NSD. Overexpression of full-length FAN enhanced nSMase activity in TNF-treated cells, whereas truncated mutants of FAN produced dominant negative effects. FAN, however, did not interfere with any of the other TNF responses signaled by the death domain. Taken together, the data suggest that distinct cytoplasmic domains of TNF-R55 initiate independent signaling pathways by binding different adapter proteins [52].

Although the functional regulation of the downstream events is understood in some detail [46], and the formation of the death domain adapter protein complexes appears independent of ceramide, emerging data suggest that its ability to confer apoptosis may depend on coordinated signaling via ceramide [31]. Deletions of the death domain region of the TNF-R55, as well as overexpression of dominant negative FADD blocked ligand induced ceramide generation and apoptosis. Furthermore, it has been reported that treatment with ceramide analogs can bypass the anti-apoptotic effect of the dominant-negative FADD mutants and restore apoptosis [31]. In addition, it has been recently demonstrated that exogenous, as well as endogenous ceramide facilitates TNFR1-activated signal transduction by increasing TRADD recruitment to the DISC complex and caspase 8-activation [53].

Downstream from the death receptors, the apoptotic pathway involves the activation of proximal caspases, changes in mitochondrial function, the release of cytochrome C (cyt C), the activation of effector (distal, or executioner) caspases and the induction of the subsequent hallmarks of apoptosis, as detailed below.

3.2. Caspases

The caspases are cysteine proteases with specificity for aspartic acid residues [54] that are activated during apoptosis. The caspases are divided functionally into initiator caspases, such as caspase 1, 2, and 8, which couple to cytokine receptors of the TNF superfamily and link to effector caspases, which commit the cell to undergo death (Figure 4). The final steps of cell death are coordinated by the distal caspases (called effector or executioner caspases) out of which caspase 3 is the major executioner.

Distal effector caspases, such as caspase 3, appear to operate downstream from ceramide [55–59]. On the other hand, proteases that belong to the caspase 8, or initiator caspase family [49, 60, 61] which are inhibited by the viral protein CrmA, function upstream of ceramide and may control stress-activated ceramide generation by SM hydrolysis. In turn, exogenous ceramides can activate the distal, but not the proximal caspases, which suggests a role for endogenous ceramide upstream of DNA fragmentation and distal caspase action. This is further supported by studies examining the relationship between ceramide and the antiapoptotic protein, Bcl2. The latter does not interfere with ceramide generation but does inhibit the ability of exogenous ceramides to activate the distal executioner caspases and to induce apoptosis [62]. On the other hand, some other reports demonstrated that caspase 1 inhibitors do not block stress-induced ceramide production [63–64], whereas Takeda et al suggested that caspase 3 has a direct role in activating the Mg^{+2}-dependent nSMase [65]. In addition to caspase inhibitors, small serine-protease inhibitors like TPCK have shown to inhibit SM hydrolysis [66] through inhibition of a neutral [17, 67] but not acidic SMase [68]. Taken together, these data suggest that ceramide generation occurs downstream from a protease(s) that remains to be identified.

The possible activation of a SMase by a protease seems to be also evolutionary conserved, since ceramide generation in *Drosophila* cells is controlled by a proteolytic event that can be inhibited by ICE-like inhibitors such as z-VAD-fmk [69, 70]. Even though it is hypothesized that SMase itself is activated after proteolysis, or, alternatively, an additional protein that negatively couples to SMase may be cleaved by the protease, thereby turning into an activator, more work is still required to elucidate the characteristics of the protease that targets SM hydrolysis.

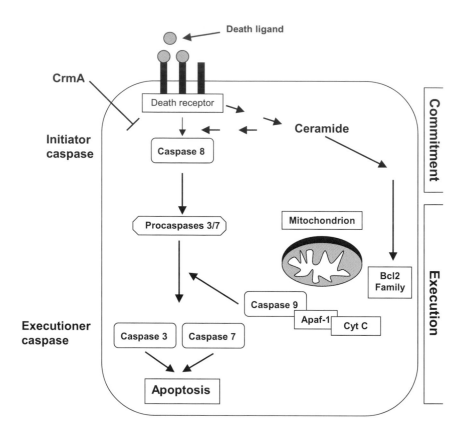

Figure 4. The framework of apoptotic pathways leading to the activation of caspases and mitochondrion involvement.

3.3. Mitochondrial Pathways

Pro-apoptotic cell stimuli induce the activation of the pro-apoptotic members of the Bcl2 family, which target the mitochondria and induce the release of proteins that reside in the space between the inner and outer mitochondrial membranes. One of these is cyt C, which mediates the execution phase of apoptosis (Figure 4). This phase is centered on the activation of caspase 9. The initiator caspase 9 is activated following the release of mitochondrial cyt C to form the apoptotic protease activating factor -1 (Apaf[-1]) complex. Then, the activated caspase 9 converges with caspase 8 on the proteolytic activation of caspase 3 [45]. On the other hand, the anti-apoptotic members of the Bcl2 family block the release of cyt C from the mitochondria [71] and can inhibit ceramide production in cells treated with DNA damaging agents [72].

Bcl2 overexpression blocked cell-permeant ceramide- as well as daunorubicin- induced apoptosis [73]. Nevertheless, activation of a nSMase was not affected. Similar results were shown for TNFα [61] and ceramide-mediated [56, 74–76] apoptosis. It therefore appears that Bcl2 operates downstream from ceramide. Another study reported that overexpression of Bcl2 in PC12 cells resulted in protection against Hypoxia-induced cell death through a decrease in SM hydrolysis and ceramide generation [55]. In contrast, overexpression of Bcl-xL in MCF7 cells has been shown to prevent ceramide generation and apoptosis induced by TNFα, thereby placing Bcl-xL upstream of ceramide creation [77]. However, this does not fit the study that no inhibition by Bcl-xL on anti-immunoglobulin-induced ceramide generation could be observed [78]. Therefore, ceramide generation in respect to mitochondria signals and Bcl2 members requires additional

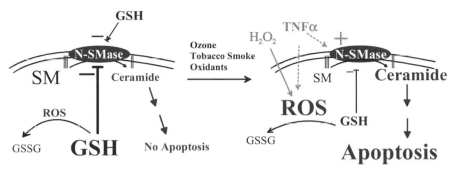

Figure 5. Oxidative stress [Reactive Oxygen Species (ROS)]-mediated ceramide generation and apoptosis.

studies, and now seems to vary in different cells.

3.4. Protein Kinase C (PKC)

Previous studies [79, 80] demonstrated that PKC activation through DAG or phorbol esters (TPA) inhibited the induction of apoptosis by cell-permeable ceramides. These studies suggested that PKC is an important negative regulator of ceramide-induced apoptosis (Figure 2). Furthermore, TPA inhibited ceramide generation and apoptosis in H_2O_2-treated epithelial cells [81], which is consistent with the observation that PKC inhibitors trigger a nSMase, suggesting that PKC may also play a key role in regulating basal SMase activity [82, 83]

4. CERAMIDE-MEDIATED OXIDATIVE STRESS AND APOPTOSIS

Very little is presently known about the regulation of SMases [41]. We have demonstrated that H_2O_2-mediated oxidative stress generates ceramide and induces apoptosis in airway epithelial cells, and that H_2O_2-induced generation of ceramide is a critical and obligatory event in the H_2O_2 induction of the apoptotic cascade in airway epithelial cells [80, 81, 84, 85].

Studies in a cell free system, devoid of nuclei, demonstrated that H_2O_2 activates a Mg^{+2}-dependent nSMase localized to the plasma membrane [80, 81]. Subsequently, treatment of A549 cells with glutathione (GSH) resulted in loss of their ability to produce ceramide in a time and dose-dependent manner, whereas depletion of intracellular GSH by DL-buthionine-[S,R]-sulfoximine (BSO) induced ceramide levels and apoptosis [84, 85]. These results substantiate the observation that physiologic levels of GSH in airway epithelial cells completely inhibit nSMase, also implying that a sharp drop in cellular levels of GSH may alleviate this inhibition and cause activation of nSMase (Figure 5).

The tripeptide GSH functions as an antioxidant, and depletion of reduced GSH cellular levels often occurs at the initial stages of apoptosis. GSH has been shown to inhibit the neutral, Mg^{+2}-dependent SMase in-vitro [86]. The importance of reactive oxygen species in cytokine (TNFα, IL1β) mediated SM hydrolysis was demonstrated in brain cells by the inhibition of cytokine-induced SM degradation via N-acetylcysteine [87]. In addition, exposure to thiol-depleting agents or to H_2O_2 resulted in elevated SM breakdown [86–88]. Similarly, we observed that H_2O_2-induced ceramide generation in lung epithelial cells was inhibited by GSH and followed by a decrease in apoptosis [84, 85]. It is therefore proposed [84, 85] that oxidant-mediated depletion of GSH during cellular injury may play a regulatory role in the activation of nSMase, thus resulting in an increase in ceramide, and GSH-depletion may be the link between oxidative stress and ceramide-mediated apoptosis (Figure 5). Further elucidation of the molecular mechanisms linking oxidative stress to apoptotic signaling pathways will improve pharmacological intervention in the signaling processes that regulate oxidant-mediated inflammatory diseases.

5. CERAMIDE GENERATION AND APOPTOSIS IN IMMUNE-MEDIATED DISEASES

Ceramide pathway and apoptosis have been suggested to play a role in diseases such as rheumatoid arthritis (RA) [89–91], Systemic Lupus Erythematosus (SLE) [92–95], atherosclerosis [96–98], cystic fibrosis (CF) [99] and asthma [100]. However, the molecular mechanism(s) underlying the pathobiochemistry, as well as the genes that may be modulated by ceramide are unknown.

The possible connection between ceramide and caspases in both Fas- and HLA class I- apoptosis pathways was examined [64]. The results point toward activation of caspases upstream and downstream of ceramide production, leading to reduction of mitochondrial transmembrane potential and subsequent propagation of the death signal. The data support a close relationship between caspases and ceramide in the signaling of apoptosis mediated by Fas and HLA class I molecules.

A positive correlation between Bcl2 levels and SLE activity was suggested. It is possible that the self-reactive lymphocytes, which may be triggering autoimmunity, avoid apoptosis by the overexpression of Bcl2 [92]. It was also hypothesized that in SLE defective Fas-mediated apoptosis of host lymphocytes could result in failure of self-tolerance [95]. However, both the expression and function of Fas and its ligand are normal in SLE. In fact, far from being a disease of too little apoptosis, the evidence is that SLE is the opposite. Deficient phagocyte-mediated clearance of intact apoptotic cells leads to their fragmentation and the release of intracellular antigens (to which the immune system is not tolerant) in a form that can trigger an immune response [94].

Marked proliferation of synovial cells is a primary feature of RA. This led to an early hypothesis that the RA synovial cells have defects in apoptotic processes. However, it was demonstrated that ceramide induces apoptosis of RA synovial cells [89–91]. Moreover, these cells have similar sensitivity to ceramide- induced apoptosis as the dermal fibroblast [89]. Thus, the effect of ceramide is not specific for RA synovial cells, suggesting that apoptosis signal transduction downstream of ceramide is intact in RA synovial cells.

6. ATHEROSCLEROSIS AS AN AUTOIMMUNE DISEASE

Atherosclerosis is characterized by the appearance of mononuclear cells in the vessel wall at arterial branching points. Initial lesions are characterized by the formation of foam cells, which constitute macrophages that uptake oxidized low-density lipoproteins (oxLDLs) by their scavenger receptors, leading to their overloading with lipids and ultimate deposition of extracellular cholesterol. This constitutes cushion-like lesions, called fatty streaks, which lead to atherosclerotic plaques. With progression of lesions, smooth muscle cells (SMCs) immigrate into the intima from the media. Upon proliferation at the intima collagen fibers are deposited, which leads to thickening and hardening of the arteries (arteriosclerosis).

The occurrence of macrophages, endothelial cells and activated lymphocytes in the atherosclerotic plaque has brought up the idea of atherosclerosis as an inflammatory disorder [101]. It has been known that both humoral and cellular immune reactions take place in atherosclerotic lesions. However, it has not been obvious whether these routes were primary or secondary in nature. Evidence for the participation of the immune system in the evolvement of the atherosclerotic lesion is reviewed in refs [102–104].

The study of murine models of atherosclerosis has contributed much to the progress of understanding the role of inflammatory mediators. Several transgenic knockout mice that develop atherosclerosis have been produced [105–107]. The apolipoprotein E (apoE) knockout mouse spontenasouly develops hypercholesterolemia followed by atherosclerosis [105, 106]. The low-density lipoprotein (LDL) receptor-deficient mouse develops extensive atherosclerosis only when fed a high fat diet. The lesions of these transgenic mice contain immunopotent cells (CD4 and CD8 lymphocytes), and treatment of these mice with blocking monoclonal antibodies to CD4 lymphocytes or to TNFα reduced atherosclerosis [104]. Furthermore, crossing the apoE mouse with IFNγ receptor knockout mice yields a double knockout mouse relatively protected from atherosclerosis, suggesting that IFNγ has a pro-atherogenic role [101].

The atherosclerotic lesions from both experimental animals and humans contain inflammatory cells and cross reactive antigens that may mount an autoimmune response. Several autoantigens have been already proposed to affect atherosclerosis, such as the microbial substances, heat shock protein 60/65, some modified forms of LDL, and β2-glycoprotein I (β2GPI: a circulating protein that serves as a target for antiphospholipid antibodies).

Heat shock proteins are highly conserved. HSP60, the mammalian form, and HSP65, the bacterial form, cross react. An HSP65-induced immune response (towards bacteria) may also turn on against our own self-expressed HSP60. Furthermore, induction of an immune reaction against HSP65 in rabbits and mice [108, 109] resulted in enhanced atherosclerotic plaques.

OxLDL displays different functional properties from LDL such as activation of endothelial cells and stimulation of SMC proliferation. Therefore it has been suggested that oxLDL plays a major role in the initiation and progression of atherosclerosis [110]. Although generation of antibodies to oxLDL by immunization with the oxLDL protects animals against atherosclerosis [111–113], antibodies to oxLDL correlate with atherosclerosis [114]. OxLDL is immunogenic and autoantibodies to its modified targets are associated with the extent of atherosclerosis and may predict future myocardial infractions and subsequent Restenosis [114–117]. Furthermore, oxLDL (but not LDL) induces in-vitro the secretion of pro-inflammatory cytokines.

George and Shoenfeld [118] hypothesized that antiphospholipid antibodies (aPLs) that are known to inflict a thrombotic trend are also pro-atherogenic. These antibodies activate endothelial cells and platelets. aPLs bind to phospholipids or to co-factors that associate with phospholipids [119]. The most likely target of aPLs is the phospholipid-binding protein β2GPI [120]. Antibodies that bind β2GPI are of autoimmune nature and are associated with prothrombotic predisposition [119]. The term "antiphospholipid syndrome" covers the increased frequency of thrombotic events together with the presence of autoimmune-type aPLs [120, 121]. SLE is associated with antiphospholipid syndrome, and patients with SLE experience premature atherosclerosis [118].

Early atherosclerosis in either LDL-receptor deficient mice or apoE-deficient mice was enhanced by immunization with β2GPI with no change in their lipid profile [122, 123]. Moreover, β2GPI was found to be expressed in subendothelial regions of human atherosclerotic plaques [124], which led to the hypothesis that the immune response against β2GPI is involved in increasing the inflammation in the atherosclerotic plaques. Furthermore, it has been recently found that SLE patients, who develop atherosclerosis, display elevated levels of anti-oxLDL, anti-HSP65 and anti-β2GPI antibodies, which suggests a multifactorial role of autoimmune factors in atherogenesis [125]. However, the immune response against oxLDL seems protective, whereas the reaction against the protective proteins (HSP60 and β2GPI) appears pro-atherogenic.

In sum, the formation of atherosclerotic lesions involves initial endothelial dysfunction, chemokine production leading to expression of adhesion molecules by endothelial cells, and intimal infiltration by cells of the immune system, especially monocytes. These cells can collect lipids or modified lipoproteins mostly by their scavenger receptors. The lipids accumulate intracellularly as cholesterol esters and lead to the generation of foam cells characteristic of the fatty streak, which is one of the first noticeable changes of atherogenesis. However, most of the molecular mechanisms and signaling pathways involved in the development of these lesions are still unknown.

7. ATHEROSCLEROSIS INFLAMMATION AND MITOGENESIS

Inflammation plays a critical role in atherogenesis, yet the mediators linking inflammation to specific atherogenic processes remain to be elucidated. One such mediator may be secretory sphingomyelinase (S-SMase), a product of the acid sphingomyelinase gene.

The secretion of S-SMase by cultured endothelial cells is induced by inflammatory cytokines, and in vivo data have implicated S-SMase in subendothelial lipoprotein aggregation, macrophage foam cell formation, and possibly other atherogenic processes [126–128]. In addition, there is evidence for S-SMase regulation in vivo during a physiologically relevant inflammatory response. The data show regulation of S-SMase activity in vivo and raise the possibility that local stimulation of S-SMase may contribute to the effects of inflammatory cytokines in atherosclerosis [129].

Several groups have shown that SMC proliferation could be directly affected by oxLDL [16, 130–133]. This mitogenic effect is dependent on the generation of sphingolipids. Chatterjee et al [134–137] have shown that oxLDL-induced proliferation of SMC can be initiated by the production of lactosylceramide. Since ceramide can be converted to other bioactive metabolites, such as the mitogen sphingosine–1-phosphate (S-1-P) [138], it has been investigated whether additional sphingomyelin metabolites could be involved in the oxLDL-induced SMC proliferation. It has been shown that cellular sphingosine and S-1-P levels were increased upon incubation of rabbit SMC with oxLDL [139]. These findings suggest that S-1-P is a key mediator of the mitogenic effect of oxLDL on SMC. The mechanism of this effect is still unknown, but may involve calcium mobilization, activation of phospholipase D and generation of phosphatidic acid as a second messenger, and activation of the transcription factor AP-1 as most of these results have been observed when cells were exposed to either oxLDL or to S-1-P [140–143]. It is also possible that oxLDL activates growth factor receptors such as EGF receptor [144] in SMC or endothelial cells, and therefore it is likely that growth factor receptors also participate in the generation of S-1-P.

Whereas experimental data have clearly implicated ceramide in TNFα induced adhesion of blood cells to the endothelium [145, 146], or in oxidized LDL-induced SMC proliferation [17, 134] further studies are needed to identify the different pathways leading to the activation of the enzymes responsible for ceramide generation as well as the investigation of its localization and its mechanism of activation. In some instances, the identity of the sphingolipid involved in the signaling still remains to be determined [17, 134] .

8. ATHEROSCLEROSIS, CERAMIDE AND APOPTOSIS

Apoptosis has been recently shown to play a major role in modulating the generation of atherosclerotic lesions in vascular cells [96–98]. Exogenously added ceramides or intracellular SMase overexpression have been shown to induce apoptosis in various cell types of the vascular wall, including endothelial cells [66, 147–150], SMC [151] or macrophages [152]. Furthermore, ceramide can inhibit the Akt–activated cell surviving pathway in endothelial cells [149]. Therefore, it is believed that apoptotic agents induce their effect in vascular cells via ceramide generation as described in many other cell types [27, 31, 41, 151].

OxLDLs promote chronic inflammatory responses in the vasculature and give rise to atherosclerotic plaques [147]. We have provided evidence that oxLDL, but not native LDL, induced rapid increase in ceramide in mouse peritoneal macrophages [153]. The elevation of ceramide paralleled the induction of apoptosis. Elevation of ceramide with exogenous membrane-permeant ceramide analogs was sufficient for induction of apoptosis with the same characteristics and in the same time frame, suggesting that the formation of ceramide from sphingomyelin in the plasma membrane is a key event in oxLDL-induced apoptosis in peritoneal macrophages. In addition, ex-*vivo* studies showed that oxLDL, but not native LDL, increased ceramide levels in aortas of inbred C57BL/6J mice, while aortas from apoE-deficient mice did not respond with ceramide elevation to oxLDL. This could suggest that resistance to ceramide signaling in apoE-deficient tissues accompanied by diminished apoptosis might be linked to the enhanced development of atherosclerosis in these tissues.

We have also demonstrated that oxLDL, but not native LDL, induced rapid sphingomyelin hydrolysis to ceramide in endothelial cells. Moreover, both ceramide generation and apoptosis induction by oxLDL were inhibited by β2GPI, suggesting that the β2GPI contributes to the development of atherosclerosis by diminishing apoptosis [153]. Indeed, β2GPI, a highly glycosylated plasma protein that binds to negatively charged phospholipids and acts as a major antigenic target for autoimmune type antiphospholipid antibodies [122, 124, 154, 155], has been recently suggested by George et al [156] to enhance atherosclerosis in apoE-deficient mice.

OxLDLs induce an early activation of the ceramide pathway in human endothelial cells [66, 147, 157, 158]. However, when data originated in different studies are compared, the implication of ceramide generation in the oxLDL-induced apoptotic response is inconsistent. Harada-Shiba et al showed that oxLDL-induced apoptosis involved superoxide dismutase activation, which led to the downstream activation of caspase 1 and caspase 3 [147]. In addition, these investigators observed that inhibition of aSMase blocked both ceramide generation and apoptosis induced by oxLDL [147]. In contrast, Escargueil-Blanc et al showed that the activation of nSMase and ceramide pathway by oxLDL can be inhibited with no observed effect on the apoptosis induced by oxLDL [66].

9. FUTURE DIRECTIONS

The variety of the cellular changes observed during atherogenesis is related not only to the combination of various cellular events, which involve both vascular cells and circulating blood cells, but is also due to differences in the ability of distinctive cell types to modulate sphingolipid-regulated pathways.

The studies on cellular signaling in vascular cells are very recent, and it is very likely that similar sphingolipid signaling pathways are activated in vascular cells as in other cell types, such as lymphoid cell lines or fibroblasts. This is demonstrated by the MAPK activation in S-1-P-induced proliferation of SMC or 3T3 fibroblasts [17, 140, 159, 160], or the activation of caspases during ceramide-induced apoptosis of endothelial cells [27, 31, 39, 147].

The overall SM turnover in mammalian cells is modulated by different SM-cleaving enzymes situated in separate subcellular compartments. However, it is still unknown whether one SMase or more than one and which SMase is involved in cell signaling [41, 161–163]. Whereas the contribution of the lysosomal aSMase is controversial [163], other SMases wait for their purification and cloning to make possible animal studies with targeted interruption of the genes encoding theses enzymes.

Demonstrating the characteristics of the signaling SMase(s) and their regulatory mechanism(s) will be an essential milestone in understanding the routes that involve sphingolipids. In addition, the problem of the topology of the generation of SM-derived signaling products waits to be addressed. The importance of SMase(s) in signaling is underscored by the fact that not only ceramide acts as a second messenger but also other sphingolipids [28, 158, 164, 165]. Activation of SMase may thus serve as the initial point of a cascade that leads to the generation of bioactive lipids such as sphingosine, S-1-P and ceramide-1-phosphate. Resolving these matters will offer essential information to the pathobiology of animal and human diseases.

When the genes of the sphingolipid modulating enzymes become available, these issues will be addressed through in-vivo studies with knockout animals. This is yet to lead to the development of drugs containing the sphingolipid backbone aiming to affect diseases with undesired cell activation and apoptosis such as atherogenesis and atherosclerosis.

REFERENCES

1. Goldkorn T, Dressler KA, Muindi J, Radin NS, Mendelsohn J, Menaldino D, Liotta D, and Kolesnick RN. Ceramide stimulates epidermal growth factor receptor phosphorylation in A431 human epidermoid carcinoma cells. Evidence that ceramide may mediate sphingosine action. J Biol Chem 1991;266(24):16092–7.

2. Schutze S, Potthoff K, Machleidt T, Berkovic D, Wiegmann K, and Kronke M. TNF activates NF-kappa B by phosphatidylcholine-specific phospholipase C-induced "acidic" sphingomyelin breakdown. Cell 1992;71(5):765–76.

3. Dressler KA, Mathias S, and Kolesnick RN. Tumor necrosis factor-alpha activates the sphingomyelin signal transduction pathway in a cell-free system. Science 1992;255(5052):1715–8.

4. Dbaibo GS, Obeid LM, and Hannun YA. Tumor necrosis factor-alpha (TNF-alpha) signal transduction through ceramide. Dissociation of growth inhibitory effects of TNF-alpha from activation of nuclear factor-kappa B. J Biol Chem 1993;268(24):17762–6.

5. Wiegmann K, Schutze S, Machleidt T, Witte D, and Kronke, M. Functional dichotomy of neutral and acidic sphingomyelinases in tumor necrosis factor signaling. Cell 1994;78(6):1005–15.

6. Ballou LR, Chao CP, Holness MA, Barker SC, and Raghow R. Interleukin-1-mediated PGE2 production and sphingomyelin metabolism. Evidence for the regulation of cyclooxygenase gene expression by sphingosine and ceramide. J Biol Chem 1992;267(28):20044–50.

7. Mathias S, Younes A, Kan CC, Orlow I, Joseph C, and Kolesnick RN. Activation of the sphingomyelin signaling pathway in intact EL4 cells and in a cell-free system

by IL-1 beta. Science 1993;259(5094):519–22.

8. Kim MY, Linardic C, Obeid L, and Hannun Y. Identification of sphingomyelin turnover as an effector mechanism for the action of tumor necrosis factor alpha and gamma-interferon. Specific role in cell differentiation. J Biol Chem 1991;266(1):484–9.

9. Okazaki T, Bell RM, and Hannun YA. Sphingomyelin turnover induced by vitamin D3 in HL-60 cells. Role in cell differentiation. J Biol Chem 1989;264(32):19076–80.

10. Dobrowsky RT, Werner MH, Castellino AM, Chao MV, and Hannun YA. Activation of the sphingomyelin cycle through the low-affinity neurotrophin receptor. Science 1994;265(5178):1596–9.

11. Boucher LM, Wiegmann K, Futterer A, Pfeffer K, Machleidt T, Schutze S, Mak TW, and Kronke M. CD28 signals through acidic sphingomyelinase. J Exp Med 1995;181(6):2059–68.

12. Chan G, and Ochi A. Sphingomyelin-ceramide turnover in CD28 costimulatory signaling. Eur J Immunol 1995;25(7):1999–2004.

13. Segui B, Andrieu-Abadie N, Adam-Klages S, Meilhac O, Kreder D, Garcia V, Bruno AP, Jaffrezou JP, Salvayre R, Kronke M, and Levade T. CD40 signals apoptosis through FAN-regulated activation of the sphingomyelin-ceramide pathway. J Biol Chem 1999;274(52):37251–8.

14. Cifone MG, De Maria R, Roncaioli P, Rippo MR, Azuma M, Lanier LL, Santoni A, and Testi R. Apoptotic signaling through CD95 (Fas/Apo-1) activates an acidic sphingomyelinase. J Exp Med 1994;180(4):1547–52.

15. Tepper CG, Jayadev S, Liu B, Bielawska A, Wolff R, Yonehara S, Hannun YA, and Seldin MF. Role for ceramide as an endogenous mediator of Fas-induced cytotoxicity. Proc Natl Acad Sci USA 1995;92(18):8443–7.

16. Auge N, Andrieu N, Negre-Salvayre A, Thiers JC, Levade T, and Salvayre R. The sphingomyelin-ceramide signaling pathway is involved in oxidized low density lipoprotein-induced cell proliferation. J Biol Chem 1996;271(32):19251–5.

17. Auge N, Escargueil-Blanc I, Lajoie-Mazenc I, Suc I, Andrieu-Abadie N, Pieraggi MT, Chatelut M, Thiers,JC, Jaffrezou JP, Laurent G, Levade T, Negre-Salvayre,A, and Salvayre R. Potential role for ceramide in mitogen-activated protein kinase activation and proliferation of vascular smooth muscle cells induced by oxidized low density lipoprotein. J Biol Chem 1998;273(21):12893–900.

18. Jaffrezou JP, Maestre N, de Mas-Mansat V, Bezombes C, Levade T, and Laurent G. Positive feedback control of neutral sphingomyelinase activity by ceramide. Faseb J 1998;12(11):999–1006.

19. Hannun YA, Loomis CR, Merrill AH Jr., and Bell RM.

20. Okazaki T, Bielawska A, Domae N, Bell RM, and Hannun YA. Characteristics and partial purification of a novel cytosolic, magnesium-independent, neutral sphingomyelinase activated in the early signal transduction of 1 alpha,25-dihydroxyvitamin D3-induced HL-60 cell differentiation [published erratum appears in J Biol Chem 1994 Jun 10;269(23):16518]. J Biol Chem 1994;269(6):4070–7.

Sphingosine inhibition of protein kinase C activity and of phorbol dibutyrate binding in vitro and in human platelets. J Biol Chem 1986;261(27):12604–9.

21. Kolesnick RN, Goni FM, and Alonso A. Compartmentalization of ceramide signaling: physical foundations and biological effects. J Cell Physiol 2000;184(3):285–300.

22. Segui B, Bezombes C, Uro-Coste E, Medin JA, Andrieu-Abadie N, Auge N, Brouchet A, Laurent G, Salvayre R, Jaffrezou JP, and Levade T. Stress-induced apoptosis is not mediated by endolysosomal ceramide. Faseb J 2000;14(1):36–47.

23. Andrieu-Abadie N, Carpentier S, Salvayre R, and Levade T. The tumour necrosis factor-sensitive pool of sphingomyelin is resynthesized in a distinct compartment of the plasma membrane. Biochem J 1998;333(Pt 1):91–7.

24. Obeid LM, and Hannun YA. Ceramide: a stress signal and mediator of growth suppression and apoptosis. J Cell Biochem 1995;58(2):191–8.

25. Mathias S, Pena LA, and Kolesnick RN. Signal transduction of stress via ceramide. Biochem J 1998;335(Pt 3):465–80.

26. Perry DK, and Hannun YA. The role of ceramide in cell signaling. Biochim Biophys Acta 1998;1436(1–2):233–43.

27. Hannun YA. Functions of ceramide in coordinating cellular responses to stress. Science 1996;274(5294):1855–9.

28. Spiegel S, and Merrill AH Jr.. Sphingolipid metabolism and cell growth regulation. Faseb J 1996;10(12):1388–97.

29. Testi R. Sphingomyelin breakdown and cell fate. Trends Biochem Sci 1996;21(12):468–71.

30. Ballou LR, Laulederkind SJ, Rosloniec EF, and Raghow R. Ceramide signalling and the immune response. Biochim Biophys Acta 1996;1301(3):273–87.

31. Kolesnick RN, and Kronke M. Regulation of ceramide production and apoptosis. Annu Rev Physiol 1998;60643–65.

32. Obeid LM, Linardic CM, Karolak LA, and Hannun YA. Programmed cell death induced by ceramide. Science 1993;259(5102):1769–71.

33. Hannun YA, and Obeid LM. Ceramide: an intracellular signal for apoptosis. Trends Biochem Sci

1995;20(2):73–7.

34. Haimovitz-Friedman A, Kolesnick RN, and Fuks Z. Ceramide signaling in apoptosis. Br Med Bull 1997;53(3):539–53.

35. Burow ME, Weldon CB, Collins-Burow BM, Ramsey N, McKee A, Klippel A, McLachlan JA, Clejan S, and Beckman BS. Cross-talk between phosphatidylinositol 3-kinase and sphingomyelinase pathways as a mechanism for cell survival/death decisions. J Biol Chem 2000;275(13):9628–35.

36. Olivera A, Buckley NE, and Spiegel S. Sphingomyelinase and cell-permeable ceramide analogs stimulate cellular proliferation in quiescent Swiss 3T3 fibroblasts. J Biol Chem 1992;267(36):26121–7.

37. Bielawska A, Linardic CM, and Hannun YA. Modulation of cell growth and differentiation by ceramide. FEBS Lett 1992;307(2):211–4.

38. Spiegel S, Foster D, and Kolesnick R. Signal transduction through lipid second messengers. Curr Opin Cell Biol 1996;8(2):159–67.

39. Luberto C, and Hannun YA. Sphingolipid metabolism in the regulation of bioactive molecules. Lipids 1999;34(Suppl): S5–11.

40. Kolesnick R, and Hannun YA. Ceramide and apoptosis. Trends Biochem Sci 1999;24(6):224–5; discussion 227.

41. Levade T, and Jaffrezou JP. Signalling sphingomyelinases: which, where, how and why? Biochim Biophys Acta 1999;1438(1):1–17.

42. Auge N, Negre-Salvayre A, Salvayre R, and Levade T. Sphingomyelin metabolites in vascular cell signaling and atherogenesis. Prog Lipid Res 2000;39(3):207–29.

43. Chatterjee S. Sphingolipids in atherosclerosis and vascular biology. Arterioscler Thromb Vasc Biol 1998;18(10):1523–33.

44. Ashkenazi A, and Dixit VM. Death receptors: signaling and modulation. Science 1998;281(5381):1305–8.

45. Green DR. Apoptotic pathways: the roads to ruin. Cell 1998;94(6):695–8.

46. Borner C, Monney L, Olivier R, Rosse T, Hacki J, and Conus, S. Life and death in a medieval atmosphere. Cell Death Differ 1999;6(2):201–6.

47. Adam D, Wiegmann K, Adam-Klages S, Ruff A, and Kronke M. A novel cytoplasmic domain of the p55 tumor necrosis factor receptor initiates the neutral sphingomyelinase pathway. J Biol Chem 1996;271(24):14617–22.

48. Adam-Klages S, Adam D, Wiegmann K, Struve S, Kolanus W, Schneider-Mergener J, and Kronke M. FAN, a novel WD-repeat protein, couples the p55 TNF-receptor to neutral sphingomyelinase. Cell 1996;86(6):937–47.

49. Schwandner, R, Wiegmann, K, Bernardo, K, Kreder, D, and Kronke, M. TNF receptor death domain-associated proteins TRADD and FADD signal activation of acid sphingomyelinase. J Biol Chem 1998;273(10):5916–22.

50. Wiegmann K, Schwandner R, Krut O, Yeh WC, Mak TW, and Kronke M. Requirement of FADD for tumor necrosis factor-induced activation of acid sphingomyelinase. J Biol Chem 1999;274(9):5267–70.

51. Chinnaiyan AM, Tepper CG, Seldin MF, O'Rourke K, Kischkel FC, Hellbardt S, Krammer PH, Peter ME, and Dixit VM. FADD/MORT1 is a common mediator of CD95 (Fas/APO-1) and tumor necrosis factor receptor-induced apoptosis. J Biol Chem 1996;271(9):4961–5.

52. Adam-Klages S, Schwandner R, Adam D, Kreder D, Bernardo K, and Kronke M. Distinct adapter proteins mediate acid versus neutral sphingomyelinase activation through the p55 receptor for tumor necrosis factor. J Leukoc Biol 1998;63(6):678–82.

53. De Nadai C, Sestili P, Cantoni O, Lievremont JP, Sciorati C, Barsacchi R, Moncada S, Meldolesi J, and Clementi E. Nitric oxide inhibits tumor necrosis factor-alpha-induced apoptosis by reducing the generation of ceramide. Proc Natl Acad Sci USA 2000;97(10):5480–5.

54. Wolf BB, and Green DR. Suicidal tendencies: apoptotic cell death by caspase family proteinases. J Biol Chem 1999;274(29):20049–52.

55. Yoshimura S, Banno Y, Nakashima S, Takenaka K, Sakai H, Nishimura Y, Sakai N, Shimizu S, Eguchi Y, Tsujimoto Y, and Nozawa Y. Ceramide formation leads to caspase-3 activation during hypoxic PC12 cell death. Inhibitory effects of Bcl-2 on ceramide formation and caspase-3 activation. J Biol Chem 1998;273(12):6921–7.

56. Smyth MJ, Perry DK, Zhang J, Poirier GG, Hannun YA, and Obeid LM. prICE: a downstream target for ceramide-induced apoptosis and for the inhibitory action of Bcl-2. Biochem J 1996;316(Pt 1):25–8.

57. Tepper AD, Cock JG, de Vries E, Borst J, and van Blitterswijk WJ. CD95/Fas-induced ceramide formation proceeds with slow kinetics and is not blocked by caspase-3/CPP32 inhibition. J Biol Chem 1997;272(39):24308–12.

58. Cuvillier O, Rosenthal DS, Smulson ME, and Spiegel S. Sphingosine 1-phosphate inhibits activation of caspases that cleave poly(ADP-ribose) polymerase and lamins during Fas- and ceramide- mediated apoptosis in Jurkat T lymphocytes. J Biol Chem 1998;273(5):2910–6.

59. Laethem RM, Hannun YA, Jayadev S, Sexton CJ, Strum JC, Sundseth R, and Smith GK. Increases in neutral, Mg2+-dependent and acidic, Mg2+-independent sphingomyelinase activities precede commitment to apoptosis and are not a consequence of caspase 3-like activity in Molt-4 cells in response to thymidylate synthase inhibition by GW1843. Blood 1998;91(11):4350–60.

60. Gamard, CJ, Dbaibo, GS, Liu, B, Obeid, LM, and Hannun, YA. Selective involvement of ceramide in

cytokine-induced apoptosis. Ceramide inhibits phorbol ester activation of nuclear factor kappaB. J Biol Chem 1997;272(26):16474–81.

61. Dbaibo GS, Perry DK, Gamard CJ, Platt R, Poirier GG, Obeid LM, and Hannun YA. Cytokine response modifier A (CrmA) inhibits ceramide formation in response to tumor necrosis factor (TNF)-alpha: CrmA and Bcl-2 target distinct components in the apoptotic pathway. J Exp Med 1997;185(3):481–90.

62. Hannun YA, and Luberto C. Ceramide in the eukaryotic stress response. Trends Cell Biol 2000;10(2):73–80.

63. Monney L, Olivier R, Otter I, Jansen B, Poirier GG, and Borner C. Role of an acidic compartment in tumor-necrosis-factor-alpha-induced production of ceramide, activation of caspase-3 and apoptosis. Eur J Biochem 1998;251(1–2):295–303.

64. Genestier L, Prigent AF, Paillot R, Quemeneur L, Durand I, Banchereau J, Revillard JP, and Bonnefoy-Berard N. Caspase-dependent ceramide production in Fas- and HLA class I-mediated peripheral T cell apoptosis. J Biol Chem 1998;273(9):5060–6.

65. Takeda Y, Tashima M, Takahashi A, Uchiyama T, Okazaki T. Ceramide generation in nitric oxide-induced apoptosis. Activation of magnesium dependent neutral sphingomyelinase via caspase-3. J Biol Chem. 1999;274(15):10654–60.

66. Escargueil-Blanc I, Andrieu-Abadie N, Caspar-Bauguil S, Brossmer R, Levade T, Negre-Salvayre A, and Salvayre R. Apoptosis and activation of the sphingomyelin-ceramide pathway induced by oxidized low density lipoproteins are not causally related in ECV- 304 endothelial cells. J Biol Chem 1998;273(42):27389–95.

67. Mansat V, Bettaieb A, Levade T, Laurent G, and Jaffrezou JP. Serine protease inhibitors block neutral sphingomyelinase activation, ceramide generation, and apoptosis triggered by daunorubicin. Faseb J 1997;11(8):695–702.

68. Machleidt T, Wiegmann K, Henkel T, Schutze S, Baeuerle P, and Kronke M. Sphingomyelinase activates proteolytic I kappa B-alpha degradation in a cell-free system. J Biol Chem 1994;269(19):13760–5.

69. Pronk GJ, Ramer K, Amiri P, and Williams LT. Requirement of an ICE-like protease for induction of apoptosis and ceramide generation by REAPER. Science 1996;271(5250):808–10.

70. Bose R, Chen P, Loconti A, Grullich C, Abrams JM, and Kolesnick RN. Ceramide generation by the Reaper protein is not blocked by the caspase inhibitor, p35. J Biol Chem 1998;273(44):28852–9.

71. Kluck RM, Bossy-Wetzel E, Green DR, and Newmeyer DD. The release of cytochrome c from mitochondria: a primary site for Bcl-2 regulation of apoptosis [see comments]. Science 1997;275(5303):1132–6.

72. Tepper,AD, de Vries E, van Blitterswijk WJ, and Borst J. Ordering of ceramide formation, caspase activation, and mitochondrial changes during CD95- and DNA damage-induced apoptosis [published erratum appears in J Clin Invest 1999 May;103(9):1363]. J Clin Invest 1999;103(7):971–8.

73. Allouche M, Bettaieb A, Vindis C, Rousse A, Grignon C, and Laurent G. Influence of Bcl-2 overexpression on the ceramide pathway in daunorubicin-induced apoptosis of leukemic cells. Oncogene 1997;14(15):1837–45.

74. Fang W, Rivard JJ, Ganser JA, LeBien TW, Nath KA, Mueller DL, and Behrens TW. Bcl-xL rescues WEHI 231 B lymphocytes from oxidant-mediated death following diverse apoptotic stimuli. J Immunol 1995;155(1):66–75.

75. Karsan A, Yee E, and Harlan JM. Endothelial cell death induced by tumor necrosis factor-alpha is inhibited by the Bcl-2 family member, A1. J Biol Chem 1996;271(44):27201–4.

76. Geley S, Hartmann BL, and Kofler Rc. Ceramides induce a form of apoptosis in human acute lymphoblastic leukemia cells that is inhibited by Bcl-2, but not by CrmA. FEBS Lett 1996;400(1):15–8.

77. El-Assaad W, El-Sabban M, Awaraji C, Abboushi N, and Dbaibo GS. Distinct sites of action of Bcl-2 and Bcl-xL in the ceramide pathway of apoptosis. Biochem J 1998;336(Pt 3):735–41.

78. Wiesner DA, Kilkus JP, Gottschalk AR, Quintans J, and Dawson G. Anti-immunoglobulin-induced apoptosis in WEHI 231 cells involves the slow formation of ceramide from sphingomyelin and is blocked by bcl-XL. J Biol Chem 1997;272(15):9868–76.

79. Jarvis WD, Turner AJ, Povirk LF, Traylor RS, and Grant S. Induction of apoptotic DNA fragmentation and cell death in HL-60 human promyelocytic leukemia cells by pharmacological inhibitors of protein kinase C. Cancer Res 1994;54(7):1707–14.

80. Chan C, and Goldkorn T. Ceramide path in human lung cell death. Am J Respir Cell Mol Biol 2000;22(4):460–8.

81. Goldkorn T, Balaban N, Shannon M, Chea V, Matsukuma K, Gilchrist D, Wang H, and Chan C. H2O2 acts on cellular membranes to generate ceramide signaling and initiate apoptosis in tracheobronchial epithelial cells. J Cell Sci 1998;111(Pt 21):3209–20.

82. Chmura SJ, Nodzenski E, Weichselbaum RR, and Quintans J. Protein kinase C inhibition induces apoptosis and ceramide production through activation of a neutral sphingomyelinase. Cancer Res 1996;56(12):2711–4.

83. Chmura SJ, Mauceri HJ, Advani S, Heimann R, Beckett MA, Nodzenski E, Quintans J, Kufe DW, and Weichselbaum RR. Decreasing the apoptotic threshold of tumor cells through protein kinase C inhibition and sphingo-

myelinase activation increases tumor killing by ionizing radiation. Cancer Res 1997; 57(19):4340–7.

84. Lavrentiadou S, Chan C, Rasooly R, van der Vliet A, Kawcak T, and Goldkorn T. Ceramide path in lung epithelial cell is regulated by glutathione. 2000;submitted.

85. Goldkorn T, Lavrentiadou S, Chan C, Rassooly R, van der Vliet A, and Kawcak T. Glutathione regulation of ceramide pathway in lung epithelial cells. Am. J. Respir. Crit. Care Medicine 2000;161(3): A242.

86. Liu B, and Hannun YA. Inhibition of the neutral magnesium-dependent sphingomyelinase by glutathione. J Biol Chem 1997;272(26):16281–7.

87. Singh I, Pahan K, Khan M, and Singh AK. Cytokine-mediated induction of ceramide production is redox-sensitive. Implications to proinflammatory cytokine-mediated apoptosis in demyelinating diseases. J Biol Chem 1998;273(32):20354–62.

88. Furuke K, and Bloom ET. Redox-sensitive events in Fas-induced apoptosis in human NK cells include ceramide generation and protein tyrosine dephosphorylation. Int Immunol 1998;10(9):1261–72.

89. Mizushima N, Kohsaka H, and Miyasaka N. Ceramide, a mediator of interleukin 1, tumour necrosis factor alpha, as well as Fas receptor signalling, induces apoptosis of rheumatoid arthritis synovial cells. Ann Rheum Dis 1998;57(8):495–9.

90. Hayashida K, Shimaoka Y, Ochi T, and Lipsky PE. Rheumatoid arthritis synovial stromal cells inhibit apoptosis and up- regulate Bcl-xL expression by B cells in a CD49/CD29-CD106-dependent mechanism. J Immunol 2000;164(2):1110–6.

91. Ichinose Y, Eguchi K, Migita K, Kawabe Y, Tsukada T, Koji T, Abe K, Aoyagi T, Nakamura H, and Nagataki S. Apoptosis induction in synovial fibroblasts by ceramide: in vitro and in vivo effects. J Lab Clin Med 1998;131(5):410–6.

92. Miret C, Font J, Molina R, Garcia-Carrasco M, Filella X, Ramos M, Cervera R, Ballesta A, and Ingelmo M. Bcl-2 oncogene (B cell lymphoma/leukemia-2) levels correlate with systemic lupus erythematosus disease activity. Anticancer Res 1999;19(4B):3073–6.

93. Caricchio R, and Cohen PL. Spontaneous and induced apoptosis in systemic lupus erythematosus: multiple assays fail to reveal consistent abnormalities. Cell Immunol 1999;198(1):54–60.

94. Salmon M, and Gordon C. The role of apoptosis in systemic lupus erythematosus. Rheumatology (Oxford) 1999;38(12):1177–83.

95. Sakata K, Sakata A, Vela-Roch N, Espinosa R, Escalante A, Kong L, Nakabayashi T, Cheng J, Talal N, and Dang H. Fas (CD95)-transduced signal preferentially stimulates lupus peripheral T lymphocytes. Eur J Immunol 1998;28(9):2648–60.

96. Stehbens WE. The significance of programmed cell death or apoptosis and matrix vesicles in atherogenesis. Cell Mol Biol (Noisy-le-grand) 2000;46(1):99–110.

97. Kockx MM, and Herman AG. Apoptosis in atherosclerosis: beneficial or detrimental? Cardiovasc Res 2000;45(3):736–46.

98. Kockx MM, and Knaapen MW. The role of apoptosis in vascular disease. J Pathol 2000;190(3):267–80.

99. DiMango E, Ratner AJ, Bryan R, Tabibi S, and Prince,A. Activation of NF-kappaB by adherent Pseudomonas aeruginosa in normal and cystic fibrosis respiratory epithelial cells. J Clin Invest 1998;101(11):2598–605.

100. Jayaraman S, Castro M, O'Sullivan M, Bragdon MJ, and Holtzman MJ. Resistance to Fas-mediated T cell apoptosis in asthma. J Immunol 1999;162(3):1717–22.

101. Ross R. Atherosclerosis--an inflammatory disease [see comments]. N Engl J Med 1999;340(2):115–26.

102. Libby P, and Hansson GKc. Involvement of the immune system in human atherogenesis: current knowledge and unanswered questions. Lab Invest 1999;64(1):5–15.

103. Wick G, Schett G, Amberger A, Kleindienst R, and Xu Q. Is atherosclerosis an immunologically mediated disease? Immunol Today 1995;16(1):27–33.

104. George J, Harats D, Gilburd B, and Shoenfeld Y. Emerging cross-regulatory roles of immunity and autoimmunity in atherosclerosis. Immunol Res 1996;15(4):315–22.

105. Plump AS, Smith JD, Hayek T, Aalto-Setala K, Walsh A, Verstuyft JG, Rubin EM, and Breslow JL. Severe hypercholesterolemia and atherosclerosis in apolipoprotein E- deficient mice created by homologous recombination in ES cells. Cell 1992;71(2):343–53.

106. Zhang SH, Reddick RL, Piedrahita JA, and Maeda N. Spontaneous hypercholesterolemia and arterial lesions in mice lacking apolipoprotein E. Science 1992;258(5081):468–71.

107. Ishibashi S, Brown MS, Goldstein JL, Gerard RD, Hammer RE, and Herz J. Hypercholesterolemia in low density lipoprotein receptor knockout mice and its reversal by adenovirus-mediated gene delivery [see comments]. J Clin Invest 1993;92(2):883–93.

108. Xu Q, Dietrich H, Steiner HJ, Gown AM, Schoel B, Mikuz G, Kaufmann SH, and Wick G. Induction of arteriosclerosis in normocholesterolemic rabbits by immunization with heat shock protein 65. Arterioscler Thromb 1992;12(7):789–99.

109. George J, Shoenfeld Y, Afek A, Gilburd B, Keren P, Shaish A, Kopolovic J, Wick G, and Harats D. Enhanced fatty streak formation in C57BL/6J mice by immunization with heat shock protein-65. Arterioscler Thromb Vasc Biol 1999;19(3):505–10.

110. Witztum\ JL, and Steinberg D. Role of oxidized low density lipoprotein in atherogenesis. J Clin Invest

1991;88(6):1785–92.

111. Palinski W, Miller E, and Witztum JL. Immunization of low density lipoprotein (LDL) receptor-deficient rabbits with homologous malondialdehyde-modified LDL reduces atherogenesis. Proc Natl Acad Sci USA 1995;92(3):821–5.

112. George J, Afek A, Gilburd B, Levkovitz H, Shaish A, Goldberg I, Kopolovic Y, Wick G, Shoenfeld Y, and Harats D. Hyperimmunization of apo-E-deficient mice with homologous malondialdehyde low-density lipoprotein suppresses early atherogenesis. Atherosclerosis 1998;138(1):147–52.

113. Freigang S, Horkko S, Miller E, Witztum JL, and Palinski W. Immunization of LDL receptor-deficient mice with homologous malondialdehyde-modified and native LDL reduces progression of atherosclerosis by mechanisms other than induction of high titers of antibodies to oxidative neoepitopes. Arterioscler Thromb Vasc Biol 1998;18(12):1972–82.

114. Salonen JT, Yla-Herttuala S, Yamamoto R, Butler S, Korpela H, Salonen R, Nyyssonen K, Palinski W, and Witztum JL. Autoantibody against oxidised LDL and progression of carotid atherosclerosis [see comments]. Lancet 1992;339(8798):883–7.

115. Bergmark C, Wu R, de Faire U, Lefvert AK, and Swedenborg J. Patients with early-onset peripheral vascular disease have increased levels of autoantibodies against oxidized LDL. Arterioscler Thromb Vasc Biol 1995;15(4):441–5.

116. Puurunen M, Manttari M, Manninen V, Tenkanen L, Alfthan G, Ehnholm C, Vaarala O, Aho K, and Palosuo T. Antibody against oxidized low-density lipoprotein predicting myocardial infarction [published erratum appears in Arch Intern Med 1995;155(8):817]. Arch Intern Med 1994;154(22):2605–9.

117. George J, Harats D, Bakshi E, Adler Y, Levy Y, Gilburd B, and Shoenfeld Y. Anti-oxidized low density lipoprotein antibody determination as a predictor of restenosis following percutaneous transluminal coronary angioplasty. Immunol Lett 1999;68(2–3):263–6.

118. George J, and Shoenfeld Y. The anti-phospholipid (Hughes) syndrome: a crossroads of autoimmunity and atherosclerosis [editorial]. Lupus 1997;6(7):559–60.

119. Matsuura E, Igarashi Y, Fujimoto M, Ichikawa K, Suzuki T, Sumida T, Yasuda T, and Koike T. Heterogeneity of anticardiolipin antibodies defined by the anticardiolipin cofactor. J Immunol 1992;148(12):3885–91.

120. Shoenfeld Y, Gharavi A, and Koike,T. Beta2GP-I in the anti phospholipid (Hughes') syndrome--from a cofactor to an autoantigen--from induction to prevention of antiphospholipid syndrome. Lupus 1998;7(8):503–6.

121. Hughes GR. The antiphospholipid syndrome: ten years on [see comments]. Lancet 1993;342(8867):341–4.

122. George J, Afek A, Gilburd B, Blank M, Levy Y, Aron-Maor A, Levkovitz H, Shaish A, Goldberg I, Kopolovic J, Harats D, and Shoenfeld Y. Induction of early atherosclerosis in LDL-receptor-deficient mice immunized with beta2-glycoprotein I. Circulation 1998;98(11):1108–15.

123. Afek A, George J, Shoenfeld Y, Gilburd B, Levy Y, Shaish A, Keren P, Janackovic Z, Goldberg I, Kopolovic J, and Harats D. Enhancement of atherosclerosis in beta-2-glycoprotein I-immunized apolipoprotein E-deficient mice. Pathobiology 1999;67(1):19–25.

124. George J, Harats D, Gilburd B, Afek A, Levy Y, Schneiderman J, Barshack I, Kopolovic J, and Shoenfeld Y. Immunolocalization of beta2-glycoprotein I (apolipoprotein H) to human atherosclerotic plaques: potential implications for lesion progression. Circulation 1999;99(17):2227–30.

125. George J, Harats D, Gilburd B, Levy Y, Langevitz P, and Shoenfeld Y. Atherosclerosis-related markers in systemic lupus erythematosus patients: the role of humoral immunity in enhanced atherogenesis. Lupus 1999;8(3):220–6.

126. Marathe S, Kuriakose G, Williams KJ, and Tabas I. Sphingomyelinase, an enzyme implicated in atherogenesis, is present in atherosclerotic lesions and binds to specific components of the subendothelial extracellular matrix. Arterioscler Thromb Vasc Biol 1999;19(11):2648–58.

127. Schissel SL, Keesler GA, Schuchman EH, Williams KJ, and Tabas I. The cellular trafficking and zinc dependence of secretory and lysosomal sphingomyelinase, two products of the acid sphingomyelinase gene. J Biol Chem 1998;273(29):18250–9.

128. Marathe S, Schissel SL, Yellin MJ, Beatini N, Mintzer,R, Williams KJ, and Tabas I. Human vascular endothelial cells are a rich and regulatable source of secretory sphingomyelinase. Implications for early atherogenesis and ceramide-mediated cell signaling. J Biol Chem 1998;273(7):4081–8.

129. Wong ML, Xie B, Beatini N, Phu P, Marathe S, Johns,A, Gold PW, Hirsch E, Williams KJ, Licinio J, and Tabas I. Acute systemic inflammation up-regulates secretory sphingomyelinase in vivo: A possible link between inflammatory cytokines and atherogenesis [In Process Citation]. Proc Natl Acad Sci USA 2000;97(15):8681–6.

130. Chatterjee S. Role of oxidized human plasma low density lipoproteins in atherosclerosis: effects on smooth muscle cell proliferation. Mol Cell Biochem 1992;111(1–2):143–7.

131. Auge N, Pieraggi MT, Thiers JC, Negre-Salvayre A, and Salvayre R. Proliferative and cytotoxic effects of mildly oxidized low-density lipoproteins on vascular smooth-

muscle cells. Biochem J 1995;309(Pt 3):1015–20.

132. Chatterjee S, and Ghosh N. Oxidized low density lipoprotein stimulates aortic smooth muscle cell proliferation. Glycobiology 1996;6(3):303–11.

133. Balagopalakrishna C, Bhunia AK, Rifkind JM, and Chatterjee S. Minimally modified low density lipoproteins induce aortic smooth muscle cell proliferation via the activation of mitogen activated protein kinase. Mol Cell Biochem 1997;170(1–2):85–9.

134. Chatterjee S, Bhunia AK, Snowden A, and Han H. Oxidized low density lipoproteins stimulate galactosyltransferase activity, ras activation, p44 mitogen activated protein kinase and c- fos expression in aortic smooth muscle cells. Glycobiology 1997;7(5):703–10.

135. Chatterjee S. Lactosylceramide stimulates aortic smooth muscle cell proliferation. Biochem Biophys Res Commun 1991;181(2):554–61.

136. Bhunia AK, Han H, Snowden A, and Chatterjee S. Lactosylceramide stimulates Ras-GTP loading, kinases (MEK, Raf), p44 mitogen-activated protein kinase, and c-fos expression in human aortic smooth muscle cells. J Biol Chem 1996;271(18):10660–6.

137. Bhunia AK, Han H, Snowden A, and Chatterjee S. Redox-regulated signaling by lactosylceramide in the proliferation of human aortic smooth muscle cells. J Biol Chem 1997;272(25):15642–9.

138. Zhang H, Desai NN, Olivera A, Seki T, Brooker G, and Spiegel S. Sphingosine-1-phosphate, a novel lipid, involved in cellular proliferation. J Cell Biol 1991;114(1):155–67.

139. Auge N, Nikolova-Karakashian M, Carpentier S, Parthasarathy S, Negre-Salvayre A, Salvayre R, Merrill AH Jr., and Levade T. Role of sphingosine 1-phosphate in the mitogenesis induced by oxidized low density lipoprotein in smooth muscle cells via activation of sphingomyelinase, ceramidase, and sphingosine kinase. J Biol Chem 1999;274(31):21533–8.

140. Spiegel S, Cuvillier O, Edsall LC, Kohama T, Menzeleev R, Olah Z, Olivera A, Pirianov G, Thomas DM, Tu Z, Van Brocklyn JR, and Wang F. Sphingosine-1-phosphate in cell growth and cell death. Ann N Y Acad Sci 1998;84511–8.

141. Spiegel S. Sphingosine 1-phosphate: a prototype of a new class of second messengers. J Leukoc Biol 1999;65(3):341–4.

142. Parthasarathy S, Santanam N, and Auge N. Oxidized low-density lipoprotein, a two-faced Janus in coronary artery disease? Biochem Pharmacol 1998;56(3):279–84.

143. Parthasarathy S, and Santanam N. Mechanisms of oxidation, antioxidants, and atherosclerosis. Curr Opin Lipidol 1994;5(5):371–5.

144. Suc I, Meilhac O, Lajoie-Mazenc I, Vandaele J, Jurgens G, Salvayre R, and Negre-Salvayre A. Activation of EGF

receptor by oxidized LDL. Faseb J 1998;12(9):665–71.

145. Bhunia AK, Arai T, Bulkley G, and Chatterjee S. Lactosylceramide mediates tumor necrosis factor-alpha-induced intercellular adhesion molecule-1 (ICAM-1) expression and the adhesion of neutrophil in human umbilical vein endothelial cells. J Biol Chem 1998;273(51):34349–57.

146. Xia P, Gamble JR, Rye KA, Wang L, Hii CS, Cockerill P, Khew-Goodall Y, Bert AG, Barter PJ, and Vadas MA. Tumor necrosis factor-alpha induces adhesion molecule expression through the sphingosine kinase pathway. Proc Natl Acad Sci USA 1998;95(24):14196–201.

147. Harada-Shiba M, Kinoshita M, Kamido H, and Shimokado K. Oxidized low density lipoprotein induces apoptosis in cultured human umbilical vein endothelial cells by common and unique mechanisms. J Biol Chem 1998;273(16):9681–7.

148. Ackermann EJ, Taylor JK, Narayana R, and Bennett CF. The role of antiapoptotic Bcl-2 family members in endothelial apoptosis elucidated with antisense oligonucleotides. J Biol Chem 1999;274(16):11245–52.

149. Fujikawa K, de Aos Scherpenseel I, Jain SK, Presman E, Christensen RA, and Varticovski L. Role of PI 3-kinase in angiopoietin-1-mediated migration and attachment-dependent survival of endothelial cells [published erratum appears in Exp Cell Res 2000;255(1):133]. Exp Cell Res 1999;253(2):663–72.

150. Gupta K, Kshirsagar S, Li W, Gui L, Ramakrishnan S, Gupta P, Law PY, and Hebbel RP. VEGF prevents apoptosis of human microvascular endothelial cells via opposing effects on MAPK/ERK and SAPK/JNK signaling. Exp Cell Res 1999;247(2):495–504.

151. Chatterjee S, Han H, Rollins S, and Cleveland T. Molecular cloning, characterization, and expression of a novel human neutral sphingomyelinase. J Biol Chem 1999;274(52):37407–12.

152. Ohta H, Sweeney EA, Masamune A, Yatomi Y, Hakomori S, and Igarashi Y. Induction of apoptosis by sphingosine in human leukemic HL-60 cells: a possible endogenous modulator of apoptotic DNA fragmentation occurring during phorbol ester-induced differentiation. Cancer Res 1995;55(3):691–7.

153. Lavrentiadou S, George J, Gilburd B, Harats D, Shoenfeld Y, Barak A, and Goldkorn T. OxLDL induces ceramide and apoptosis in macrophages but not in aortas of ApoE-deficient mice. 6th Annual Meeting of the Oxygen Society. Free Radical Biology & Medicine 1999;27(Sup.1): S114.

154. Visvanathan S, and McNeil HP. Cellular immunity to beta 2-glycoprotein-1 in patients with the antiphospholipid syndrome. J Immunol 1999;162(11):6919–25.

155. Pittoni V, Ravirajan CT, Donohoe S, MacHin SJ, Lydyard PM, and Isenberg DA. Human monoclonal anti-phos-

pholipid antibodies selectively bind to membrane phospholipid and beta2-glycoprotein I (beta2-GPI) on apoptotic cells. Clin Exp Immunol 2000;119(3):533–43.

156. George J, Shoenfeld Y, and Harats D. The involvement of beta2-glycoprotein I (beta2-GPI) in human and murine atherosclerosis. J Autoimmun 1999;13(1):57–60.

157. Escargueil-Blanc I, Salvayre R, and Negre-Salvayre A. Necrosis and apoptosis induced by oxidized low density lipoproteins occur through two calcium-dependent pathways in lymphoblastoid cells. Faseb J 1994;8(13):1075–80.

158. Riboni L, Viani P, Bassi R, Prinetti A, and Tettamanti G. The role of sphingolipids in the process of signal transduction. Prog Lipid Res 1997;36(2–3):153–95.

159. Pyne S, Chapman J, Steele L, and Pyne NJ. Sphingomyelin-derived lipids differentially regulate the extracellular signal-regulated kinase 2 (ERK-2) and c-Jun N-terminal kinase (JNK) signal cascades in airway smooth muscle. Eur J Biochem 1996;237(3):819–26.

160. Spiegel S, Cuvillier O, Edsall L, Kohama T, Menzeleev R, Olivera A, Thomas D, Tu Z, Van Brocklyn J, and Wang F. Roles of sphingosine-1-phosphate in cell growth, differentiation, and death. Biochemistry (Mosc) 1998;63(1):69–73.

161. Merrill AH Jr., and Jones DD. An update of the enzymology and regulation of sphingomyelin metabolism. Biochim Biophys Acta 1990;1044(1):1–12.

162. Koval M, and Pagano RE. Intracellular transport and metabolism of sphingomyelin. Biochim Biophys Acta 1991;1082(2):113–25.

163. Hofmann K, and Dixit VM. Ceramide in apoptosis – does it really matter? Trends Biochem Sci 1998;23(10):374–7.

164. Hannun YA, and Bell RM. Functions of sphingolipids and sphingolipid breakdown products in cellular regulation [see comments]. Science 1989;243(4890):500–7.

165. Desai NN, and Spiegel S. Sphingosylphosphorylcholine is a remarkably potent mitogen for a variety of cell lines. Biochem Biophys Res Commun 1991;181(1):361–6.

Atherosclerosis and Autoimmunity
Y. Shoenfeld, D. Harats and G. Wick, editors

α-Defensins: Potential Link between Inflammation, Thrombosis and Atherosclerosis

Abd Al-Roof Higazi[1,2], Douglas B. Cines[2] and Khalil Bdeir[2]

[1]Department of Clinical Biochemistry, Hebrew University-Hadassah Medical Center, Jerusalem, Israel IL-91120; [2]Department of Pathology and Laboratory Medicine, University of Pennsylvania, Philadelphia, PA 19104, USA

1. INFLAMMATION AND ATHEROSCLEROSIS

Interest in the contribution of chronic vascular inflammation to the pathogenesis of atherosclerosis has been revived by several recent observations (reviewed in [1,2]). The involvement of macrophages, the cellular and humoral immune systems, cytokine networks and regulation of integrin function have been examined through elegant *in vitro* studies, epidemiological approaches [3–5], and novel murine models (reviewed in [6–8]). Clinical correlation between systemic markers of inflammation, endothelial cell activation, and response to therapeutic intervention have converged to focus interest on the sequence of inflammatory events responsible for lesion progression and plaque instability [9–12]. Thus, the way in which inflammation orchestrates the development of atherosclerotic lesions has become of prime importance.

It is likely that vascular inflammation affects the progression of atherosclerosis through diverse mechanisms. One pathway may involve the enhancement of lipoprotein retention. It has been estimated that 30–50% of the risk of symptomatic coronary artery disease involves factors that complement hypercholesterolemia and other identified abnormalities of lipid metabolism [13, 14].

Part of this variability appears to result from factors that act locally to alter lipoprotein metabolism. The rate of lipoprotein transport into vessel walls considerably exceeds their rate of accumulation (reviewed in [15]). This indicates that retention is the rate-limiting step in lipoprotein accumulation. Retained lipoproteins are subject to oxidation, aggregation and other modifications that promote lipid accumulation and vascular injury (reviewed in [16]). Consistent with this idea is the finding that reduction of vascular retention time may help to prevent oxidant-induced vascular injury [17]. Yet, surprisingly little is known about the factors that mediate lipoprotein retention in vessel walls. Among these, there is evidence that alterations in the composition of the proteoglycan matrix of vessels that accompany the development of atherosclerosis may participate in this process [18–20].

Inflammation also contributes to lesion progression by activating the coagulation system. There is extensive literature demonstrating the presence of fibrin both in native atherosclerotic lesions (reviewed in [21]) and in the accelerated atherosclerosis that develops in allografts (reviewed in [22]). Involvement of the fibrinolytic system in lesion development has been demonstrated through the analysis of mice with targeted deletions in one or more of the genes that encode for plasminogen activators and their inhibitors (reviewed in [23]) and through the analysis of mice that overexpress Lp(a) [24]. Immunohistochemical studies indicate that monocyte adherence to the endothelial cells [25] precedes and promotes fibrin deposition along the vascular intima [26]. Coagulation may be initiated when tissue factor is induced on these infiltrating macrophages [27] or on resident vascular cells [28, 29].

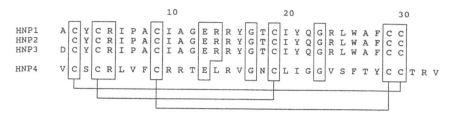

Figure 1. Amino acid sequences of human neutrophil α-defensins (HNP 1-4). The pairing of the invariant cysteine bonds is indicated. HNP refers to human neutrophil peptide.

In turn, fibrin may promote the retention of Lp(a) in fatty streaks. Lp(a) may compete with plasminogen for binding to fibrin and thereby impede fibrinolysis [30, 31]. Loss of plasmin-mediated activation of transforming growth factor-β also permits smooth muscle cell proliferation in response to various mitogens to go unchecked [32, 33]. In this way, persistent inflammation within the vessel wall may link the processes of coagulation and lipoprotein accumulation.

2. STRUCTURAL BIOLOGY OF DEFENSINS

Complex, multi-cellular organisms have evolved a system of innate host defense that provides rapid protection against microbial invasion prior to the development of a high affinity, cognate immune response, a process to which antimicrobial peptides contribute. These peptides are highly conserved in nature from plants through insects to mammals. Certain classes of antimicrobial peptides are constitutively expressed on epithelial surfaces where they come in direct contact with microorganisms, while others are sequestered and their expression is induced by mediators of inflammation (reviewed in [34]).

Defensins constitute one such family of antimicrobial peptides that are expressed by mammals. Defensins are cationic peptides composed of 29–32 amino acids (Figure 1) arranged in three antiparallel β-sheets that are stabilized by three canonical intramolecular disulfide bonds (Figure 2) [34,35]. α-defensins (human neutrophils peptides 1-4; HNP-1-4) are sequestered in the granules of neutrophils where they constitute 5% of the total cellular protein [36] and in the granules of Paneth cells (HNP 5 and 6) (reviewed in [37, 38], whereas

the β-defensins have been identified on mucosal and epithelial surfaces. The α-defensins and β-defensins differ in the pattern of pairing of these disulfide bonds. This review will focus on certain effects of neutrophil α-defensins on the vasculature. The reader is referred elsewhere for more recent studies on β-defensins (reviewed in [39]).

It is generally accepted that defensins exert their antibacterial, antiviral, antiprotozoal and antifungal activity by polymerizing in prokaryotic membranes as a result of their amphiphilic properties, opening ion channels and eventuating in cell lysis [40]. The structure of defensins, as revealed by NMR and crystallography, provides insight into the basis of this pore-forming activity. It is generally held that α-defensins exist in solution as dimers, having a three-dimensional structure resembling a basket or a cup bounded on one side by a hydrophobic surface which is assumed to insert into the phospholipid bilayer of microbes, while the open end of the basket is bounded by the polar residues contributed by the amino- and carboxy-termini of the molecule [40,41] (Figure 2) . Defensin is found in concentrations approaching 30 μM in the blood of patients with bacterial septicemia and meningitis [42], conditions that predispose to thrombosis. Even higher levels are found in empyema fluid where they make contribute to the accumulation of fibrin that may lead to permanent reduction in lung capacity [43].

Sequestration of α-defensins within granules limits potentially deleterious interactions with host cells. High concentrations of α-defensins are cytotoxic for certain mammalian cells [44]. α-defensins are also chemotactic for monocytes and T-cells, activate neutrophils, stimulate the release of IL-8, stimulate proliferation of epithelial cells and fibroblasts, induce histamine release by mast cells and increase airway hyperresponsiveness to histamine (reviewed

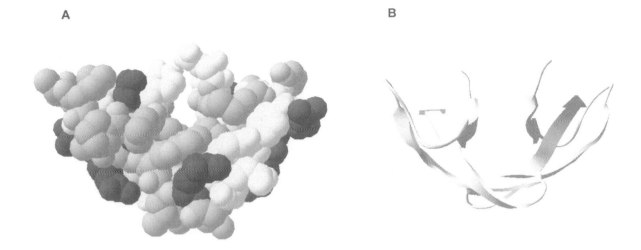

Figure 2. Panel A. Solution structure of the α-defensin dimer of HNP-3. Arginine residues are shaded black, hydrophobic residues gray and other polar amino acids are shown in white. Panel B. Ribbon diagram of the HNP-3 dimer. The hydrophobic surface is shown facing the bottom. The polar residues are shown contributing to the sides of the cup-like structure.

$$67 \quad \text{Y C R I P A C I A G E R R Y G T C I Y Q G R L W A F C} \quad 93$$

$$330 \quad \text{Y C R N P D G D V G G P W C Y T - T N P R K L Y D Y C} \quad 555$$

Figure 3. Sequence similarity of α-defensin and plasminogen kringle 5. Comparison of the amino acid sequence of α-defensin (top) with part of the sequence of kringle 5 of plasminogen (bottom). The dots indicate conservative substitutions. Published with permission from the Journal of Biological Chemistry 1995;270:9472–7.

in [45]), and inhibit HLA-DR-restricted T cell proliferation by binding to MHC class II molecules and restricting access to antigen [46]. More recently α-defensins have been reported to promote both Th-1 and Th-2 mediated immune responses to tumor antigens *in vitro* and to inhibit tumor growth *in vivo* [47].

Analysis of the structure of defensins reveals additional properties that may be relevant to the pathogenesis of thrombosis and atherosclerosis. For example, α-defensin shares certain structural similarities with proteins involved in fibrinolysis and lipid metabolism. Comparison of the amino acid sequences of α-defensin and plasminogen revealed a 54% similarity with portions of the internal loop of plasminogen kringle-5 (Figure 3) [48]. Similarities in the amino acid sequence and distribution of charged residues and hydrophobicity between the defensin and tissue type plasminogen activator (tPA) kringle 2 are evident as well. The region of greatest

similarity is with the portion of the kringles that are involved in the binding of lysine and have been implicated in their interactions with other molecules and cell surfaces. These structural similarities between α-defensin and the kringles of fibrinolytic proteins are likely to be of pathophysiological relevance (*vide infra*).

3. DEFENSINS INHIBIT PLASMINOGEN ACTIVATION *IN VITRO*

We began to investigate the potential involvement of α-defensin in atherosclerosis based on the well-described association between inflammation and thrombosis. To do so, we tried to understand the basis for the deposition of fibrin that is characteristic of delayed hypersensitivity reactions [49,50]. The extent of induration invoked by inflammatory stimuli is reduced in patients with afibrinogenemia

[51] and individuals who are being treated with anti-coagulants [52]. The purpose of this fibrin deposition is uncertain. It has been proposed that fibrin helps to immobilize the irritant [53], acts as a chemoattractant and provides a provisional scaffolding for macrophages and other leukocytes [54–56] and contributes to vascular wound healing [57].

To appreciate this phenomenon, it is important to recognize that the fibrinolytic system prevents appreciable accretion of fibrin in most circumstances. Fibrin not only acts as a substrate of this proteolytic system, but also acts as a cofactor that increases the efficiency of plasmin production from plasminogen by tPA. Thus, finding that fibrin accumulates in inflammatory lesions suggests that in addition to activation of the coagulation system, it is likely that the activity of the plasminogen activator system has been impeded in a coordinate manner. Such inhibition not only serves to confine the provocative agent, but also limits the release of thrombin and fibrinogen degradation products that are chemotactic and mitogenic for inflammatory cells [58–60].

It is known that clots infiltrated with neutrophils are resistant to fibrinolysis [61]. Therefore, we investigated mechanism by which neutrophils help to stabilize fibrin at sites of inflammation by inhibiting plasminogen activation. An unexpected finding was that greater than 95% of the plasminogen activator inhibitor activity isolated from neutrophil lysates migrated as a single 4 kDa protein band on SDS-PAGE, which on N-terminal sequencing was identified as the most prevalent α-defensin, human neutrophil peptide 2 (HNP-2). Subsequent studies demonstrated that neutrophil α-defensins (HNP 1-3), individually and collectively, inhibit tPA-mediated plasminogen activation by fibrin (Figure 4). α-defensins bind to fibrin and at pathophysiologic (μmolar) concentrations encountered *in vivo* act as competitive inhibitors of tPA binding. The capacity of α-defensin to compete with plasminogen and tPA can be explained by the similarities in sequence and charge distribution with kringle-2 of tPA[62], which is known to bind to fibrin.

α-defensins also inhibit the binding of plasminogen to fibrin through a somewhat more complex mechanism. At the lower end of the effective range of concentrations (1–5 μM), defensins stimulate the binding of plasminogen to fibrin, whereas higher

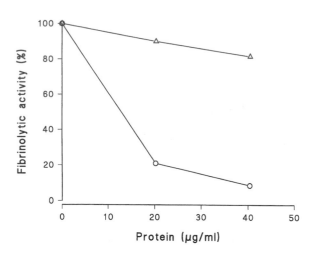

Figure 4. Defensin inhibits tPA-mediated fibrinolysis. ^{125}I-fibrin clots were incubated with 6.6 IU/mL tPA (O) or urokinase (△), 80 μg/ml plasminogen and the indicated concentrations of α-defensin for 2 hours at 37 °C and the released radioactivity was measured. The data are expressed relative to maximal fibrinolysis. Published with permission from the Journal of Biological Chemistry 1995;270:9472–7.

concentrations of α-defensins inhibit plasminogen binding [62]. This biphasic effect is best explained by the observation that α-defensins bind to plasminogen in solution, likely through one or more of its kringles. Plasminogen-defensin complexes bind to fibrin through sites shared with defensin. These sites are occupied preferentially by unbound defensin when it is present at high concentrations. The finding that defensin inhibits plasminogen activation even at concentrations at which plasminogen binding is enhanced is reminiscent of the behavior of Lp(a) [63]. It is likely that plasminogen bound to defensin, like Lp(a), is less susceptible to activation by tPA. Thus, α-defensins bind to fibrin, inhibit plasminogen binding and activation and impair fibrinolysis.

α-defensins have a similar effect on cell-mediated fibrinolysis. α-defensins bind specifically to cultured human umbilical vein endothelial cells and smooth muscle cells (half-maximal binding 3 μM), concentrations well within the range encountered in inflammatory settings. α-defensins inhibit tPA-mediated fibrinolysis on cultured cells in a dose-dependent manner through the same paradigm observed on the surface of fibrin (Figure 5), i.e.

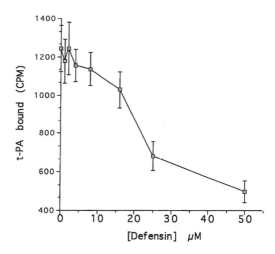

Figure 5. Defensin inhibits the binding of tPA to fibrin. ^{125}I-tPA (15 nM) was incubated with fibrin in the presence of the indicated concentrations of α-defensin and the bound radioactivity was measured. The mean ± S.D. of three experiments is shown. Identical results were obtained when binding of tPA to cultured human umbilical vein endothelial cells in the presence of α-defensin was measured. Published with permission from the Journal of Biological Chemistry 1996;271:17650–17655.

competitive inhibition of tPA binding and a biphasic effect on plasminogen binding [62]. Although beneficial for the immediate containment of microbial organisms within the vessel wall, delay of fibrinolysis may promote the progression of atherosclerosis and thrombotic vascular occlusion.

4. α-DEFENSINS REGULATE THE METABOLISM OF Lp(a) AND LDL *IN VITRO*

Several epidemiological studies have revealed a correlation between leukocytosis ([64–66], among others) and the prevalence of atherosclerosis. Neutrophil activation has been implicated in the initial stages of intimal thickening in certain experimental models of vascular injury [67], through the release of proteolytic enzymes [68] and by stimulating the release of PDGF from IL-1β treated endothelial cells [69]. However, little is known with respect to the effect of neutrophil activation on lipoprotein metabolism by vascular cells.

The likelihood that α-defensins bind to the krin-gles of plasminogen suggests that these peptides may similarly affect the binding properties of Lp(a). Lp(a) contains a variable, genetically determined number of kringle IV-type 2 repeats, a single kringle-V type moiety and a protease-like domain which cannot be cleaved by plasmin to a two-chain active enzyme. Accumulation of Lp(a) in atherosclerotic lesions has been attributed to their interaction with fibrin, proteoglycans and fibronectin [70–72], but the regulation of this process has not been described in detail. α-defensins stimulate the binding of Lp(a) to cultured human vascular endothelial and smooth muscle cells approximately 4 fold and 6 fold (Figure 6), respectively. α-defensins form stable complexes with Lp(a) detected by gel filtration, surface plasmon resonance and immunoelectron microscopy [76]. High affinity binding of α-defensin to natural and recombinant apo(a) affirmed the hypothesis that their effect is mediated through interactions with the kringles. These complexes bind to cellular sites that are capable of binding α-defensin itself, as was observed with plasminogen. α-defensins also stimulate the binding of Lp(a) to fibrin, suggesting that synthesis of novel cellular binding sites is not required. Of interest, accumulation of defensin/Lp(a) was not accompanied by a comparable increase in lipoprotein degradation. A series of experiments was then conducted to examine potential mechanisms for this increase in Lp(a) acquisition by vascular cells.

Early in the development of atherosclerosis, lipoproteins accumulate in sub-endothelial matrix. Therefore, we examined the effect of α-defensin on the binding of Lp(a) to matrix prepared from cultured endothelial cells and smooth muscle cells [73]. Binding of Lp(a) to each matrix is enhanced almost 40 fold in the presence of α-defensin. Lp(a)/defensin complexes show little elution from the matrix, resulting in a marked net accumulation of lipoprotein (Figure 7). Binding of defensin/Lp(a) complexes to matrix is inhibited by very low concentrations of heparin. Part of this effect is attributable to competition with cellular proteoglycans, as binding of the complexes was reduced approximately one-third when matrix from cells lacking heparan- and chondroitin sulfate was studied. The remainder was mediated by an interaction of defensin/Lp(a) with fibronectin, which contains a heparin binding motif. Thus, α-defensin causes large amounts of

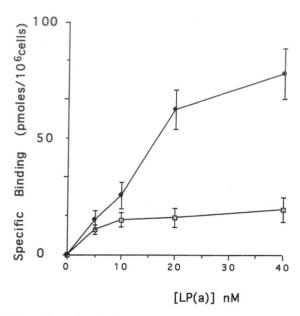

Figure 6. Defensin stimulates the binding of Lp(a) to cultured human endothelial cells (HUVEC). Cells were incubated with 0–40 nM ^{125}I-Lp(a) alone or in the presence of 3 μM α-defensin for 4 hours at 4°C and the specific binding was determined. Binding of Lp(a) in the absence (□) and in the presence (♦) of defensin. The mean ± S.D. of three experiments is shown. Published with permission from Blood 89:4290–8, 1997.

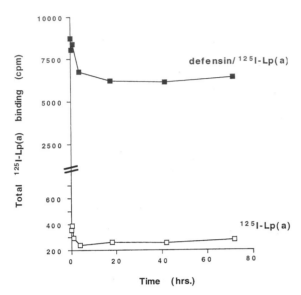

Figure 7. Lp(a) and defensin/Lp(a) bind tightly to HUVEC matrix. ^{125}I-Lp(a) (10 nM; □) or 2.5 μM defensin/10 nM ^{125}I-Lp(a) (■) was incubated with HUVEC matrix for 1 hour at 37°C. The matrix was extensively washed, buffer was added and the bound radioactivity was measured at the indicated times. The mean of two experiments performed in triplicate is shown. Published with permission from Blood 94:2007–19, 1999.

Lp(a) to be retained in vascular matrix where is would be susceptible to oxidative and other modifications [73]. Furthermore, defensin/Lp(a) complexes are internalized inefficiently if at all by endothelial cells. Rather they remain predominantly in the form of complexes on and between the cells as viewed by confocal microscopy [73] (Figure 8).

α-defensin also binds saturably to LDL, although with somewhat lower affinity than it does to Lp(a). α-defensin stimulates the binding of LDL to endothelial, smooth muscle and fibroblast cells approximately 7 fold [74]. One surprise was the finding that in the presence of defensin, LDL binds to fibroblasts lacking the LDL-receptor (LDL-R) to the same extent as to wild type cells. This outcome suggests not only that the binding of defensin/LDL is independent of LDL-R, but that LDL-R appears unable to bind LDL when defensin is present. Subsequent studies using fibroblasts lacking LDL-receptors and anti-LDL receptor antibodies affirmed this hypothesis, indicating that defensin binds to LDL-R

and inhibits its capacity to bind LDL. Several pieces of evidence indicate that the complexes between α-defensin and LDL bind to cellular proteoglycans: i) Binding is inhibited by low concentrations of heparin; ii) α-defensin/LDL complexes bind less well to cells lacking heparan sulfate-containing proteoglycans (HSPGs); and iii) Enhanced binding of the complexes is observed to cells overexpressing syndecan 1 heparan sulfate [74].

The diversion of LDL from LDL-R to HSPGs would be predicted to inhibit the efficient receptor-mediated pathway of endocytosis and degradation while promoting binding to a high capacity pathway through which the lipoprotein is degraded far more slowly. In agreement with this hypothesis, α-defensin shifted the $t_{1/2}$ of endocytosis by wild type fibroblasts from minutes to hours, consistent with the degradation of LDL by fibroblasts from a patient with familial hypercholesterolemia which lack LDL-R. The extent of internalization of LDL/defensin varied in direct proportion to the level of HSPG expression. α-defensins may act on the

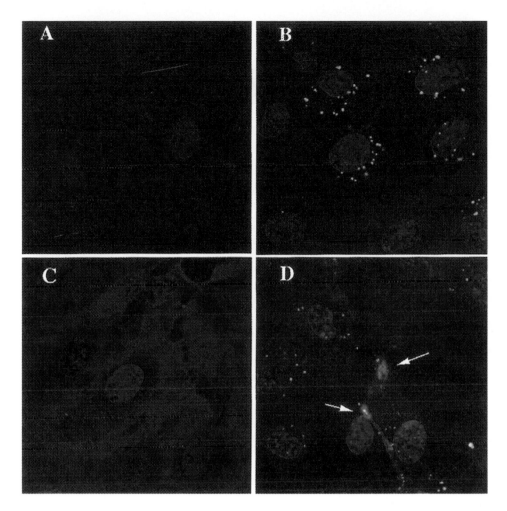

Figure 8. Subcellular distribution of defensin, Lp(a) and Lp(a)/defensin complexes in HUVECs as assessed by confocal microscopy. HUVECs were incubated with either Lp(a) (50 nM; Panel b) defensin (10 μM; Panel c), or co-incubated with defensin and Lp(a) (Panel d) for 30 min at 37 °C, and then analyzed by confocal microscopy using polyclonal Lp(a) antibodies followed by FITC-conjugated anti-rabbit IgG (detected as green) and/or a monoclonal anti-human defensin followed by rhodamine TRITC-conjugated donkey anti-mouse IgG (detected as red). Normal rabbit IgGs served as controls, as shown in (a). Cell nuclei were stained with DAPI (detected as blue). Colocalization of defensin and Lp(a) was assessed by double staining (d) and results in a yellow color (arrows). Published with permission from Blood 1999;94:2007–19.

degradation of Lp(a) by vascular cells in a similar manner. α-defensins enhance Lp(a) accumulation on the cell surface, retard its endocytosis, and with prolonged incubation, promote the esterification of cholesterol from Lp(a) by a macrophage cell line [74].

5. VASCULAR LOCALIZATION OF α-DEFENSINS *IN VIVO*

Our *in vitro* studies indicate that α-defensins regulate the interaction of atherogenic lipoproteins with components of the blood vessel wall. To begin to address the biologic relevance of these findings, the distribution of defensin in the human vasculature was examined by immunohistochemistry using antibodies that recognize α-defensin but not β-defensin. Human epicardial coronary arteries were examined

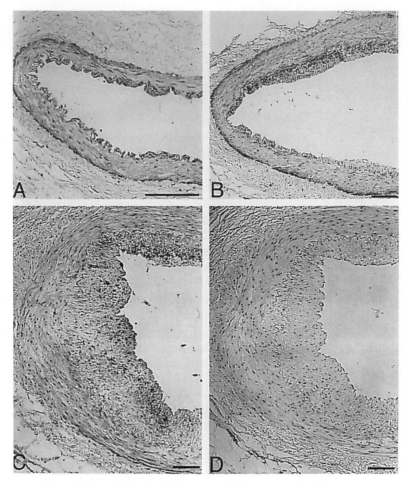

Figure 9. Localization of defensin in histologically normal and atherosclerotic coronary arteries. Samples of epicardial coronary arteries were taken from a donor heart with histologically normal-appearing vessels (A), from a patient with idiopathic dilated cardiomyopathy but with early atherosclerotic changes in the intima (B), and from a patient with extensive atherosclerotic disease (C). Sections were stained with monoclonal anti-α-defensin antibody (C) or an equal concentration of a normal mouse isotype control (D). Antibodies were detected using a peroxidase conjugated secondary antibody. Original magnification ×100. Bar, 100 μM. Published with permission from American Journal of Pathology 1997;150:1009–20.

for the presence of α-defensin [75]. α-defensin was identified in the intima of vessels lacking morphologic evidence of atherosclerosis as well as in those with minimal intimal thickening. Prominent staining was also seen along the external elastic lamina but was less intense in the media (Figure 9).

Staining for α-defensin was more prominent in arteries showing more extensive intimal hyperplasia and medial hypertrophy. α-defensin was found focally in the endothelium and in association with intimal and medial smooth muscle cells. In some of the most severely affected vessels, staining for α-defensin was most pronounced in acellular regions

of the plaque compared with neighboring areas of intense smooth muscle proliferation.

The relationship between the distribution of α-defensin and Lp(a) in vessels affected by atherosclerosis was then examined [76]. Atherosclerotic and non-atherosclerotic arteries from the circle of Willis obtained from 28 patients were studied. Again, staining for α-defensin and Lp(a) was most prominent in vessels involved with atherosclerosis, and the intensity of staining correlated closely with the severity of the atherosclerotic changes. In areas where the endothelium was intact and little or no intimal thickening was apparent, little α-defensin was apparent. In contrast, prominent deposition of α-defensin and Lp(a) was found in the endothelium and subendothelial regions of vessels containing complex plaques, cholesterol clefts and significant medial hyperplasia. In acellular areas, the co-localization of defensin and Lp(a) was less precise, consistent with the proteins having separate metabolic pathways.

6. PERSPECTIVE: MODEL OF DEFENSIN ACTIVITY

Our studies over the past several years indicate that α-defensins can regulate several biological pathways that have been implicated in the development of atherosclerosis. For example, α-defensins inhibit fibrinolysis both in solution and on cell surfaces. α-defensins also stimulate binding of LDL and Lp(a) to vascular cells and subcellular matrix. Moreover, α-defensins inhibit the ability of vascular cells to utilize pathways that have evolved to remove and degrade these potentially atherogenic lipoproteins efficiently, diverting them to matrix proteins or to cell surface proteoglycans. This has the net effect of prolonging the retention of lipoproteins in matrices and on cell surfaces where they are subject to oxidative and other modifications that have been implicated in the pathogenesis of atherosclerosis.

Our data also provide insight into the mechanisms that underlie these activities. The arginines on the polar face of α-defensins may mimic certain behaviors exhibited by specific lysine residues in the kringles of plasminogen and tPA. α-defensins may thereby help to retain plasminogen in the closed conformation, which is less susceptible to activation. α-defensins may also inhibit plasminogen activation by competing with kringle 2 of tPA for binding to fibrin and cell surfaces, which is necessary for optimal catalytic activity. These same properties may mediate the binding of α-defensins to one or more kringles in Lp(a).

In addition to these specific effects, we hypothesize that α-defensins impart cationic charges onto the proteins to which they bind. Cationization of proteins, e.g. ferritin containing Fe^{3+} compared with Fe^{2+}, promotes their interaction with high capacity, lower affinity anionic sites that are widely expressed on cell surfaces. Through this mechanism, the clearance of a wide variety of proteins is enhanced which may affect their internalization and degradation [77].

α-defensins exhibit this capacity to bind to the large reservoir of cell surface proteoglycans through their cationic surface (Figure 10). Furthermore, through unoccupied charged residues or through the exposed hydrophobic face, α-defensin may interact simultaneously with additional proteins. The combination of these two properties permits α-defensins to facilitate the transfer of diverse reactants to cell surface proteoglycans. Some of these ligands may then be internalized and degraded relatively slowly through the as yet only partially characterized proteoglycan-dependent endocytic pathway [15].

However, in the case of lipoproteins such as LDL and Lp(a) that interact with their cognate receptors through cationic residues, α-defensins may compete for receptor binding, divert the ligands towards proteoglycans, and thereby impede their normal pathway of rapid clearance.

Through this combination of activities, α-defensins may also modulate the physiologic functions of the proteoglycans themselves, including binding and activation of various cationic growth factors and cytokines, binding of apoE and the function of cell surface lipases [78–80] The high concentrations of α-defensin attained during inflammation would be expected to magnify these effects. In this manner, neutrophils that are activated or undergo apoptosis within the vasculature may change the behavior of the surrounding cells. Furthermore, α-defensins may modify the endocytosis and processing of microbial or host antigens by antigen presenting cells at sites of inflammation through a similar mechanism.

Thus, α-defensins may be viewed as a specialized example of molecules, such as C-reactive protein and serum amyloid protein, that are expressed in high concentrations during inflammation and that link diverse ligands, including modified lipoproteins, with proteoglycans, extracellular matrix proteins and other components of the vasculature [81] (Figure 10) with beneficial or deleterious consequences depending on the nature of the ligand. Other cationic peptides expressed during the course of inflammatory reactions may compete for binding to proteoglycans or to such cell surface receptors because, unlike α-defensins, they lack the capacity

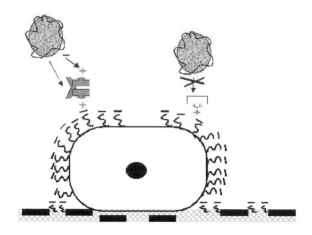

Figure 10. Model of α-defensin-ligand interaction with vascular matrix. The α-defensin dimer (left side) contains both cationic (+) and hydrophobic (indentation) regions that may permit its interaction with lipoproteins. α-defensin may bind simultaneously through unoccupied cationic regions serving as a bridge between the lipoproteins or other particles and cell surface or matrix. Other cationic proteins (right side) may bind in a similar manner to proteoglycans but lack the ability to bind (lipo)proteins simultaneously and thereby serve to block their binding to cell surfaces or matrix.

to bind simultaneously to the cationic ligand and thereby serve a bridging function (Figure 10). Additional studies will be needed to explore the ramifications of defensin deposition in the vasculature.

REFERENCES

1. Ross R. Atherosclerosis – An inflammatory Disease. N Engl J Med 1999;320:115–126.
2. Tracy RP. Epidemiological evidence for inflammation in cardiovascular disease. Thromb Haemost 1999;82:826–831.
3. Xu Q, Kiechl S, Mayr M, et al. Association of serum antibodies to heat-shock protein 65 with carotid atherosclerosis. Clinical significance determined in a follow-up study. Circulation 1999;100:1169–1174.
4. Ridker PM, Cushman M, Stampfer MJ, Tracy RP, Hennekens CH. Inflammation, aspirin, and the risk of cardiovascular disease in apparently healthy men. N Engl J Med 1997;336:973–979.
5. Kearney, JF. Immune recognition of OxLDL in atherosclerosis. J Clin Invest 2000;105:1683–1685.
6. Rader DJ, Fitzgerald GA. State of the art: Atherosclerosis in a limited edition. Nat Med 1998;4:899–900.
7. Fuster V, Poon M, Willerson JT. Learning from the transgenic mouse. Endothelium, adhesive molecules and neointimal formation. Circulation 1998;97:16–18.
8. Kearney JF. Immune recognition of OxLDL in atherosclerosis. J Clin Invest 2000;105:1683–1685.
9. van der Wal AC, Becker AE, van der Loos CM, Das PK. Site of intimal rupture or erosion of thrombosed coronary atherosclerotic plaques is characterized by an inflammatory process irrespective of the dominant plaque morphology. Circulation 1994;89:36–44.
10. Berliner JA, Navab M, Fogelman AM, et al. Atherosclerosis: Basic mechanisms. Oxidation, inflammation, and genetics. Circulation 1995;91:2488–2496.
11. Ridker PM. Inflammation, infection, and cardiovascular risk. How good is the clinical evidence? Circulation 1998;97:1671–1674.
12. Shah PK. Circulating markers of inflammation for vascular risk prediction. Are they ready for prime time? Circulation 2000;105:1758–1759.
13. Crouse III JR. Progress in coronary artery risk-factor research: What remains to be done? Clin Chem 1984;30:1125–1127.
14. Schreiner PJ, Heiss G, Tyroler HA, Morrisett JD, Davis CE, Smith R. Race and gender differences in the association of Lp(a) with carotid artery wall thickness. The Atherosclerosis Risk in Communities (ARIC) study. Arterioscler Thromb Vasc Biol 1996;16:471–478.
15. Williams KJ, Tabas I. The response-to-retention hypothesis of early atherogenesis. Arterioscler Thromb Vasc Biol 1995;15:551–558.
16. Steinberg D. Low density lipoprotein oxidation and its pathobiological significance. J Biol Chem 1997;272:20963–20966.
17. Fruebis J, Steinberg D, Dresel HA, Carew TE. A comparison of the antiatherogenic effects of Probucol and of a structural analogue of Probucol in low density lipoprotein receptor-deficient rabbits. J Clin Invest 1994;94:392–398l.
18. Manley G, Hawksworth J. Distribution of mucopolysaccharides in the human vascular tree. Nature 1965;206:1152–1153.
19. Wight TN, Curwen KD, Litrenta MM, Alonso DR, Minick CR. Effect of endothelium on glycosaminoglycan accumulation in injured rabbit aorta. Am J Pathol 1983;113:156–164.
20. Cardosoe LEM, Mourao PAS. Glycosaminoglycan fractions from human arteries presenting diverse susceptibilities to atherosclerosis have different binding affinities to plasma LDL. Arterioscl Thrombos 1994;1:115–124.
21. Smith EB, Thompson WD. Fibrin as a factor in atherogenesis. Thromb Res 1993;73:1–19.
22. Weis M, Scheidt v. Coronary artery disease in the transplanted heart. Annu Rev Med 2000;51:81–100.

23. Carmeliet P, Collen D. Development and disease in proteinase-deficient mice: Role of the plasminogen matrix metalloproteinase and coagulation system. Thromb Res 1998;91:255–285.

24. Hughes SD, Lou XJ, Ighani S, et al. Lipoprotein(a) vascular accumulation in mice. In vivo analysis of the role of lysine binding sites using recombinant adenovirus. J Clin Invest 1997;100:1493–1500.

25. Adams DH, Wyner LR, Steinbeck MJ, Karnovsky MJ. Inhibition of graft arteriosclerosis by modulation of the inflammatory response. Transplant Proceedings 1993;25:2092–2094.

26. Faulk WP, Labarrere C. Vascular immunopathology and atheroma development in human allografted organs. Arch Pathol Lab Med 1992;116:1337–1342.

27. Wilcox JN, Smith KM, Schwartz SM, Gordon D. Localization of tissue factor in the normal vessel wall and in the atherosclerotic plaque. Proc Natl Acad Sci USA 1989;86:2839–2843.

28. Thiruvikraman SV, Guha A, Roboz J, Taubman MB, Nemerson Y, Fallon JT. In situ localization of tissue factor in human atherosclerotic plaques by binding of digoxigenin-labeled factors VIIa and X. Lab Invest 1996;75:451–461.

29. Hatakeyama K, Asada Y, Marutsuka K, Sato Y, Kamikubo Y, Sumiyoashi A. Localization and activity of tissue factor in human aortic atherosclerotic lesions. Atherosclerosis 1997;133:213–219.

30. Miles LA, Plow EF. Lp(a): An interloper into the fibrinolytic system? Thromb Haemost 1990;63:331–335.

31. Miles LA, Fless GM, Scanu AM, et al. Interaction of Lp(a) with plasminogen binding sites on cells. Thromb Haemost 1995;73:458–465.

32. Grainger DJ, Kirschenlohr HL, Metcalfe JC, Weissberg PL, Wade DP, Lawn RM. Proliferation of human smooth muscle cells promoted by lipoprotein(a). Science 1993;260:1655–1658.

33. Grainger DJ, Kemp PR, Liu AC, Lawn RM, Metcalfe JC. Activation of transforming growth factor-β is inhibited in transgenic apolipoprotein(a) mice. Nature 1994;370:460–462.

34. Kagan BL, Ganz T, Lehrer RI. Defensins: a family of antimicrobial and cytotoxic peptides. Toxicol 1994;87:131–149.

35. Ganz T, Selsted ME, Lehrer RI. Defensins [Review] [85 refs]. Eur J Haematol 1990;44:1–8.

36. Ganz T. Extracellular release of antimicrobial defensins by human polymorphonuclear leukocytes. Infect Immun 1987;55:568–571.

37. Oulette AJ, Selsted ME. Paneth cell defensins: Endogenous peptide components of intestinal host defense. FASEB J 1996;10:1280–1289.

38. Bevins CL, Martin-Porter E, Ganz T. Defensins and innate host defense of the gastrointestinal tract. Gut 1999;45:911–916.

39. Diamond G, Bevins CL. beta-Defensins. Endogenous antibiotics of the innate host defense response. Clin Immunol Immunopathol 1998;88:221–225.

40. Hill CP, Yee J, Selsted ME, Eisenberg D. Crystal structure of defensin HNP-3, an amphiphilic dimer: Mechanisms of membrane permeabilization. Science 1991;251:1481–1485.

41. Pardi A, Zhang XL, Selsted ME, Skalicky JJ, Yip PF. NMR studies of defensin antimicrobial peptides. 2. Three-dimensional structures of rabbit NP-2 and human HNP-1. Biochemistry 1992;31:11357–11364.

42. Panyutich AV, Panyutich EA, Krapivin VA, Baturevich EA, Ganz T. Plasma defensin concentrations are elevated in patients with sepsis or bacterial meningitis. J Lab Clin Med 1993;122:202–207.

43. Ashitani J, Mukae H, Nakazato M, et al. Elevated pleural fluid levels of defensins in patients with empyema. Chest 1998;113:788–794.

44. Okrent DG, Lichtenstein AK, Ganz T. Direct cytotoxicity of polymorphonuclear leukocyte granule proteins to human lung-derived cells and endothelial cells. Am Rev Resp Dis 1990;141:179–185.

45. van Wetering S, Sterk PJ, Rabe KF, Hiemstra PS. Defensins: Key players or bystanders in infection, injury, and repair in the lung? J Allergy Clin Immunol 1999;104:1131–1138.

46. Halder TM, Bluggel M, Heinzel S, Pawelec G, Meyer HE, Kalbacher H. Defensins are dominant HLD-DR-associated self-peptides from CD34- peripheral blood mononuclear cells of different tumor patients (plasmacytoma, chronic myeloid leukemia). Blood 2000;95:2890–2896.

47. Tani K, Murphy WJ, Chertov O, et al. Defensins act as potent adjuvants that promote cellular and human immune responses in mice to a lymphoma idiotype and carrier antigens. Int Immunol 2000;12:691–700.

48. Higazi AA-R, Barghouti II, Abu-Much R. Identification of an inhibitor of tissue-type plasminogen activator-mediated fibrinolysis in human neutrophils. J Biol Chem 1995;270:9472–9477.

49. Colvin RB, Dvorak HF. Role of the clotting system in cell-mediated hypersensitivity. II. Kinetics of fibrinogen/fibrin accumulation and vascular permeability changes in tuberculin and cutaneous basophil hypersensitivity reactions. J Immunol 1975;114:377–387.

50. Colvin RB, Johnson RA, Mihm Jr. MC, Dvorak HF. Role of the clotting system in cell-mediated hypersensitivity. I. Fibrin deposition in delayed skin reactions in man. J Exp Med 1973;138:686–698.

51. Colvin RB, Mosesson MW, Dvorak HF. Delayed-type hypersensitivity skin reactions in congenital afibrino-

genemia lack fibrin deposition and induration. J Clin Invest 1979;63:1302–1306.

52. Edwards RL, Rickles FR. Delayed hypersensitivity in man: effect of systemic anticoagulation. Science 1978;200:541–543.

53. Menkin V. Physiol Reviews 1938;18:366–392.

54. Ciano PS, Colvin RB, Dvorak AM, McDonagh J, Dvorak HF. Macrophage migration in fibrin gel matrices. Lab Invest 1986;54:62–70.

55. Castellucci M, Montesano R. Phorbol ester stimulates macrophage invasion of fibrin matrices. Anat Rec 1988;220:1–10.

56. Herijgers N, Vettel U, Schaefer B, Spring H, Todd III RF, Kramer MD. Cell surface-bound urokinase-type plasminogen activator facilitates infiltration of freshly isolated granulocytes into fibrin. Immunobiol 1995;194:363–375.

57. Carmeliet P, Moons L, Ploplis V, Plow E, Collen D. Impaired arterial neointimal formation in mice with disruption of the plasminogen gene. J Clin Invest 1997;99:200–208.

58. Perdue JF, Lubenskyi W, Kivity E, Sonder SA, Fenton II JW. Protease mitogenic response of chick embryo fibroblasts and receptor binding/processing of human alpha-thrombin. J Biol Chem 1981;256:2767–2776.

59. Senior RM, Skogen WF, Griffin GL, Wilner GD. Effects of fibrinogen derivatives upon the inflammatory response. Studies with human fibrinopeptide B. J Clin Invest 1986;77:1014–1019.

60. Bar-Shavit R, Kahn A, Fenton II JW. Monocyte chemotaxis: stimulation by specific exosite region in thrombin. Science 1983;220:728–731.

61. Schulman G, Fogo A, Gung A, Badr K, Hakim R. Complement activation retards resolution of acute ischemic renal failure in the rat. Kidney Int 1991;40:1069–1074.

62. Higazi AA-R, Ganz T, Kariko K, Cines DB. Defensin modulates tPA and plasminogen binding to fibrin and endothelial cells. J Biol Chem 1996;271:17650–17655.

63. Liu J, Harpel PC, Gurewich V. Fibrin-bound lipoprotein(a) promotes plasminogen binding but inhibits fibrin degradation by plasmin. Biochemistry 1994;33:2554–2560.

64. Weijenberg MP, Feskens EJM, Kromhout D. White blood cell count and the risk of coronary heart disease and all-cause mortality in elderly men. Arterioscler Thromb Vasc Biol 1996;16:499–503.

65. Grau AJ, Buggle F, Becher H, Werle E, Hacke W. The association of leukocyte count, fibrinogen and C-reactive protein with vascular disease risk factors and ischemic vascular diseases. Thromb Res 1996;82:245–255.

66. Held C, Hjemdahl P, Rehnqvist N, et al. Haemostatic markers, inflammatory parameters and lipids in male and female patients in the Angina Prognosis Study in Stockholm (APSIS). A comparison with healthy controls. J Intern Med 1997;241:59–69.

67. van Put DJM, van Osselaer N, De Meyer GRY, et al. Role of polymorphonuclear leukocytes in collar-induced intimal thickening in the rabbit carotid artery. Arterioscler Thromb Vasc Biol 1998;18:915–921.

68. Elneihoum AM, Falke P, Hedblad B, Lingarde F, Ohlsson K. Leukocyte activation in atherosclerosis: correlation with risk factors. Atherosclerosis 1997;131:79–84.

69. Totani L, Cumashi A, Piccoli A, Lorenzet R. Polymorphonuclear leukocytes induce PDGF release from IL-1β-treated endothelial cells. Role of adhesion molecules and serine proteases. Arterioscler Thromb Vasc Biol 1998;18:1534–1540.

70. Miles LA, Fless GM, Levin EG, Scanu AM, Plow EF. A potential basis for the thrombotic risks associated with lipoprotein(a). Nature 1989;339:301–302.

71. Hajjar KA, Gavish D, Breslow JL, Nachman RL. Lipoprotein(a) modulation of endothelial cell surface fibrinolysis and its potential role in atherosclerosis. Nature 1989;339:303–305.

72. Loscalzo J, Weinfeld M, Fless GM, Scanu AM. Lipoprotein(a), fibrin binding, and plasminogen activation. Arteriosclerosis 1990;10:240–245.

73. Bdeir K, Cane W, Canziani G, et al. Defensin promotes the binding of Lp(a) to vascular matrix. Blood 1999;

74. Higazi AA-R, Nassar T, Ganz T, et al. α-defensins stimulate proteoglycan-dependent catabolism of low density lipoprotein by vascular cells: A new class of inflammatory apolipoprotein and a possible contributor to atherogenesis. Blood (In press)

75. Barnathan ES, Raghunath PN, Tomaszewski JE, Ganz T, Cines DB, Higazi AA-R. Immunohistochemical localization of defensin in human coronary vessels. Am J Pathol 1997;150:1009–1020.

76. Higazi AA-R, Lavi E, Bdeir K, et al. Defensin stimulates the binding of Lp(a) to human vascular endothelial and smooth muscle cells. Blood 1997;89:4290–4298.

77. Basu SK, Goldstein JL, Anderson RG, Brown MS. Degradation of cationized low density lipoprotein and regulation of cholesterol metabolism in homozygous familial hypercholesterolemia fibroblasts. Proc Natl Acad Sci USA 1976;73:3178–3182.

78. Williams KJ, Fuki IV. Cell-surface heparan sulfate proteoglycans: dynamic molecules mediating ligand catabolism. Curr Opin Lipidol 1997;8:253–262.

79. Mahley RW, Ji Z-S. Remnant lipoprotein metabolism: key pathways involving cell-surface heparan sulfate proteoglycans and apolipoprotein E. J Lipidol 1999;40:1–16.

80. Iozzo R. The biology of the small leucine-rich proteoglycans. J Biol Chem 1999;274:18843–18846.

81. Bhakdi S, Torzewski M, Klouche N, Hemmes M. Com-

plement and atherogenesis. Binding of CRP to degraded, nonoxidized LDL enhances complement activation. Arterioscler Thromb Vasc Biol 1999;19:2348–2354.

Lipids and Immunity

Steven M. Watkins[1], J. Bruce German[2], Yehuda Shoenfeld[3] and M. Eric Gershwin[4]

[1]FAME Analytics, Inc., 2545 Boatman Avenue, West Sacramento, CA 95691, USA; [2]Department of Food Science & Technology, University of California at Davis, Davis, CA 95616, USA; [3]Department of Medicine, Research Unit of Autoimmune Diseases, Chaim Sheba Medical Center, Tel-Hashomer, Israel, 52621.; [4]Division of Rheumatology/Allergy and Clinical Immunology, University of California at Davis, Davis, CA, 95616, USA

Abbreviations: Cardiovascular Disease (CVD), Cholesterol Ester Transfer Protein (CETP), Conjugated Linoleic Acids (CLA), High-Density Lipoprotein (HDL), Interferon-γ (IF-γ), Interleukin-1 (IL-1), Lecithin:Cholesterol Acyltransferase (LCAT), Leukotrienes (LT), Lipopolysaccharide (LPS), Lipoxygenase (LO), Low-Density Lipoprotein (LDL), Non-Steroidal Anti-Inflammatory Drugs (NSAIDS), Phosphatidylcholine (PC), Phophatidylethanolamine (PE), Rheumatoid Arthritis (RA) , Systemic Lupus Erythematosus (SLE), Triacylglyceride (TAG), Tumor Necrosis Factor-α (TNF-α), Very-Low Density Lipoprotein (VLDL),

1. INTRODUCTION

Fatty acids are unique among the major macronutrients in that they survive digestion intact, remodeling the composition of tissues and fluids so that they, to a large extent, reflect dietary intake. Because the specific structures of fatty acids influence their physiological and biochemical properties in cells, nutrition and specifically the intake of dietary lipids have major implications for metabolic regulation and have important effects on the prevention and treatment of disease. The role lipids play in modulating metabolic processes is tied to their physical structure. Lipids, in contrast to proteins, do not have activities, but rather exert their biochemical influence by changing the physical structure of membranes and other lipid-containing assemblies. Perhaps more importantly for immunology, fatty acids are substrates for the production of several classes of bioactive chemical mediators, molecules that signal a diverse array of physiological actions.

Although some fatty acids are synthesized *de novo*, polyunsaturated fatty acids (PUFA) are derived almost exclusively from the diet. As PUFA act as substrates for the synthesis of bioactive lipids, including eicosanoids, significant and directed modulation of physiology is achievable through diet. Thus, an understanding of fatty acid structure and metabolism is key to making rational decisions about the use of dietary lipids in the treatment or prevention of disease.

2. FATTY ACID METABOLISM

The following is a brief review of fatty acid metabolism and nomenclature intended to aid the reader in understanding the biochemistry of fatty acids.

2.1. Nomenclature

Fatty acids are hydrocarbon chains of varying lengths that contain a terminal carboxylic acid and that often contain one or several double bonds. These double bonds are inserted enzymatically by desaturase enzymes. The systematic method for naming fatty acids includes information on the chain length of the fatty acid and the number and position of the unsaturated bonds. A sixteen carbon satu-

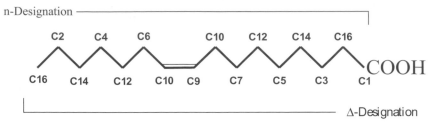

Figure 1. The systematic naming of palmitoleic acid. The sixteen-carbon fatty acid has its double bond at the 7th carbon when named using the n-designation system (16:1n7) and at the 9th carbon when named by the Δ-designation system (16:1 Δ9).

rated fatty acid (palmitic acid) would be given the numerical name 16:0, because it contains sixteen carbons and no double bonds. The insertion of a single double bond into this fatty acid would change the numerical designation to 16:1 (palmitoleic acid). There are two distinct systems for describing the location of the double bond, the n-designation or the Δ-designation. Using the n-designation, the position of the double bond is identified by counting the carbons from the methyl end of the fatty acid to the double bond (Fig. 1). Using the Δ-designation, the position of the double bond is identified by counting the carbons from the carboxylic acid to the double bond (Fig. 1). The Δ-designation system typically identifies the position of all double bonds in the fatty acid. Thus, linoleic acid is named 18:2 Δ9, 12 by the Δ-designation system. Alternatively, the n-designation system typically identifies only the carbon involved in the first occurrence of a double bond, counted from the methyl end of the fatty acid. Thus, linoleic acid is named 18:2n6 by the n-designation system. Although not explicitly, this system still identifies the position of all of the double bonds, because double bonds, with few exceptions, are inserted into a fatty acid with a spacing of three carbons. Thus, the name 18:2n6 identifies the position of the double bonds as n-6 and n-9. The reason for maintaining two systems of nomenclature arises from the distinct needs of nutritionists and biochemists. As metabolic modifications of fatty acids all occur stereospecifically from the carboxylic terminus, the Δ-designation is useful for describing the activity of enzymes such as the Δ9 desaturase. The n-designation is particularly useful for nutritionists. Because all human desaturases act on the carboxylic acid side of the Δ9 carbon, humans can not alter the double bonds on the methyl side of the Δ9 carbon. Thus, the n-designation of any unsaturated

fatty acid consumed in the diet will remain constant, no matter what further modification are made to the fatty acid after consumption. Because of this constant property of dietary fatty acids, individual fatty acids can be grouped by their n-designation "family". This property also explains why humans have requirements for both n-6 and n-3 fatty acids, as the two types of fatty acid families are not inter-convertible. Figure 2 depicts the metabolism of dietary PUFA by humans.

2.2. De Novo Biosynthesis of Fatty Acids

2.2.1. De novo synthesis

De novo fatty acid synthesis occurs predominantly in the liver. The combined action of a group of enzymes known as fatty acid synthase produce saturated fatty acids by subsequent reaction cycles, with each cycle adding an acetate group to the growing acyl chain. Thioesterases specific for fatty acid chain length remove the fatty acids from this cyclic synthesis. The dominant product of *de novo* fatty acid synthesis is palmitic acid (16:0). Other fatty acids including stearic acid (18:0) and myristic acid (14:0) are also produced by fatty acid synthase but at much lower concentrations.

2.2.2. Desaturation/elongation

Desaturation of fatty acids serves an important functional purpose in lipid metabolism. It is the physical properties of fatty acids that allow lipid molecules to serve as membranes, micelles, bulk energy storage components (triacylglycerides) and emulsions in biological systems. In hydrophobic regions, these physical properties are dominated by van der Waals forces, which cause an attraction between adjacent

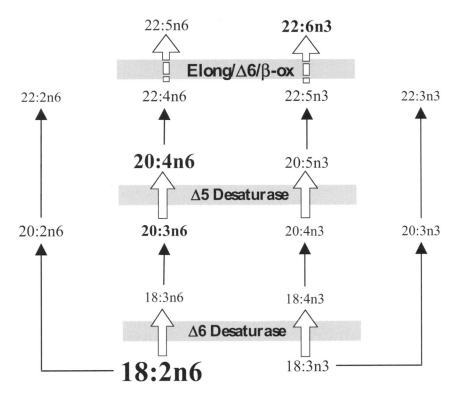

Figure 2. The metabolism of diet-derived unsaturated fatty acids in humans. The weight of the text approximates the concentration of the fatty acid found in human plasma.

fatty acid molecules. Van der Waals forces cause adjacent fatty acids to align along their carbon chains and thereby form a relatively stable but reversible bond. The degree to which adjacent fatty acids can align determines the relative strength of this interaction. The carbon chain of a saturated fatty acid is composed entirely of single (sigma) bonds that are free to rotate 180° around the bond. Thus, saturated fatty acids are free to adopt any configuration necessary to strengthen the interaction with an adjacent fatty acid. In contrast, unsaturated fatty acids have one or more double (pi) bonded carbons that do not rotate about the bond, and which therefore, impart a "kink" or un-resolvable rigidity to the fatty acid. These "kinks" do not allow adjacent fatty acids to associate as closely with one another. Because van der Waals forces are acutely sensitive to distance, unsaturated fatty acids do not form associations that are as stable as ones formed among saturated fatty acids.

The primary desaturase in *de novo* lipogenesis is the Δ9 or steroyl CoA-desaturase. This desaturase is common to both plants and animals, and is unfailingly the first desaturase to act on a saturated fatty acid. The conservation of this enzyme among plants and animals and the specific role it plays in *de novo* lipogenesis are no accident. As most fatty acids synthesized *de novo* are sixteen or eighteen carbons long, a Δ9 desaturase provides the maximal physical benefit to desaturation by introducing the bond in the center of the molecule rather than at either end. Subsequent desaturations on either side of the Δ9 desaturation have progressively diminishing effects on the physical properties of the fatty acid.

2.3. Metabolism of Dietary Fatty Acids

Dietary fatty acids can be grouped into two very general categories: those that can also be produced *de novo* by humans and those that can not. The fatty acids that can not be produced by *de novo* synthesis include the n-3 and n-6 fatty acids. These fatty acids are considered essential because one or more of the fatty acids belonging to these families (see Fig. 2) is

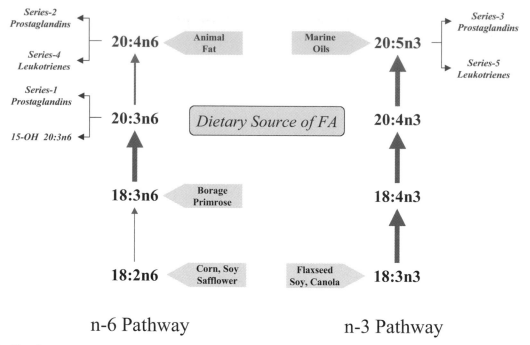

Figure 3. The dietary source and metabolism of polyunsaturated fatty acids and the production of their corresponding eicosanoids.

required for health. The desaturases that act on dietary unsaturated fatty acids include the Δ6 and Δ5 desaturases. Figure 3 shows the metabolic pathways that convert essential fatty acids. Until recently, it was assumed that the insertion of a double bond in the Δ4 position of a 22-carbon fatty acid (i.e., 22:6n3 and 22:5n6) was catalyzed by a Δ4 desaturase. Now it is known that this double bond is inserted via a multi-step process involving a chain elongation, a Δ6 desaturase and a two-carbon chain shortening via peroxisomal oxidation [1, 2]. The metabolism of dietary unsaturated fatty acids is critically important to immune function as the functional role of desaturation in fatty acid metabolism is not limited to changing the physical properties of fatty acids. Enzymes recognize fatty acids by the number and the position of their double bonds. Thus, the type of fatty acid consumed in the diet and the metabolic properties of an individual define the ways in which fatty acids get utilized *in vivo*. Science is just beginning to understand how to manipulate the dietary fat composition to control the addition of fatty acids as substrate for metabolism, and in turn, how metabolism and diet can interact to modify physiology.

3. LIPIDS AS IMMUNOLOGICAL SIGNALING MOLECULES

3.1. Eicosanoids

Eicosanoids are a group of oxygenated fatty acids with diverse and potent biological activity, produced via the action of the cyclooxygenase, lipoxygenase and epoxygenase pathways. Because the predominant substrate for these pathways is arachidonic acid (20:4n6), the pathways producing eicosanoids are termed the "arachidonate cascade". Although 20:4n6 is the primary substrate for the arachidonate cascade, other fatty acids including 20:3n6 and 20:5n3 can be converted into active eicosanoids. The variety of eicosanoid products and their correspondingly diverse physiological effects have been well characterized, and probably represent the best-understood relationship between lipids and biological function.

3.1.2. Prostanoids

Prostanoids are a diverse group of fatty acids oxygenated by the enzyme cyclooxygenase (COX-1 and

COX-2). The first committed step in the production of prostaglandins from 20:4n6 involves the addition of oxygen to 20:4n6 via cyclooxygenase. The oxygenated fatty acid (prostaglandin G_2; PGG_2) is then acted on by a peroxidase, producing prostaglandin H_2 (PGH_2). PGH_2 serves as the substrate for the production of a wide variety of prostanoids, including thromboxane A_2 (TxA_2), prostaglandin D_2 (PGD_2), prostaglandin E_2 (PGE_2), prostaglandin I_2 (PGI_2) and prostaglandin G_2 (PGG_2). The presence and distribution of active prostanoid resulting from the enzymatic conversion of PGH_2 are cell-specific.

The primary prostanoid in immune function is PGE_2, which is associated with redness, edema, heat and pain. The pro-inflammatory PGE_2 is produced primarily by leukocytes that migrate into the area of the inflammation, yet the production of PGE_2 is not regulated in a simple fashion. There are two distinct isoforms of cyclooxygenase (COX-1 and COX-2). The first isoform, COX-1, is constitutively expressed in most cells and does not appear responsive to external stimuli [3]. Considerable scientific interest is focused on the second isoform, COX-2, as COX-2 is expressed in response to stimuli and has thus been implicated in the production of inflammatory prostanoids [3]. It is the operational assumption of a large pharmaceutical initiative that the selective inhibition of COX-2 allows for normal prostanoid synthesis while decreasing the harmful and excessive production of prostanoids associated with inflammation. In adjuvant-induced inflammation in rats, the inhibition of COX-2 by the specific inhibitor SC-58125 not only decreased PGE_2 concentrations and reduced swelling; it also decreased the expression of COX-2 [4]. As positive results emerge from the large populations consuming COX-2 inhibitors, the selective inhibition of COX-2 as a pharmacological target is becoming increasingly accepted. It remains undetermined whether dietary lipids exert any COX-2 specific effects.

Individual prostaglandins belong to families of prostanoids that are grouped by the fatty acid substrate from which the prostaglandin is synthesized. Prostaglandins produced from 20:4n6 include PGH_2, PGD_2, PGE_2, $PGF_{2\alpha}$ and PGI_2 and are termed the series-2 prostaglandins. The prostaglandins produced from 20:3n6 and 20:5n3 are termed the series-1 and series-3 prostaglandins, respectively. The primary series-1 and series-3 prostaglandins related to inflammation are PGE_1 and PGE_3.

3.1.2. Leukotrienes

Leukotrienes (LT) are a class of eicosanoids produced via the action of a lipoxygenase (LO) enzyme. Like prostanoids, leukotrienes have potent biological activity. The first committed step in the formation of leukotrienes from 20:4n6 is the action of a 5-LO. The lipoxygenases relevant to human physiology include 5-LO, 12-LO and 15-LO. Although leukotrienes are synthesized in many cell types, they are most notably the major products of the arachidonate cascade in immune cells.

Immune cell-derived leukotrienes are predominantly synthesized via the action of the 5-LO. Upon release from membranes, 20:4n6 is converted to 5-hydroperoxy-6,8,11,14-eicosatetraenoic acid (5-HpETE) by 5-LO [3, 5]. This enzyme further catalyzes the formation of leukotriene A_4 from 5-HpETE [3, 5]. Leukotriene A_4 is thus the substrate for the formation of a variety of enzymatically and non-enzymatically produced leukotriene products. In macrophage and neutrophils, LTA_4 is converted to LTB_4 via LTA_4 hydrolase, whereas in eosinophils, LTA_4 is converted to LTC_4 by LTC synthase [5]. Other cell types such as blood monocytes produce both LTB_4 and LTC_4.

Like prostaglandins, leukotrienes are grouped by the fatty acid substrate from which they are formed. Leukotrienes produced from 20:4n6 include LTA_4, LTB_4, LTC_4, LTD_4 and LTE_4 and are thus termed series-4 leukotrienes. Leukotrienes produced from 20:5n3 include LTA_5, LTB_5, LTC_5, LTD_5 and LTE_5 and are termed series-5 leukotrienes.

3.2. Regulation of Eicosanoid Synthesis

3.2.1. Incorporation of fatty acids into membrane substrate pools

The primary substrate for eicosanoid synthesis, 20:4n6, is prevalent in the diet and is actively produced *de novo* from other n-6 fatty acids, most notably linoleic acid (18:2n6). Other fatty acids used directly or converted into substrate for eicosanoid synthesis are listed in Table 1. Because inflammatory cells do not possess the biochemical machin-

Table 1. Fatty acids and their eicosanoid products relevant to inflammation

Fatty Acid	Dietary Source	Concentration in Human Plasma[1]	Pertinent Metabolic Products	Primary Eicosanoid Products
18:2n6	Corn, Safflower, Soybean Oils	1267 ± 360	20:3n6, 20:4n6	–
18:3n6	Primrose, Borage, Perilla Oil	21 ± 10	20:3n6, 20:4n6	–
18:3n3	Linseed, Canola, Soybean Oil	25 ± 10	20:5n3	–
20:3n6	Animal Foods	64 ± 23	20:4n6	PGE_1, 15-OH-DGLA
20:4n6	Animal Foods	310 ± 95	–	PGE_2, LTB_4, TxA_2
20:5n3	Marine Oils	23 ± 15	–	PGE_3, LTB_5
22:6n3	Marine Oils	66 ± 31	20:5n3	–

[1] Expressed in micrograms per milliliter ± SD; unpublished data from FAME Analytics, Inc., West Sacramento, CA, 95691.

ery to synthesize 20:4n6 from precursor, plasma 20:4n6 represents the entire pool of 20:4n6 available for incorporation. Table 1 also reports the average concentration of 20:4n6 and other fatty acids in non-fasted human plasma.

Most cells, including inflammatory cells acquire fatty acids from plasma lipoproteins. The mechanism for incorporating 20:4n6 is of particular interest because of both the role of 20:4n6 in physiology and the fact that 20:4n6 is a fatty acid that, ultimately, must be acquired from the diet. As 20:4n6 is highly unsaturated, the primary plasma lipid pools of 20:4n6 are PL and cholesterol esters. Therefore, inflammatory cells are unlikely to acquire 20:4n6 via the traditional lipoprotein lipase pathway. In human fibroblasts, the inhibition of low-density lipoprotein (LDL) uptake from plasma was demonstrated to completely eliminate the incorporation of 20:4n6 [6]. The inhibition of LDL uptake also eliminated the production of prostaglandins. The accumulation of 20:4n6 by immune cells is similarly dependent on the uptake of lipoprotein lipids. Arachidonic acid present in the phosphatidylinositol of chylomicrons (particles largely responsible for distributing dietary lipids to tissues) is transferred to high-density lipoproteins in plasma [7]. Recent data demonstrates that human monocytes are able to acquire lipoprotein phospholipids intact by endocytosis via the action of the scavenger receptor BI [8]. Thus, it now appears that inflammatory cells acquire 20:4n6 at least in part as intact phospholipid, obtained by the

uptake of plasma lipoproteins. This is interesting in light of the fact that the uptake of damaged LDL by macrophage is implicated as a seminal event in the progression of atherosclerosis [9, 10].

Mammalian cells and immune cells in particular regulate the concentration and distribution of 20:4n6 with apparently considerable control. In fact, unique and highly selective phospholipid molecular species exist, acting, in-as-much as is known, solely as membrane pools for 20:4n6 fated to eicosanoid synthesis. These unique membrane molecules include phospholipids with alkyl and alky-1-enyl linked fatty acids in the sn-1 position [11]. Although these phospholipid species are highly enriched with 20:4n6, the distribution of newly incorporated 20:4n6 follows a pattern typical of many cell types. As a general rule in lipid metabolism, newly incorporated fatty acids are found first in phosphatidylcholine (PC). After a short time, the fatty acids are redistributed among phospholipids, only then reflecting the expected acyl-specific distributions. This dynamic remodeling of lipid membranes also occurs in inflammatory cells after the initial incorporation of 20:4n6. In neutrophils treated with exogenous fatty acid for 5 minutes, 20:4n6 was incorporated into phosphatidylinositol and PC to the virtual exclusion of other lipid classes [12]. After 120 minutes of treatment, 20:4n6 was found in 1-alkyl-acyl-and 1-alk-1-enyl-acyl-sn-glycero-3 PC and -phosphatidylethanolamine (PE) molecular species [12]. The cause of this dynamic remodeling of membranes is a difference in how fatty acids get incorporated into different phospholipid classes. Early work by Lands and colleagues [13] demonstrated that 20:4n6 was not used for *de novo* synthesis of phospholipids, but instead acylated into lysophospholipids. As 20:4n6 is incorporated into cells, it is converted to an acyl-CoA thioester, and in this form acts as substrate for CoA-dependant acyltransferase. CoA-dependant acyltransferase catalyzes the esterification of fatty acid CoA esters into lysophospholipids, predominantly at the endoplasmic reticulum. Thus, the initial incorporation of 20:4n6 into membranes follows the Lands pathway of acyl "remodeling" rather than biosynthesis. Because lysoPC is the predominant acceptor molecule for CoA-dependant acyl transferase, PC accumulates most of the newly incorporated 20:4n6. Following the accretion of 20:4n6 by PC, other enzymes catalyze the movement of esterified 20:4n6 to alkyl- and alk-1-enyl phospholipids. In a series of publications, Chilton and colleagues (reviewed in [11]) described the action of a CoA-independent transacylase that shuttles 20:4n6 from PC to 1-alkyl-2-arachidonoyl- and alk-1-enyl-2-arachidonoyl-PE. This reaction does not require the release of 20:4n6 by phospholipase, nor does it require the formation of arachidonoyl-CoA thioesters. The alkyl- and alk-1-enyl phospholipids formed serve as the membrane pool of 20:4n6 for eicosanoid synthesis. The dynamic distribution of 20:4n6 among phospholipid species is thus the result of several distinct transferase enzymes.

This section provides only a cursory review of 20:4n6 metabolism, and the reader should be aware that many more enzyme activities and lipid species are involved in regulating membrane 20:4n6 composition. For a review of the subject, the reader is referred to reference [11].

3.2.2. *Induction of eicosanoid synthesis*

Inflammatory cells are induced to synthesize eicosanoids by a variety of extracellular stimuli, including eicosanoids themselves. Other extracellular stimuli that induce eicosanoid production include hormones such as bradykinin [14], angiotensin II [15-17] and estradiol [18] as well as a variety of non-specific stressors acting through the NFkB pathway [19]. The specific mechanism of induction by these medi-

ators varies, but they all induce the action of phospholipases and the selective release of 20:4n6 from membranes [20-22]. The phospholipase most closely associated with eicosanoid production is phospholipase A_2, which catalyzes the hydrolysis of the sn-2 position of phospholipids. Arachidonic acid, like other unsaturated fatty acids, is esterified to the sn-2 position of phospholipids. Yet the hydrolysis of 20:4n6 from membranes occurs in response to inflammatory stimulation to the virtual exclusion of other unsaturated fatty acids, suggesting that pool- and purpose-specific phospholipases A_2 exist. In fact, the hydrolytic cleavage of 20:4n6 from membranes appears in and of itself to be carried out by a variety of phospholipases acting on numerous 20:4n6-containing phospholipid pools. Fonteh and Chilton [23] observed that upon the stimulation of mast cells, free 20:4n6 and 20:4n6 utilized for leukotriene synthesis arose from the distinct membrane pools.

4. LIPIDS AND IMMUNE DYSFUNCTION

4.1. Plasma Lipid Changes Associated with Inflammation

Chronic inflammation is a strong risk factor for progressive cardiovascular disease (CVD), yet the mechanism of this association is just now emerging. In general, inflammation causes a modulation of lipoprotein metabolism that mirrors changes in lipoprotein profiles associated with increased risk for CVD. However, the molecular basis for this metabolic shift in response to inflammation is largely unknown. For a current and thorough examination of this topic, the reader is directed to an excellent review [24].

4.1.1. *Plasma VLDL*

The hallmark changes in lipoprotein profiles associated with inflammation include an increased very-low density lipoprotein (VLDL) concentration and a decreased high-density lipoprotein (HDL) concentration [24]. As VLDL contains predominantly triacylglyceride (TAG), TAG concentrations are also increased in plasma during inflammation [25, 26]. Attention has focused on determining whether increasing VLDL concentrations are the result of increased production of VLDL or decreased clearance. Grunfeld, Feingold and colleagues [24, 27, 28] demonstrated increased *de novo* lipogenesis and decreased TAG clearance in patients with HIV infection. These observations were also correlated with plasma interferon-γ (IF-γ) concentrations, suggesting that IF-γ may mediate this effect. Further, the same group demonstrated that low doses of lipopolysaccharide (LPS, a surrogate for microbial infection) increase *de novo* lipogenesis, increase fatty acid mobilization from adiposites and decrease hepatic fatty acid catabolism [27, 29]. The inflammatory cytokines tumor necrosis factor-α (TNF-α) and interleukin-1 (IL-1) also elevate plasma TAG concentrations. In response to TNF-α, *de novo* lipogenesis and VLDL secretion are increased [30–32]. The TAG elevating effect of TNF-α is not linked to a decreased clearance of TAG from the plasma by lipoprotein lipase [31, 33]. Interestingly, the VLDL produced *de novo* during inflammation contain increased concentrations of sphingomyelin [30]. Sphingolipids are a class of phospholipid with diverse biological function, and may cause the inhibition of VLDL clearance.

4.1.2. *Plasma LDL*

The overall concentration of LDL decreases during inflammation, but the concentration of a particularly atherogenic subclass of LDL, the small, dense LDL particles, increases [24]. Small dense LDL are more atherogenic than normal LDL due to their increased uptake by interstitial macrophage. The increased uptake by macrophage may result from an increased susceptibility to oxidation [34] or an association with proteoglycans [35, 36]. The clearance of small dense LDL is also diminished relative to normal LDL because of a decreased affinity of LDL-receptor for small dense particles [37]. Compounding these pro-atherogenic factors is the possibility that chronic inflammation could itself cause an increase in the oxidation of LDL particles. LDL from Syrian hamsters treated with LPS contained more conjugated dienes (a marker for the oxidation of PUFA) and were more susceptible to copper-induced oxidation than controls [38]. Inflammation is by nature an oxidant generating condition, and it is not unlikely that this increased oxidant stress could modify LDL par-

ticles. Moreover, the increased synthesis of lipoprotein particles without an accompanying increase in particle clearance means that the circulating particles themselves are necessarily older than rapidly cleared particles. Lipoprotein particle age is correlated with the oxidizability of the particle [39]. It is not clear what compositional or conformational changes in the lipoprotein particles mediate this increase in oxidizability.

Increased hepatic synthesis of lipid is also reflected in the composition of LDL during inflammation. In parallel with VLDL compositions, the concentration of TAG and free cholesterol are increased in LDL from animals stimulated with LPS [40]. Perhaps more importantly, the concentration of sphingomyelin in LDL is increased during inflammation as a result of increased hepatic palmitoyltransferase activity, which catalyzes the rate-limiting step in *de novo* sphingomyelin synthesis [41]. Lipopolysaccharide and IL-1 each induced an increase in hepatic palmitoyltransferase activity in Syrian hamsters that in turn caused an increase in the sphingomyelin concentration of plasma LDL particles [41]. Hydrolysis of sphingomyelin by endogenous enzymes yields the highly bioactive ceramide and sphingosine compounds. Ceramide in particular is produced from sphingomyelin by sphingomyelinase at the arterial endothelial cell wall [42]. In a series of reports, Tabas and colleagues [42–48] demonstrated the critical role of LDL sphingomyelin in atherogenesis. Co-incubation of lipoprotein particles with lipoprotein lipase and sphingomyelinase lead to a massive accumulation of the LDL particles on a bovine endothelial cell layer *in vitro* [43]. This accumulation required the activity of both enzymes. Further studies demonstrated that LDL found in lesions was ten- to fifty-fold enriched with ceramide relative to LDL found in plasma [46]. The ceramide found in lesional LDL was almost exclusively found in aggregated particles, with very low concentrations of ceramide observed in unaggregated lesional particles [46]. Thus, the hydrolysis of LDL sphingomyelin is intimately involved in the aggregation and deposition of LDL particles that represents the seminal event in the progression of atherosclerosis. In addition to compositional changes in LDL, several cell types found in atherosclerotic lesions contained increased concentrations of sphingomyelinase [42, 48]. Clearly, the up-regulation of hepatic sphingomyelin synthesis by inflammation is a key factor in the link between immune dysfunction and CVD, and much more investigation will continue in this area.

4.1.3. Plasma HDL

The lipid composition of HDL is dominated by phospholipids and cholesterol esters [49]. A primary function of HDL is to transport cholesterol from tissues back to the liver in the form of cholesterol esters. This function of HDL also helps to remove excess cholesterol from vascular lesions. This process is often referred to as "reverse cholesterol transport" and is the basis for the assumption that HDL is the "good" cholesterol. Like other lipoproteins, HDL concentrations are responsive to inflammation and infection. In animal models, plasma concentrations of HDL are decreased as the result of surrogate-induced inflammation [40, 50]. In humans, HDL concentrations are diminished in patients with disorders involving chronic inflammation, including systemic lupus erythematosus (SLE) [51] and rheumatoid arthritis (RA) [52]. As low concentrations of HDL are linked with an increased risk for CVD, the pro-atherogenic effects of inflammation may be in part mediated by HDL concentrations. A diminished HDL concentration could inhibit reverse cholesterol transport or even increase the oxidation of LDL particles, as HDL contains enzymes that help prevent LDL oxidation [24].

Specific changes in the lipid composition of HDL are associated with chronic inflammation. In parallel with VLDL and LDL, HDL from LPS-stimulated hamsters contained increased concentrations of sphingolipids [41]. The plasma HDL cholesterol ester concentrations of green monkeys treated with LPS were significantly lower than controls [53]. Similar results were obtained in cynomolgus monkeys injected with LPS and TNF-α, as HDL from the treated group contained less cholesterol ester and more free cholesterol than controls [26].

The effects of inflammation on HDL composition are caused by changes in the activity of several key metabolic enzymes. The movement of cholesterol out of cells and into HDL is partially aided by the enzyme lecithin:cholesterol acyltransferase (LCAT). Lecithin:cholesterol acyltransferase converts free cholesterol, which is soluble almost exclu-

sively in phospholipid, to cholesterol ester, thereby facilitating the movement of cholesterol into the core of the HDL particle. Additionally, the conversion of free cholesterol to cholesterol ester maintains the gradient required to move free cholesterol from cells to the HDL particles. Inflammation reduces not only the activity of LCAT in plasma, but also the expression of LCAT mRNA in the liver [26, 54]. Once cholesterol is transferred into HDL and converted to cholesterol ester, the HDL particle is subsequently depleted of cholesterol ester by one of several mechanisms. The first mechanism involves an equilibration reaction between HDL, which donate a cholesterol ester, and VLDL or chylomicrons, which donate a TAG. The enzyme responsible for this exchange activity is cholesterol ester transfer protein (CETP). Under LPS stimulation, plasma CETP activity in Syrian hamsters was significantly reduced relative to controls [55]. Additionally, the expression of CETP mRNA in adipose, heart and muscle was depleted following LPS stimulation [55]. It is plausible that the diminished CETP expression was secondary and responsive to the decreased HDL concentrations, as CETP is responsible for depleting the core contents of HDL. Regardless, a reduction in CETP activity would substantially diminish effectiveness of HDL to conduct reverse cholesterol transport. Taken together, diminished LCAT and CETP activities could severely cripple reverse cholesterol transport and may in large part be responsible for the pro-atherogenic activity of chronic inflammation.

High-density lipoprotein particles are important to the successful clearance of a variety of foreign particles from circulation including LPS. In plasma, LPS is bound by HDL and, in vitro, the uptake of LPS by macrophages is pro-inflammatory if ingested without HDL but not if initially bound to HDL [56]. Furthermore, in vivo HDL protects mice from septic shock apparently via this mechanism [57].

4.2. Rheumatoid Arthritis

Lipoprotein metabolism is altered in patients with RA. The plasma concentrations of HDL and apoA1 protein were lower in RA patients than in controls [52], and lipoprotein (a), a marker for many inflammatory diseases, was increased in RA patients relative to controls [52, 58, 59]. These differences were more pronounced in patients with active RA relative to controls than in patients with inactive RA relative to controls [60]. The apoA1-lowering effect of RA was also observed in juvenile chronic arthritis, suggesting that it is a hallmark of the disease [61] consistent among varying age groups. In one major epidemiological study following 52,800 individuals over approximately 21 years, serum cholesterol concentrations were closely related to the incidence of RA; however, the relationship was clearly different between men and women [62]. Serum cholesterol was positively associated with rheumatoid factor-positive RA in women and rheumatoid factor-negative RA in men. No association was observed between rheumatoid factor-negative women or rheumatoid factor positive men and serum cholesterol.

There are also indications that the type and the amount of plasma lipids influence or are reflective of RA. Both the concentration and composition of circulating plasma free fatty acids significantly modulated T-lymphocyte proliferation when these conditions were reproduced *in vitro* [63]. Thus, assuming these observations hold true *in vivo*, inflammatory responses may be modulated by diet, state of fasting and other factors influencing the concentration of free fatty acids in the plasma, such as diabetes and obesity. Notably, a trial of 21 recently diagnosed and 21 chronic RA patients found that the concentrations 18:2n6 and 18:2n3 in plasma PC were significantly lower in RA patients than in controls [64]. Linoleic and linolenic acids are biosynthetic precursors to fatty acids used as substrate for eicosanoid formation, and are the predominant PUFA consumed in the diet. Interestingly, the concentration of these fatty acids continued to drop with disease duration and correlated well with acute phase proteins orosomucoid and C-reactive protein. No attempt was made to determine whether these fatty acids were unusually distributed among lipid classes (only PC was measured), converted to products, consumed in lower quantities by the patient population or more actively catabolized.

Other metabolic changes observed in RA patients may also manifest themselves as an altered plasma lipid profile. Circulating carnitine concentrations were significantly lower in RA patients than in controls [65]. Carnitine is intimately involved in coordinating energy production with lipid catabolism, and

fluctuations in carnitine concentrations are associated with altered lipid compositions and degenerative diseases including aging [66, 67]. Additionally, the concentration of monomeric lipoprotein lipase, a competitive inhibitor of active dimeric lipoprotein lipase, is negatively correlated with inflammatory variables, including orosomucoid and C-reactive protein [68]. Thus, the composition and the concentration of plasma lipids stand to be significantly altered by the inflammation caused by RA. These changes parallel changes associated with the degenerative processes of CVD.

4.3. Systemic Lupus

Systemic lupus erythematosus is a complex immunological disorder that may be triggered by multiple stimuli [69], follow at least three distinct patterns of disease activity and lead to myriad distinct physiological outcomes [70]. Premature CVD is common in SLE patients [71, 72], and often occurs as early as childhood. The underlying cause of this early onset CVD may be chronic inflammation resulting from SLE or corticosteroid use or both. Both inflammation and corticosteroid use are hypothesized to mediate CVD by causing a dysregulation of lipoprotein metabolism [71, 73]. In a trial of one hundred and thirty-four SLE patients, 40% expressed sustained hypercholesterolemia and 35% expressed intermittent hypercholesterolemia [74]. The dose of steroid treatment and the age of SLE onset were well correlated with the incidence of hypercholesterolemia [74]. Further, intervention by the diminishment of steroidal therapy and the management of hypertension among SLE patients improved CVD outcome [75]. The specific alterations in fasted-state lipoprotein metabolism associated with SLE include elevated TAG and VLDL-C and low concentrations of HDL-C (not defined) [51]. These alterations are accentuated in active disease relative to inactive SLE [51]. Dysregulation of lipid metabolism in the liver may be secondary to SLE; however, the lipoprotein profiles described above are consistent even when excluding patients with any non-lipid signs of liver dysfunction [51]. Each of these particles and their lipid components is synthesized largely in the liver, yet it is not clear how SLE affects de novo lipid synthesis. Studies on the concentration of de novo synthesized fatty acids in plasma have not been reported. Alternative to a dysregulation of de novo lipogenesis, elevated circulating lipids could result from a decreased clearance of lipid from the blood. In one interesting study, labeled, synthetic chylomicron analogues were injected into SLE patients and their healthy, age and sex-matched controls. By following the decay of signal from the blood of the test subjects, the authors determined that patients with SLE had decreased lipolysis and decreased lipoprotein remnant clearance from plasma, suggesting that the utilization of plasma lipids was altered in patients with SLE [76].

4.4. Inflammatory Bowel Disease

Inflammatory bowel disease (IBD) encompasses several disorders, including Crohn's disease and ulcerative colitis. The tissue damage observed in most IBD patients is the result of a secondary inflammatory response rather than the initiating event itself [77]. This secondary inflammation is associated with a significant elevation of prostaglandin formation in the lower bowel [77]. In a series of studies by Rask-Madsen et al. [78–80], patients with IBD had bowel concentrations of eicosanoids specific for and reflective of individual inflammatory disorders. Patients with Crohn's disease had significantly elevated rectal concentrations of PGE_2 during active disease [78]. As patients with inactive disease did not also express this difference, elevated PGE_2 rectal concentrations were predictive of a Crohn's flare-up. In patients with ulcerative colitis, an increase in both PGE_2 and thromboxane B_2 was observed independent of disease severity [79]. The LTB_4 and 5-OH 20:4n6 concentration of intestinal mucosa is also elevated in IBD patients relative to controls. The obvious contribution of inflammatory eicosanoids to the progression of IBD is interesting in light of the fact that non-steroidal anti-inflammatory drugs (NSAIDs) exacerbate the inflammation (reviewed in Krause and DuBois [77]).

Diet clearly influences the appearance and progression of IBD, although the exact modulatory agents are not yet apparent. In a questionnaire trial, patients with active IBD had consumed significantly more sucrose, animal fat and cholesterol than control patients. Very few studies have quantified differences in circulating lipid metabolites in active

or inactive IBD. In one study, circulating cholestanol (a precursor of cholesterol) was increased in IBD patients relative to controls [81]. This finding was linked to a dysfunction of cholesterol elimination. The fatty acid composition of plasma is also reported to change in response to IBD. The plasma acyl composition of patients with IBD contained increased saturated fatty acids and decreased monounsaturated fatty acids [81]. Inflammatory bowel disease patients also have elevated n-3 fatty acids and decreased n-6 fatty acids in plasma relative to controls [81]. This difference persists even in inactive IBD [81].

The accumulation and release of 20:4n6 is altered in the intestinal tissue of IBD patients. Surgically resected intestinal sections from patients with Crohn's disease and ulcerative colitis displayed an increased activity of the phospholipase A_2 responsible for hydrolyzing 20:4n6 from plasmenylethanolamine relative to control patients [82]. The concentration of the phospholipase A_2 responsible for general membrane PC hydrolysis (not associated with eicosanoid synthesis) was not altered [82]. Additionally, the acyl composition of plasmenylethanolamine from IBD patients contained more 20:4n6 than that from control patients [83, 84].

5. TREATMENT OF INFLAMMATION WITH DIETARY LIPIDS

Eicosanoids are potent chemical mediators of inflammation, and are invariably produced by the conversion of diet-derived fatty acids by specific enzymes. Consequently, attempts to modulate the production of eicosanoids must target either the enzyme activities responsible for synthesizing eicosanoids or the concentration of fatty acid substrate entering the biological system through the diet. Ultimately, these two approaches are more similar than different in that they both aim to change the eicosanoid metabolite profile. However, there are distinct problems and benefits associated with modulating inflammation by controlling the dietary substrate. The encouraging data are many, if controversial, and describe how dietary fatty acid composition influences eicosanoid production in ways that current pharmacological practice does not. For instance, a typical treatment of inflammation involves the prescription of NSAIDs that achieve apparent benefits of managing the phenotypic hallmarks of inflammation. However, the specific nature of the pharmacological intervention is an inhibition of the COX enzyme, and no reduction in 5-LO activity is obtained via NSAID treatment. Thus, the production of LTB_4, a potent pro-inflammatory leukotriene is not greatly affected by the treatment. Alternatively, substrate manipulation via dietary choice is capable of altering the very pools from which the fatty acid for both prostaglandin and leukotriene production are drawn. Therefore, diet is capable of modulating eicosanoid metabolism upstream of the current pharmacological intervention. Additionally, manipulating the lipid substrate pool offers the possibility of changing the final product in a way not currently possible by enzyme inhibition. Apart from the eicosanoid products discussed above, novel eicosanoids with unknown biological activity can be formed from non-20:4n6 substrate [85]. Therefore, diet, at least in theory, may prove as or more useful than pharmacological interventions in the management of chronic inflammation.

In practice the results have been less promising. Despite years of research, it is still not clear what doses of dietary fatty acids are needed to produce significant changes in appropriate membrane pools. In part, this uncertainty arises from methodological hurdles, as few dietary or metabolic studies have been conducted in a truly quantitative fashion. Additionally, dietary manipulation of substrate pools must overcome the endogenous preferences of lipid metabolism enzymes, whereas pharmacology simply modifies them. For instance, 20:4n6 is clearly a preferred substrate for many metabolic activities, and the manipulation of 20:4n6 concentrations in tissues has proven difficult. Finally, dietary fatty acids are ubiquitous in foods and therefore compete significantly with any attempt to manipulate fat intakes through specific foods [86]. To modify pool-specific 20:4n6 concentrations with selected fatty acids may require a combinatorial approach, where some activities are inhibited, while the diet is carefully chosen.

5.1. Experimental Trials

Clinical and experimental trials testing the efficacy of diet on the progression of inflammatory diseases have focused primarily on how diet modulates tissue and plasma 20:4n6 content. Arachidonic acid is an obvious target for manipulation because of its role in the production of inflammatory eicosanoids. However, the incorporation of other fatty acids into important membrane pools has important physiological effects apart from diminishing the concentration of 20:4n6. Dietary oils as common as olive and fish oil show promise as anti-inflammatory agents. Likewise, oils previously considered boutique or obscure, e.g., borage, flax or primrose oil, are gaining prominence on the basis of their ability to inhibit inflammatory metabolism.

The choice of placebo has remained a pervasive controversy in trials testing the efficacy of dietary lipids in controlling inflammatory diseases. Essentially, the controversy arises from the inescapable fact that all lipids exert some physiological effect, and that, therefore, no traditional dietary lipid is an appropriate placebo. In circumventing this dilemma some researchers have used paraffin or other non-digestible lipid analogue. However, it seems only logical that future studies should focus on comparative analyses rather than isolating the effects of individual oils. In the real world, people have choices, and for an individual suffering from a chronic disease, it is relevant to know that a specific oil is more effective in treating the condition than another. Because we already know that choosing an ideal diet for all individuals and conditions is an impossibility (note the widespread recommendation for increased consumption of 18:2n6 on the basis that it lowers circulating LDL concentrations, despite the known detrimental effects of 18:2n6 on auto-immunity and cancer), individualized prescription and treatment will be the future of nutrition and medicine. To accomplish this goal, considerable information will need to be obtained about the individual responses to dietary fatty acids. A general overview of current knowledge about dietary lipids and the inhibition of inflammation follows.

5.1.1. Eicosapentaenoic and docosahexaenoic acids

Eicosapentaenoic (20:5n3) and docosahexaenoic (22:6n3) acids are found primarily in oils of marine origin. Although most closely associated with fish oil, the 20:5n3 and 22:6n3 in fish are actually the products of algal lipid synthesis. Fish oil has received a tremendous amount of attention as a dietary supplement for the treatment of inflammatory disorders. The basis for the professed effects of fish oil are the high concentrations of the n-3 PUFA 20:5n3 and 22:6n3. Interest focuses on 20:5n3 in particular because it is directly competitive with 20:4n6 for incorporation into and release from critical membrane pools, and for conversion to eicosanoids. Eicosapentaenoic acid, however, does not produce highly inflammatory eicosanoids, but rather gives rise to series-3 prostaglandins and series-5 leukotrienes that do not elicit a strong inflammatory response. The role dietary 22:6n3 plays in attenuating inflammation production is less clear. Docosahexaenoic acid is not directly converted into any major eicosanoid product, but may increase tissue concentrations of 20:5n3 via a fatty acid retro-conversion reaction. However, increasing evidence points towards a unique and independent role for 22:6n3 in modulating inflammation, unrelated to its properties as substrate for 20:5n3 production. The data relating fish oil fatty acids to inflammation are the subject of numerous of reviews [87-90], and it is not the intention of the current authors to cover all of the topics relevant to this subject. The following is only a brief summary of the physiological properties of dietary 20:5n3 and 22:6n3.

The 20:5n3 and 22:6n3 content of fish oil varies from 6–20% and 5–25% by weight, respectively [91]. Although the 22:6n3 content of some fish oils can reach 25%, it is most unusual to find 22:6n3 in greater proportion than 20:5n3. Fish oil is also a good source of 20:4n6, although the concentrations can range from nearly 0 to 15% 20:4n6 by weight [91]. Fish oil also contains minor amounts of very unusual fatty acids, including odd-chain fatty acids and fatty acids belonging to the n-4, n-5 and n-10 fatty acids. Although 22:6n3, 20:5n3 and 20:4n6 have been extensively investigated, very little attention has been paid to these unusual minor components.

The primary research interest in fish oil has been in how eicosanoids produced from 20:5n3 influence inflammation and other eicosanoid-related physiology. The incorporation of 20:5n3 into cell membranes modulates the production of pro-inflammatory eicosanoids in several ways. Eicosapentaenoic acid is a good substrate for acyla-

tion into arachidonate-containing membrane pools and for both COX and LO enzymes. The competition for acylation into similar membrane pools allows 20:5n3 to essentially dilute the concentration of 20:4n6 in these active pools. Therefore, simply by its presence, 20:5n3 can reduce the concentration of n-6-derived COX and LO products. Additionally, the conversion of 20:5n3 to eicosanoids results in less inflammatory products [92]. The conversion of 20:5n3 to a prostaglandin via COX activity produces PGE_3, a prostanoid with pro-inflammatory properties similar to PGE_2; however, PGE_3 is produced with a low efficiency [93]. The conversion of 20:5n3 to leukotriene via the 5-LO pathway produces LTB_5, a leukotriene with minimal pro-inflammatory activity. Thus, the ability of 20:5n3 to dilute 20:4n6-containing membrane pools and its relative inability to act as substrate for pro-inflammatory eicosanoids provide a partial basis for the anti-inflammatory properties of fish oil.

The cytokines TNF-α and IL-1β act as pro-inflammatory agents and are associated in many chronic inflammatory disorders with joint and tissue destruction [92, 94]. Dietary fish oil suppressed the production of TNF-α and IL-1β by immune cells in healthy men [95, 96] and women [97] and in RA patients [98]. The active agent in fish oil has not been identified, although it is suspected that, like the inhibition of pro-inflammatory eicosanoid synthesis, 20:5n3 exerts the strongest anti-TNF-α and IL-1β action.

The effects of fish oil fatty acids on inflammation may extend beyond the modulation of inflammatory mediators. *In vitro* studies of fish oil fatty acids and immune function indicate that 20:5n3 and 22:6n3 inhibit inflammatory response by inhibiting the expression and presentation of surface antigens by human monocytes. Hughes and colleagues [99] found that 20:5n3 inhibits the expression of HLA-DR (a major histocompatability complex class II protein; MHC class II) and ICAM-1 on normal human monocytes in culture. Interestingly, 22:6n3 induced the opposite effect, increasing the proportion of cultured monocytes expressing these proteins. In studying the effects of these fatty acids on IF-γ activated monocytes, both 20:5n3 and 22:6n3 diminished the proportion of cultured cells expressing HLA-DR [99]. Further studies combined the fatty acids (12 μM 20:5n3 and 8 μM 22:6n3) in a proportion typically found in dietary fish oil, and found that the mixture also inhibited antigen presentation [100]. In unstimulated, cultured monocytes, the fatty acid mixture decreased the proportion of cells expressing ICAM-1 and CD-58. In IF-γ activated monocytes, the expression of HLA-DR, HLA-DP, ICAM-1 and CD-58 were decreased relative to controls in response to the 20:5n3/22:6n3 mixture [100]. The increased expression of MHC class II and ICAM-1 expression is a characteristic feature of joint inflammation in RA patients. The attenuation of joint pain observed in RA patients in response to high doses of fish oil may be mediated by a diminished expression of cell surface antigens.

Chronic inflammation is associated with an increase in the production of oxygen radicals. These highly reactive chemical species are partially responsible for the tissue degradation observed in patients with inflammatory disease. Dietary oils rich in 18:2n6 exacerbate this oxidant state by increasing the concentration of *in vivo* free radicals, and by reducing the expression of the key anti-inflammatory cytokines IL-2 and TGF-β [101]. In contrast, dietary fish oil increased the expression of antioxidant enzymes and IL-2 in mouse autoimmune disease models [102, 103]. In humans, dietary 20:5n3 and 22:6n3 reduced the normally high concentrations of plasma hydroperoxides and nitric oxide present in SLE patients [104]. Additionally, the depressed concentration of superoxide dismutase and glutathione reductase present in SLE patients was restored by supplementation with fish oil [104]. These changes in oxidant concentration and enzyme expression were associated with an increased incidence of remission.

Numerous studies have addressed a role for fish oil in the treatment of inflammatory disease. These studies are far to numerous to review in this space. The reader is directed to several excellent reviews and books on this subject [105–107]

5.1.2. α-linolenic acid

α-Linolenic acid (18:3n3) is the metabolic precursor to the n-3 fatty acid family, which includes the long chain PUFAs 20:5n3 and 22:6n3. α-Linolenic acid is the product of plant fatty acid synthesis, and includes unsaturated bonds at each of the metabolically possible positions (higher plants express only

Δ9, Δ12 and Δ15 desaturases). In general, the consumption of 18:3n3 has dramatically decreased as the result of modern agriculture [108]. The very properties advantageous for the growth of agriculture and the stability of the food supply have led to the selection of 18:2n6-rich commodities over 18:3n3-rich commodities. Linoleic acid is typically found in high abundance in seed oils (which are not only processed into food, but also feed to livestock, compounding the accumulation of n-6 fatty acids in the food supply), whereas 18:3n3 is found in the leafy portions of plants. Estimates of the ratio of n-6 to n-3 fatty acids consumed throughout human evolution range from 1:1 to 2:1 [106, 108]. In stark contrast to this balanced intake, the ratio of n-6 to n-3 fatty acids consumed in today's diet ranges from 20 to 50:1. Because n-6 fatty acids serve as direct or indirect precursors to the arachidonate cascade, the monumental shift in the dietary n-6 to n-3 ratio likely has much to do with rising rates of CVD and auto-immunity.

A primary dietary source of 18:3n3 is canola oil, which contains 18:3n3 as 10–15% of its fatty acid composition [91]. Canola oil is produced from rapeseed by solvent extraction. Canola oil also contains about twice as much 18:2n6 as 18:3n3 [91]. Another major source of 18:3n3 in the diet is soybean oil, which contains as much as 10% 18:3n3 [91]. However, soybean oil typically also contains 18:2n6 at approximately 50–60% of its fatty acids. Thus, although soybeans probably contribute the majority of 18:3n3 consumed in the diet, the resulting consumption of 18:3n3 is swamped by the high concentration of co-consumed 18:2n6. The dietary oil yielding both the highest concentration of 18:3n3 and the smallest n-6 to n-3 ratio is linseed, or flaxseed oil [91]. Flaxseed oil contains up to 60% of its fatty acids as 18:3n3 and contains only about 15–20% 18:2n6 [91]. Flaxseed therefore represents one of the few seed oils rich in 18:3n3. In accordance with its increased degree of unsaturation, flaxseed oil is far less stable than other dietary oils, and its production for consumption has remained largely a cottage industry. In fact, the rapid oxidation and polymerization of flaxseed oil is the basis for its inclusion in common paint.

The main action of dietary 18:3n3 on inflammation is not as a direct inhibitor of 20:4n6 metabolism, but rather as a substrate for the endogenous production of 20:5n3. Eicosapentaenoic acid in turn is converted to relatively non-active inflammatory eicosanoids in competition with 20:4n6. Dietary 18:3n3 is converted to longer chain n-3 fatty acids *in vivo*; however, the degree of conversion is dependant on other dietary components [105]. The main interaction affecting the conversion of 18:3n3 to 20:5n3 and 22:6n3 occurs with dietary 18:2n6 [105]. In doubling the 18:2n6 concentration of a test diet from 4.7 to 9.3% of total calories, the conversion of 18:3n3 to longer chain PUFA was diminished by approximately 50% [109]. These data suggest a competition between 18:3n3 and 18:2n6 for either elongation/desaturation, or esterification into glycerolipid pools. They also indicate that the efficacy of dietary 18:3n3 in treating inflammatory disorders is complicated by other dietary factors. However, increasing the dietary consumption of 18:3n3 by substituting 18:3n3 oils into a typical Western diet led to the increased accumulation of 20:5n3 in plasma lipids and, importantly, neutrophil phospholipids [110]. Therefore, 18:3n3 may be a useful dietary agent for modulating inflammation, particularly among vegetarians, whose diets do not contain longer chain PUFA.

Dietary 18:3n3 can influence the production of bioactive chemical mediators of inflammation at a number of levels. In one intriguing study, high concentrations of dietary 18:3n3 in the form of perilla oil reduced the concentration of alkyacyl-linked PC in rat kidney membranes when compared to corn oil [52]. The alkylacyl glycerolipids are an active substrate pool of 20:4n3 for the synthesis of eicosanoids. Therefore, dietary n-3 fatty acids may be able to change the size of the eicosanoid substrate pool. No subsequent experiments have corroborated this result. The synthesis of eicosanoids in animals fed n-3 fatty acids is also altered. In rats fed various forms of n-3 and n-6 fatty acids, dietary 18:3n3 suppressed prostaglandin production in a dose-dependant fashion, but not as efficiently as longer chain n-3 PUFA [111]. Similar results were obtained in BALB/c mice, as dietary 18:3n3 reduced the production of both prostaglandins and leukotrienes in *ex vivo* splenocytes [112]. In humans, the consumption of 18:3n3 also inhibits the expression of certain cytokines. Caughey and colleagues [95] demonstrated that dietary flaxseed oil led to a significant reduction in plasma TNF-α and IL-1

concentrations. Additionally, the proliferation of peripheral blood mononuclear cells in response to concanavalin-A and phytohemagglutinin-P was suppressed in subjects fed flaxseed oil as compared with controls [113].

Although not nearly as extensively investigated as longer chain n-3 fatty acids or 18:3n6, several investigators have examined the utility of dietary 18:3n3 as an anti-inflammatory agent in immune dysfunction. Dietary flaxseed oil was investigated as a potential therapeutic agent in the treatment of lupus nephritis. The glomerular filtration rate was increased and the onset of proteinuria was delayed in mice fed 15% flaxseed oil for 14 weeks relative to control mice [114]. Additionally, flaxseed oil-fed mice had significantly longer lifespans than mice fed a control diet. The beneficial effects of dietary flaxseed oil on lupus nephritis in mice led to a small clinical trial in humans. Increasing doses of flaxseed oil decreased platelet platelet aggregation factor-induced aggregation, diminished proteinuria, depressed serum creatine concentrations and decreased CD11b expression on blood neutrophils [115]. All of these effects support a role for flaxseed oil in the effective treatment of lupus nephritis. However, the size of this clinical trial was extremely small (8 participants), and it is curious that follow-up studies were not performed. Two experiments indicate a utility for 18:3n3 in the treatment of IBD. In mice with experimental IBD, the administration of perilla oil (rich in 18:3n3) increased colonic phospholipid 20:5n3 concentrations and decreased colonic phospholipid 20:4n6 concentrations [84]. Accordingly, the production of LTB$_4$ and subjective colon damage scores were diminished in the perilla oil-infused group relative to the controls group [83]. Although promising in the treatment of IBD and lupus nephritis, the use of flaxseed oil in the treatment of RA has not met with great success [116].

5.1.3. γ-linolenic and dihomo-γ-linolenic acid

γ-Linolenic acid (18:3n6) is an uncommon fatty acid produced in low abundance by lower plants. The formation of 18:3n6 requires the activity of a $\Delta 6$ desaturase, and thus can not be produced by standard agricultural crop plants. The primary sources of 18:3n6 in the diet are evening primrose oil and borage oil. Evening primrose oil is derived from the seeds of *Oenothera sp.* by pressing or solvent extraction. The rationale for its use as a dietary supplement and as an anti-inflammatory agent is its high concentration of γ-linolenic acid (18:3n6). Depending on the species and the growth conditions, evening primrose oil can contain as much as 16% 18:3n6 acid by weight [91]. Industrial applications exist for enriching the oil with 18:3n6 after extraction. Borage oil is obtained in a similar fashion from the starflower plant and also contains high concentrations of 18:3n6. Dietary 18:3n6 increases the tissue and plasma concentration of dihomo-γ-linolenic acid (20:3n6), which serves as substrate for the formation of series-1 prostaglandins (PGE$_1$) and 15-OH 20:3n6 [117]. Although PGE$_1$ causes swelling, redness and pain, it inhibits chemotaxis and other inflammatory responses in immune cells [118]. The 15-OH 20:3n6 formed from 20:3n6 also blocks the formation of leukotrienes from 20:4n6 [117, 119, 120]. The anti-inflammatory properties of series-1 prostaglandins and 15-OH 20:3n6 are the primary basis for the use of dietary primrose oil as an anti-inflammatory agent. However, the metabolism of 18:3n6 and the influence of 18:3n6 on 18:2n6 metabolism may be worthy of investigation as well. Although it seems counterintuitive, dietary 18:3n6 does not lead to the *de novo* synthesis of 20:4n6, a downstream product of 18:3n6. In fact, dietary 18:3n6 may suppress the formation of 20:4n6 from endogenous substrate. Although the exact mechanism is unclear at present, the ultra-low concentrations of 18:3n6 found in animal tissues indicate a coupled reaction process that produces 20:4n6 from 18:2n6 in a rapid fashion [121]. Even in rats, conspicuous for their elevated elongase/desaturase activity, orally administered radiolabeled 20:3n6 is converted to 20:4n6 very slowly [122]. The concentration of plasma and tissue 20:4n6 is not greatly affected by either dietary 18:3n6 or its immediate elongation product, 20:3n6 [121, 123, 124]. Thus, dietary 18:3n6 may inhibit the initial desaturation of 18:2n6 through a feedback inhibition of the Δ6 desaturase, and thereby reduce the production of 20:4n6 *de novo*. Because 18:3n6 is not rapidly converted to 20:4n6, the presence of 18:3n6 in the diet could inhibit the arachidonate cascade by limiting the conversion of substrate to 20:4n6. This is a less explored aspect of

the anti-inflammatory properties of dietary 18:3n6. The lack of metabolic conversion of 18:3n6 stands in stark contrast to the metabolism of its n-3 homologue, 18:3n3, which is actively converted to its downstream products 20:5n3 and 22:6n3 by the same set of metabolic enzymes.

Some researchers have hypothesized that enrichment of macrophage membranes with 20:3n6 at the expense of 20:4n6 could alter the physical properties of the membranes, thereby changing cell activity. It is unlikely that the relatively small incorporation of 20:3n6 into membranes observed in nutritional trials exerts such an effect, as its structure differs from 20:4n6 only by the exclusion of a Δ5 double bond. As described above, increasing the number of *pi* bonds in a fatty acid returns diminishing physical effect, and 20:3n6 already contains three *pi* bonds. However, the enzymes that distribute fatty acids among phospholipid pools can be variably specific for fatty acid structure, and it is more likely that any effect 20:3n6 exerts would be attributable to it competitive properties for key membrane fatty acid pools.

The accumulation of 20:3n6 in immune cell lipids following the consumption of 18:3n6 is well documented. Feeding dietary borage oil significantly increased murine macrophage 20:3n6 concentrations [125, 126]. Dietary primrose oil has also been shown to increase human plasma [127, 128], epidermal [129], and neutrophil [129, 130] 20:3n6 concentrations. The effect of this modification of fatty acid composition is manifested in alterations in the profile of eicosanoids produced by inflammatory cells. More than 20 years ago, it was observed that 20:3n6 and 20:4n6 were competitive substrates for prostaglandin synthase activity [131]. Subsequently, many experiments have defined the changes in eicosanoid production that result from consuming a diet rich in 18:3n6. In guinea pigs supplemented with 18:3n6 in the form of borage oil, LTB$_4$ production was reduced [132] and production of the anti-inflammatory compound 15-OH γ-20:3n6 was increased [133]. Dietary borage and primrose oils also increased the production of PGE$_1$ in mice when compared to dietary corn oil [134]. In rats, borage oil inhibited the production of LTB$_4$, LTC$_4$, LTD$_4$, and thromboxane B$_2$ in response to endotoxin relative to rats fed corn oil [135]. Interestingly, the effect of dietary 18:3n6 on modulating chemical mediators is not limited to eicosanoids. In rats supplemented with 18:3n6, serum concentrations of IF-γ and monocyte chemotactic protein-1 were significantly decreased while TNF-α concentrations were significantly increased relative to controls [136]. In humans, dietary 18:3n6 decreased the production of LTB_4 [130, 137], PGE_2 and LTC_4 in *ex vivo* stimulated monocytes [137]. Plasma PGE_2 concentrations were also reduced with 18:3n6 supplementation [138]. Some evidence exists that dietary 18:3n6 alters the expression of eicosanoid-producing enzymes. Dietary evening primrose oil elevated the expression of COX-1 mRNA in the nerve and retinal tissue of diabetic rats [139]. Thus, dietary 18:3n6 is capable of modulating the concentration of a wide range of immunoactive compounds and may be of use in the treatment of human inflammatory disorders.

Early investigations of the beneficial effects of dietary 18:3n6 in humans focused on disorders commonly associated with RA. Patients with Sjögrens syndrome were given 135 mg of dietary 18:3n6 a day in the form of Efamol for three weeks and classical phenotypic tests were administered. The treatment group showed improvement in the Schirmer test (which measures tear fluid production) relative to the control group, but did not show improvement in any other phenotypic assessment [140]. Further studies have been even less conclusive [141]. Belch and colleagues [142, 143] studied the effects of dietary primrose oil on patients with Raynaud's phenomenon. Patients were administered 540 mg 18:3n6 in the form of Efamol for 11 weeks after a two- week placebo wash out. In response to dropping climactic temperatures, the control group experienced more vasospastic attacks than the treatment group [143]. The severity of the vasospastic attacks was also reduced in the 18:3n6-supplemented group. Both of the studies described above utilized less than 30 patients, and thus, despite the encouraging results, more research is need to determine whether long-term 18:3n6 supplementation is a viable treatment for Raynaud's phenomenon and Sjögrens syndrome.

Rheumatoid arthritis presents difficult challenges for describing and quantifying the phenotypic severity of the disease. In several studies, investigators measured the subjective reduction of NSAIDs taken by the patients in response to dietary oils. In a double-blind design, 16 patients were given 540 mg 18:3n6 per day, 15 patients were given 240 mg 20:5n3 and 450 mg 18:3n6 per day, and 18 patients were given a placebo for 12 months, and the daily dose of NSAIDs was recorded [144]. After 12 months, both of the treatment groups had reduced their dose of NSAIDs relative to controls. The severity of RA did not change with the reduced NSAID dose [144]. In a study of 56 patients with active RA, dietary 18:3n6 in both free and esterified form (as evening primrose oil) reduced the clinical severity of RA [145]. After a six-month double-blind supplementation with 2.8 grams of 18:3n6 per day, patients consuming 18:3n6 showed significant signs of improvement relative to control patients as assessed by clinical evaluation [145]. The joint damage in RA patients induced by inflammatory cells may also be ameliorated by dietary 18:3n6. The proliferation of human synovial cells stimulated with IL-1 *in vitro* was significantly diminished in medium containing 20:3n6 relative to medium containing 20:4n6 [146]. Additionally, the production of PGE_1 increased in the 20:3n6-supplemented cells. Similar results were obtained by measuring the proliferation of murine spleen lymphocytes following dietary evening primrose oil. High doses of evening primrose oil diminished the *ex vivo* proliferation of splenic lymphocytes in response to concanavalin-A by 60% relative to controls [147]. Thus, dietary 18:3n6, when taken at an appropriate dose, may aid in diminishing the severity of RA.

γ-Linolenic and 20:3n6 have shown promise as anti-inflammatory agents in skin disorders. In patients with atopic eczema who demonstrated a clear increase in plasma 20:3n6 concentration following a 24-week supplementation with borage oil (500 mg daily), there was a significant decrease in self-applied skin treatments relative to control groups [148]. However, increased plasma 20:3n6 was not evident in all borage oil consumers, and for these patients, supplementation was not an effective treatment. It is not clear whether metabolic differences or non-compliance among the trial participants caused this difference in plasma composition [148]. The basis for the ameliorative effects of dietary 18:3n6 on skin disorders may be an increase in the production of anti-inflammatory eicosanoids by the epidermis. The epidermal tissue of guinea pigs supplemented with ethyl esters of borage oil demonstrated both a significant accumulation of 20:3n6 in phospholipids and increased 15-OH 20:3n6 production [133]. Alternatively, dietary 18:3n6 may ameliorate atopic eczema by providing necessary metabolic substrate. Atopic eczema is closely linked with a defect in $\Delta 6$ desaturase activity, and some researchers have postulated that the uncommon $\Delta 6$ bond in 18:3n6 may therefore act to compensate for this deficiency (reviewed in [149]).

5.1.4. Oleic acid

In many parts of the world, particularly in Mediterranean and Middle Eastern areas, olive oil comprises most of the oil consumed in the diet. The production and consumption of olive oil in North America has increased steadily over the past few decades. Olive oil is conspicuous among the dietary oils for its high concentration of oleic acid (18:1n9). Some olive oils contain 18:1n9 at concentrations as high 85% (by wt) of their fatty acids [91]. Oleic acid is the direct $\Delta 9$-desaturation product of 18:0, and is produced in high concentrations by *de novo* synthesis in animals. Other components of olive oil relevant to inflammation include 18:2n6 and 18:3n3, which account for 2–20% and < 1.5% of fatty acids in olive oil, respectively. On average, PUFA account for less than 10% of the fatty acids in olive oils. Thus, most of the composition of olive oil can be produced *de novo* by animals.

Two trials have suggested that the consumption of olive oil has beneficial effects for RA patients [98, 150]. In a clinical trial, dietary olive oil decreased the production of IL-1 [98] in RA patients. Subsequently, Linos et al. [150] found an inverse correlation between reported dietary olive oil consumption and the incidence of RA. The biochemical mechanism by which olive oil or its primary component, 18:1n9, would influence RA is not known.

5.1.5. Unusual fatty acids

Conjugated linoleic acids (CLA) are isomers of linoleic acid produced by chemical modification of linoleic acid or the desaturation of *trans*-oleic acid. These fatty acids are of considerable interest to nutritionists as they occur in foods at a low concentration and appear to have potent biological actions. Although not well characterized for their influence

on the immune system, some evidence suggests that dietary CLA can modulate inflammatory processes. In chicks, the consumption of CLA decreased the concentration of 20:4n6 in foot pads and suppressed the growth-inhibitory effects of injected LPS [151]. Splenocytes from mice fed a diet containing 1% of its fatty acids as CLA isomers displayed an increased proliferation in response to concanavalin-A [152]. The splenocytes from these mice also produced more IL-2 than mice fed control diets [152]. A role for CLA in modulating the phenotypic outcomes of inflammation remains untested.

The highly unusual fatty acid 20:3 $\Delta 5,11,14$ is found in ancient plants such as *Platycladus* and has unique metabolic properties. 20:3 $\Delta 5,11,14$ acid is an analogue of 20:4n6 that lacks a $\Delta 8$ double bond. Thus, it is a rare example of a fatty acid wherein the double bonds are not found at every third carbon. When fed to NZB mice, 20:3 $\Delta 5,11,14$ very effectively competed for acylation into plasma and tissue lipid pools typically associated with 20:4n6 [153]. However, because its structure does not contain a $\Delta 8$ double bond, it can not be converted into any traditionally defined eicosanoid. Thus, 20:3 $\Delta 5,11,14$ may act as an arachidonate cascade "cork" by occupying membrane pools typically occupied by 20:4n6, yet not serving as a suitable substrate for eicosanoid metabolism. Mice fed 20:3 $\Delta 5,11,14$ showed a substantial and significant delay in both the onset and the titer of the Coombs' test relative to mice fed either fish or safflower oil [153]. More research is needed to determine both the physiological effects and the safety of dietary 20:3 $\Delta 5,11,14$.

6. CONCLUSION

Fatty acids are often viewed as members of structural groups, and are assumed to have actions attributable to these groupings. For instance, it is common to observe in both the scientific and the popular literature recommendations for increasing the intake of n3 fatty acids relative to n6 fatty acids. Unfortunately, this simplistic approach doesn't begin to describe the complexity of lipid metabolism, or even the role of lipid metabolism in specific physiological processes such as inflammation. As described above, the n6 fatty acid 20:3n6 has potent anti-inflammatory properties that stand in stark contrast to its metabolic product and n6 family member 20:4n6. What 20:3n6 shares in common with 20:4n6 is only a metabolic pathway, and the potential for inter-conversion. Thus, fatty acids must be viewed as unique entities with distinct physiological actions. The study of lipid metabolism must begin to embrace the individual properties of lipid metabolites rather than try to group and oversimplify them. The pathways for fatty acid metabolism are largely known, and yet attempts to identify dysregulation of lipid metabolism in specific diseases are disappointingly non-descriptive. Fortunately, genomics has taught us the value of the large dataset, and the future study of lipid metabolism is likely to look very similar to other informatic analyses. Armed with enough quantitative data, a highly defined role for dietary lipids in the prevention and treatment of immune dysfunction will emerge.

REFERENCES

1. Sprecher H, Chen Q. Polyunsaturated fatty acid biosynthesis: a microsomal-peroxisomal process. Prostaglandins Leukotrienes Essential Fatty Acids 1999;60(5-6):317–321.
2. Voss A, Reinhart M, Sankarappa S, Sprecher H. The metabolism of 7,10,13,16,19-docosapentaenoic acid to 4,7,10,13,16,19-docosahexaenoic acid in rat liver is independent of a 4-desaturase. J Biol Chem 1991;266(30):19995–20000.
3. Ziboh VA. Nutritional modulation of inflammation by polyunsaturated fatty acids/eicosanoids. In: Gershwin M, German J, Keen C, editors. Nutrition and Immunology: Principals and Practice. Totowa, New Jersey: Humana Press; 2000. p. 157–170.
4. Anderson GD, Hauser SD, McGarity KL, Bremer ME, Isakson PC, Gregory SA. Selective inhibition of cyclooxygenase (COX)-2 reverses inflammation and expression of COX-2 and interleukin 6 in rat adjuvant arthritis. J Clin Invest 1996;97(11):2672–2679.
5. Smith W, Borgeat P, Fitzpatrick F. The eicosanoids: cyclooxygenase, lipoxygenase and epoxygenase pathways. In: Vance D, Vance J, editors. Biochemistry of Lipids, Lipoproteins and Membranes. Amsterdam: Elsevier; 1991. p. 297–323.
6. Habenicht AJ, Salbach P, Goerig M, Zeh W, Janssen-Timmen U, Blattner C, et al. The LDL receptor pathway delivers arachidonic acid for eicosanoid formation in cells stimulated by platelet-derived growth factor [published erratum appears in Nature 1990 Aug

9;346(6284):589]. Nature 1990;345(6276):634–6.
7. Nilsson A, Chen Q, Dahlman E. Metabolism of chylomicron phosphatidylinositol in the rat: fate in vivo and hydrolysis with lipoprotein lipase and hepatic lipase in vitro. J Lipid Res 1994;35(12):2151–60.
8. Urban S, Zieseniss S, Werder M, Hauser H, Budzinski R, Engelmann B. Scavenger receptor BI transfers major lipoprotein associated phospholipids into the cells. J Biol Chem 2000:M004031200
9. Sparrow CP, Parthasarathy S, Steinberg D. A macrophage receptor that recognizes oxidized low density lipoprotein but not acetylated low density lipoprotein. J Biol Chem 1989;264(5):2599–604.
10. Parthasarathy S, Fong LG, Otero D, Steinberg D. Recognition of solubilized apoproteins from delipidated, oxidized low density lipoprotein (LDL) by the acetyl-LDL receptor. Proc Natl Acad Sci USA 1987;84(2):537–40.
11. Chilton FH, Fonteh AN, Surette ME, Triggiani M, Winkler JD. Control of arachidonate levels within inflammatory cells. Biochim Biophys Acta 1996;1299(1):1–15.
12. Chilton FH, Murphy RC. Remodeling of arachidonate-containing phosphoglycerides within the human neutrophil. J Biol Chem 1986;261(17):7771–7.
13. Hill E, Lands W. In: Wakil S, editor. Lipid Metabolism. New York: Academic Press; 1970. p. 185
14. Vasta V, Meacci E, Romiti E, Farnararo M, Bruni P. A role for phospholipase D activation in the lipid signalling cascade generated by bradykinin and thrombin in C2C12 myoblasts. Biochim Biophys Acta 1998;1391(2):280–6.
15. Shinoda J, Kozawa O, Suzuki A, Watanabe-Tomita Y, Oiso Y, Uematsu T. Mechanism of angiotensin II-induced arachidonic acid metabolite release in aortic smooth muscle cells: involvement of phospholipase D. Eur J Endo 1997;136(2):207–12.
16. Baines RJ, Brown C, Ng LL, Boarder MR. Angiotensin II-stimulated phospholipase C responses of two vascular smooth muscle-derived cell lines. Role of cyclic GMP. Hypertension 1996;28(5):772–8.
17. Jacobs LS, Douglas JG. Angiotensin II type 2 receptor subtype mediates phospholipase A2-dependent signaling in rabbit proximal tubular epithelial cells. Hypertension 1996;28(4):663–8.
18. Periwal SB, Farooq A, Bhargava VL, Bhatla N, Vij U, Murugesan K. Effect of hormones and antihormones on phospholipase A2 activity in human endometrial stromal cells. Prostaglandins 1996;51(3):191–201.
19. Renard P, Raes M. The proinflammatory transcription factor NFkappaB: a potential target for novel therapeutical strategies. Cell Biology and Toxicology 1999;15(6):341–4.
20. Tanaka Y, Amano F, Kishi H, Nishijima M, Akamatsu Y. Degradation of arachidonyl phospholipids catalyzed by

two phospholipases A2 and phospholipase C in a lipopol-ysaccharide-treated macrophage cell line RAW264.7. Arch Biochem Biophys 1989;272(1):210–8.

21. Walsh CE, Dechatelet LR, Chilton FH, Wykle RL, Waite M. Mechanism of arachidonic acid release in human polymorphonuclear leukocytes. Biochim Biophys Acta 1983;750(1):32–40.

22. Yamada K, Okano Y, Miura K, Nozawa Y. A major role for phospholipase A2 in antigen-induced arachidonic acid release in rat mast cells. Biochem J 1987;247(1):95–9.

23. Fonteh AN, Chilton FH. Mobilization of different arachidonate pools and their roles in the generation of leukotrienes and free arachidonic acid during immunologic activation of mast cells. J Immunol 1993;150(2):563–570.

24. Khovidunkit W, Riaz M, Feingold K, Grunfeld C. Infection and inflammation-induced proatherogenic changes of lipoproteins. J Infectious Dis 2000;181(Suppl 3):S462–72.

25. Gallin JI, Kaye D, O'Leary WM. Serum lipids in infection. New England J Med 1969;281(20):1081–6.

26. Ettinger WH, Miller LD, Albers JJ, Smith TK, Parks JS. Lipopolysaccharide and tumor necrosis factor cause a fall in plasma concentration of lecithin: cholesterol acyltransferase in cynomolgus monkeys. J Lipid Res 1990;31(6):1099–107.

27. Memon RA, Grunfeld C, Moser AH, Feingold KR. Tumor necrosis factor mediates the effects of endotoxin on cholesterol and triglyceride metabolism in mice. Endocrinology 1993;132(5):2246–53.

28. Hellerstein MK, Grunfeld C, Wu K, Christiansen M, Kaempfer S, Kletke C, et al. Increased de novo hepatic lipogenesis in human immunodeficiency virus infection. J Clin Endocrinology Met 1993;76(3):559–65.

29. Memon RA, Feingold KR, Moser AH, Doerrler W, Adi S, Dinarello CA, et al. Differential effects of interleukin-1 and tumor necrosis factor on ketogenesis. Am J Physiol 1992;263(2 Pt 1):E301–9.

30. Krauss RM, Grunfeld C, Doerrler WT, Feingold KR. Tumor necrosis factor acutely increases plasma levels of very low density lipoproteins of normal size and composition. Endocrinology 1990;127(3):1016–21.

31. Feingold KR, Serio MK, Adi S, Moser AH, Grunfeld C. Tumor necrosis factor stimulates hepatic lipid synthesis and secretion. Endocrinology 1989;124(5):2336–42.

32. Feingold KR, Grunfeld C. Tumor necrosis factor-alpha stimulates hepatic lipogenesis in the rat in vivo. J Clin Invest 1987;80(1):184–90.

33. Grunfeld C, Gulli R, Moser AH, Gavin LA, Feingold KR. Effect of tumor necrosis factor administration in vivo on lipoprotein lipase activity in various tissues of the rat. J Lipid Res 1989;30(4):579–85.

34. Chait A, Brazg RL, Tribble DL, Krauss RM. Susceptibility of small, dense, low-density lipoproteins to oxidative modification in subjects with the atherogenic lipoprotein phenotype, pattern B [see comments]. Am J Med 1993;94(4):350–6.

35. Hurt-Camejo E, Camejo G, Rosengren B, Lopez F, Wiklund O, Bondjers G. Differential uptake of proteoglycan-selected subfractions of low density lipoprotein by human macrophages. J Lipid Res 1990;31(8):1387–98.

36. Camejo G, Hurt-Camejo E, Rosengren B, Wiklund O, López F, Bondjers G. Modification of copper-catalyzed oxidation of low density lipoprotein by proteoglycans and glycosaminoglycans. J Lipid Res 1991;32(12):1983–91.

37. Nigon F, Lesnik P, Rouis M, Chapman MJ. Discrete subspecies of human low density lipoproteins are heterogeneous in their interaction with the cellular LDL receptor. J Lipid Res 1991;32(11):1741–53.

38. Memon RA, Staprans I, Noor M, Holleran WM, Uchida Y, Moser AH, et al. Infection and inflammation induce LDL oxidation in vivo [see comments]. Arteriosclerosis Thrombosis Vascular Biol 2000;20(6):1536–42.

39. Walzem RL, Watkins S, Frankel EN, Hansen RJ, German JB. Older plasma lipoproteins are more susceptible to oxidation: a linking mechanism for the lipid and oxidation theories of atherosclerotic cardiovascular disease. Proc Natl Acad Sci U S A 1995;92(16):7460–7464.

40. Feingold KR, Hardardottir I, Memon R, Krul EJ, Moser AH, Taylor JM, et al. Effect of endotoxin on cholesterol biosynthesis and distribution in serum lipoproteins in Syrian hamsters. J Lipid Res 1993;34(12):2147–58.

41. Memon RA, Holleran WM, Moser AH, Seki T, Uchida Y, Fuller J, et al. Endotoxin and cytokines increase hepatic sphingolipid biosynthesis and produce lipoproteins enriched in ceramides and sphingomyelin. Arteriosclerosis Thrombosis Vascular Biol 1998;18(8):1257–65.

42. Marathe S, Schissel SL, Yellin MJ, Beatini N, Mintzer R, Williams KJ, et al. Human vascular endothelial cells are a rich and regulatable source of secretory sphingomyelinase. Implications for early atherogenesis and ceramide-mediated cell signaling. J Biol Chem 1998;273(7):4081–8.

43. Tabas I, Li Y, Brocia RW, Xu SW, Swenson TL, Williams KJ. Lipoprotein lipase and sphingomyelinase synergistically enhance the association of atherogenic lipoproteins with smooth muscle cells and extracellular matrix. A possible mechanism for low density lipoprotein and lipoprotein(a) retention and macrophage foam cell formation. J Biol Chem 1993;268(27):20419–32.

44. Xu XX, Tabas I. Sphingomyelinase enhances low density lipoprotein uptake and ability to induce cholesteryl ester accumulation in macrophages. J Biol Chem 1991;266(36):24849–58.

45. Schissel SL, Jiang X, Tweedie-Hardman J, Jeong T, Camejo EH, Najib J, et al. Secretory sphingomyelinase, a product of the acid sphingomyelinase gene, can hydrolyze atherogenic lipoproteins at neutral pH. Implications for atherosclerotic lesion development. J Biol Chem 1998;273(5):2738–46.

46. Schissel SL, Tweedie-Hardman J, Rapp JH, Graham G, Williams KJ, Tabas I. Rabbit aorta and human atherosclerotic lesions hydrolyze the sphingomyelin of retained low-density lipoprotein. Proposed role for arterial-wall sphingomyelinase in subendothelial retention and aggregation of atherogenic lipoproteins. J Clin Invest 1996;98(6):1455–64.

47. Schissel SL, Keesler GA, Schuchman EH, Williams KJ, Tabas I. The cellular trafficking and zinc dependence of secretory and lysosomal sphingomyelinase, two products of the acid sphingomyelinase gene. J Biol Chem 1998;273(29):18250–9.

48. Schissel SL, Schuchman EH, Williams KJ, Tabas I. Zn2+-stimulated sphingomyelinase is secreted by many cell types and is a product of the acid sphingomyelinase gene. J Biol Chem 1996;271(31):18431–6.

49. Fielding PE, Fielding CJ. Dynamics of lipoprotein transport in the circulatory system. In: Vance DE, Vance J, editors. Biochemistry of Lipids, Lipoproteins and Membranes. Amsterdam: Elsevier Science Publishers B.V.; 1991. p. 427–459.

50. Cabana VG, Siegel JN, Sabesin SM. Effects of the acute phase response on the concentration and density distribution of plasma lipids and apolipoproteins. J Lipid Res 1989;30(1):39–49.

51. Borba EF, Bonfá E. Dyslipoproteinemias in systemic lupus erythematosus: influence of disease, activity, and anticardiolipin antibodies. Lupus 1997;6(6):533–9.

52. Park JH, Park EJ, Kim KS, Yeo YK. Changes in ether-linked phospholipids in rat kidney by dietary alpha-linolenic acid in vivo. Lipids 1995;30(6):541–6.

53. Auerbach BJ, Parks JS. Lipoprotein abnormalities associated with lipopolysaccharide-induced lecithin: cholesterol acyltransferase and lipase deficiency. J Biol Chem 1989;264(17):10264–70.

54. Ly H, Francone OL, Fielding CJ, Shigenaga JK, Moser AH, Grunfeld C, et al. Endotoxin and TNF lead to reduced plasma LCAT activity and decreased hepatic LCAT mRNA levels in Syrian hamsters. J Lipid Res 1995;36(6):1254–63.

55. Hardardóttir I, Moser AH, Fuller J, Fielding C, Feingold K, Grünfeld C. Endotoxin and cytokines decrease serum levels and extra hepatic protein and mRNA levels of cholesteryl ester transfer protein in syrian hamsters. J Clin Invest 1996;97(11):2585–92.

56. Grunfeld C, Marshall M, Shigenaga JK, Moser AH, Tobias P, Feingold KR. Lipoproteins inhibit macrophage activation by lipoteichoic acid. J Lipid Res 1999;40(2):245–252.

57. Lamping N, Dettmer R, Schröder NW, Pfeil D, Hallatschek W, Burger R, et al. LPS-binding protein protects mice from septic shock caused by LPS or gram-negative bacteria. J Clin Invest 1998;101(10):2065–71.

58. Asanuma Y, Kawai S, Aoshima H, Kaburaki J, Mizushima Y. Serum lipoprotein(a) and apolipoprotein(a) phenotypes in patients with rheumatoid arthritis. Arthritis and Rheumatism 1999;42(3):443–7.

59. Rantapää-Dahlqvist S, Wållberg-Jonsson S, Dahlén G. Lipoprotein (a), lipids, and lipoproteins in patients with rheumatoid arthritis. Ann Rheumatic Dis 1991;50(6):366–8.

60. Situnayake RD, Kitas G. Dyslipidemia and rheumatoid arthritis [comment]. Ann Rheumatic Dis 1997;56(6):341–2.

61. Bakkaloglu A, Kirel B, Ozen S, Saatçi U, Topalo*glu, Be*sba*s N. Plasma lipids and lipoproteins in juvenile chronic arthritis. Clin Rheum 1996;15(4):341–5.

62. Heliövaara M, Aho K, Knekt P, Reunanen A, Aromaa A. Serum cholesterol and risk of rheumatoid arthritis in a cohort of 52 800 men and women. Brit J Rheum 1996;35(3):255–7.

63. Fraser DA, Thoen J, Bondhus S, Haugen M, Reseland JE, Djøseland O, et al. Reduction in serum leptin and IGF-1 but preserved T-lymphocyte numbers and activation after a ketogenic diet in rheumatoid arthritis patients. Clin Exper Rheum 2000;18(2):209–14.

64. Jacobsson L, Lindgärde F, Manthorpe R, Akesson B. Correlation of fatty acid composition of adipose tissue lipids and serum phosphatidylcholine and serum concentrations of micronutrients with disease duration in rheumatoid arthritis. Ann Rheumatic Dis 1990;49(11):901–5.

65. Kiziltunc A, Cogalgil S, Cerrahoglu L. Carnitine and antioxidants levels in patients with rheumatoid arthritis. Scand J Rheum 1998;27(6):441–5.

66. Hagen TM, Wehr CM, Ames BN. Mitochondrial decay in ageing: Reversal through supplementation of acetyl-L-carnitine and N-tert-Butyl-alpha-phenyl-nitrone. In:? 1998. p. 214–223.

67. Shigenaga MK, Hagen TM, Ames BN. Oxidative damage and mitochondrial decay in aging. Proc Natl Acad Sci U S A 1994;91(23):10771–10778.

68. Wållberg-Jonsson S, Dahlén G, Johnson O, Olivecrona G, Rantapää-Dahlqvist S. Lipoprotein lipase in relation to inflammatory activity in rheumatoid arthritis. J Intern Med 1996;240(6):373–80.

69. Pisetsky DS. Systemic lupus erythematosus. A. Epidemiology, pathology and pathogenesis. In: Klippel JH, editor. Primer on the Rheumatic Diseases. 11 ed.

Atlanta: Arthritis Foundation; 1997. p. 246–251.

70. Gladman DD, Urowitz MB. Systemic lupus erythematosus. B. Clinical and laboratory features. In: Klippel JH, editor. Primer on the Rheumatic Diseases. 11 ed. Atlanta: Arthritis Foundation; 1997. p. 251–257.

71. Ilowite NT. Hyperlipidemia and the rheumatic diseases. Cur Opin Rheum 1996;8(5):455–8.

72. Urowitz MB, Gladman DD. Accelerated atheroma in lupus-background. Lupus 2000;9(3):161–5.

73. Ilowite NT. Premature atherosclerosis in systemic lupus erythematosus. J Rheum 2000;27 Suppl 58(11):15–9.

74. Bruce IN, Urowitz MB, Gladman DD, Hallett DC. Natural history of hypercholesterolemia in systemic lupus erythematosus. J Rheum 1999;26(10):2137–43.

75. Bruce IN, Gladman DD, Urowitz MB. Detection and modification of risk factors for coronary artery disease in patients with systemic lupus erythematosus: a quality improvement study. Clin Exper Rheum 1998;16(4):435–40.

76. Borba EF, Bonfá E, Vinagre CG, Ramires JA, Maranhão RC. Chylomicron metabolism is markedly altered in systemic lupus erythematosus. Arthritis and Rheumatism 2000;43(5):1033–40.

77. Krause W, DuBois RN. Eicosanoids and the large intestine. Prostaglandins and Other Lipid Mediators 2000;61(3-4):145–61.

78. Lauritsen K, Laursen LS, Bukhave K, Rask-Madsen J. Use of colonic eicosanoid concentrations as predictors of relapse in ulcerative colitis: double blind placebo controlled study on sulphasalazine maintenance treatment. Gut 1988;29(10):1316–21.

79. Lauritsen K, Laursen LS, Bukhave K, Rask-Madsen J. In vivo profiles of eicosanoids in ulcerative colitis, Crohn's colitis, and Clostridium difficile colitis. Gastroenterology 1988;95(1):11–7.

80. Lauritsen K, Laursen LS, Bukhave K, Rask-Madsen J. Inflammatory intermediaries in inflammatory bowel disease. Int J Colorectal Dis 1989;4(2):75–90.

81. Esteve M, Navarro E, Klaassen J, Abad-Lacruz A, González-Huix F, Cabré E, et al. Plasma and mucosal fatty acid pattern in colectomized ulcerative colitis patients. Digestive Dis Sciences 1998;43(5):1071–8.

82. Morita H, Nakanishi K, Dohi T, Yasugi E, Oshima M. Phospholipid turnover in the inflamed intestinal mucosa: arachidonic acid-rich phosphatidyl/plasmenylethanolamine in the mucosa in inflammatory bowel disease. J Gastroenterology 1999;34(1):46–53.

83. Inui K, Fukuta Y, Ikeda A, Kameda H, Kokuba Y, Sato M. The effect of alpha-linolenic acid-rich emulsion on fatty acid metabolism and leukotriene generation of the colon in a rat model with inflammatory bowel disease. Ann Nut Metab 1996;40(3):175–82.

84. Inui K, Fukuta Y, Ikeda A, Kameda H, Kokuba Y, Sato M. The nutritional effect of a-linolenic acid-rich emulsion with total parenteral nutrition in a rat model with inflammatory bowel disease. Ann Nut Metab 1996;40(4):227–33.

85. Hammarström S. Conversion of dihomo-gamma-linolenic acid to an isomer of leukotriene C3, oxygenated at C-8. J Biol Chem 1981;256(15):7712–4.

86. German JB, Dillard CJ, Whelan J. Biological effects of dietary arachidonic acid. Introduction. J Nutr 1996;126(4 Suppl):1076S-80S.

87. Woods RK, Thien FC, Abramson MJ. Dietary marine fatty acids (fish oil) for asthma. Cochrane Database Syst Rev 2000;38(2):CD001283.

88. McCarthy GM, Kenny D. Dietary fish oil and rheumatic diseases. Sem Arthritis Rheumatism 1992;21(6):368–75.

89. Ziboh VA. Omega 3 polyunsaturated fatty acid constituents of fish oil and the management of skin inflammatory and scaly disorders. World Review of Nutrition and Dietetics 1991;66(2):425–35.

90. Kinsella JE, Lokesh B, Broughton S, Whelan J. Dietary polyunsaturated fatty acids and eicosanoids: potential effects on the modulation of inflammatory and immune cells: an overview. Nutr 1990;6(1):24–44; discussion 59–62.

91. Padley F, Gunstone F, Harwood J. Occurence and characteristics of oils and fats. In: Gunstone F, Harwood J, Padley F, editors. The Lipid Handbook. 2nd ed. London: Chapman & Hall; 1986. p. 47–223.

92. James MJ, Gibson RA, Cleland LG. Dietary polyunsaturated fatty acids and inflammatory mediator production. Am J Clin Nutr 2000;71(1 Suppl):343S-8S.

93. Hawkes JS, James MJ, Cleland LG. Separation and quantification of PGE3 following derivatization with panacyl bromide by high pressure liquid chromatography with fluorometric detection. Prostaglandins 1991;42(4):355–68.

94. Arend WP, Dayer JM. Inhibition of the production and effects of interleukin-1 and tumor necrosis factor alpha in rheumatoid arthritis. Arthritis and Rheumatism 1995;38(2):151–60.

95. Caughey GE, Mantzioris E, Gibson RA, Cleland LG, James MJ. The effect on human tumor necrosis factor alpha and interleukin 1 beta production of diets enriched in n-3 fatty acids from vegetable oil or fish oil. Am J Clin Nutr 1996;63(1):116–22.

96. Endres S, Ghorbani R, Kelley VE, Georgilis K, Lonnemann G, van der Meer JW, et al. The effect of dietary supplementation with n-3 polyunsaturated fatty acids on the synthesis of interleukin-1 and tumor necrosis factor by mononuclear cells. New England J Med 1989;320(5):265–71.

97. Meydani SN, Endres S, Woods MM, Goldin BR, Soo

C, Morrill-Labrode A, et al. Oral (n-3) fatty acid supplementation suppresses cytokine production and lymphocyte proliferation: comparison between young and older women. J Nutr 1991;121(4):547–55.

98. Kremer JM, Lawrence DA, Jubiz W, DiGiacomo R, Rynes R, Bartholomew LE, et al. Dietary fish oil and olive oil supplementation in patients with rheumatoid arthritis. Clinical and immunologic effects. Arthritis and Rheumatism 1990;33(6):810–20.

99. Hughes DA, Southon S, Pinder AC. (n-3) Polyunsaturated fatty acids modulate the expression of functionally associated molecules on human monocytes in vitro. J Nutr 1996;126(3):603–10.

100. Hughes DA, Pinder AC. n-3 polyunsaturated fatty acids inhibit the antigen-presenting function of human monocytes. Am J Clin Nutr 2000;71(1 Suppl):357S-60S.

101. Fernandes G. Dietary lipids and risk of autoimmune disease. Clin Immunol Immunopathol 1994;72(2):193–197.

102. Fernandez G, Chandrsekar B, Luan X, Troyer DA. Modulation of antioxidant enzymes and programmed cell death by n-3 fatty acids. Lipids 1996;31(Suppl):S91-S96

103. Fernandes G, Bysani C, Venkatraman JT, Tomar V, Zhao W. Increased TGF-beta and decreased oncogene expression by omega-3 fatty acids in the spleen delays onset of autoimmune disease in B/W mice. J Immunol 1994;152(12):5979–5987.

104. Mohan IK, Das UN. Oxidant stress, anti-oxidants and essential fatty acids in systemic lupus erythematosus. Prostaglandins Leukotrienes Essential Fatty Acids 1997;56(3):193–8.

105. Simopoulos AP. Essential fatty acids in health and chronic disease. Am J Clin Nutr 1999;70(3 Suppl):560S-569S.

106. Simopoulos AP. Evolutionary aspects of omega-3 fatty acids in the food supply. Prostaglandins Leukotrienes Essential Fatty Acids 1999;60(5-6):421–9.

107. Kinsella J, editor. Seafoods and Fish Oils in Human Health and Disease. New York: Marcel Dekker, Inc; 1987.

108. Crawford MA. Fatty-acid ratios in free-living and domestic animals. Possible implications for atheroma. Lancet 1968;1(7556):1329–33.

109. Emken EA, Adlof RO, Gulley RM. Dietary linoleic acid influences desaturation and acylation of deuterium-labeled linoleic and linolenic acids in young adult males. Biochim Biophys Acta 1994;1213(3):277–88.

110. Mantzioris E, James MJ, Gibson RA, Cleland LG. Dietary substitution with an alpha-linolenic acid-rich vegetable oil increases eicosapentaenoic acid concentrations in tissues. Am J Clin Nutr 1994;59(6):1304–9.

111. Hwang DH, Boudreau M, Chanmugam P. Dietary linolenic acid and longer-chain n-3 fatty acids: comparison of effects on arachidonic acid metabolism in rats. J Nutr 1988;118(4):427–37.

112. Fritsche KL, Johnston PV. Modulation of eicosanoid production and cell-mediated cytotoxicity by dietary alpha-linolenic acid in BALB/c mice. Lipids 1989;24(4):305–11.

113. Kelley DS, Branch LB, Love JE, Taylor PC, Rivera YM, Iacono JM. Dietary alpha-linolenic acid and immunocompetence in humans. Am J Clin Nutr 1991;53(1):40–6.

114. Hall AV, Parbtani A, Clark WF, Spanner E, Keeney M, Chin-Yee I, et al. Abrogation of MRL/lpr lupus nephritis by dietary flaxseed. American Journal of Kidney Diseases 1993;22(2):326–32.

115. Clark WF, Parbtani A, Huff MW, Spanner E, de Salis H, Chin-Yee I, et al. Flaxseed: a potential treatment for lupus nephritis. Kidney Int 1995;48(2):475–80.

116. Nordström DC, Honkanen VE, Nasu Y, Antila E, Friman C, Konttinen YT. Alpha-linolenic acid in the treatment of rheumatoid arthritis. A double-blind, placebo-controlled and randomized study: flaxseed vs. safflower seed. Rheum Int 1995;14(6):231–4.

117. Belch JJ, Hill A. Evening primrose oil and borage oil in rheumatologic conditions. Am J Clin Nutr 2000;71(1 Suppl):352S-6S.

118. Weissmann G, Smolen JE, Korchak H. Prostaglandins and inflammation: receptor/cyclase coupling as an explanation of why PGEs and PGI2 inhibit functions of inflammatory cells. Adv Prostaglandin Thromboxane Res 1980;8(4):1637–53.

119. Voorhees JJ. Leukotrienes and other lipoxygenase products in the pathogenesis and therapy of psoriasis and other dermatoses. Arch Derm 1983;119(7):541–7.

120. Chapkin RS, Miller CC, Somers SD, Erickson KL. Ability of 15-hydroxyeicosatrienoic acid (15-OH-20:3) to modulate macrophage arachidonic acid metabolism. Biochem Biophys Res Commun 1988;153(2):799–804.

121. Horrobin DF, Ells KM, Morse-Fisher N, Manku MS. The effects of evening primrose oil, safflower oil and paraffin on plasma fatty acid levels in humans: choice of an appropriate placebo for clinical studies on primrose oil. Prostaglandins Leukotrienes Essential Fatty Acids 1991;42(4):245–9.

122. Hassam AG, Crawford MA. The incorporation of orally administered radiolabeled dihomo gamma-linolenic acid (20 : 3 omega 6) into rat tissue lipids and its conversion of arachidonic acid. Lipids 1978;13(11):801–3.

123. Stone KJ, Willis AL, Hart WM, Kirtland SJ, Kernoff PB, McNicol GP. The metabolism of dihomo-gamma-linolenic acid in man. Lipids 1979;14(2):174–80.

124. Yoshimoto-Furuie K, Yoshimoto K, Tanaka T, Saima S, Kikuchi Y, Shay J, et al. Effects of oral supple-

mentation with evening primrose oil for six weeks on plasma essential fatty acids and uremic skin symptoms in hemodialysis patients. Nephron 1999;81(2):151–9.

125. Chapkin RS, Somers SD, Schumacher L, Erickson KL. Fatty acid composition of macrophage phospholipids in mice fed fish or borage oil. Lipids 1988;23(4):380–3.

126. Chapkin RS, Somers SD, Erickson KL. Dietary manipulation of macrophage phospholipid classes: selective increase of dihomogammalinolenic acid. Lipids 1988;23(8):766–70.

127. Jäntti J, Seppälä E, Vapaatalo H, Isomäki H. Evening primrose oil and olive oil in treatment of rheumatoid arthritis. Clin Rheum 1989;8(2):238–44.

128. Schalin-Karrila M, Mattila L, Jansen CT, Uotila P. Evening primrose oil in the treatment of atopic eczema: effect on clinical status, plasma phospholipid fatty acids and circulating blood prostaglandins. Brit J Derm 1987;117(1):11–9.

129. Schäfer L, Kragballe K. Supplementation with evening primrose oil in atopic dermatitis: effect on fatty acids in neutrophils and epidermis. Lipids 1991;26(7):557–60.

130. Ziboh VA, Fletcher MP. Dose-response effects of dietary gamma-linolenic acid-enriched oils on human polymorphonuclear-neutrophil biosynthesis of leukotriene B4. Am J Clin Nutr 1992;55(1):39–45.

131. Srivastava KC. Metabolism of arachidonic acid by platelets: utilization of arachidonic acid by human platelets in presence of linoleic and dihomo-gamma-linolenic acids. Zeitschrift fur Ernahrungswissenschaft 1978;17(4):248–61.

132. Fletcher MP, Ziboh VA. Effects of dietary supplementation with eicosapentaenoic acid or gamma-linolenic acid on neutrophil phospholipid fatty acid composition and activation responses. Inflammation 1990;14(5):585–97.

133. Miller CC, Tang W, Ziboh VA, Fletcher MP. Dietary supplementation with ethyl ester concentrates of fish oil (n-3) and borage oil (n-6) polyunsaturated fatty acids induces epidermal generation of local putative anti-inflammatory metabolites. J Investigative Derm 1991;96(1):98–103.

134. Fan YY, Chapkin RS. Mouse peritoneal macrophage prostaglandin E1 synthesis is altered by dietary gamma-linolenic acid. J Nutr 1992;122(8):1600–6.

135. Mancuso P, Whelan J, DeMichele SJ, Snider CC, Guszcza JA, Karlstad MD. Dietary fish oil and fish and borage oil suppress intrapulmonary proinflammatory eicosanoid biosynthesis and attenuate pulmonary neutrophil accumulation in endotoxic rats. Critical Care Medicine 1997;25(7):1198–206.

136. Dirks J, van Aswegen CH, du Plessis DJ. Cytokine levels affected by gamma-linolenic acid. Prostaglandins Leukotrienes Essential Fatty Acids 1998;59(4):273–7.

137. Pullman-Mooar S, Laposata M, Lem D, Holman RT, Leventhal LJ, DeMarco D, et al. Alteration of the cellular fatty acid profile and the production of eicosanoids in human monocytes by gamma-linolenic acid. Arthritis and Rheumatism 1990;33(10):1526–33.

138. Arisaka M, Arisaka O, Yamashiro Y. Fatty acid and prostaglandin metabolism in children with diabetes mellitus. II. The effect of evening primrose oil supplementation on serum fatty acid and plasma prostaglandin levels. Prostaglandins Leukotrienes Essential Fatty Acids 1991;43(3):197–201.

139. Fang C, Jiang Z, Tomlinson DR. Expression of constitutive cyclo-oxygenase (COX-1) in rats with streptozotocin-induced diabetes; effects of treatment with evening primrose oil or an aldose reductase inhibitor on COX-1 mRNA levels. Prostaglandins Leukotrienes Essential Fatty Acids 1997;56(2):157–63.

140. Manthorpe R, Hagen Petersen S, Prause JU. Primary Sjögren's syndrome treated with Efamol/Efavit. A double-blind cross-over investigation. Rheum Int 1984;4(4):165–7.

141. Oxholm P, Manthorpe R, Prause JU, Horrobin D. Patients with primary Sjögren's syndrome treated for two months with evening primrose oil. Scand J Rheum 1986;15(2):103–8.

142. Belch J, Shaw B, O'Dowd A, Curran L, Forbes C, Sturrock R. Evening primrose oil (Efamol) as a treatment for cold-induced vasospasm (Raynaud's phenomenon). Prog Lipid Res 1986;25:335–40.

143. Belch JJ, Shaw B, O'Dowd A, Saniabadi A, Leiberman P, Sturrock RD, et al. Evening primrose oil (Efamol) in the treatment of Raynaud's phenomenon: a double blind study. Thrombosis and Haemostasis 1985;54(2):490–4.

144. Belch JJ, Ansell D, Madhok R, O'Dowd A, Sturrock RD. Effects of altering dietary essential fatty acids on requirements for non-steroidal anti-inflammatory drugs in patients with rheumatoid arthritis: a double blind placebo controlled study. Ann Rheumatic Dis 1988;47(2):96–104.

145. Zurier RB, Rossetti RG, Jacobson EW, DeMarco DM, Liu NY, Temming JE, et al. gamma-Linolenic acid treatment of rheumatoid arthritis. A randomized, placebo-controlled trial. Arthritis and Rheumatism 1996;39(11):1808–17.

146. Baker DG, Krakauer KA, Tate G, Laposata M, Zurier RB. Suppression of human synovial cell proliferation by dihomo-gamma-linolenic acid. Arthritis and Rheumatism 1989;32(10):1273–81.

147. Peterson LD, Thies F, Calder PC. Dose-dependent effects of dietary gamma-linolenic acid on rat spleen lymphocyte functions. Prostaglandins Leukotrienes Essential Fatty Acids 1999;61(1):19–24.

148. Henz BM, Jablonska S, van de Kerkhof PC, Stingl G,

Blaszczyk M, Vandervalk PG, et al. Double-blind, mul-ticentre analysis of the efficacy of borage oil in patients with atopic eczema. Brit J Derm 1999;140(4):685–8.

149. Kerscher MJ, Korting HC. Treatment of atopic eczema with evening primrose oil: rationale and clinical results. Clin Investigator 1992;70(2):167–71.

150. Linos A, Kaklamani VG, Kaklamani E, Koumantaki Y, Giziaki E, Papazoglou S, et al. Dietary factors in relation to rheumatoid arthritis: a role for olive oil and cooked vegetables? Am J Clin Nutr 1999;70(6):1077–82.

151. Cook ME, Miller CC, Park Y, Pariza M. Immune modu-lation by altered nutrient metabolism: nutritional con-trol of immune-induced growth depression. Poultry Sci 1993;72(7):1301–5.

152. Hayek MG, Han SN, Wu D, Watkins BA, Meydani M, Dorsey JL, et al. Dietary conjugated linoleic acid influ-ences the immune response of young and old C57BL/6NCrlBR mice. J Nutr 1999;129(1):32–8.

153. Lai LT, Naiki M, Yoshida SH, German JB, Gershwin ME. Dietary Platycladus orientalis seed oil suppresses anti-erythrocyte autoantibodies and prolongs survival of NZB mice. Clin Immun Immunopath 1994;71(3):293–302.

INFECTIONS, IMMUNITY AND ATHEROSCLEROSIS

Atherosclerosis and Autoimmunity
Y. Shoenfeld, D. Harats and G. Wick, editors

Immune Activation Augments Infection-Dependent Atherogenesis

Giovanni Ricevuti[1] and Christian J. Wiedermann[2]

[1]Section of Internal Medicine and Nephrology, Department of Internal Medicine and Therapeutics, University of Pavia, IRCCS Policlinico San Matteo, Piazzale Golgi 4, I-27100 Pavia, Italy; [2]Department of Internal Medicine, University of Innsbruck, Anichstrasse 35, A-6020 Innsbruck, Austria

1. INTRODUCTION

Evidence has accumulated that implicates chronic infection and inflammation in the etiology of atherosclerosis. Chronic inflammatory mediators are believed to contribute to the atherogenic process including C-reactive protein, proinflammatory cytokines and various growth factors [1, 2].

A direct link between infection and atherosclerosis has not been rapidly forthcoming. One hypothesis proposed direct vascular invasion by pathogens such as chlamydial organisms [3], but recent studies show that the causal relation between serological evidence of infection with *C. pneumoniae* and arteriosclerosis may be weak [4, 5]. Systemic inflammatory mediators may arise in response to infections at distant sites, but nonetheless promote coronary or carotid plaque development. Consistent with this hypothesis, recent epidemiologic evidence confirms a role of common chronic (bacterial) infections in human atherogenesis [6]. Systemic inflammatory mediators that have marked atherogenic effects on endothelium may be potential pathophysiological links [7]. Thus, it appears probable that some infectious agents contribute to the disease by maintaining a heightened state of inflammatory response.

Whether systemic inflammation is an epiphenomenon of atherosclerosis or whether it is in the atherosclerosis causal pathway requires further study. In a recent prospective study by Schratzberger et al. [7], endothelial monolayers were activated for transmigration of leukocytes more potently by plasma from subjects with carotid artery plaques than subjects without it; increased endothelial activation with plasma was prospectively associated with the development of new atherosclerotic lesions during a period of five years [7]. Thus, plasma from subjects with prevalent atherosclerosis of carotid arteries activates endothelium for leukocyte transmigration suggesting the presence of systemic proinflammatory mediators; epidemiological survey follow-up data on new lesion formation after five years indicate that plasma-mediated endothelium activation for interaction with leukocytes preceeds the development of atherosclerotic lesions.

2. INFLAMMATORY MEDIATORS IN BACTERIAL INFECTION

Infection produces a large array of mediators capable of initiating and maintaining the inflammatory and immune responses. Unmethylated bacterial deoxyribonucleic acid containing the CpG motif is a potent immunostimulant; bacterial heat-shock proteins can activate macrophages and also stimulate production of antibodies [8]. These antibodies frequently cross-react with human heat-shock proteins and are often invoked as etiologic in autoimmune or autoimmune-like conditions. However, the prototypical inflammatory bacterial product is endotoxin. Endotoxin possesses a multitude of biologic effects and is one of the most potent biologic response modifiers currently recognized. The interaction with its specific receptor stimulates the production of cytokines, chemokines, interferons, eicosanoids and free radicals leading to a wave of adhesion and signaling molecules in a variety of cell types [9].

In a recent study, plasma endotoxin levels were measured and incident atherosclerosis and cardiovascular disease assessed at follow-up [10]. Results demonstrated that endotoxemia constitutes a strong blood circulating risk factor of atherogenesis and atherosclerotic disease [10]. One may speculate that such proinflammatory activity of plasma contributes to the atherogenic endothelial activating activity such as uncovered recently [7]. Design of the studies and observed associations of endothelial activation by plasma with some of the parameters of inflammation that were obtained [7, 10], however, do not allow any conclusions as to the precise nature of the circulating factors responsible for the transendothelial migration of leukocytes.

3. ROLE OF IMMUNE ACTIVATION IN ENDOTOXEMIA-ASSOCIATED ATHEROGENESIS

Although it was previously identified that the risk for atherosclerosis is associated with elevated (highest decile) plasma levels of endotoxin [10], it is still difficult to firmly establish what place endotoxin assumes in the etiology of this disease [8]. Uncertainty arises from the inability to discern any trend toward risk at blood levels of endotoxin lower than the highest decile and from an apparent lack of risk with elevated endotoxin in the absence of risk factors, smoking and/or infection [9]. Thus, the relation between endotoxemia and vascular disease appears complex.

3.1. Endotoxin Hyperresponsiveness

The ability for endotoxin to promote disease may depend on its ability to initiate an inflammatory response. This effect may be controlled by additional regulatory factors. It is known from animal studies that endotoxin hypersensitivity may be induced by live or killed Gram-negative and Gram-positive bacteria, which is characterized by an overproduction of proinflammatory cytokines in response to endotoxin [11]. The induction of endotoxin hypersensitivity by bacteria appears to be mediated by interferon-γ [12, 13].

3.2. Neopterin, Endotoxin and Atherosclerosis

In vitro studies revealed that human monocytes/macrophages produce neopterin when stimulated by interferon-γ [14]. As neopterin is also closely correlated with the extent of carotid and coronary atherosclerosis [15, 16], interferon-γ or other neopterin-inducing activities may play an augmenting role in endotoxin-induced atherogenesis. Consistent with such mechanism is a recent *in vitro* observation of synergy between endotoxin, interferon-γ and C-reactive protein in increasing monocyte/macrophage tissue factor production [17].

The potential of interferon-induced immune activation – reflected by circulating neopterin – as a possible explanation for the strong effect modification seen in atherosclerosis between endotoxin and infection has been most recently investigated [18]. Elevated baseline plasma levels of neopterin (> median) with low levels of endotoxin (< highest decile) or, vice versa, low baseline plasma levels of neopterin (< median) high levels of endotoxin (upper decile) were not predictive of new carotid artery lesion formation during five years; however, in combination when both neopterin and endotoxin were increeased in plasma, the risk of lesion progression and new lesion formation was markedly increased [18]. These observations suggest that neopterin and endotoxin syergize in the pathophysiology of atherogenesis.

4. CONCLUSIONS

Epidemiologic data convincingly demonstrate risk for atherosclerotic disease associated with bacterial infection and endotoxin [9]; however, the independent contributions to disease and pathogenic mechanisms of endotoxin remained elusive. Further investigation into this relation tested the correlation between endotoxin and neopterin, and indicated that neopterin functions as effect modifying factor on the effects of endotoxin [18]. Until now, interferon-γ could not be associated with atherosclerosis risk [19, 20]. Since neopterin is the typical product of immune-activated macrophages, with interferon-γ as principal stimulatory agent, it may well be that this lymphokine gives rise to the array of effects that chronic infections impart in atherogenesis. Synergistic effects of interferon-γ and endotoxin on atherosclerosis-related hemostasis have been observed by others [17] and strongly support our proposed hypothesis.

REFERENCES

1. Anderson JL, Carlquist JF, Muhlestein JB, Horne BD, Elmer SP. Evaluation of C-reactive protein, an inflammatory marker, and infectious serology as risk factor for coronary artery disease and myocardial infarction. J Am Coll Cardiol 1998;32:35–41.

2. Koenig W. Heart disease and the inflammatory response. BMJ 2000;321:187–188.

3. Jackson LA, Campbell LA, Schmidt RA, Kuo C-C, Cappuccio AL, Grayston JT. Specificity of detection of Chlamydia pneumoniae in cardiovascular tissues: evaluation of innocent bystander hypothesis. Am J Pathol 1997;150:1785–1790.

4. Wald NJ, Law MR, Morris JK, Zhou X, Wong Y, Ward MF. Chlamydia pneumoniae infection and mortality from ischemic heart disease: large prospective study. BMJ 2000;321:204–207.

5. Danesh J, Whincup P, Walker M, Lennon L, Thomson A, Appleby P, et al. Chlamydia pneumoniae IgG titres and coronary heart disease: prospective study and meta-analysis. BMJ 2000;321:208–213.

6. Kiechl S, Egger G, Mayr M, Wiedermann CJ, Bonora E, Oberhollenzer F, et al. Chronic infections and the risk of carotid atherosclerosis: prospective results from a large population study. Circulation 2000; 102: submitted (in revision).

7. Schratzberger P, Kiechl S, Dunzendorfer S, Kähler CM, Patsch JR, Willeit J, Wiedermann CJ. Plasma-induced endothelial activation associated with incident atherosclerosis: prospective results from the Bruneck study. J Cardiovasc Risk 2000;7:285–291.

8. Carlquist JF. Endotoxin: another phantom menace? J Am Coll Cardiol 1999;34:1982–1984.

9. Raetz CR, Ulevitch RJ, Wright SD, Sibley CH, Ding A, Nathan CF. Gram-negative endotoxin: an extraordinary lipid with profound effects on eukaryotic signal transduction. FASEB J 1991;5:2652–2660.

10. Wiedermann CJ, Kiechl S, Dunzendorfer S, Schratzberger P, Egger G, Oberhollenzer F, Willeit J. Association of endotoxemia with carotid atherosclerosis and cardiovascular disease: prospective results from the Bruneck Study. J Am Coll Cardiol 1999;34:1975–1981.

11. Freudenberg MA, Merlin T, Gumenscheimer M, Sing A, Galanos C. Bacteria-induced hypersensitivity to endotoxin. J Endotox Res 1999;5:231–238.

12. Kamijo R, Le J, Shapiro D, Havell EA, Huang S, Aguet M, et al. Mice that lack the interferon-gamma receptor have profoundly altered responses to infection with Bacillus Calmette-Guerin and subsequent challenge with lipopolysaccharide. J Exp Med 1993;178:1435–1440.

13. Freudenberg MA, Kopf M, Galanos C. Lipopolysaccharide-sensitivity of interferon-γ-receptor deficient mice. J Endotoxin Res 1996;3:291–295.

14. Fuchs D, Weiss G, Wachter H. Neopterin, biochemistry and clinical use as a marker for cellular immune reactions. Int Arch Allergy Immunol 1993;101:1–6.

15. Weiss G, Willeit J, Kiechl S, Fuchs D, Jarosch E, Oberhollenzer F, et al. Increased concentrations of neopterin in carotid atherosclerosis. Atherosclerosis 1994;106:263–271.

16. Garcia-Moll X, Coccolo F, Cole D, Kaski JC. Serum neopterin and complex stenosis morphology in patients with unstable angina. J Am Coll Cardiol 2000;35:956–962.

17. Nakagomi A, Freedman SB, Geczy CL. Interferon-gamma and lipopolysaccharide potentiate monocyte tissue factor induction by C-reactive protein: relationship with age, sex, and hormone replacement treatment. Circulation 2000;101:1785–1791.

18. Wiedermann CJ, Kiechl S, Schratzberger P, Dunzendorfer S, Weiss G, Willeit J. The role of immune activation in endotoxin-induced atherogenesis. J Endotox Res, in press.

19. Zhou YF, Shou M, Guetta E, Guzman R, Unger EF, Yu ZX, et al. Cytomegalovirus infection of rats increases the neointimal response to vascular injury without consistent evidence of direct infection of the vascular wall. Circulation 1999;100:1569–1575.

20. Wilson AC, Schaub RG, Goldstein RC, Kuo PT. Suppression of aortic atherosclerosis in cholesterol-fed rabbits by purified rabbit interferon. Arteriosclerosis 1990;10:208–214.

Host Response Differences to Infection May Affect Disease Susceptibility in Atherosclerotic Patients

Jianhui Zhu, Yi Fu Zhou, Stephen E. Epstein

Cardiovascular Research Institute, Washington Hospital Center, Washington, DC 20010, USA

1. INTRODUCTION

Inflammation plays a major role in atherogenesis. However, the stimuli responsible for triggering the inflammatory process are not entirely known. Infectious agents may be one class of such stimuli based on evidence for infectious associations with atherosclerosis [1–7]. If infection is a risk factor, a perplexing problem that recurs in the infection/atherosclerosis literature is the inconsistency of the associations between a given pathogen and atherosclerosis--some studies show positive associations [8–20], some negative [21–24]. One of the issues we have focused on to explain this conundrum is the host-pathogen interaction--in particular, previous studies indicate that infection-related atherogenesis is a process related to host-mediated inflammatory and immune responses targeted to the pathogen and, importantly, that these responses vary among individuals. In this chapter we focus on recent evidence relating to these responses, and discuss the concept that differences in the host responses to infection may affect host susceptibility to infection-induced atherosclerosis.

2. THE ROLE OF INFLAMMATION IN INFECTION-RELATED ATHEROSCLEROSIS

2.1. C-Reactive Protein

Studies indicating that C-reactive protein (CRP) is a marker of underlying inflammation have stimulated inquiries into the issue of whether the level of inflammatory activity a given pathogen elicits in a given host (as reflected by CRP levels), influences the risk posed by a pathogen to the development of atherosclerosis.

CRP is a member of the pentraxin protein family (formed from five identical subunits). It was named by Tillet and Francis in 1930 because it reacts with the somatic C polysaccharide of *Streptococcus pneumonia*. CRP is normally present in trace amounts in human serum. Among normal healthy subjects, 95% have serum CRP levels less than 0.5mg/dL and 99% less than 1.0 mg/dL [*Abbott Laboratories Diagnostic Division, List No. 9550, January 1996*]. However, it increases rapidly in infection and inflammation as a consequence of increased synthesis in hepatocytes.

Although CRP binds to bacterial surface polysaccharides, its biological function is not clear. It may be involved in regulation of complement function [25, 26], but no demonstrable antimicrobal activity has been found. CRP is regulated by proinflammatory cytokines, especially IL-6, and some studies suggest its levels are altered by anti-inflammatory drugs [27]. CRP has been widely used as an indicator of infection and various other diseases in which inflammation plays a role.

2.2. CRP and Atherosclerosis

Elevated levels of CRP have been consistently found in patients with cardiovascular disease, such as unstable angina and myocardial infarction [28, 29]. Among patients with coronary artery disease (CAD), an elevated CRP level is a predictor of coronary events in both patients with stable and unstable angina [30, 31]. An elevated CRP is also associated with risk of coronary death in smokers with multiple risk factors for atherosclerosis [32]. Recently, studies by Ridker et al. [27] showed that the baseline plasma concentration of CRP is a predictor of increased risk for future major cardiac events (myocardial infarction or stroke) in apparently healthy male physicians with no known CAD. In addition, although CRP has been found in atherosclerotic lesions [33–36], it is not known what direct role, if any, it plays in the pathophysiology of atherosclerosis.

2.3. Infection as an Inducer of Inflammation in Atherosclerosis

As indicated above, although infection has been proposed to play a role in atherosclerosis, the data are not entirely consistent [8–24]. Of possible relevance to this dilemma are two considerations: 1) substantial evidence now exists indicating that inflammation contributes to the atherogenic process; 2) individuals vary in their response to infection. It is possible that a similar variation occurs in response to infection, with only certain individuals developing an inflammatory response (as reflected by elevated CRP levels), and therefore only a certain subset of infected individuals being susceptible to atherogenic effects of the infectious agents.

We studied the possible relationship of cytomegalovirus (CMV) infection and CRP levels on the risk of CAD in a cross-sectional study, and examined the hypothesis that *the likelihood of CMV infection predisposing to CAD is importantly dependent on the development of an inflammatory response* [7]. Blood samples were tested for CMV IgG antibodies and CRP levels from patients being evaluated for CAD by coronary angiography ($\geq$ 50% stenoses). Age, male gender, race, cigarette smoking, diabetes, hypercholesterolemia and hypertension were also studied as covariables. In this population, as found in other studies, an elevated CRP level (>0.5 mg/dL) was a significant predictor of CAD, even after adjustment for traditional risk factors (odds ratio 2.4, P=0.02).

Of note, CMV seropositivity was significantly associated with increased CRP levels, a relationship that retained statistical significance by using multivariate analysis. However, there was consider-

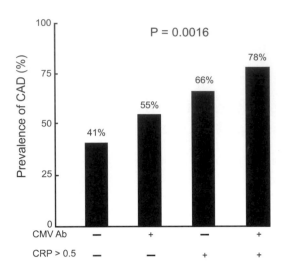

Figure 1. Prevalence of CAD among subgroups with variation in inflammation and CMV infection [7]. When adjustment for CAD risk factors, the odds ratios for CAD were 1.3 (95% CI, 0.4 to 4.4; P=0.7) in the subgroup with CMV seropositivity alone, 2.3 (95% CI, 0.7 to 7.5; P=0.2) in the subgroup with elevated CRP levels alone, and 4.3 (95% CI, 1.4 to 13.1; P=0.01) in the subgroup with combined CMV seropositivity and elevated CRP levels. Overall liner trend achieves significance even after adjustment for CAD risk factors (P=0.0016). CMV Ab+ or CMV Ab-: CMV antibody response positive or negative, respectively; CRP>0.5+ or CRP>0.5-: CRP levels>0.5 mg/dL or CRP levels≤0.5 mg/dL, respectively.

able variation in the host's inflammatory response (judged by elevated CRP levels) to CMV infection. Thus, whereas the majority of CMV seropositive individuals had elevated CRP levels, 27% *did not*. This variability allowed us to test whether the presence or absence of an inflammatory response in seropositive individuals influenced the risk for CAD. When adjusted for CAD risk factors, the odds ratios for CAD were 1.3 (95% CI 0.4 to 4.4) in the subgroup with CMV seropositivity alone, 2.3 (95% CI 0.7 to 7.5) in the subgroup with elevated CRP levels alone, and 4.3 (95% CI 1.4 to 13.1) in the subgroup with combined CMV seropositivity and elevated CRP levels (Figure 1). The overall stepwise increase in CAD prevalence remained significant by multiple logistic regression analysis (P=0.0016).

Our results therefore provide a potential explanation for the conflicting evidence relating to the role of CMV in atherosclerosis; considerable host variability exists in the inflammatory response to

CMV infection, and it appears that susceptibility to the atherogenic effects of CMV depends, at least in part, on the capacity of the host to suppress CMV-induced inflammatory activity. This conclusion implies that studies assessing whether CMV infection (or probably any infectious agent) is associated with CAD must take into consideration the frequency with which infection leads to inflammation in the particular cohort being studied. It could be anticipated that on the basis of genetic, environmental, or selection factors, different populations being studied may exhibit different dominant modes of responding to a specific infection – the dominant response of one population may be to develop an inflammatory response, whereas such a response may be absent in another population.

These considerations may relate to the apparently discordant results between our study, which demonstrated a significant association between CMV seropositivity and elevated CRP levels, and the lack of such a significant association in the study published by Anderson and co-workers [37]. They reported on the relation between seropositivity to three pathogens – CMV, *Chlamydia pneumoniae*, and *Helicobacter pylori* – and elevated CRP levels. They found, concordant with the results of many other studies, that CRP levels were significantly higher in individuals with CAD vs. those without. However, in contrast to our results, they found no significant association between elevated CRP levels and any of the pathogens. On the basis of the above discussion it is possible that the disparate results between our study and that of Anderson and associates may partly relate to inherent differences in the populations studied. In addition, whereas patients with recent myocardial infarction were excluded from our study, Anderson and co-workers did admit to study patients with recent infarction. Myocardial infarction by itself can cause substantial increases in CRP levels. It is therefore possible that the presence of this independent factor leading to increased CRP levels exerted confounding influences accounting for the failure to establish a significant association between CMV seropositivity and elevated CRP levels.

3. THE ROLE OF IMMUNE RESPONSES IN INFECTION-RELATED ATHEROSCLEROSIS

Infectious agents have two possible pathogenetic effects in the development of atherosclerosis: infection of the arterial wall with the local activity of the pathogen directly at the site of the developing atheroma influencing lesion development, and indirect effects of the pathogen on lesion development resulting from systemic effects of infection-triggered inflammation/immune reactions, with the pathogen residing at sites distant from the vessel [20]. Our recent studies investigating the effects of CMV infection on the neointimal response to acute vascular injury in rats bears on these two mechanisms. These studies showed that CMV infection increased the neointimal response to vascular injury; however, this effect occurred without the presence of virus in the vessel wall. Of note, serum levels of IL-2, IL-4 and IFNγ were increased in the infected rats [38, 39]. These findings suggested that systemic reactions to infection, such as immune and inflammatory responses, can also be pathogenically important in the vascular response to injury, and therefore in restenosis/atherosclerosis.

3.1. Cytomegalovirus

CMV is a large DNA virus (150–200 nm in diameter) and belongs to the family of *Herpetoviriae*. The entire viral genome has been sequenced and has the capacity to code for about 200 different proteins. Some of the viral proteins, such as CMV immediate-early (IE) proteins, have been demonstrated to play important roles in regulation of CMV gene expression and virus-host cell interactions. Since the virus can persist in the host for life and has a complex biological interaction with the cells that it infects, the immune response to CMV is quite complex.

3.2. Immune Responses to CMV

There are two lines of immune defense against CMV: the innate and the adaptive defense. The innate defense restricts the early stages of infection and delays spread of virus. It includes interferon and NK cells. The adaptive defense, including humoral (antibody) and cell-mediated immune responses, takes several days to develop, as T and B lymphocytes must encounter viral antigen, proliferate, and differentiate into effector cells. Following an infection, hosts will develop IgM, IgA and IgG antibodies against CMV. These antibodies may persist for a lifetime, dependent on the status of infection. The humoral immune response plays a protective but imperfect role in host defense against CMV infection. In contrast, the cellular response, including cytokine production and the proliferation and activation of CD4+ and CD8+ T cells, plays a bigger role than humoral immunity in eliminating CMV and providing the host with a protective immunity.

3.3. Immune Responses to CMV in Atherosclerosis

The link between infection and atherosclerosis has traditionally been assessed by identifying infected individuals through the presence or absence of antibodies directed at the pathogen. This issue is considerably more complex, however, since 1) evidence is beginning to emerge suggesting that the type of immune response (humoral or cellular) mounted by the host to a specific pathogen may be one of the factors determining whether infection with that pathogen contributes to the atherogenic process, and 2) the relative intensities of the humoral and cellular immune responses generated by an infectious agent depends upon multiple factors, including the specific pathogen and on the genetic determinants of the individual host.

Recently, we examined the hypothesis *the type of immune response mounted by the host to CMV contributes to susceptibility or resistance to CMV-associated CAD* in a group of patients undergoing diagnostic coronary angiography (63% men, 71% white, the mean age 57) [40]. Each individual was tested for anti-CMV IgG antibodies (Ab) and for proliferation of T lymphocytes (Tc) from peripheral blood mononuclear cells in response to CMV antigens. We found, for example, that there were four types of immune response patterns to CMV infection in our study population. Some individuals had neither a humoral (antibody) nor T-cell response to CMV antigens (Ab-/Tc- subgroup), suggesting they were either never exposed to CMV, or they were successful in clearing the virus and at the time of testing had

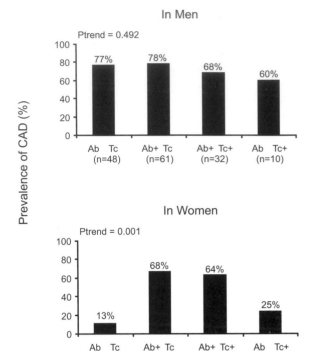

Figure 2. Prevalence of CAD in men and in women with different types of immune response to CMV infection [40]. Ab+ and Ab-: antibody response positive and negative, respectively; Tc+ and Tc-: T lymphocyte proliferative response positive and negative, respectively.

no immunologic evidence of prior infection. Others, all of whom demonstrated immunologic evidence of prior infection, had either a dominant humoral phenotype (Ab+/Tc- subgroup), a dominant cellular phenotype (Ab-/Tc+ subgroup), or a combined response (Ab+/Tc+ subgroup). The most common was a Ab+/Tc- response, and the least common was a Ab-/Tc+ response. Most importantly, we found that the type of immune response to CMV influences CAD risk. As shown in Figure 2, CAD prevalence was 5 times higher in Ab+/Tc- (P=0.0005) and in Ab+/Tc+ women (P=0.003) than in Ab-/Tc- women (those with no immunologic evidence of prior CMV infection). CAD prevalence in women with a cellular response (Ab-/Tc+) was not different from the Ab-/Tc- group, but was significantly lower than that of Ab+/Tc- group (P=0.016). There were no differences in age, smoking, diabetes, hypercholesterolemia or hypertension among these study subjects with different types of immune response to

CMV infection (all P>0.1).

There are at least two possible explanations, not mutually exclusive, to account for the findings in women that susceptibility to CMV-associated CAD occurs in the humoral response subgroups, whereas resistance is observed in the cellular responders. First, it is possible that a cellular response to CMV, an intracellular pathogen, conveys greater control of viral activity than a humoral response. This explanation implies the cellular response is primary in determining outcome. If this were the sole explanation, however, it might have been expected that greater control of viral activity would be accompanied by lower CRP levels, and that women with a combined humoral and cellular response would have a lower prevalence of CAD than women with a humoral response who lacked a cellular response. These were not observed.

The alternative explanation focuses on the humoral immune response as the major player. Thus, it is possible that the humoral response to CMV is a reflection of antibody-induced autoimmune disease. In this regard, there is now growing evidence that autoimmune responses may play a role in atherosclerosis [41–45]. Even more relevant to our concept that the antibody response to CMV infection may predispose to atherosclerosis through autoimmune mechanisms are the many examples of immunopathology triggered by the host's immune response to viral infection. Perhaps the best studied potential mechanism for infection-induced immunopathology is that of molecular mimicry, which is based on the invading pathogen having peptides highly homologous to host peptides. The immune response targeted to the infectious pathogen would, through molecular mimicry, effectively result in the development of autoantibodies or auto-aggressive T cells to host peptides.

4. PATHOGEN-HOST INTERACTION IN HOST SUSCEPTIBILITY TO INFECTION-RELATED CAD

Because of the marked influence of gender on susceptibility to CAD, and because of the presumed roles of inflammatory and immune responses in CAD, after we completed the above studies we then postulated that overall susceptibility or resistance to CMV-induced CAD will be determined by gender-related heterogeneity of the inflammatory and immune responses to CMV infection. We therefore investigated possible gender differences in the associations among CMV, CRP and CAD [40].

We found that the prevalence of anti-CMV IgG antibodies in men with CAD was similar as those without CAD. However, mean CRP was significantly higher in CAD than non-CAD patients, with a high proportion of men with CAD having elevated CRP levels (>0.5 mg/dL). When adjusted for traditional CAD risk factors (age, smoking, diabetes, hypertension and hypercholesterolemia) and CMV seropositivity, elevated CRP level was a significant independent predictor of CAD (odds ratio 3.1, 95%CI 1.21–7.97). Interestingly, there were no positive CMV sero-association and no influence of the type of immune responses (immunodominant humoral vs cellular) to CMV on CAD prevalence in men. However, CMV seropositivity was significantly and independently associated with elevated CRP levels, by both univariate and multivariate analysis.

In contrast, in women, patients with CAD had a significantly higher prevalence of anti-CMV IgG antibodies than those without CAD. After adjustment for traditional CAD risk factors, the presence of CMV seropositivity was a highly significant predictor of CAD (odds ratio 41.8, P=0.0016). Also contrasting with the data in men, CPR levels did not correlate independently with CAD risk; although the levels tended to be higher in women with CAD than in those without, the differences did not reach statistical significance. And, as indicated above, although the type of immune response mounted by men (humoral vs. cellular) did not influence CAD risk, it did in women (Figure 2).

These results indicate that multiple mechanisms exist whereby CMV infection, and perhaps infection by other pathogens, contribute to CAD. They also indicate that the relative contribution of these mechanisms to atherogenesis is gender-determined, and is influenced by whether or not the host mounts an inflammatory response to CMV infection, as well as by the nature of the immune response. The data suggest that CMV, at least in men, may contribute to CAD insofar as it induces an inflammatory response (although it must be emphasized that insofar as an inflammatory response contributes to CAD, CMV can be considered only one possible factor). In women, however, CMV infection is an independent predictor of CAD risk, but not CRP, and the type of immune response generated by the host appears to significantly contribute to the pro-atherogenic effects of CMV.

In addition to the information relating to potential mechanisms by which CMV, and presumably other pathogens, contribute to atherogenesis, these gender-related data may also help to explain the conflicting epidemiological evidence relating to the possible role of infectious agents in atherosclerosis. Although some studies have found an association between CMV and atherosclerosis or restenosis based on analysis of CMV seropositivity, other studies have questioned such a relationship. This controversy may be due to the paucity of women in these studies, in whom a direct association between CMV seropositivity and CAD is observed, and to the failure to analyse, concomitantly, an index of inflammation, such as CRP elevations.

5. SUMMARY

In the past years, epidemiological studies for infections in human populations have shown the associations between atherosclerotic disease and positive serology. Despite not all authors reported positive associations, such studies have made essential contributions to the totality of evidence. Basic researches have demonstrated pathogen antigens or nucleic acids in arterial tissues taken from patients undergoing vascular operation or autopsy. These data supported the epidemiological findings, and provided direct observation of what actually happens in human. Although a clear mechanism for the infection in the development atherosclerosis has not been established, numerous investigations that have attempted to link atherosclerosis in humans with infection with various pathogens, such as CMV, *Chlamydia pneumoniae* and *Helicobacter pylori,* have led to the suggestion that infection-related cardiovascular disease is an inflammation and immune reaction-mediated process. The susceptibility to the atherogenic effects of infectious agents depend, at least in part, on the capacity of the host to pathogen-induced inflammatory activity or immunr responses. Therefore, it is likely that a complete understand-

ing of the potential role of infection in atherosclerosis will be achieved only after the more complex interrelations between a pathogen and the host's response to the pathogen are elucidated.

REFERENCES

1. Frothingham C. The relation between acute infectious diseases and arterial lesions. Arch Intern Med 1911;8:153–162.
2. Ophuls W. Arteriosclerosis and cardiovascular disease: their relation to infectious diseases. JAMA 1921;76:700–701.
3. Fabricant CG, Fabricant J, Litrenta MM, Minik CR. Virus-induced atherosclerosis. J Exp Med 1978;148:335–340.
4. Adam E, Probtsfield JL, Burek J, McCollum CH, Melnick JL, Petrie BL, Bailey KR, Debakey ME. High levels of cytomegalovirus antibody in patients requiring vascular surgery for atherosclerosis. Lancet 1987;2:291–293.
5. Saikku P, Leinonen M, Mattila K, Ekman MR, Nieminen MS, Makela PH, Huttunen JK, Valtonen V. Serological evidence of an association of a novel chlamydia, TWAR, with chronic coronary heart disease and acute myocardial infarction. Lancet 1988;2:983–986.
6. Mendall MA, Goggin PM, Molineaux N, Levy J, Toosy T, Strachan D, Camm AJ, Northfield TC. Relation of *Helicobacter pylori* infection and coronary heart disease. Br Heart J 1994;71:437–439.
7. Zhu J, Quyyumi AA, Norman JE, Csako G, Epstein SE. Cytomegalovirus in the pathogenesis of atherosclerosis: the role of inflammation, as reflected by elevated C-reactive protein levels. JACC 1999;34:1738–1743.
8. Grattan MT, Moreno-Cabral CE, Starnes VA, Oyer PE, Stinson EB, Shumway NE. Cytomegalovirus infection is associated with cardiac allograft rejection and atherosclerosis. JAMA 1989;261:3561–3566.
9. Nieto FJ, Adam E, Sorlie P, Farzadegan H, Melnick JL, Comstock GW, Szklo M. Cohort study of cytomegalovirus infection as a risk factor for carotid intimal-medial thickening, a measure of subclinical atherosclerosis. Circulation 1996;94:922–927.
10. Zhou YF, Leon MB, Waclawiw MA, Popma JJ, Yu ZX, Finkel T, Epstein SE. Association between prior cytomegalovirus infection and the risk of restenosis after coronary atherectomy. N Engl J Med 1996;335:624–630.
11. Thom DM, Grayston JT, Siscovitch DS, Wang SP, Weiss NS, Daling JR. Association of prior infection with *Chlamydia pneumoniae* and angiographically demonstrated coronary artery disease. JAMA

1992;268:68–72.

12. Miettinen H, Lehto S, Saikku P, Haffner SM, Ronnemaa T, Pyorala K, Laakso M. Association of *Chlamydia pneumoniae* and acute coronary heart disease events in non-insulin dependent diabetic and non-diabetic subjects in Finland. Eur Heart 1996;17:682–688.

13. Cook PJ, Honeybourne D, Lip GY, Beevers DG, Wise R. *Chlamydia pneumoniae* and acute arterial thrombotic disease. Circulation 1995; 92:3148–3149.

14. Morgando A, Sanseverino P, Perotto C, Molono F, Gai V, Ponzetto A. *Helicobacter pylori* seropositivity in myocardial infarction. Lancet 1995;345:1380.

15. Pasceri V, Cammarota G, Patti G, Cuoco L, Gasbarrini A, Grillo RL, Fedeli G, Gasbarrini G, Maseri A. Association of virulent *Helicobacter pylori* strains with ischemic heart disease. Cirulation 1998;97:1675–1679.

16. Folsom AR, Nieto FJ, Sorlie P, Chambless LE, Graham DY, for the Atherosclerosis Risk in Communities (ARIC) Study Investigators. *Helicobacter pylori* seropositivity and coronary heart disease incidence. Circulation 1998;98:845–850.

17. Sorlie PD, Adam E, Melnick SL, Folsom A, Skelton T, Chambless LE, Barnes R, Melnock JL. Cytomegalovirus/herpesvirus and carotid atherosclerosis: the ARIC study. J Med Virol 1994;42:33–37.

18. Chiu B, Viira E, Tucker W, Fong IW. *Chlamydia pneumoniae*, cytomegalovirus, and herpes simplex virus in atherosclerosis of the carotid artery. Circulation 1997;96:2144–2148.

19. Zhu J, Quyyumi AA, Norman JE, Casko G, Waclawiw MA, Shearer GM, Epstein SE. Effects of total pathogen burden on coronary artery disease risk and C-reactive protein levels. Am J Cardiol 2000;85:140–146.

20. Danesh J, Collins R, Peto R. Chronic infections and coronary heart disease: Is there a link? Lancet 1997;350:430–436.

21. Havlik RJ, Blackwelder WC, Kaslow R, Castelli W. Unlikely association between clinically apparent herpesvirus infection and coronary incidence at older ages. Arteriosclerosis 1989;9:877–880.

22. Adler SP, Hur JK, Wang JB, Vetrovec GW. Prior infection with cytomegalovirus is not a major risk factor for angiographically demonstrated coronary artery atherosclerosis. J Infect Dis 1998;177:209–212.

23. Weiss SW, Roblin PM, Gaydos CA, Cummings P, Patton DL, Schulhoff N, Shani J, Frankel R, Penney K, Quinn TC, Hammerschlag MR, Schachter J. Failure to detect *Chlamydia pneumoniae* in coronary atheromas of patients undergoing atherectomy. J Infect Dis 1996;173:957–963.

24. Ridker PM, Hennekens CH, Buring JE, Kundsin R, Shih J. Baseline IgG antibody titers to *Chlamydia pneumoniae*, *Helicobacter pylori*, herpes simplex virus, and

cytomegalovirus and the risk for cardiovascular disease in women. Ann intern Med 1999;131:573–577.

25. Volanakis JE. Complement activation by C-reactive protein complexes. Ann NY Acad Sci 1982;89:235–238.

26. Wolbink GJ. CRP-mediated activation of complement in vivo. J Immunol 1996;157:473–479.

27. Ridker PM, Cushman M, Stampfer MJ, Tracy RP, Hennekens CH. Inflammation, aspirin, and the risk of cardiovascular disease in apparently healthy men. N Engl J Med 1997;336:973–979.

28. de Beer FC, Hind CR, Fox KM, Allan RM, Maseri A, Pepys MB. Measurement of serum C-reactive protein concentration in myocardial ischemia and infarction. Br Heart J 1982;47:239–243.

29. Berk BC, Weintraub WS, Alexander RW. Elevation of C-reactive protein in "active" coronary artery disease. Am J Cardiol 1990;65:168–172.

30. Liuzzo G, Biasucci LM, Gallimore JR, Grillo RL, Rebuzzi AG, Pepys MB, Maseri A. The prognostic value of C-reactive protein and serum amyloid A protein in severe unstable angina. N Engl J Med 1994;331:417–424.

31. Toss H, Lindahl B, Siegbahn A, Wallentin L. Prognostic influence of increased fibrinogen and c-reactive protein levels in unstable coronary artery disease. Circulation 1997;96:4204–4210.

32. Kuller LH, Tracy RP, Shaten J, Meilahn EN. Relation of C-reactive protein and coronary heart disease in the MRFIT nested case-control study. Am J Epidemiol 1996;144:537–547.

33. Vlaicu R, Rus HG, Niculescu F, Cristea A. Immunoglobulins and complement components in human aortic atherosclerotic intima. Atherosclerosis 1985;55:35–50.

34. Reynolds GD, Vance RP. C-reactive protein immunohistochemical localization in normal and atherosclerotic human aortas. Arch Pathol Lab Med 1987;111:265–269.

35. Hatanaka K, Li XA, Masuda K, Yutanii C, Yamamoto A. Immunohistochemical localization of C-reactive protein binding sites in human aortic lesions by modified streptavidin-biotin-staining method. Pathol Int 1995;45:635–642.

36. Torzewski J, Torzewski M, Bowyer DE, Frohlich M, Koenig W, Walterberger J, Fitzsimmons C, Hombach V. C-reactive protein frequently colocalizes with the terminal complement complex in the intima of early atherosclerotic lesions of human coronary arteries. Arterioscler Thromb Vasc Biol 1998;18:1386–1392.

37. Anderson J, Carlquist JF, Muhlestein JB, Horne BD, Elmer SP. Evaluation of C-reactive protein, an inflammatory marker, and infectious serology as risk factors for coronary artery disease and myocardial infarction.

JACC 1998;32:35–41.

38. Zhou YF, Shou M, Guetta E, Guzman R, Unger EF, Yu ZX, Zhang J, Finkel T, Epstein SE. Cytomegalovirus infection of rats increases the neointimal response to vascular injury without consistent evidence of direct infection of the vascular wall. Circulation 1999;100:1569–1575.

39. Zhou YF, Shou M, Harrell RF, Yu ZX, Unger EF, Epstein SE. Chronic non-vascular cytomegalovirus infection: effects on the neointimal response to experimental vascular injury. Cardiovascular Research 2000;45:1019–1025.

40. Zhu J, Shearer GM, Norman JE, Pinto LA, Marincola FM, Prasad A, Waclawiw MA, Csako G, Quyyumi AA, Epstein SE. Host response to cytomegalovirus infection as a determinant of susceptibility to coronary artery disease: Gender-based differences in inflammation and type of immune response. Circulation 2000;102:2491–2496.

41. Fujinami RS, Oldstone MBA. Molecular mimicry as a mechanism for virus-induced autoimmunity. Immunol Res 1989;8:3–15.

42. Wick G, Schett G, Amberger A, Kleindienst R, Xu Q. Is atherosclerosis an immunologically mediated disease? Immunol Today 1995;16:27–33.

43. George J, Harats D, Gilburd B, Levy Y, Langevitz P, Shoenfeld Y. Atherosclerosis-related markers in systemic lupus erythematosus patients: the role of humoral immunity in enhanced atherogenesis. Lupus 1999;8:220–226.

44. Krause I, Blank M, Shoenfeld Y. The induction of experimental vascular diseases by immunization with pathogenic autoantibodies. Clin Exp Rheumatol 2000;18:257–261.

45. George J, Afek A, Gilburd B, Harats D, Shoenfeld Y. Autoimmunity in atherosclerosis: lessons from experimental models. Lupus 2000;9:223–227.

Atherosclerosis and Autoimmunity
Y. Shoenfeld, D. Harats and G. Wick, editors

The Role of Chronic Infection in Atherosclerosis

Sandeep Gupta[1] and Amarjit Sethi[2]

[1]Whipps Cross and St. Bartholomew's Hospitals, London EC1A 7BE, UK; [2]Department of Experimental Therapeutics, The William Harvey Research Institute, London EC1M 6BQ, UK

1. INTRODUCTION

Established risk factors for atherosclerosis (such as hypercholesterolaemia, smoking, hypertension and diabetes mellitus) fail to fully explain the extent and/or severity of coronary artery disease (CAD) in up to 50% of patients [1]. Other causative agents and processes that may be involved in the pathogenesis of atherosclerosis have hence been sought. Chronic infection is one possibility – both by initiating atherogenesis and/or as a 'modulating' factor in plaque progression and instability [2, 3]. Conversely, infective organisms may merely represent 'innocent bystanders' in atheroma, transported to sites of inflammation within the vascular wall.

Sir William Osler first proposed the role of infection in the pathogenesis of atherosclerosis in 1908 [4]. Interest re-emerged in the 1970's and within the last decade increasing evidence links various infective agents with human atherosclerosis. This chapter aims to review the evidence for the role of chronic infections in the aetiology of atherosclerosis, with a particular focus on *Chlamydia pneumoniae* as evidence for the role of this particular organism is stronger than for other infective agents.

2. CHLAMYDIA PNEUMONIAE

2.1. Diagnosis of Chronic Infection

Chlamydia pneumoniae, an obligatory intracellular pathogen, is a common cause of mild respiratory symptoms [5], but can also result in bronchitis, sinusitis, tonsillitis and pneumonia [6]. Antibody prevalence to *C. pneumoniae* increases with age and is about 50% in middle-aged adults in various populations world-wide. Chronic infection and recurrent infections are both well documented [5].

The diagnosis of *C. pneumoniae* infection is hampered by difficulties in culturing the organism. There has hence been reliance on indirect serological tests, which are unable to distinguish between persistent chronic infection and past exposure to the organism. The criteria for defining infection are controversial, but persistently raised specific IgA and IgG levels are generally accepted to reflect chronic infection [7]. The established microimmunofluorescence test is dependent on the interpretation by expert microscopists and as yet is inadequately standardised [8]. Variable antibody titre cut-offs have been used to define seropositivity and there is also debate on whether the height of antibody titres reflects chronic infection or mere previous exposure to the organism. Newer diagnostic tests for detecting chronic *C. pneumoniae* infection are emerging, especially using polymerase chain reaction (PCR) techniques to identify the organism within peripheral blood mononuclear cells [9]. Such methods require further validation and evaluation in the clinical settings.

2.2. Serological Association of Chronic C Pneumoniae Infection and Atherosclerosis

The first evidence of an association between *C. pneumoniae* and CAD was reported in 1988 [10]. Saikku et al found that 68% of patients with myocardial infarction (MI) and 50% of patients with chronic CAD had elevated IgG (>1/128) or IgA

Table 1. Prospective studies of Chlamydia pneumoniae IgG titres and coronary heart disease. Black squares indicate the odds ratio in each study, with the square size proportional to the number of cases and horizontal lines representing 99% confidence intervals. The combined odds ratio and its 95% confidence interval are indicated by a diamond. Degree of adjustment for possible confounders is denoted as +++ for age, sex, smoking, and some other classic vascular risk factors, and ++++ for these plus markers of socioeconomic status (or studies done in socially homogeneous groups). BMJ 2000;321:199–204, with permission from the BMJ Publishing Group. All studies referenced in same article.

Study	No of cases	Degree of adjustment	Odds ratio and confidence intervals
Wald et al[7]	647	++++	
Present study	496	++++	
Ridker et al[8]	343	++++	
Strachan et al[9]	278	++++	
Tavendale et al[10]	252	++++	
Nieto et al[11]	246	++++	
Ridker et al[12]	85	++++	
Miettinen et al[13]	202	+++	
Haider et al[14]	199	+++	
Saikku et al[15]	102	+++	
Siscovik et al[16]	100	+++	
Glader et al[17]	78	+++	
von Hertzen et al[18]	67	+++	
Ossewarde et al[19]	54	+++	
Gupta et al[20]	20	+++	
Total	3169		1.15 (95% CI 0.97 to 1.36)

0.25   0.5   1   2   4   8

(>1/32) antibodies against *C. pneumoniae* compared with only 17% of controls. The investigators postulated that acute MI might be linked to an exacerbation of chronic *C. pneumoniae* infection. Several workers from North America, UK and Europe soon corroborated the findings [11–13]. In patients undergoing coronary angiography, an increased IgG antibody titre against *C. pneumoniae* was associated with a twofold increase in having angiographically detectable CAD [11]. In the Helsinki Heart Study, an association was found between elevated IgA titres to C. pneumoniae and the presence of immune complexes containing chlamydial lipopolysaccharide antigen with the development of a cardiac event 6 months later [13]. In a meta-analysis of 18 published sero-epidemiological studies [14], a raised anti-*C. pneumoniae* antibody titre was associated with a 2 to 4 fold increased prevalence of CAD.

Wong et al. went on to critically review 27 studies that have investigated *C. pneumoniae* antibodies and atherosclerosis [7]. Twenty-one of the 27 studies were associated with a positive link. To date, the association between CAD and *C. pneumoniae* antibody seropositivity has been verified in 30 studies in eight different countries [15]. However, prospective data is limited and weaken any association (Table 1). In the Caerphilly prospective heart disease study, plasma specimens were collected from men aged 45–59 years over a 13 year period and tested for IgG and IgA antibody to *C. pneumoniae* [16]. An association was found between IgA antibodies (but not IgG) to *C. pneumoniae* and subsequent risk of death from CAD. In the most recent review, Danesh et al. showed little association between *C. pneumoniae* IgG titres and incident CAD [17]. However, this study and the subsequent meta-analysis were limited by the diagnosis of chronic infection being made on only one serum sample taken many years prior to any coronary events.

There has been recent interest in the role of low grade systemic inflammation in CAD [18], as measured by elevated levels of C-reactive protein (CRP) in patients developing non fatal myocardial infarction or dying from CAD. The reason for this low grade inflammation is not clear but chronic infection leading to a systemic inflammatory response remains a possibility. Evidence for this remains in the balance at the present time – with studies showing both positive and negative associations [19, 20]. Interestingly, there is some preliminary evidence for an association between antibodies to *Chlamydia*-specific lipopolysaccharide and patients with acute coronary syndromes [21]. This finding suggests that infection with *Chlamydia* could lead to disruption of vulnerable plaques in patients with acute coronary syndromes, possibly by initiating an inflammatory process within the coronary vasculature.

In addition to an association between *C. pneumoniae* antibodies and CAD, there may also be an association between *C. pneumoniae* and development of aortic disease [22], peripheral arterial and cerebrovascular atherosclerotic disease [23].

The main limitation with epidemiological antibody studies rest in defining the meaning of the various types and titres of antibodies measured and their significance relating to past exposure, current chronic infection or the endovascular presence of the organism. Chronic infection of arterial walls leading to local inflammation and cytokine production, for example, could lead to a low-grade systemic inflammatory response without a systemic antibody response.

2.3. Chronic Infection within Arterial Tissue

In 1992, Shor et al. were the first to identify *C. pneumoniae* within coronary artery tissue [24]. Since then, numerous studies using immunocytochemistry (Figure 1) and PCR (Figure 2) techniques have

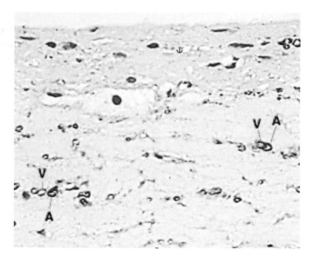

Figure 1. Photomicrograph of an Early Atherosclerotic Lesion of the Aorta Positive for Chlamydia pneumoniae by Polymerase Chain Reaction. The smooth muscle cells are histochemically stained for smooth muscle actin (brown) and counterstained with hematoxylin to show evidence of vacuolation, caused by C. pneumoniae. A indicates smooth muscle cell actin; V, vacuoles (original magnification 400x). With permission from JAMA Dec 1 1999, vol 282, no 21: 2071–2073. Copyrighted © 1999, American Medical Association.

shown *C. pneumoniae* located within plaque tissue. In an analysis of 17 studies published examining for *C. pneumoniae* in vascular tissue, all but 2 studies showed the presence of the organism in atherosclerotic tissue[25]. *Chlamydia pneumoniae* can be identified in about 50% of atheromatous lesions examined, compared with only 5% in non-atheromatous arterial samples [26]. In an autopsy study of Alaskan Natives, a strong relationship was found between increased *C. pneumoniae* antibodies (taken over 8.8 years prior to death) and increasing severity of coronary atherosclerotic lesions [27]. Conversely, other studies have found no association with increasing severity of atherosclerosis: the organism was just as likely to be found in mildly diseased lesions as in fatal plaques with acute thrombosis, rupture or haemorrhage [28]. There are some 50 reported studies of *C. pneumoniae* in atherosclerotic tissue and all but 4 demonstrated the organism in atheroma [29]. These studies clearly demonstrate that *C. pneumoniae* is found frequently in atheromatous lesions but whether this establishes a causal link between infection and atherogenesis remains

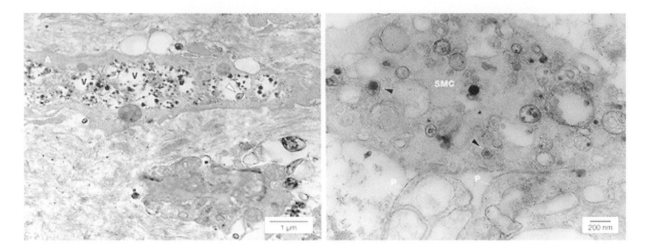

Figure 2. Transmission Electron Micrograph of Smooth Muscle Cells in an Early Atherosclerotic Lesion of the Aorta Positive for Chlamydia pneumoniae by Polymerase Chain Reaction. Left, one smooth muscle cell contains vacuoles (V) and C pneumoniae elementary bodies (arrowhead); the other is fragmenting. A indicates actin filaments. Right, macrophage pseudopodia (P) in contact with a fragment of smooth muscle cell (SMC) containing C pneumoniae (arrowheads). PERMISSION PENDING from JAMA Dec 1 1999, vol 282, no 21: 2071–2073. Copyrighted © 1999, American Medical Association.

controversial and unclear.

Recently, 'live' viable organisms have been cultured from atherosclerotic lesions obtained from endarterectomy and restenotic bypass samples [30]. This may indicate that venous grafts from some patients can be infected by *C. pneumoniae* and this could possibly lead to the development of vein graft disease. Studies are underway to investigate whether patients undergoing coronary artery bypass surgery may benefit from antibiotic therapy to prevent vein graft disease. The presence of replicating viable organisms within plaque do favour a pathogenetic role for *C. pneumoniae* in atherosclerosis.

2.4. In Vitro and Animal Studies

Chlamydia pneumoniae can replicate and maintain infection in human macrophages, endothelial cells and aortic smooth muscle cells [31, 32]. Infection can stimulate a fourfold increase in the expression of tissue factor and platelet adhesion [33] and human umbilical vein endothelial cells (HUVEC) infected with *C. pneumoniae* stimulate smooth muscle cell replication in a time-and dose-dependent fashion [34]. Such findings suggest that the cells involved in atherogenesis are susceptible to infection by *C. pneumoniae* and this may lead to a procoagulant state.

Animal models of infection-induced atherosclerosis are emerging. Apolipoprotein E-deficient transgenic mice (which spontaneously develop atherosclerosis) can be inoculated with intra-nasal *C. pneumoniae* and the organism can subsequently be detected within atherosclerotic regions of the aorta using PCR and immunocytochemical techniques [35]. In other mouse models however, C57BL/6J mice inoculated with *C. pneumoniae* developed inflammatory changes in the heart and aorta but no evidence of atherosclerotic lesions [36]. In another study [37], repeated *C. pneumoniae* infection in apolipoprotein-E knockout mice produced endothelial dysfunction but no intimal thickening after 6 weeks of infection.

Chlamydia pneumoniae infection of the respiratory tract of rabbits fed a non-cholesterol diet induces atherosclerotic-like changes in the aorta [38]. Furthermore, treatment with azithromycin (an antibiotic effective against *Chlamydial* infections) after infectious exposure in rabbits prevents such lesion formation [39]. Whether studies that induce atherogenesis in animals can be translated into the pathogenesis of human atherosclerosis remains unclear. These studies are also limited by small sample size.

3. CYTOMEGALOVIRUS

Studies have shown that antibodies against Cytomegalovirus (CMV) are elevated in patients with CAD compared with control subjects [40] and CMV DNA has been found in the arterial walls of patients with CAD. Cytomegalovirus infection has been associated with high levels of lipoprotein (a) and fibrinogen [41].

Further evidence for the role of CMV in the development of thrombosis comes from in vitro and animal work. Human endothelial cells infected with CMV have shown increased adherence of leukocytes and platelets to these cells [42] and CMV infection of rat aorta has been shown to induce synthesis of procoagulant activity [43]. In a prospective study of patients undergoing coronary angioplasty and stent placement, a positive CMV IgG titre was associated with an increased rate of death, nonfatal Q-wave myocardial infarction and urgent reintervention during a 30-day follow up period. Hence, previous CMV infection may increase the risk of coronary thrombotic events after stent   placement [44].

However, a recent study showed that CMV could not be detected in the arterial wall at the time of bypass surgery [45] and recent meta-analyses show no strong association between CMV and CAD [46]. Although CMV has been linked with the pathogenesis of CAD, the overall evidence remains weak, as most of the studies are observational and have not adequately controlled for confounding by other risk factors [14].

4. HELICOBACTER PYLORI

Original case-control studies found an association between seropositivity to *Helicobacter pylori* and CAD [47, 48]. A recent study suggests that the association of chronic *H. pylori* infection with myocardial infarction is restricted to certain more virulent strains of *H. pylori* bearing the cytotoxin associated gene-A (cagA) antigen [49]. However, larger prospective studies and meta-analyses have not found a strong association [50–52]. Lower socio-economic status remains the major confounding variable.

5. OTHER CHRONIC INFECTIONS

Evidence for the role of other viruses in atherogenesis is scarce and the studies are limited by small sample sizes [53]. There is some limited evidence for the role of other chronic bacterial infections. Dental sepsis [54] and chronic bronchitis [55] have been associated with CAD. However, confounding factors weaken the associations and prospective data is limited.

6. THE INTERACTION OF CHRONIC INFECTION WITH TRADITIONAL RISK FACTORS

It is possible that a complex interaction exists between chronic infection and established risk factors for CAD, leading to atherogenesis and disease progression. Furthermore, this association may only be valid in certain genetically susceptible individuals [56]. Patients with combined positive serology for *H. pylori* and *C. pneumoniae* are characterised by greater age, lower social class and higher body mass index [57]. It is postulated that obesity might be a marker not only for lower social class but also a greater than normal susceptibility to such infections.

Altered lipid profiles have been noted in chronic *C. pneumoniae* infection. Serum triglyceride and total cholesterol are higher in subjects with a chronic *C. pneumoniae* infection than in subjects without evidence of infection [58], while HDL cholesterol is significantly decreased in such subjects. Whether low-level production of TNF and IL-1 within atherosclerotic lesions lead to the altered lipid profile (possibly by effects on cholesterol transport or lipoprotein lipase) or whether subjects with altered serum lipid profile have an increased susceptibility to *C. pneumoniae* infection remains unclear.

Interestingly, Hu et al showed that in mice with low-density lipoprotein receptor deficiency that are fed a high cholesterol diet, a super-imposed infection with *C. pneumoniae* significantly exacerbated the hypercholesterolaemia-induced atherosclerosis [59]. Hence, supporting evidence for a 'modulating' role of infection.

Chlamydia pneumoniae has also been associated with cigarette smoking [60], hypertension [61] and

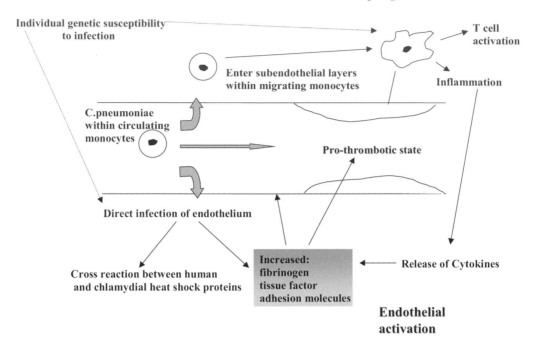

Chronic Macrophage infection

Figure 3. *C. pneumoniae* and possible mechanisms of atherogenesis. With permission from Thrombus 2000;4:1–4.

plasma fibrinogen levels [62].

7. CHRONIC INFECTION AND MECHANISMS OF ATHEROGENESIS

Atherosclerosis results from an excessive inflammatory response to different forms of vessel injury [63]. An initial insult to the arterial wall may trigger atherogenesis and plaque formation. Such stimuli may include modified low-density lipoproteins (LDL) [64] and intracellular pathogens such as *C. pneumoniae* [26]. There are several possible mechanisms by which *C. pneumoniae* could either initiate or exacerbate atherogenesis (Figure 3). Two key events in atherogenesis include the formation of foam cells from macrophages and the oxidation of LDL. In vitro, the presence of *C. pneumoniae* causes macrophage foam cell formation and lipid oxidation with murine and human cells cocultured in the presence of LDL [65]. This is mediated by chlamydial lipopolysaccharide, which causes macrophages to develop into foam cells in the presence of LDL, and the 60-kDa chlamydial heat shock pro-

tein, which contributes to the oxidation of LDL in the presence of macrophages.

Chlamydia pneumoniae may enter the circulation via the respiratory tract and replicate within alveolar macrophages [66]. Systemic spread within circulating monocytes leading to infection of the coronary artery endothelium may form the basis of an inflammatory response and development or destabilisation of a mature atheromatous plaque.

Chlamydial infection may induce chronic immune activation mediated by cytokines and stimulate the synthesis of acute phase proteins such as fibrinogen [12]. There may also be an enhanced procoagulant state with increased risk of coronary thrombosis. Alternatively, chronic bacterial infection may enhance T cell activation contributing to destabilisation of the intimal cap and plaque rupture. Other proposed mechanisms are an immune cross-reactivity between human and *chlamydial* heat shock proteins [67] and endothelial activation and the expression of adhesion molecules [68]. Finally, *C. pneumoniae* may contribute to plaque instability by triggering apoptosis leading to plaque cap thinning, rupture and an acute coronary event [69].

The mechanisms by which the above effects are mediated are gradually becoming clearer. Monocyte infiltration, regulated by the chemokine monocyte chemotactic protein-1 (MCP-1), is thought to play a key part in atherogenesis. Recently, *C. pneumoniae* infection of human umbilical vein endothelial cells has been shown to increase the expression of MCP-1 [70]. This effect involved the activation of nuclear factor-kappa beta (NF-KB).

It still remains possible that *C. pneumoniae* may simply reside within the macrophage as a 'secondary passenger'. Indeed, its distribution in the body is widespread, being found in arthritic joints [71], cerebrospinal fluid [72], aortic valves [73] and hepatic vessels [74]. At the present time, a direct causal link between *C. pneumoniae* and atherosclerosis still lacks definitive evidence.

8. TREATING CHRONIC INFECTION AND ATHEROSCLEROSIS

If infection does play a role in the pathogenesis of atherosclerosis, it can be surmised that *C. pneumoniae* antibiotic therapy may be protective against cardiovascular events. The new generation macrolide antibiotic, azithromycin (which has anti-Chlamydial activity), has been shown to lower levels of serum and monocyte activation markers in male survivors of MI with stable elevated anti- *C. pneumoniae* antibody titres [75]. It also reduced the number of cardiovascular events in such post-MI patients [76]. In another pilot study, the macrolide roxithromycin was given to patients with unstable angina or non-Q-wave MI [77]. After 30 days treatment and follow up, there was a reduction in severe recurrent ischaemia, MI and ischaemic death compared to placebo. However, both these preliminary studies were relatively small and the positive results could be due to chance.

More recently, preliminary findings of the ACA-DEMIC study (Azithromycin in Coronary Artery Disease: Elimination of Myocardial Infection with Chlamydia) found that tests for four markers of inflammation (CRP, IL-1, IL-6 and TNF-alpha) improved at 6 months in patients randomised to azithromycin compared with placebo. However, no difference was seen in the antibody titre or clinical events at 6 months [78]. The two-year follows up

results are awaited.

A large case-control study showed that patients treated with tetracycline or quinolone antibiotics in the community were less likely to have a first-time acute MI compared to matched controls [79]. However, antibiotics may only be useful if given at specific times to selected patients. More recently, roxithromycin was found to have no effect on restenosis rate, early thrombotic complications or clinical outcomes 8 months after coronary stenting [80]. Currently, a number of large-scale prospective antibiotic intervention trials are in progress and they should help to clarify the potential use of antibiotics in patients with CAD [26]. There is an obvious concern for the use of broad-spectrum antibiotics in the community and the risk-benefit ratio will need to be addressed.

Other unresolved issues include the optimal antibiotic regimen, duration of therapy, the timing of therapy and the defining of eradication of infection. It is possible that antibiotics will be targeted to those with evidence of chronic infection and inflammation (perhaps those with elevated *C. pneumoniae* antibodies, positive PCR in mononuclear cells and/or elevated C-reactive protein). With the limited data and unresolved issues, such antibiotic use in CAD remains in the research arena.

9. SUMMARY

Inflammation plays an important role in atherogenesis and plaque destabilisation. Whether antigens from infective agents can initiate this inflammation is as yet uncertain [81]. Sero-epidemiological studies show an association between infection and CAD. However, these studies cannot distinguish between a causal relationship and secondary infection. There are difficulties in diagnosing chronic infection and regimens for antibiotic therapy are not established. When to initiate therapy, for whom and for how long remains unclear. Ultimately, it may be possible to identify a sub-group of patients with CAD in whom infection is the cause or modulator of atherogenesis. It may also be possible to identify infections as the 'culprit' in the development of acute coronary syndromes. If the large-scale antibiotic trials in progress establish a role for macrolide antibiotics in the secondary prevention of CAD, this will have a major effect on public health strategies world-wide [82].

REFERENCES

1. Farmer JA, Gotto AM Jr,. Dyslipidaemia and other risk factors for coronary artery disease. In: Braunwald E, editor. Heart Disease. A Textbook of Cardiovascular Medicine, 5th edn. Philadelphia: Saunders, 1997;1121–60.

2. Gupta S, Camm AJ. Is there an infective aetiology to atherosclerosis? Drugs and Aging 1991;13:1–7.

3. Libby P, Egan D, Skarlatos S. Roles of Infectious Agents in Atherosclerosis and Restenosis. Circulation 1997;96:4091–4103.

4. Osler W. Diseases of the arteries. In: Osler W, ed. Modern medicine: its practice and theory. Philadelphia: Lea and Febiger, 1901;421–47.

5. Aldous MB, Grayston JT, Wang S, and Foy HM. Seroepidemiology of Chlamydia pneumoniae TWAR Infection in Seattle Families, 1961–1979. J Infect Dis 1991;161:646.

6. Geberding JL, Sande MA. Infectious Diseases of The Lung. In Textbook of Respiratory Medicine Vol 1, 2nd Ed. (Murray and Nadel) 1991;32:1077.

7. Wong Y-K, Gallagher PJ, Ward ME. Chlamydia pneumoniae and atherosclerosis. Heart 1991;81:231–238.

8. Wang SP, Grayston JT. Microimmunofluorescence serology in Chlamydia trachomatis. In: de la Moza LM, editor. The 1983 Internetional Symposium on Medical Virology. New York: Elsevier, 1984:81–118.

9. Bowman J, Söderberg S, Forsberg J, et al. High prevalence of Chlamydia pneumoniae DNA in peripheral blood mononuclear cells in patients with cardiovascular disease and in middle aged blood donors. J Infect Dis 1991;178:271–7.

10. Saikku P, Mattila K, Nieminen S, et al. Serological Evidence of an Association of a Novel Chlamydia, TWAR, with Coronary Heart Disease and Acute MI. Lancet 1981;1:981–5.

11. Thom DH, Grayston T, Siscovick DS, et al. Association of Prior Infection with Chlamydia pneumoniae and Angiographically Demonstrated Coronary Artery Disease. JAMA 1991;268(1):61–72.

12. Patel P, Mendall MA, Carrington D, Strachan DP, Leatham EW, Molineaux N, et al. Association of Helicobacter pylori and Chlamydia pneumoniae infections with coronary heart disease and cardiovascular risk factors. BMJ 1991;311:711–4.

13. Saikku P, Leiononen M, Tenkanen L, et al. Chronic Chlamydia pneumoniae Infection a Risk Factor for Coronary Heart Disease in The Helsinki Heart Study. Ann Int Med 1991;111:271–8.

14. Danesh J, Collins R, Peto R. Chronic infections and coronary heart disease: is there a link? Lancet 1991;350(9075):431–436.

15. Saikku P. Epidemiology of Chlamydia pneumoniae in atherosclerosis. Am Heart J 1991;138:S500–S503.

16. Strachan DP, Carrington D, Mendall MA, et al. Relation of Chlamydia pneumoniae serology to mortality and incidence of ischaemic heart disease over 13 years in the Caerphilly prospective heart disease study. BMJ 1991;311:1031–1039.

17. Danesh J, Whincup P, Walker M, et al. Chlamydia Pneumoniae IgG titres and coronary heart disease:prospective study and meta-analysis. BMJ 2001;321:201–13.

18. Danesh J, Whincup P, Walker M, et al. Low grade inflammation and coronary heart disease: prospective study and updated meta-analysis. BMJ 2001;321:191–204.

19. Roivainen M, Viik-Kajander M, Palosuo T, et al. Infections, Inflammation, and the Risk of Coronary Heart Disease. Circulation 2000;101:251–257.

20. Hoffmeister A, Rothenbacher D, Wanner P, et al. Seropositivity to Chlamydia Lipopolysaccharide and Chlamydia pneumoniae, Systemic Inflammation and Stable Coronary Artery Disease. JACC 2000;35(1):111–8.

21. Shimada K, Mokuno H, Watanabe Y, Sawano M, Diada H, Yamaguchi H. High prevalence of seropositivity for antibodies to Chlamydia-specific lipopolysaccharide in patients with acute coronary syndromes. J Cardiovasc Risk 2001;1:201–213.

22. Lindholt JS, Juul S, Vammen S, Lind I, Fasting H, Henneberg EW. Immunoglobin A antibodies Chlamydia pneumoniae are associated with expansion of abdominal aortic aneurysm. British Journal of Surgery 1991;86(5):631–8.

23. Cook PJ, Honeybourne D, Lip GY, Beevers DG, Wise R, Davis P. Chlamydia pneumoniae antibody titres are significantly associated with a cute stroke and transient cerebral ischaemia: the West Birmingham Stroke Project. Stroke 1991;29(2):401–10.

24. Shor A, Kuo CC, Patton DC. Detection of Chlamydia pneumoniae in coronary artery fatty streaks and atheromatous plaques. South African Med J 1991;82(3):151–61.

25. Taylor-Robinson D. Chlamydia pneumoniae in vascular tissue. Atherosclerosis 1991;140(S1):S21–4.

26. Gupta S. Chronic infection in the aetiology of atherosclerosis – focus on Chlamydia pneumoniae. [The John French Memorial Lecture] Atherosclerosis 1991;141:1–6.

27. Davidson M, Kuo CC, Middaugh JP, et al. Confirmed previous infection with Chlamydia pneumoniae (TWAR) and its presence in early coronary atherosclerosis. Cir-

culation 1991;98(7):621–33.

28. Thomas M, Wong Y-K, Thomas D, et al. Direct detection of Chlamydia pneumoniae DNA at multiple sites in human coronary arteries post mortem and its relationship to the histological severity (Stary grade) of associated atherosclerotic plaque. In Stephens RS, Byrne GI, Christiansen G, et al, eds. Chlamydial infections. Proceedings of the ninth international symposium on human chlamydial infection. International Chlamydia Symposium, San Francisco, 1991:191–202.

29. Grayston JT. Does Chlamydia pneumoniae cause atherosclerosis? Arch Surg 1991;134(9): 931–934.

30. Maas M, Bartelin C, Engel PM, et al. Endovascular Presence of Viable Chlamydia pneumoniae is a Common Phenomenon in Coronary Artery Disease. J Am Coll Cardiol 1991;31(4):821–32.

31. Gaydos CA, Summersgill JT, Sahney NN, et al. Replication of Chlamydia pneumoniae in vitro in human macrophages, Endothelial Cells and Aortic Artery Smooth Muscle Cells. Infect Immun 1991;61:1611–20.

32. Godzick KL, O'Brien ER, Wang S and Kuo CC. In Vitro Susceptibility of Human Vascular Wall Cells to Infection with Chlamydia pneumoniae. J Clin Microbiol 1991;31:2411–3.

33. Fryer RH, Schworbe EP, Woods ML and Rogers GM. Chlamydia species Infect Human Vascular Endothelial Cells and Induce Procoagulant Activity. J Invest Med 1991;41:161–74.

34. Coombes BK, Mahoney JB, Chlamydia pneumoniae infection of human endothelial cells induces proliferation of smooth muscle cells via an endothelial cell derived soluble factor(s). Inf Immun 1991;67(6):2901–15.

35. Moazed TC, Kuo CG, Grayston JT and Campbell LA. Murine Models of Chlamydia pneumoniae Infection and Atherosclerosis. J Infect Dis 1991;171:881–90.

36. Blessing E, Lin T-M, Campbell LA, Rosenfeld ME, Lloyd D, Kuo C-C. Chlamydia pneumoniae Induces Inflammatory Changes in the Heart and Aorta of Mormocholesterolaemic C57BL/6J Mice. Inf Immun 2001;68(8):4761 8.

37. Liuba P, Karnani P, Pesonen E, et al. Endothelail Dysfunction After Repeated Chlamydia pneumoniae Infection in Apolipoprotein E-Knockout Mice. Circulation 2001;101:1039.

38. Fong IW, Chiu B, Viira E, Jang D, Mahoney JB. De Novo Induction of Atherosclerosis by Chlamydia pneumoniae in a rabbit model. Infect Immun 1991;67(11):6041–55.

39. Muhlestein JB, Anderson JL, Hammond EH, et al. Infection with Chlamydia pneumoniae accelerates the development of atherosclerosis and treatment with azithromycin prevents it in a rabbit model. Circulation 1991;97(7):631–6.

40. Adam E, Melnick JL, Probtsfield JL, et al. High level of cytomegalovirus antibody in patients requiring vascular surgery for atherosclerosis. Lancet 1981;1:291–3.

41. Nieto FJ, Sorlie P, Comstock GW, et al. Cytomegalovirus infection, Lipoprotcin (a), and Hypercoagulability: An Atherogenic Link? Arterioscl Thromb Vasc Biol 1991;17(9):1781–85.

42. Mehta JL, Saldeen TGP, Rand K. Interactive Role of Infection, Inflammation and Traditional Risk Factors in Atherosclerosis and Coronary Artery Disease. J Am Coll Cardiol 1998;31:1211–25.

43. Van Dam-Mieras MC, Bruggeman CA, Muller AD, Debie WH & Zwaal RF. Induction of endothelial cell procoagulant activity by cytomegalovirus infection. Thrombosis Res 1981;41:61–75.

44. Neumann F-J, Kastrati A, Miethke T, Pogatsa-Murray G, Seyfarth M, Schömig A. Circulation 2001;101:11–13.

45. Bartels C, Maas M, Bein G, et al. Association of Serology With the Endovascular Presence of Chlamydia pneumoniae and Cytomegalovirus in Coronary Artery and Vein. Graft Disease Circulation 2001;101:137.

46. Danesh J. Coronary heart disease, Helicobacter pylori, dental disease, Chlamydia pneumoniae, and cytomegalovirus: Meta-amalyses of prospective studies. Am Heart J 1991;138:S434-S437.

47. Mendall MA, Goggin PM, Molineaux N, et al. Relation of Helicobacter pylori infection and coronary artery disease. Br Heart J 1991;71:431–9.

48. Martin-de-Argila C, Boixeda D, Canton R, et al. High seroprevalence of Helicobacter pylori infection in coronary heart disease (Letter). Lancet 1991;341:310.

49. Gunn M, Stephens JC, Thompson JR, Rathbone BJ, Samani NJ. Significant association of cagA positive Helicobacter pylori strains with risk of premature myocardial infarction. Heart 2000;81:261–271.

50. Murray LJ, Bamford KB, O'Reilly DP, et al. Helicobacter pylori infection: relation with cardiovascular risk factors, ischaemic heart disease, and social class. Br Heart J 1991;71:491–50.

51. Whincup PH, Mendall MA, Perry IJ, et al. Prospective relations between Helicobacter pylori, coronary heart disease and stroke in middle aged men. Heart 1991;71:561–72.

52. Wald NJ, Law MR, Morris JR, Bagnall AM. Helicobacter pylori infection and mortality from ischaemic heart disease: negative result from a large prospective study. BMJ 1991;311:1191–201.

53. Nieto FJ. Viruses and atherosclerosis: a critical review of the epidemiologic evidence. Am Heart J 1999;138:S453-S460.

54. Mattila KJ, Nieminen MS, Valtonen VV, et al. Association between dental health and acute myocardial infarction. BMJ 1981;291:771–82.

55. Jousilahti P, Vartianinen E, Tacomilekhot T, et al. Symp-

toms of chronic bronchitis and risk of coronary disease. Lancet 1991;341:561–72.

56. Dahlen GH, Bowman J, Birgander LS, Lindholm B. Lipoprotein(a), IgG, IgA and IgM antibodies to Chlamydia pneumoniae and HLA class II genotype in early coronary artery disease. Atherosclerosis 1991;111:161–74.

57. Ekesbo R, Nilsson PM, Lindholm LH, Persson K, Wadström T. Combined seropositivity for H. pylori and C. pneumoniae is associated with age obesity and social factors. Cardiovasc Risk 2001;1:191–195.

58. Laurila A, Bloigu A, Nayha S, Hassi J, Leinonen M, Saikku P. Chronic Chlamydia pneumoniae infection is associated with a Serum Lipid Profile Known to be a Risk Factor for Atherosclerosis. Arterioscler Thromb Vasc Biol 1991;17(11):2911–13.

59. Hu H, Pierce GN, Zhong G. The atherogenic effects of Chlamydia are dependent on serum cholesterol and specific to Chlamydia pneumoniae. J Clin Investigation 1999;103(5):741–53.

60. Hahn DL, Golub jatnikov R. Smoking as a potential confounder of the Chlamydia pneumoniae – coronary artery disease association. Arterioscler Thromb 1991;11:251–60.

61. Cook PJ, Lip GY, Davies P, Beevers DG, Wise R. Chlamydia pneumoniae antibodies in severe essential hypertension. Hypertension 1991;31:581–94.

62. Toss H, Gnarpe J, Gnarpe A, et al. Increased fibrinogen levels are associated with persistent Chlamydia pneumoniae infection in unstable coronary artery disease. Eur Heart J 1991;11:571–7.

63. Ross R. The Pathogenesis of Atherosclerosis: a perspective for the 1990's. Nature 1993;362:801–9.

64. Steinberg D, Parthasarathy S, Carew T, et al. Modification of low-density lipoprotein that increases its atherogenicity. New Engl J Med 1981;321:911–24.

65. Byrne GI, Kalayoglu MV. Chlamydia pneumoniae and atherosclerosis: links to the disease process. Am Heart J 1991;138(5 Pt 2): S481–90.

66. Black CM, Perez R. Chlamydia pneumoniae multiplies within human pulmonary macrophages (abstract). 90th Annual Meeting ASM, Washington DC, American Society of Microbiology 1990, D1:80.

67. Mayr M, Metzler B, Kiechl S, et al. Endothelial cytotoxicity mediated by serum antibodies to Heat Shock Proteins of Escherichia coli and Chlamydia pneumoniae: Immune Reactions to Heat Shock Proteins as a Possible Link Between Infection and Atherosclerosis. Circulation 1991;99(12):1561–66.

68. Kol A, Bourcier T, Lichtman AH, Libby P. Chlamydial and human heat shock protein 60s activate human vascular endothelium, smooth muscle cells and macrophages. J Clin Invest 1991;103(4):571–77.

69. Sethi A, Gupta S. Apoptosis, infection and atherosclerosis: partners in crime? Int J Cardiol 2000 (in press).

70. Molestina RE, Miller Rd, Lentsch AB, Ramirez JA, Summersgill JT. Requirement for NF –kB in Transcriptional Activation of Monocyte Chemotactic Protein 1 by Chlamydia pneumoniae in Human Endothelial Cells. Infec Immun 2001;68(7):4281–8.

71. Braun J, Laitkos S, Treherne J, et al. Chlamydia pneumoniae – a new causative agent of reactive arthritis and undifferentiated oligoarthritis. Ann Rheum Dis 1991;51:101–5.

72. Socan M, Beovic B. Chlamydia pneumoniae and meningoencephalitis. N Engl J Med 1991;331:406.

73. Juvonen J, Laurila A, Juvonen T, et al. Detection of Chlamydia pneumoniae in human nonrheumatic stenotic aortic valves. J Am Coll Cardiol 1991;21:1051–9.

74. Ong G, Thomas BJ, Mansfield AO, et al. Detection and widespread distribution of Chlamydia pneumoniae in the vascular system and its possible implications. J Clin Pathol 1991;41:101–6.

75. Gupta S. Chlamydia pneumoniae, monocyte activation and antimicrobial therapy in coronary heart disease. MD Thesis. University of London 1999.

76. Gupta S, Leatham EW, Carrington D, et al. Elevated Chlamydia pneumoniae antibodies, cardiovascular events and azithromycin in male survivors of myocardial infarction. Circulation 1991;91:401–7.

77. Gurfinkel E, Bozovich G, Daroca A, et al. Randomised Trial of Roxithromycin in non-Q-wave Coronary Syndromes: ROXIS pilot study. Lancet 1991;351:401–7.

78. Anderson JL, Muhlestein JB, Carlquist J, et al. Randomised Secondary Prevention Trial of azithromycin in Patients With Coronary Artery disease and Serological Evidence for Chlamydia pneumoniae Infection: The Azithromycin in Coronary Artery Disease: Elimination of Myocardial Infection with Chlamydia (ACADEMIC) Study. Circulation 1991;99(12):1541–7.

79. Meier CR, Derby LE, Jick SS, Vasilakis C, Jick H. Antibiotics and risk of subsequent first-time acute myocardial infarction. JAMA 1991;281(5):421–31.

80. Neumann FJ. Roxithromycin for prevention of restenosis after stenting. JACC 2000;35:2 (Suppl 1).

81. Gupta S, Kaski JC. Chlamydia causes coronary heart disease: an inflammatory idea? Acute Coronary Syndromes 1991;1:41–8.

82. Gupta S. Camm AJ. Chronic infection, Chlamydia and coronary heart disease. [Book] Kluwer Academic Publishers, ISBN 1–7921–5791–3, June 1999.

ATHEROSCLEROSIS RELATED AUTOANTIBODIES

Atherosclerosis and Autoimmunity
Y. Shoenfeld, D. Harats and G. Wick, editors

Atherosclerosis: Evidence for the Role of Autoimmunity

Yehuda Shoenfeld[1], Jacob George[1], Yaniv Sherer[1] and Dror Harats[2]

[1]Department of Medicine B and the Research Unit of Autoimmune Diseases, Sheba Medical Center, Tel-Hashomer, and Sackler Faculty of Medicine, Tel-Aviv University, Israel; [2]Institute of Lipid and Atherosclerosis Research, Sheba Medical Center, Tel-Hashomer, Israel

1. INTRODUCTION

Atherosclerosis is a histopathological condition that entails accumulation of lipid laden lesions in the vessel walls at sites of shear stress [1]. The complications of atherosclerosis are tremendous, being the major cause of mortality (over 50%) in the Western world [1].

Recent data implies that the immune system plays a dominant role in atherogenesis, as manifested by the observation of T cells and immunoglobulins within lesions [2]. Further evidence stems from creation of knockout mouse models simulating human atherogenesis that have manipulated immunologically to result in various effects on atherogenesis. Further exciting realms within this field holds that autoimmune processes contribute significantly to the evolution of the mature plaque [3,4].

Classical autoimmune diseases are recognized by autoreactivity against distinct antigens expressed in the host. Identification of the specific autoantigen, aids in establishing the diagnosis of the disorder, and subsequently furnishes tools by which to manipulate the immune system in the intention of treatment.

Common denominators by which to establish the diagnosis of autoimmune diseases have been formulated by the *Rose and Witebsky* criteria. The principal experimental support relies on the isolation of a target autoantigen, specific for a given disease. Subsequently, when used for immunization, the autoantigen leads to production of antibodies and signs of the respective autoimmune disease. Our observations combined with others, follow this paradigm

with respect to three candidate autoantigens.

2. HEAT SHOCK PROTEINS AS AUTOANTIGENS

Heat shock proteins are a family of approximately 25 molecules, with highly conserved structures that serve protective roles [5]. However, HSPs, (i.e. HSP-65) has been implicated as a target autoantigen in several autoimmune diseases (i.e. diabetes, arthritis, etc.). The realization that HSP-65 autoimmunity may be involved in atherosclerosis came from the laboratory of G. Wick in the early 90s [3]. It has been shown that normocholesterolemic rabbits can be triggered to develop arteriosclerotic lesions when immunized with HSP-65 or alternatively, with HSP-65 rich suspension of heat killed Mycobacterium tuberculosis (MT) bacteria [6]. We have recently obtained, for the first time, evidence to support the role of HSP-65 in atherosclerosis progression in mice [6]. Unlike rabbits, mice are more resistant to atherosclerosis for reasons that have not been completely resolved. The strain most susceptible to fatty streak formation is the C57BL/6 which tends to develop early lesions only when fed a high fat diet for 14 weeks. Thus, we sought to investigate whether we can influence the progression of the early atherosclerotic lesions by immunization with MT or with the recombinant HSP-65. We have found that an immunization protocol similar to the one applied by Xu et al. [6] did not induce fatty streak formation in mice fed a normal chow-diet [7]. However, when challenging the mice with a high fat diet, mice immunized with MT or with HSP-65 developed maturer atherosclerotic lesion.

We have subsequently reinforced these findings in LDL receptor deficient mice showing that immunization with HSP65 and MT led an increase in fatty streak size [8].

Thus, the autoimmune response towards HSP-60/65 concomitant with the expression of HSP-60/65, may result in local activation of the immune system within the atherosclerotic plaque thereby contributing to lesion progression.

3. OXIDIZED LDL AS A POSSIBLE AUTOANTIGEN

The oxidative modification LDL is considered contributory to the progression of atherosclerosis [9].

Interesting observations follow the study of induced immune responses to oxLDL. *Palinski et al* [10] were the first to report on the effects of homologous oxLDL immunization showing that rabbits that were immunized with oxLDL developed anti-oxLDL antibodies and developed reduced atherosclerosis. No mechanism has been provided to explain this intriguing effect. A subsequent study by *Ameli et al* [11] came with essentially similar results in rabbits.

We have recently reinforced these findings showing that immunization of apo-E deficient mice with homologous modified LDL resulted in a significant delay of fatty streak formation [12]. This effect was associated with production of a sustained and specific humoral immune response to oxLDL.

The cumulative data from the above lines suggests that an induced autoimmune response to oxLDL may play a role in protection against atherosclerosis.

4. β2GPI AS AN AUTOANTIGEN IN ATHEROSCLEROSIS

Antiphospholipid antibodies (aPL) are a heterogeneous group of antibodies which can be found in the sera of patients with infections, autoimmune diseases and normal subjects. An intensive research in this field has brought to the finding of two major subgroups of aPL:

1) Antibodies which react negatively charged phospholipids (the prototypes of which are cardiolipin and phosphatidylserine). These antibodies are usually provoked by the occurrence of infections and not related to autoimmune diseases.

2) aPL which react with plasma proteins ('cofactors') bound to negatively charged surfaces/phospholipids. The principal protein that has been shown to bind negatively charged structures and to allow for subsequent aPL binding is β2-glycoprotein I (β2GPI). Although still under investigation, β2GPI (also termed apoprotein-H for its structural resemblance with plasma apolipoproteins) associates with plasma lipoproteins and displays *in vitro* anticoagulant properties. Reactivity of aPL with β2GPI is present among patients with autoimmune disease and is strongly associated with a prothrombotic tendency. When anti-β2GPI antibodies are present in patients with recurrent fetal loss and arterial/venous thromboembolic events, they define the primary antiphospholipid syndrome (APS) [13].

SLE patients, 50% of whom are aPL positive suffer from the consequences of accelerated atherosclerosis [14]. The lipid abnormalities and medications do not fully account for the effect of atherosclerosis. Thus, we hypothesized that aPL may play a role in speeding the atherosclerotic process. Furthermore, aPL which have been shown to possess endothelial cell activating properties [15], can influence in a similar manner, the progression of atherosclerosis. This hypothesis gained further strength by in vitro studies showing that aPL are capable of enhancing the influx of oxLDL into macrophages [16].

We employed the method of idiotypic manipulation to generate aPL in mice [17]. Using this method, immunization of an animal with a given antibody (Ab1) leads to idiotypic dysregulation culminating in the production of anti-idiotypic antibodies (Ab2), which further extends to elicit anti-anti-idiotypic antibodies (Ab3) [18]. These latter antibodies (Ab3) of mouse origin may mimic Ab1 in their binding specificities. Thus, we have used IgG from a patient with APS (rich in aPL) to immunize the atherosclerosis prone LDL-receptor deficient (LDL-RD) mice [17]. We have found that mouse aPL generated in the mice were associated with increased early atherosclerotic lesions. The humoral response was not cross-reactive with oxLDL as has been suggested in other contexts and was independent of β2GPI binding.

Aiming to extend the findings to β2GPI-reactive antibodies (so called autoimmune aPL), we immunized mice of similar genetic background with human β2GPI [19]. A single immunization with β2GPI was sufficient to evoke a sustained and specific humoral and cellular immune response to β2GPI. Immunohistochemical study of the lesions from the β2GPI immunized mice revealed dense subaortic infiltration of CD4 lymphocytes raising the possibility that they may have taken an important role in mitigating of the fatty streak formation. These findings were also evident in an additional mouse model (the apo-E knockout mouse) employing a similar immunization protocol with human β2GPI [20].

When attempting to explore the mechanisms mediating the proatherogenic properties of â2GPI immunization we have made cell transfer experiments. Accordingly, we have observed that anti-â2GPI lymphocytes were able to transfer susceptibility to atherosclerosis to non-treated mice by intraperitoneal injection [21].

5. CONCLUSIONS

The conclusions from the above studies indicate that terms by which define autoimmune disorders can be discerned with mice:
1. Suggested autoantigens are expressed within atherosclerotic lesions.
2. Immunization with the given autoantigens elicits an immune response that influences lesion progression
3. Atherosclerosis susceptiblity can be transferred by autoantigen sensitized lymphocytes from immunized animals.

REFERENCES

1. Ross R. Atherosclerosis-an inflammatory condition. N Eng J Med 1999;340:115–126.
2. Libby P, Hansson GK. Involvement of the immune system in human atherogenesis: Current knowledge and unanswered questions. Lab Invest 1991;64:5–11.
3. Wick G, Schett G, Amberger A, Kleindienst R, Xu Q. Is atherosclerosis an immunologically mediated disease? Immunol Today 1995;16:27–33.
4. George J, Harats D, Gilburd B, Shoenfeld Y. Emerging cross-regulatory roles of immunity and autoimmunity in atherosclerosis. Immunol Res 1996;155:315–322.
5. Benjamin IJ, McMillan DR. Stress (heat shock) proteins. Molecular chaperones in cardiovascular biology and disease. Circ Res 1998;83:117–132.
6. Xu Q, Dietrich H, Steiner HJ, Gown AM, Schoel B, Mikuz G, Kaufman SHE, Wick G. Induction of arteriosclerosis in normocholesterolemic mice rabbits by immunization with heat shock protein 65. Arterioscler Thrombosis 1992;12:789–799.
7. George J, Shoenfeld Y, Afek A, Gilburd B, Keren P, Shaish A, Kopolovic Y, Harats D. Accelerated fatty streak formation C57BL/6J mice by immunization with heat shock protein 65. Arterioscler Thromb Vasc Biol. In press.
8. Afek, J. George, B. Gilburd..D. Harats, Y. Shoenfeld. Immunization with heat shock protein 65 enhances early atherosclerosis in low-density lipoprotein receptor deficient mice. J. Autoimmunity. In press.
9. Witztum JL. The oxidation hypothesis of atherosclerosis. Lancet 1994;344:793–795.
10. Palinski W, Miller E, Witztum JL. Immunization of low density lipoprotein (LDL) receptor-deficient rabbits with homologous malondialdehyde-modified LDL reduces atherogenesis. Proc Natl Acad Sci USA 1995;92: 821–825.
11. Ameli S, Hultgardh-Nilsson A, Regnstrom J, Calara F, Yano J, Cercek B, Shah PK, Nilsson J. Effect of immunization with homologous LDL and oxidized LDL on early atherosclerosis in hypercholesterolemic rabbits. Arterioscler Thromb Vasc Biol 1996;16:1074–1079.
12. George J, Afek A, Gilburd B, Levy Y, Levkovitz H, Shaish A, Goldberg I, Kopolovic Y, Wick G, Shoenfeld Y, Harats D. Hyperimmunization of ApoE deficient mice with homologous oxLDL suppresses early atherogencis. Atherosclerosis 1998;138:147–152.
13. The Antiphospholipid syndrome. Eds; Ascherson RA, Cervera R, Piette JC, Shoenfeld Y. CRC press, 1997.
14. Jonsson H, Nived O, Sturfelt G. Outcome of systemic lupus erythematosus: a prospective study of patients from a defined population. Medicine (Baltimore) 1989;68:141–150.
15. George J, Blank M, Levy Y, Meroni PL, Damianovich M, Tincani A, Shoenfeld Y. Differential effects of anti-β2GPI antibodies on endothelial cells and on the manifestations of experimental antiphospholipid syndrome. Circulation 1998;97:900–906.
16. Hasunuma Y, Matsuura E, Makita Z, Katahira T, Nishi S, Koike T. Involvement of β2 glycoprotein I and anticardiolipin antibodies in oxidatively modified low density lipoprotein uptake by macrophages. Clin Exp

Immunol 1997;107:569–574.

17. George J, Afek A, Gilburd B, Levy Y, Blank M, Kopolovic Y, Harats D and Shoenfeld Y: Atherosclerosis in LDL receptor knockout mice is accelerated by immunization with anticardiolipin antibodies. Lupus 1997; 6:723–9.

18. Shoenfeld Y. Idiotypic induction of autoimmunity: a new aspect of the idiotypic network. FASEB J 1994;8:1296:1303.

19. George J, Afek A, Gilburd B, Aron-Maor A Shaish A, Levkovitz H, Blank M, Harats D, Shoenfeld Y. Induction of early atherosclerosis in LDL receptor deficient mice immunized with beta 2 glycoprotein I. Circulation 1998;15:1108–1115.

20. Afek A, George J, Shoenfeld Y, Gilburd B, Levy Y, Shaish A, Keren P, Goldberg I, Kopolovic J, Harats D. Enhancement of atherosclerosis in beta 2 glycoprotein I (β2GPI)- immunized apo-E deficient mice. Pathobiology 1999;67:19–25.

21. J. George, D. Harats, B. Gilburd, A. Afek, A. Shaish, Y. Levy, J. Kopolovic, Y. Shoenfeld. Adoptive transfer of â2-glycoprotein I reactive lymphocytes promotes early atherosclerosis in LDL-receptor deficient mice. Circulation 2000;102:1822–1827.

Atherosclerosis and Autoimmunity
Y. Shoenfeld, D. Harats and G. Wick, editors

Oxidized Autoantigens in Atherosclerosis

Eiji Matsuura[1], Kazuko Kobayashi[1], Junko Kasahara[1], Yehuda Shoenfeld[3] and Takao Koike[2]

[1]Department of Cell Chemistry, Institute of Cellular and Molecular Biology, Okayama University Medical School, Okayama, Japan; [2]Department of Medicine II, Hokkaido University School of Medicine, Sapporo, Japan; [3]Department of Medicine B, Research Unit of Autoimmune Diseases, Chaim Sheba Medical Center, Tel Hashomer, Israel

1. INTRODUCTION

The antiphospholipid syndrome (APS) is a thrombophilic disorder characterized by the combination of arterial and venous thromboembolic phenomena, recurrent fetal losses and thrombocytopenia [1]. This prothrombolic state is associated with the presence of antiphospholipid antibodies (aPL), such as anticardiolipin antibodies (aCL) and lupus anticoagulant (LA). It has been commonly known that β2-glycoprotein I (β2-GPI) is a major antigen for aCL induced in patients with APS [2–4]. Other blood coagulation-related proteins, such as prothrombin [5], annexin V [6], and kininogens [7], were also shown to be targeted by autoantibodies derived from the APS.

Epidemiological studies have established that an elevated plasma level of low density lipoprotein (LDL) represents one of the most important risk factors for the development of atherosclerosis [8]. A subset of chemically modified LDLs such as oxidized LDL (oxLDL) has attracted the interest of researchers as one of the causative factors underlying atherosclerosis [9, 10]. The *in vivo* oxidative modification of LDL has been proposed to play a central role in atherosclerosis [11], as suggested by the presence of oxLDL particles in the early phase of atherosclerotic plaque formation.

In 1993, it was reported that aCL in SLE patients cross-react with malonedialdehyde (MDA)-modified LDL [12]. Later on, other studies have, however, failed to show any cross-reaction between anti-β2-GPI and anti-oxLDL antibodies in the APS

patients [13]. It was also shown that anti-β2-GPI antibodies could be a marker for arterial thrombosis in SLE patients, while IgG anti-oxLDL were not associated with arterial thrombosis [14]. In contrast, we found that β2-GPI binding was specific to Cu^{2+}-oxidized plasma lipoproteins, rather than to other chemically modified LDLs and that an anti-β2-GPI autoantibodies bound to β2-GPI complexes with oxidized plasma lipoproteins [15]. Most recently, we characterized β2-GPI-specific ligands derived from Cu^{2+}-oxLDL and interaction among the ligand, β2-GPI, and anti-β2-GPI autoantibodies (submitted).

In this chapter, we review the role of oxLDL on atherogenesis of oxLDL and briefly note on our recent observations that autoantibodies could contribute to the athero-thrombosis in the APS patients, by targeting for the complex of β2-GPI and oxidized lipids as an autoantigen.

2. ATHEROGENESIS

Ross and Glomset first proposed in 1976 and renewed in 1986 and in 1993, the response-to-injury hypothesis of atherogenesis which proposes that "injury" to endothelium is the initiating event in atherogenesis [16–18].

The earliest recognizable lesion of atherosclerosis is the so-called 'fatty streak' and aggregations of lipid-rich macrophages and of T lymphocytes are observed in the intima, i.e., within the innermost layer of the artery wall. Fatty streaks precede

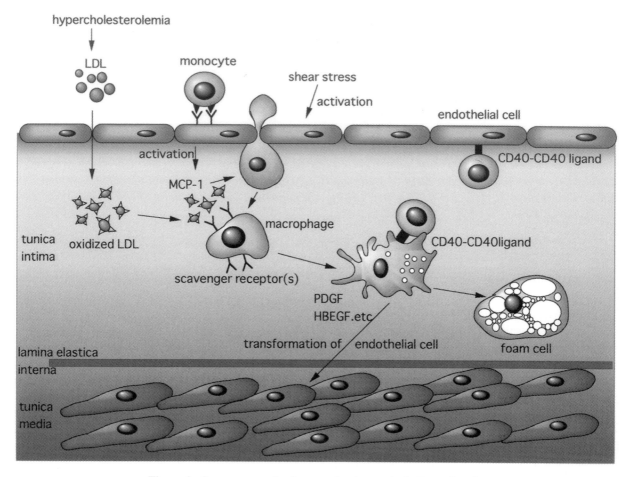

Figure 1. Consensus mechanisms on development of atherosclerosis.

the development of intermediate lesions, which are composed of layers of macrophages and smooth muscle cells and develop into fibrous plaques.

The scheme represents a current consensus on the events leading to the earliest stage of athrogenesis (Fig. 1). Hypercholesterolemia is most commonly associated with an elevation of plasma LDL and LDL is the ultimate source of the cholesterol that accumulates in developing foam cells. An increment of plasma LDL levels and/or shear stress lead to an increase in the adherence of circulating monocytes to arterial endothelial cells and also to an entry of LDL into the intima. And, these result in undergoing of the oxidative modification catalyzed by these cells locate in arterial lesions. oxLDL, different from native LDL, contains large amount of lysophosphatidylcholine and can increase adherence and penetration of monocytes, partly by stimulat-

ing release of, vascular cell adhesion molecule-1 (VCAM-1), and intracellular adhesion molecule-1 (ICAM-1) from endothelial cells [19]. Minimally oxidized LDL can also stimulate release of monocyte chemoattractant protein-1 (MCP-1) [20] and macrophage colony-stimulating factor (M-CSF) [21], which can induce differentiation of the monocyte into a cell with the phenotypic pattern of the tissue macrophage, including an increase in expression of scavenger receptor A (SRA) .

Smooth muscle cells are chemotactically migrated from tunica media to intima and proliferated by cytokines such as IFN-γ and IL-4 and by growth factors such as PDGF and heparin binding EGF-like growth factor (HB-EGF) [22], and basic fibroblast growth factor (b-FGF). These factors are released from injured endothelial cells, macrophages, accumulated T lymphocytes, and hypertrophy of the intima is finally developed. Transformation of vascular smooth muscle cells has an important role in the hypertrophy and SMemb gene regulating proliferation of smooth muscle cells. Basic transcriptional element binding protein-2 (BTEB2), as a transcriptional factor regulating the gene [23], and early growth response gene-1 (Egr-1) inducing the BTEB2 expression [24], have been recently identified. Further, it was observed that interaction between CD40 and CD40 ligand are involved in development of atherosclerosis and they are expressed on the cell surface of vascular endothelial cells [25], smooth muscle cells, T lymphocytes, and macrophages. It has also been thought that oxLDL inhibits the vasodilation that is normally induced by nitric oxide (NO) [26]. Atherogenesis, being accompanied with foam cell formation of oxLDL-uptaken macrophages, is developed under such complicated regulatory conditions.

3. OXIDATIVE MODIFICATION OF LDL

LDL particle contains about 700 molecules of phospholipids, 600 of free cholesterol, 1600 of cholesterol esters, 185 of triglycerides, and 1 of apolipoprotein B (apoB) containing 4536 amino acid residues [27]. Both the lipids and apoB are subjected to oxidation and apoB breaks down to fragments of different sizes, from 14 to over 550 kDa by oxidative attack [28]. A key feature of LDL oxidation is the breakdown of these polyunsaturated fatty acids to yield a broad array of smaller fragments including aldehydes and ketones that can become conjugated to other lipids (especially amino lipids) or to the apo B [29]. The polyunsaturated fatty acids in cholesterol esters, phospholipids, and triglycerides are subject to free radical-initiated oxidation and can participate in chain reactions that amplify the extent of damage. Recently, it was reported that two oxidized lipid components i.e., 9-, or 13-hydroxyoctadecadienoic acid (9-HODE and 13-HODE) activate peroxisome proliferator-activated receptor γ (PPARγ), a transcriptional regulator of genes linked to lipid metabolism and result in up-regulation of the scavenger receptor, CD36 [30]. Thus, the particular lipid components of oxLDL enhance the uptake of oxLDL via the PPARγ activation, thereby promoting foam cell formation. In mildly oxidized

LDL, cholesteryl hydroperoxyoctadecadienoic acid (Chol-HPODE) and cholesteryl hydroxyoctadecadienoic acid (Chol-HODE) were detected as main constituents of oxidation products [31]. Chol-HPODE was reported to inactivate platelet-derived growth factor [32]. Cholesterol is also converted to oxysterols, it is especially oxidized at the 7-position. 7-Hydroxycholesterol (both free and esterified) is the major oxysterol formed at early events in LDL oxidation, with 7-ketocholesterol dominating at later stages [33]. Recent studies indicated that elevated plasma levels of 7β-hydroxycholesterol may be associated with an increased risk of atherosclerosis [34]. At later stages in LDL oxidation, cholesteryl or 7-ketocholesteryl esters of 9-oxononanoate derived from cholesteryl linoleate [35], were detected as the most abundant fraction of oxidized cholesteryl linoleate [36, 37]. As a result of oxidation, huge numbers of oxidative structures are thus literally generated.

Cell culture studies have identified a number of enzymes, such as oxidase, 15-lipooxygenase, myeloperoxidase, which come from various cell types, i.e., endothelial cells, smooth muscle cells, monocytes, macrophages, fibroblasts, neutrophils, etc., that could play a role in the oxidation of LDL. Since oxidized LDL is present in arterial lesions at significant concentrations, it seems reasonable to assume that the cells characteristic of those lesions, i.e., endothelial cells, macrophages, and smooth muscle cells, are involved in oxidation.

Chemically modified LDL, such as MDA-modified LDL, acetylated LDL and Cu^{2+}-mediated oxLDL were widely examined as an experimental model of denatured LDL for studying the mechanisms on the development of atherosclerosis. Among these LDLs, trace amounts of Cu^{2+}-ion can induce LDL oxidation, resulting in highly reproducible LDL damage [38]. This process leads to oxidize LDL that shares many structural and functional properties with LDL oxidized by cells or LDL extracted from arterial atherosclerotic plaques. Incubation of LDL with any of several different types of cells, or with Cu^{2+}-ion even in the absence of cells, results in generating oxidatively modified LDL with similar properties [39]. There is general agreement about the use of Cu^{2+}-oxLDL as an autoantigen because oxLDL has been found in atheromatous lesions and oxLDL extracted from atherosclerotic lesions exhibits nearly all of the physicochemical and immunological properties of Cu^{2+}-oxLDL [40]. Thus, Cu^{2+}-mediated oxLDL might be a much more suitable model for physiological LDL rather than other chemically modified LDL, such as MDA-LDL. *In vivo*, LDL might be alternatively oxidized by released Cu^{2+}-ion from ceruloplasmin [41, 42].

4. RECEPTORS FOR OXLDL

Thus, it appears that oxidation of LDL plays a significant role in atherogenesis. Evidence has been obtained that cholesterol accumulation in the developing atherosclerotic region is not due to the uptake of native LDL by way of the classical LDL receptor but instead due to the uptake of some modified form of LDL by way of alternative receptors, i.e. scavenger receptors.

OxLDL can be avidly taken up by receptor-mediated endocytosis transformation into foam cells. Several different molecules, such as macrophage class A scavenger receptors, MARCO, FcγRII, CD36, scavenger receptor class B type I (SR-BI) [43], macrocialin (CD68) [44], and LOX-1 have been identified as cell-surface receptors for atherogenic oxLDL [45].

5. β2-GPI AND AUTOANTIBODIES DERIVED FROM APS

β2-GPI, a 50-kDa protein with a carbohydrate content of 17%, is present in normal human plasma at approximately 200 µg/ml and was first described in 1961 [46]. Because β2-GPI is present in the lipoprotein fractions, such as chyromicron, VLDL, and HDL, with ultracentrifugation and activated lipoprotein lipase *in vitro*, β2-GPI is also designated as apolipoprotein H (apo-H). β2-GPI binds to various anionic substances, such as phospholipids, heparin, lipoproteins, and activated platelets, and inhibits the intrinsic blood coagulation pathway, prothrombinase activity, adenosine diphosphate (ADP)-dependent aggregation [47–52]. In the most recently, we also reported that β2-GPI has an inhibitory effect on activated protein C activity [53].

Many recent studies indicated that one of the predominant antibodies considered to be aCL in the

APS patients are those against β2-GPI rather than any of anionic PLs. In 1994, we demonstrated that epitopes recognized by aCL from the APS patients could appear only when β2-GPI interacts with polyoxygenated polystyrene plates as well as with a lipid membrane containing anionic PLs [54]. Further, the antibody binding to β2-GPI on a polyoxygenated plate is not affected by the addition of highly excessive amount of fluid phase β2-GPI. From these observations, it was reasonably interpreted that such epitopes are cryptic. Besides, it has been alternatively proposed against the interpretation that binding of β2-GPI to anionic PLs increases the local concentration of β2-GPI [55, 56]. Other research groups also reported the presence of anti-β2-GPI auto-Abs directed to domain V [57] or domain I [58]. Thus, aCL, i.e., anti-β2-GPI antibodies appeared in the APS patients seem to be heterogeneous and fine specificity of these antibodies must be further characterized.

6. POSSIBLE INVOLVEMENT OF AUTOIMMUNITY IN ATHEROGENESIS

Atherosclerosis might be developed by a kind of immune dysfunctions or by autoimmunity. It was reported that antibodies against epitopes of oxLDL recognize materials in atherosclerotic lesions but not in normal arteries and the major antigenic epitopes are induced in apolipoprotein B (apo B) during the oxidative modification of LDL [59]. Malondialdehyde (MDA) is an end-product of lipid peroxidation and conjugation to the lysine residues of apo B induces the epitope for antibodies from human sera [60–62]. It was shown that aCL in SLE patients crossreact with MDA-modified LDL [12]. Later on, other studies have, however, failed to show any cross-reaction between anti-β2-GPI and anti-oxLDL antibodies in the APS patients [13] and shown that anti-β2-GPI antibodies could be a marker for arterial thrombosis in SLE patients, while IgG anti-oxLDL antibodies were not associated with arterial thrombosis [14]. In contrast, we found that β2-GPI binding was specific to Cu^{2+}-oxidized plasma lipoproteins, rather than to other chemically modified LDLs and that an anti-β2-GPI autoantibodies bound to β2-GPI complexes with oxidized plasma lipoproteins [15]. Most recently, we characterized β2-GPI-

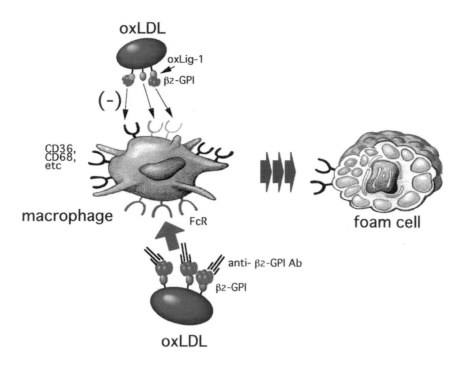

Figure 2. A possible mechanism on autoantibody-mediated oxLDL uptake by macrophages.

specific ligands derived from Cu²⁺-oxidized LDL and interaction among the ligand, β2-GPI, and anti-β2-GPI autoantibosdies. The anti-β2-GPI autoantibodies subsequently bind to β2-GPI complcxes with these oxidized lipoproteins. The ligand specific for β2-GPI, namely, oxLig-1, do not have a phosphorus / or sugar group and is an oxidative form of linolyate-esterified keto-cholesterol. It seems that the ligand is recognized by some receptor(s) via β2-GPI and might be weakly by some kinds of scavenger receptors expressed on the macrophages. In contrast, uptake of oxLig-1-liposomes by macrophages are significantly enhanced in the presence of β2-GPI and anti-β2-GPI autoantibodies (Fig. 2).

We obtained other evidences that the appearance of autoantibodies against a complex of β2-GPI and oxLig-1 in APS, especially in the secondary APS, are highly associated with a history of arterial thrombosis but not venous thrombosis. Further, plasma oxLDL positive is associated with the history of arterial one, too. It was shown that LDL-receptor-deficient mice fed a chow diet and immunized with β2-GPI had an accelerated atherosclerosis [63]. They also found that β2-GPI was abundantly expressed within subendothelial regions and intimal-medial borders of human atherosclerotic plaques, and that it co-localized with monocytes and with CD4-positive lymphocytes [64]. Thus, there is increasing circumstantial evidence that an autoimmune mechanism involving β2-GPI and oxLDL in the atherogenesis in APS.

REFERENCES

1. Hughes GRV. The anticardiolipin syndrome. Clin Exp Rheumatol 1985;3:285–286.
2. McNeil IIP, Simpsom RJ, Chesterman CN, Krilis SA. Anti-phospholipid antibodies are directed against a complex antigen that includes a lipid-binding inhibitor of coagulation: β2-glycoprotein I (apolipoprotein H). Proc Natl Acad Sci USA 1990;87:4120–4124.
3. Galli M, Comfurius P, Maassen C, Hemker HC, de Baets MH, van Breda-Vriesman PJ, Barbui T, Zwaal RF, and Bevers EM. Anticardiolipin antibodies (ACA) directed not to cardiolipin but to a plasma protein cofactor. Lancet 1990;335:1544–1546.
4. Matsuura E, Igarashi Y, Fujimoto M, Ichikawa K, Koike T. Anticardiolipin cofactor(s) and differential diagnosis of autoimmune disease. Lancet 1990;336:177–178.
5. Bevers EM, Galli M, Barbui T, Comfurius P, Zwaal RF.

147

Lupus anticoagulant IgG's (LA) are not directed to phospholipids only, but to a complex of lipid-bound human prothrombin. Thromb Haemost 1991;66:629–632.

6. Matsuda J, Saitoh N, Gohchi K, Gotoh M, Tsukamoto M. Anti-annexin V antibody in systemic lupus erythematosus patients with lupus anticoagulant and/or anticardiolipin antibody. Am J Hematol 1994;47:56–58.

7. Sugi T, McIntyre JA. Autoantibodies to phosphatidylethanolamine (PE) recognize a kininogen-PE complex. Blood 1995;86:3083–3089.

8. Brown MS, Goldstein JL. The hyperlipoproteinemias and other disorders of lipid metabolism. Harrison's Principles of Internal Medicine, 13th edition. In Isselbacher KD ed. New York: McGraw-Hill, Inc. 1994;2058–2069.

9. Witztum JL, Steinberg D. Role of oxidized low density lipoprotein in atherogenesis. J Clin Invest 1991;88:1785–1792.

10. Goldstein JL, Ho YK, Basu SK, Brown MS. Binding site on macrophages that mediates uptake and degradation of acetylated low density lipoprotein, producing massive cholesterol deposition. Proc Natl Acad Sci USA 1979;76:333–337.

11. O'Brien KD, Alpers CE, Hokanson JE, Wang S, Chait A. Oxidation-specific epitopes in human coronary atherosclerosis are not limited to oxidized low-density lipoprotein. Circulation 1996;94:1216–1225.

12. Vaarala O, Alfthan G, Jauhiainen M, Leirisalo-Repo M, Aho K, Palosuo T. Crossreaction between antibodies to oxidised low-density lipoprotein and to cardiolipin in systemic lupus erythematosus. Lancet 1993;341:923–925.

13. Tinahones FJ, Cuadrado MJ, Khamashta MA, Mujic F, Gomez-Zumaquero JM, Collantes E, Hughes GRV. Lack of cross-reaction between antibodies to β2-glycoprotein-I and oxidized low-density lipoprotein in patients with antiphospholipid syndrome. Br J Rheumatol 1998;37:746–749.

14. Romero FI, Amengual O, Atsumi T, Khamashta MA, Tinahones FJ, Hughes GRV. Arterial disease in lupus and secondary antiphospholipid syncrome: Association with anti-β2-glycoprotein I antibodies but not with antibodies against oxidized low-density lipoprotein. Br J Rheumatol 1998;37:883–888.

15. Hasunuma Y, Matsuura E, Makita Z, Katahira T, Nishi S, Koike T. Involvement of β2-glycoprotein I and anticardiolipin antibodies in oxidatively modified low-density lipoprotein uptake by macrophages. Clin Exp Immunol 1997;107:569–573.

16. Ross R, Glomset JA. The pathogenesis of atherosclerosis. N Eng J Med 1976;295:369–377.

17. Ross R. Pathogenesis of atherosclerosis - an update. New Eng I Med 1986;314:488–500.

18. Ross R. The pathogenesis of atherosclerosis: a perspective for the 1990s. Nature 1993;362:801–809.

19. Frostegard J, Wu R, Haegerstrand A, Patarroyo M, Lefvert AK, Nilsson J. Mononuclear leukocytes exposed to oxidized low density lipoprotein secrete a factor that stimulates endothelial cells to express adhesion molecules. Atherosclerosis 1993;103:213–219.

20. Cushing SD, Berliner JA, Valente AJ, Territo MC, Navab M, Parhami F, Gerrity R, Schwartz CJ, Fogelman AM. Minimally modified low density lipoprotein induces monocyte chemotactic protein 1 in human endothelial cells and smooth muscle cells. Proc Natl Acad Sci USA 1990;87:5134–5138.

21. Rajavashisth TB, Andalibi A, Territo MC, Berliner JA, Navab M, Fogelman AM, Lusis AJ. Induction of endothelial cell expression of granulocyte and macrophage colony-stimulating factors by modified low-density lipoproteins. Nature 1990;344:254–257.

22. Nakata A, Miyagawa J, Yamashita S, Nishida M, Tamura R, Yamamori K, Nakamura T, Nozaki S, Kameda-Takemura K, Kawata S, Taniguchi N, Higashiyama S, Matsuzawa Y. Localization of heparin-binding epidermal growth factor-like growth factor in human coronary arteries. Possible roles of HB-EGF in the formation of coronary atherosclerosis. Circulation 1996;94:2778–2786.

23. Watanabe N, Kurabayashi M, Shimomura Y, Kawai-Kowase K, Hoshino Y, Manabe I, Watanabe M, Aikawa M, Kuro-o M, Suzuki T, Yazaki Y, Nagai R. BTEB2, a Kruppel-like transcription factor, regulates expression of the SMemb/nonmuscle myosin heavy chain B (SMemb/NMHC-B) gene. Circ Res 1999;85:182–191.

24. Santiago FS, Lowe HC, Kavurma MM, Chesterman CN, Baker A, Atkins DG, Khachigian LM New DNA enzyme targeting Egr-1 mRNA inhibits vascular smooth muscle proliferation and regrowth after injury. Nature Med. 1999;5:1438.

25. Mach F, Schonbeck U, Sukhova GK, Atkinson E, Libby P. Reduction of athrosclerosis in mice by inhibition of CD40 signalling. Nature 1998;394:200–203.

26. Jessup W. Oxidized lipoproteins and nitric oxide. Curr Opin Lipidol 1996;7:274–280.

27. Steinberg D. Low density lipoprotein oxidation and its pathobiological significance. J Biol Chem 1997;272:20963–20966.

28. Fong LG, Parthasarathy S, Witztum JL, Steinberg D. Nonenzymatic oxidative cleavage of peptide bonds in apoprotein B-100. J Lipid Res 1987;28:1466–1477.

29. Esterbauer H, Jurgens G, Quehenberger O, Koller E. Autoxidation of human low density lipoprotein: loss of polyunsaturated fatty acids and vitamin E and generation of aldehydes. J Lipid Res 1987;28:495–509.

30. Nagy L, Tontonoz P, Alvarez JG, Chen H, Evans

RM. Oxidized LDL regulates macrophage gene expression through ligand activation of PPARγ. Cell 1998;93:229–240.

31. Kritharides L, Upston J, Jessup W, Dean RT. A method for defining the stages of low density lipoprotein oxidation by the separation of cholesterol- and cholesteryl ester-oxidation products using HPLC. Anal Biochem 1993;213:79–89.

32. van Heek M, Schmitt D, Toren P, Cathcart MK, DiCorleto PE. Cholesteryl hydroperoxyoctadecadienoate from oxidized low density lipoprotein inactivated platelet-derived growth factor. J Biol Chem 1998;273:19405–19410.

33. Brown AJ, Leong SL, Dean RT, Jessup W. 7-Hydroperoxycholesterol and its products in oxidized low density lipoprotein and human atherosclerotic plaque. J. Lipid Res. 1997;38:1730–1745.

34. Brown AJ, Jessup W. Oxysterols and atherosclerosis. Atherosclerosis 1999;142:1–28.

35. Kamido H, Kuksis A, Marai L, Myher JJ. Identification of cholesterol-bound aldehydes in copper-oxidized low density lipoprotein. FEBS Lett 1992;304:269–272.

36. Kamido H, Kuksis A, Marai L, Myher JJ. Lipid ester-bound aldehydes among copper-catalyzed peroxidation products of human plasma lipoproteins. J Lipid Res 1995;36:1876–1886.

37. Hoppe G, Ravandi A, Herrera D, Kuksis A, Hoff HF. Oxidation products of cholesteryl linoleate are resistant to hydrolysis in macrophages, form complexes with proteins, and are present in human atherosclerotic lesions. J Lipid Res 1997;38:1347–1360.

38. Kleinveld HA, Hak-Lemmers HLM, Stalenhoef AFH, Demacker PNM. Improved measurement of low-density-lipoprotein susceptibility to cooper-induced oxidation: application of a short procedure for isolating low-density lipoprotein. Clin Chem 1992;38:2066–2072.

39. Parthasarathy S, Fong LG, Quinn MT, Steinberg D. Oxidative modification of LDL: comparison between cell-mediated and copper-mediated modification. Eur Heart J 1990;11 (Suppl) E: 83–87.

40. Yla-Herttuala S, Palinski W, Rosenfeld ME, Parthasarathy S, Carew TE, Butler S, Witztum JL, Steinberg D. Evidence for presence of oxidatively modified low density lipoprotein in athcrosclerotic lesions of rabbit and man. J Clin Invest 1989;85:1086–1095.

41. Ehrenwald E, Chisolm GM, Fox PL. Intact ceruloplasmin oxidatively modifies low density lipoprotein. J Clin Invest 1994;93:1493–1501.

41. Lamb D, Leake DS. Acidic pH enables caeruloplasmin to catalyse the modification of low-density lipoprotein. FEBS Lett. 1994;338:122–126.

43. Krieger M, Acton S, Ashkenas J, Pearson A, Penman M, Resnick D. Molecular flypaper, host defense, and atherosclerosis. Structure, binding properties, and functions of macrophage scavenger receptors. J Biol Chem 1993;268:4569–4572.

44. Ramprasad MP, Fischer W, Witztum JL, Sambrano GR, Quehenberger O, Steinberg D. Cell surface expression of mouse macrosialin and human CD68 and their role as macrophage receptors for oxidized low density lipoprotein. Proc Natl Acad Sci USA 1996;93:14833–14838.

45. Sawamura T, Kume N, Aoyama T, Moriwaki H, Hoshikawa H, Aiba Y, Tanaka T, Miwa S, Katsura Y, Kita T, Masaki T. An endothelial receptor for oxidized low-density lipoproeitn. Nature 1997;386:73–77.

46. Schultze HE, Heide K, Haupt H. Uber ein bisher ubekanntes niedermolekulars β2-Globulin des Humanserums. Naturwissenschaften 1961;48:719–724.

47. Wurm H. Beta2-glycoprotein I (apolipoprotein H) interactions with phospholipid vesicles. Int J Biochem 1984;16:511–515.

48. Polz E. Isolation of a specific lipid-binding protein from human serum by affinity chromatography using heparin-Sepharose. In: Peeters H ed., Properties of Biological Fluids Pergamon Press, Oxford, 1979;102:183–186.

49. Polz E, Kostner GM. The binding of β2-glycoprotein I to human serum lipoproteins: distribution among density fraction. FEBS Lett 1979;102:183–186.

50. Nimpf J, Bevers EM, Bomans PH, Till U, Wurm H, Kostner GM, Zwaal RF. Prothrombinase activity of human platelets is inhibited by β2-glycoprotein I. Biochim Biophys Acta 1986;884:142–149.

51. Schousboe I. β2-Glycoprotein I: a plasma inhibitor of the contact activation of the intrinsic blood coagulation pathway. Blood 1985;66:1086–1091.

52. Nimpf J, Wrum H, Kostner GM. β2-Glycoprotein I (apo-H) inhibits the release reaction of human platelets during ADP-induced aggregation. Atherosclerosis 1987;63:109–114.

53. Ieko M, Ichikawa K, Triplett DA, Matsuura E, Atsumi T, Sawada K, Koike T. β2-Glycoprotein I is necessary to inhibit protein C activity by monoclonal anticardiolipin antibodies. Arthritis Rheum 1999;42:167–174.

54. Matsuura E, Igarashi Y, Yasyda T, Triplett DA, Koike T. Anticardiolipin antibodies recognize b2-glycoprotein I structure altered by interacting with an oxygen modified solid phase surface. J Exp Med 1994;179:457–462.

55. Roubey RAS. Immunology of the antiphospolipid antibody syndrome. Arthritis Rheum 1996;39:1444–1454.

56. Sheng Y, Kandiah DA, Krilis SA. Anti-β2-glycoprotein I autoantibodies from patients with the "antiphospholipid" syndrome bind to β2-glycoprotein I with low affinity: dimerization of β2-glycoprotein I induces a significant increase in anti-β2-glycoprotein I antibody affinity. J Immunol 1998;161:2038–2043.

57. Wang MX, Kandiah DA, Ichikawa K, Khamashta MA,

Hughes GRV, Koike T, Roubey RAS, Krilis SA. Epitope specificity of monoclonal anti-β2-glycoprotein I antibodies derived from patients with the antiphospholipid syndrome. J Immunol 1995;155:1629–1636.

58. Iverson GM, Victoria EJ, Marquis DM. Anti-β2-glycoprotein I (β2-GPI) autoantibodies recognize an epitope on the first domain of b2-GPI. Proc Natl Acad Sci USA 1998;95:15542–15546.

59. Palinski W, Rosenfeld ME, Yla-Herttuala S, Gurner GC, Socher SS, Butler SW, Parathasarathy S, Carew TE, Steinberg D, Witztum JL. Low density lipoprotein undergoes oxidative modification in vivo. Proc Natl Acad Sci USA 1989;86:1372–1376.

60. Palinski W, Yla-Harttuala S, Rosenfeld ME, Butler SW, Socher SA, Parathasarathy S, Curtiss LK, Witztum JL. Antisera and monoclonal antibodies specific for epitopes generated duriong oxidative modification of low density lipoproteion. Atherosclerosis 1990;10:325–335.

61. Salonen JT, Yla-Herttuala S, Yamamoto R, Butler S, korpela H, Salonen R, Nyyssonen K, Palinski W, Witztum JL. Autoantibody against oxidized LDL and progression of carotide atherosclerosis. Lancet 1992;339:883–887.

62. Puurunen M, Vaarala O, Julkunen H, Aho K, Palosuo T. Antibodies to phospholipid binding proteins and occurrence of thrombosis in patients with systemic lupus erythematosus. Clin Immunol Immunopathol 1996;80:16–22.

63. George J, Afek A, Gilburd B, Blank M, Levy Y, Aron-Maor A, Levkovitz H, Shaish A, Goldberg I, Kopolovic J, Harats D, Shoenfeld Y. Induction of early atherosclerosis in LDL-receptor-deficient mice immunized with β2-glycoprotein I, Circulation 1988;98:1108–1115.

64. George J, Harats D, Gilburd B, Afek A, Levy Y, Schneiderman J, Barshack I, Kopolovic J, Shoenfeld Y. Immunolocalization of β2-glycoprotein I (apolipoprotein H) to human atherosclerotic plaques: potential implications for lesion progression. Circulation 1999;9:2227–2230.

150

Atherosclerosis and Autoimmunity
Y. Shoenfeld, D. Harats and G. Wick, editors

Autoantibodies against Oxidized Palmitoyl Arachidonoyl Phosphocholine in Atherosclerosis

Ruihua Wu

Specialty Laboratories, Inc., Santa Monica, CA 90404, USA

1. INTRODUCTION

Accumulating studies have demonstrated that oxidative modification of low density lipoprotein contributes to the development of atherosclerosis [1, 2]. OxLDL is present in the atherosclerotic lesions and is undergone *in vivo* oxidative modification [3] in the intima of the artery wall where monocyte/macrophages and endothelial cells generate free oxygen radicals to act in the lipid oxidative reactions [4]. The oxidation can also result in transfer of phospholipid peroxides or peroxidized free fatty acids from cell membranes to lipoproteins [5] and/or through a cascade from oxidized phospholipids to another. The degree and speed of oxidation are related to amount of free oxygen radicals and LDL cholesterol [6] as well as the density of non-saturated lipids [7]. Direct auto-oxidation of phospholipids can occur in advanced atherosclerotic lesions, which frequently contain necrotic areas, abundant extra-cellular phospholipids and transition free oxygen radicals. Oxidative damage plays a major role in the pathogenesis of atherosclerosis in several ways. Oxidation induces rapid uptake of oxidized phospholipids by macrophages leading to cholesterol accumulation and development of foam cells [8]. Oxidized phospholipids are chemotactic for monocytes and inhibit macrophage motility [9]. Oxidized phospholipids cause injury to endothelial cells [10], are cytotoxic to cells, and can inhibit endothelium-dependent relaxation and adversely affect coagulation pathways [11]. OxLDL is immunogenic [12]; even mildly oxidative modifications render the native LDL more immunogenic [13]

and can alter gene expression in arterial cells (e.g., expression of colony stimulating factors, cell adhesion molecules and monocyte chemotactic protein-1 [14–16]). OxLDL can also induce circulating T cell activation [17]. T cell clones from human atherosclerotic plaques recognize oxLDL, with resultant DNA proliferation and cytokine release [18]. Peripheral blood lymphocytes from patients with active ischemic heart disease show an increased reactivity to oxLDL [19]. Autoantibodies against oxLDL (oxLDL-Ab) can be detected in human sera [20, 21]. Such antibodies recognize epitopes expressed in atherosclerotic lesions, but not in normal arteries [22, 23]. Elevated oxLDL-Ab concentrations are found in patients with manifestations of atherosclerosis [24–28]. OxLDL-Ab were independent predictors of myocardial infarction (MI) in a large prospective cohort of healthy Swedish 50-year-old men [29] and were associated with a higher risk for coronary restenosis following percutaneous transluminal coronary angioplasty [30].

Some studies have shown that oxLDL-Ab cross-react with several typical lipids and lipoproteins including cardiolipin (CL), lysophosphatidylcholine (LPC), oxidized phosphatidylcholine (PC), 1-palmitoyl-2-(5-oxovaleroyl)-sn-glycero-3-phosphatidylcholine (POVPC) and others [31–35]. Several monoclonal antibodies to oxLDL (oxLDL-mAb) are known [36–41]; a common reactive feature of these oxLDL-mAb was that recognized oxidized epitopes. The oxLDL-mAb could react with several oxidized products of phospholipids and oxidized CL [33–35, 42]. Binding of oxLDL-mAb with oxLDL could be potently inhibited by

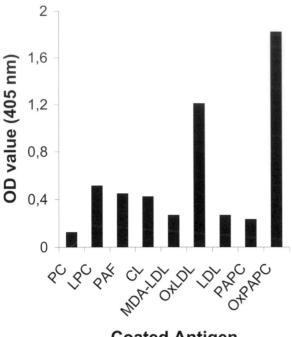

Figure 1. Reactivity of an oxLDL-mAb with oxLDL and several phospholipids. PC, LPC, PAF, CL, PAPC, oxPAPC were dissolved in ethanol and added to the bottom of 96-well microtiter plates at a concentration of 200 ng/well. The plates were dried under nitrogen at room temperature. After the plates were completely dry, the plates were washed a time with PBS containing 0.05% micro-zwitterionic detergent (lipids plate washing buffer). LDL, MDA-LDL and oxLDL were each diluted in 5 μg/mL with coating buffer (carbonate/biocarbonate buffer, 50 mmol/L, pH 9.6), and a volume of 100 μL/well to 96-well plates. The plates were incubated at 4°C overnight, then were washed with PBS containing 0.05% Tween-20 (lipoproteins plate washing buffer). Both plates blocking were accomplished with 2% bovine serum albumin in PBS for one hour at room temperature. After washing, the antigens binding with 1μg/100μL of an oxLDL monoclonal antibodies (Biodesign; Saco, MI) in 1% of BSA-PBS were detected by added 100μL of alkaline phosphatase conjugated rabbit anti-mouse IgG (1:2000 diluted) at room temperature for one hour. After washing, 100 μL of substrate/well was added. The developed color then was read in an EIA reader at 405 nm, respectively. The mean values of triplicate detection were shown in the figure.

oxidized phophatidylcholines [33] and oxidized 1-palmitoyl-2-arachidonoyl-sn-glycero-3-phospho-choline (oxPAPC) [42], strongly suggesting that oxPAPC is an important antigenic epitope of oxLDL.

2. PAPC AND OXIDATION

1-palmitoyl-2-arachidonoyl-sn-glycero-3-phospho-choline (PAPC) is a possessing phosphatidylcholine basic structure, molecular weight 782.14 Daltons non-saturation phospholipid. Native PAPC extensively presents in cells and lipoproteins *in vivo*. It has little effect on leukocytes and endothelial cells. However, oxidative stress can produce oxPAPC, which was isolated by HPLC. The analysis by fast atom bombardment-mass spectrometry indicates that oxPAPC possesses ions with a mass to charge ratio greater than PAPC by multiples of 16 Daltons, suggesting that oxPAPC contains three or four more oxygen atoms than PAPC [43]. OxPAPC and oxLDL have similar bioactivities, which could induce human aortic endothelial cells to adhere human monocytes *in vitro* and strongly induce monocyte-endothelial interaction [43].

An elegant experiment demonstrated that rapid oxidation occurs when CL is plated and exposed to air. High titer oxLDL-Ab showed a striking time-dependent increase in binding to CL that was exposed to air for increasing periods of time. But the oxLDL-Ab did not bind to a reduced CL analog that was unable to undergo peroxidation [34]. This experiment demonstrates that oxLDL-Ab are actually directed against epitopes of oxidized phospholipids. OxPAPC can be detected in fatty streak lesions from cholesterol fed rabbits and by immune reactivity with natural antibodies present in apo E null mice [44].

To identify the oxPAPC, we used a synthetic phospholipid PAPC as a surrogate for the precursor of the biologically active lipid. The lipid residue was exposed to air for 16 hours [42]. The lipid peroxide contents of oxidized PAPC and PAPC were determined by analyzing thiobarbituric acid-reactive (TBAR) substances and expressing them as malondialdehyde (MDA) equivalent [45]. The measurement values of 50 μg PAPC or oxPAPC were 1.4±0.17 and 44.2±2.02 MAD equivalents/mg protein, respectively. The result shown that lipid peroxide content of oxPAPC was more than 31-fold higher compared with PAPC.

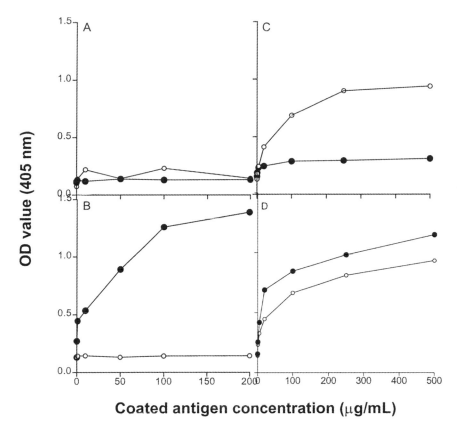

Figure 2. Reactivity of an oxLDL mAb (●) and an apo-B mAb (○) to native antigens and oxidized antigens. The plates were coated with PAPC (Figure A) or oxPAPC (Figure B) in 0, 2, 10, 50, 200, 1000 and 3000 ng/well; or LDL (Figure C) or oxLDL (Figure D) in 0, 1, 5, 20, 100, 500 and 1000 ng/well, respectively. Bound of the mAbs to thus antigens was detected by EIA as described same with figure 1. Each point represents the mean values of triplicate determination.

3. IDENTIFICATION OF OXIDIZED EPITOPE(S) ON OXLDL AND OXPAPC

A large number of reactive lipid peroxidation products are potentially generated during the oxidation of LDL [3, 37, 43, 46–48]. OxPAPC is one of the important products [43]. It had been shown that oxPAPC inhibit macrophage uptake of oxLDL and compete with oxLDL binding with the antibodies [42]. We performed a pivotal experiment to test the ability of a monoclonal antibody against oxLDL (oxLDL-mAb) to bind with several relative lipoproteins and lipids, including PC, LPC, platelet-activating factor (PAF), CL, PAPC, oxPAPC or LDL, malondialdehyde LDL (MDA-LDL), oxLDL. The data are shown in Fig. 1. Generally, oxLDL-mAb strongly bound with oxLDL. An unexpected finding was that oxLDL-mAb bound oxPAPC even stronger

than oxLDL. The oxLDL-mAb binding with other lipids and lipoproteins is weaker. The order of decreasing reactivity of oxLDL-mAb is LPC, PAF, CL, MDA-LDL, LDL, PAPC and PC.

In order to further investigate the reactivity of oxLDL-Ab, oxLDL-mAb and a monoclonal antibody against apo B protein (apoB-mAb) were reacted with increasing concentrations of native LDL or PAPC and oxLDL or oxPAPC. The results show that both monoclonal antibodies do not react with PAPC (Fig. 2A). OxLDL-mAb recognizes oxPAPC only, and the reactivity is dependent on the concentration of oxPAPC. The apoB-mAb does not react with oxPAPC (Fig. 2B). In contrast to oxPAPC, apoB-mAb reacts with LDL and the reactivity is dependent on the concentration of LDL; oxLDL-mAb does not recognize LDL (Fig. 2C). Both monoclonal antibodies bind with oxLDL and

153

amount binding with oxLDL is dependent on concentration of oxLDL coated on the plates (Fig. 2D). The data indicate that apoB-mAb could bind with antigens if it contains apo B protein, regardless of lipid oxidation state. The oxLDL-mAb bound both oxPAPC and oxLDL through common oxidized epitopes.

OxPAPC is antigenic, which possess homogeneous antigenic epitopes with oxLDL that can be recognized by oxLDL-Ab and that the antigenic epitope is induced by oxidation. Lipid peroxidation can damage the lipid bilayer of cell membranes resulting in altered immune function [49], because a functioning membrane is necessary for normal membrane metabolic activity as well as antigen reception. Several oxidation products including F2-isoprostanes, cholesterol 7 β-hydroperoxide, and phospholipids with oxidatively cleaved side chains can be detected in atherosclerotic lesions [43, 50, 51]. There are numerous lipoproteins *in vivo* that normally have different physiological functions. LDL is one of important molecule that can be a major carrier of blood cholesterol from the liver to tissues *in vivo*. However, oxidative stress can induce damage to lipoproteins and LDL can be oxidively modified *in vivo* [3]. After oxidative processing, phospholipids could produce the structural heterogeneity of the antibody-reactive products (e.g., oxidized CL [34], oxLDL [9, 52–55] and oxPAPC [43]). These products are not only antigenic, but even loss their normal functions. LDL molecules is oxidized, which can be altered from a functionary type into a bioactive type, oxLDL can deposit in vessel wall to induce a series of immuno-inflammatory responses [56, 57].

4. CHARACTERISTIC FEATURES OF OXPAPC AUTOANTIBODIES

To identify the characteristic features of oxPAPC-Ab, competition immunoassays were performed to investigate the presence of common epitopes between oxPAPC and oxLDL. Human IgG was used in the test, which was purified from a human serum pool of ten sera containing high concentrations of oxPAPC-Ab. Binding of the human IgG with oxPAPC was competed by an increasing amount of murine oxLDL-mAb. The human IgG binding with

oxPAPC was detected by adding an alkaline phosphatase-labeled goat anti-human IgG antibody. The binding of human IgG with oxPAPC decreased in a dose-dependent manner with increasing concentrations of murine oxLDL-mAb. The binding of murine oxLDL-mAb with oxPAPC was detected by adding an alkaline phosphatase-labeled rabbit anti-mouse IgG antibody. The amount of murine oxLDL-mAb binding with oxPAPC increased in a dose-dependent manner. The data is shown in Fig. 3A. The inhibitory ability of murine oxLDL-mAb was then analyzed. The maximal inhibitory capacity is about 50%. A normal murine IgG had no effect in the same test (Fig. 3B).

To investigate any immunological cross-reactivity in oxPAPC-Ab, absorptive assays were performed. Human IgG purified from a human serum pool containing 10 samples with high titers of oxPAPC-Ab at a dilution that yielded 50% of maximal binding were pre-incubated with different concentrations of oxLDL, MDA-LDL, LPC, PAF, CL, oxPAPC, PAPC and LDL for one hour at room temperature, respectively. The IgG binding to oxPAPC was determined and the percentages of inhibition were calculated. OxPAPC had very strong capacity to inhibit the IgG antibodies binding to oxPAPC-coated plates; oxLDL had an intermediate capacity to inhibit the IgG antibodies binding to oxPAPC-coated plates; MDA-LDL, LPC, CL and PAF had weaker ability in this respect; and LDL, PAPC showed no inhibitory effect.

OxPAPC-Ab mainly cross-react with oxLDL, suggesting that oxPAPC and oxLDL share the structure required for antigen recognition and that the recognition probably is specific. OxLDL only partially inhibited oxPAPC binding to the antibody even though it was used in high doses. A possible explanation is that oxLDL lacks sufficient antigenic epitopes. OxLDL molecules are a large spherical macromolecular complex of lipids and proteins with a diameter of 19–25 nm and molecular weight between $1.8–2.8 \times 10^6$ kD [58]. Many bioactive phospholpids are present in oxLDL molecules. OxPAPC is a single lipid molecule (MW about 800 kD), which is only a small component of oxLDL [43]. Another possible explanation is that the antigenic epitopes of oxLDL and oxPAPC are not completely the same. Both oxLDL and oxPAPC not only share some common antigenic structures,

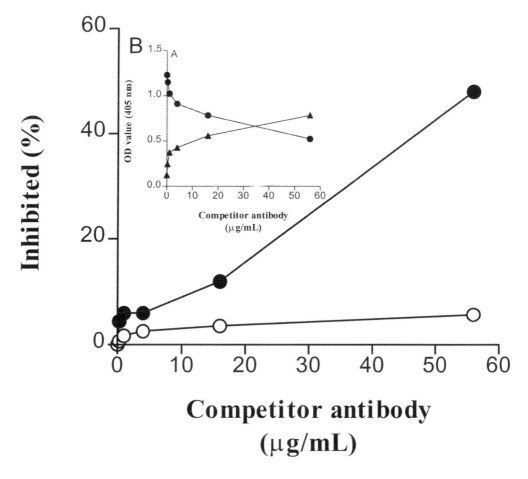

Figure 3. Competitive immunoassay shows that binding of a fixed amount of human IgG, which was purified from a human serum pool containing 10 high concentration of autoantibodies to oxPAPC, to oxPAPC-coated plates competes by an increasing concentration (0, 0.25, 1, 4, 16 and 56 µg/mL) of a murine oxLDL-mAb. The amount of antibody bound was measured with an alkaline phosphatase-labeled goat anti human IgG (●), or an alkaline phosphatase-labeled rabbit anti mouse IgG antibody (▲), respectively. The means of triplicate were shown in figure 3A. Inhibition of binding human IgG antibody with oxPAPC by two mouse IgG antibodies. Both increasing concentration (0, 0.25, 1, 4, 16 and 56 µg/mL) of a normal mouse IgG (O) and a mouse oxLDL mAb (●) completed with 5 µg/mL human IgG, which was purified from a human serum pool containing 10 high oxPAPC antibody concentrations, to bind with oxPAPC coated plates. Percentages of the inhibition are shown in figure 3B.

but are also present in different macromolecular complexes. Several molecules, CL, PAF, Lyso-PC, MDA-LDL, PAPC and LDL cross-react more weakly with oxPAPC, suggesting that the recognition is not likely specific, and the antigenic epitopes of these lipids and lipoprotein fractions are markedly heterogeneous. In contrast, the antigenic epitopes of oxPAPC and oxLDL are clearly homogeneous.

5. DETECTION OF OXPAPC AUTOANTIBODIES IN HEALTHY INDIVIDUALS AND PATIENTS WITH MANIFESTATIONS OF ATHEROSCLEROSIS (HYPERTENSION AND MYOCARDIAL INFARCTION)

The synthetic PAPC undergoes oxidative modification, has similar biological active fractions with mildly oxidized LDL, and can be recognized by the immune system [43, 59]. We have extended the oxLDL-Ab studies to test the hypothesis that there are oxPAPC autoantibodies (oxPAPC-Ab) in humans. A standardized enzyme-linked immunosorbent assay (EIA) was used to quantitatively measure antibodies against oxPAPC. The concentrations of antibodies to oxPAPC in patients with hypertension and myocardial infarction were compared with age and sex-matched controls. The data indicate that elevated concentrations of the oxPAPC autoantibodies are significantly associated with manifestation of atherosclerosis (Fig. 4).

To compare the oxPAPC-Ab and oxLDL-Ab, the concentrations of IgG oxLDL-Ab were measured in patient and control groups. Concentrations of IgG oxLDL-Ab were significantly higher, but greatly overlapping in the patients with hypertension ($p<0.001$) and in patients with MI ($p<0.05$) compared with controls. There was a correlation between oxPAPC-Ab and oxLDL-Ab in the hypertension group, MI group and controls ($R=0.332$, $p=0.0186$; $R=0.496$, $p=0.0053$; $R=0.283$, $p=0.0147$, respectively).

The concentration of oxPAPC-Ab between smokers and non-smokers was compared in all study groups. The concentrations of oxPAPC-Ab were significantly higher in the smokers than non-smokers either in patients with hypertension ($p<0.05$), patients with MI ($p<0.05$) or in healthy individuals ($p<0.001$).

The "altered antigen theory" suggests that self-substances can be modified *in vivo* and stimulate the immune response in production of autoantibodies. The presence of oxPAPC was demonstrated in atherosclerotic plaques [44]. OxPAPC might serve as antigen to induce a humoral immune response. The determined concentration of oxPAPC-Ab in serum probably could partly reflect the levels of oxPAPC *in vivo*.

Oxidative modification of phospholipids contributes to the development of atherosclerosis. The mechanism responsible for this association is still uncertain. The concentrations of oxPAPC-Ab are higher in cigarette smokers than in non-smoking subjects, which might provide some information to explain the mechanism. Cigarette smoking is one of major risk factors for atherosclerosis [60]. It has been suggested that smoking can increase numbers of circulating phagocytes and increase utilization of ascorbic acid and alpha-tocopherol; both could contribute to promoting oxidant generating systems

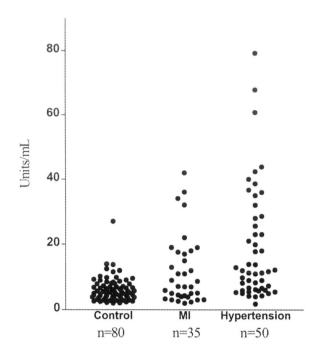

Figure 4. IgG oxPAPC-Ab in healthy individuals, patients with hypertension and patients with MI. The serum IgG oxPAPC-Ab were detected by EIA. Each point represents one individual mean value of triplicate measurement.

and decreasing plasma antioxidant capacity. Cigarette smoke exposure increases leukocyte, platelet and monocyte adhesion to endothelial cells and platelet aggregation, which might expand local inflammatory responses. A probable explanation is that elevated oxPAPC-Ab concentration in cigarette smokers likely reflects a series of oxidative responses to enhanced production of oxPAPC *in vivo*. A recent study suggested [35] apoptotic cells express oxidation-specific epitopes-including oxidized phospholipids-on their cell surface, and that these serve as ligands for recognition and phagocytosis by elicted macrophages. Oxidized lipids might inhibit phagocytosis of apoptotic cells and necrotic cells, resulting in accumulation of necrotic cells in atherosclerotic lesions.

The pathophysiologic significance and natural mechanism of the oxPAPC-Ab are not clear. In general, oxPAPC exposed on the surface of vessel endothelium might stimulate interaction of endothelial cells and immune system cells and resultant production of the autoantibodies. These autoantibodies might neutralize oxPAPC to decrease further damage, and thus play a protective role in early stages of endothelial damage. It has been indicated [61] that immunization of LDL receptor-deficient mice with homologous LDL significantly reduced progresion of atherosclerosis. The oxLDL-Ab formed *in vivo* could reduce atherosclerosis by inhibiting macrophage uptake of oxLDL to become foam cells [42]. However, formation of antigen-antibody complexes that can bind with Fc receptors and specific antibodies could block the housekeeping function of macrophages [35] resulting in accumulation of apoptotic cells, necrotic cells, macrophages and complexes to induce local complement activation, which in turn leads to the immuno-inflammatory reaction. The patients with atherosclerosis possess higher concentrations of oxPAPC-Ab, which could likely reflect a local inflammatory response *in vivo*. OxPAPC can be extracted from oxLDL and detected in atherosclerotic plaques [43, 44], oxPAPC-Ab might specifically recognize and bind to those epitopes on vessel walls. Several studies demonstrate that increasing oxLDL-Ab concentrations correlates with the extent of atherogenesis in cholesterol-fed LDL receptor-deficient mice [62]. Concentrations of the autoantibodies correlates with the degree or size of atherosclerotic lesions in humans [25]; autoantibody concentrations also positively corrrelate with incidence and mortality of future MI [29]. OxLDL or oxPAPC accumulating in atherosclerotic lesions could induce autoantibody formation, although it is also possible that the rise in concentrations of reflects increased lipid peroxidation [63, 64].

6. CONCLUSIONS

The activation of the immune system by oxidized phospholipids plays an important role in the process of developing atherosclerosis. The measurement of oxLDL-Ab could be used to investigate immune responses *in vivo*. It is known that spontaneous oxidation of LDL, as well as use of different batches of LDL possessing different susceptibilities to oxidation, leads to variations in the estimation of autoantibody concentrations. Synthesized oxPAPC might be a novel antigen to use for measurement of oxPAPC autoantibodies. Detection of oxPAPC-Ab could serve as an autoimmune marker for diagnosis

of atherosclerosis, and could suggest patients for whom anti-oxidant therapy might be appropriate. The pathophysiologic significance and natural mechanism of action of oxPAPC autoantibodies requires further investigation.

REFERENCES

1. Witztum JL, Steinberg D. Role of oxidized low density lipoprotein in atherogenesis. J Clin Invest 1991;88:1785–92.
2. Steinberg D. Modified forms of low density lipoprotein and atherosclerosis. J Intern Med 1993;233:227–32.
3. Palinski W, Rosenfeld ME, Ylä-Herttuala S, et al. Low density lipoprotein undergoes oxidative modification in vivo. Proc Natl Acad Sci USA 1989;86:1372–6.
4. Steinbrecher UP, Fisher M, Witztum JL, Curtiss LK. Immunogenicity of homologous low density lipoprotein after methylation, ethylation, acetylation, or carbamylation: generation of antibodies specific for derivatized lysine. J Lipid Res 1984;25:1109–16.
5. Holvoet P, Theilmeier G, Shivalkar B, et al. LDL hypercholesterolemia is associated with accumulation of oxidized LDL, atherosclerotic plaque growth, and compensatory vessel enlargement in coronary arteries of miniature pigs. Arterioscler Thromb Vasc Biol 1998;18:415–22.
6. Tribble DL, Holl LG, Wood PD, Krauss RM. Variations in oxidative susceptibility of LDL subtractions of differing density and particular size. Atherosclerosis 1992;93:89–95.
7. Beard CM, Barnard RJ, Robbins DC, Ordovas JM, Schaefer EJ. Effects of diet and exercise on qualitative and quantitative measures of LDL and its susceptibility to oxidation. Arterioscler Thromb Vasc Biol 1996;16:201–7.
8. Gerrity RG. The role of the monocyte in atherogenesis. I. Transition of blood-borne monocytes into foam cells in fatty lesion. II. Migration of foam cells from atherosclerotic lesions. Am J Pathol 1981;103:181–200.
9. Steinberg D, Parthasarathy S, Carew, TE, et al. Beyond cholesterol: modifications of low density lipoprotein that increase its atherogenicity. N Engl J Med 1989;320:915–24.
10. Ross R. The pathogenesis of atherosclerosis: a perspective for the 1990s. Nature 1993;362:801–9.
11. Parthasarathy S, Steinberg D, Witztum JL. The role of oxidized low-density lipoproteins in the pathogenesis of atherosclerosis. Annu Rev Med 1992;43:219–25.
12. Witztum JL, Steinbrecher UP, Fisher M, Kesaniemi A. Nonenzymatic glucosylation of homologous low

density lipoprotein and albumin render them immunogenic in the guinea pig. Proc Natl Acad Sci USA 1983;80:2757–61.

13. Berliner JA, Territo MC, Sevanian A, et al. Minimally modified low density lipoprotein stimulates monocyte endothelial interactions. J Clin Invest 1990;85:1260–6.

14. Rajavashisth TB, Andalibi A, Territo MC, et al. Induction of endothelial cell expression of granulocyte and macrophage colony-stimulating factors by modified low density lipoproteins. Nature 1990;344:254–7.

15. Cushing SD, Berliner JA, Valente AJ, et al. Minimally modified low density lipoprotein induces monocyte chemotactic protein 1 in human endothelial cells and smooth muscle cells. Proc Natl Acad Sci USA 1990;87:5134–8.

16. Frostegård J, Wu R, Haegerstrand A, et al. Mononuclear leukocytes exposed to oxidised low density lipoprotein secrete a factor that stimulates endothelial cells to express adhesion molecules. Atherosclerosis 1993;103:213–9.

17. Frostegård J, Wu R, Giscombe R, et al. Induction of T cell activation by oxidised low density lipoprotein. Arteriosclerosis and Thrombosis 1992;12:461–7.

18. Stemme S, Faber B, Holm J, et al. T lymphocytes from human atherosclerotic plaques recognize oxidized low density lipoprotein. Proc Natl Acad Sci USA 1995;92:3893–7.

19. Zurgil N, Levy Y, Deutsch M, et al. Reactivity of peripheral blood lymphocytes to oxidized low-density lipoprotein: a novel system to estimate atherosclerosis employing the cellscan. Clin Cardiol 1999;22:526–32.

20. Virella G, Virella I, Leman RB, et al. Anti-oxidized low density lipoprotein antibodies in patients with coronary heart disease and normal healthy volunteers. Int J Clin Lab Res 1993;23:95–101.

21. Wu R, Lefvert AK. Autoantibodies against oxidized low density lipoproteins (oxLDL): characterization of antibody isotype, subclass, affinity and effect on the macrophage uptake of oxLDL. Clin Exp Immunol 1995;102:174–80.

22. Haberland ME, Fong D, Cheng L. Malondialdehyde-altered protein occurs in atheroma of Watanabe heritable hyperlipidemic rabbits. Science 1988;241:215–8.

23. Yla-Herttuala S, Palinski W, Rosenfeld ME, et al. Evidence for the presence of oxidatively modified low density lipoprotein in atherosclerotic lesions of rabbit and human. J Clin Invest 1989;84:1086–95.

24. Salonen JT, Yla-Herttuala S, Yamamoto R, et al. Autoantibody against oxidized LDL and progression of carotid atherosclerosis. Lancet 1992;339:883–7.

25. Bergmark C, Wu R, de Faire U, et al. Patients with early onset of peripheral vascular disease have high levels of autoantibodies against oxidised low density lipoproteins. Arterioscler Thromb Vasc Biol 1995;15:441–5.

26. Parums DV, Brown DL, Mitchinson MJ. Serum antibodies to oxidized low-density lipoprotein and ceroid in chronic periaortitis. Arch Pathol Lab Med 1990;114:383–7.

27. Eber B, Schumacher M, Tatzber F, et al. Autoantibodies to oxidized low density lipoproteins in restenosis following coronary angioplasty. Cardiology 1994;84:310–5.

28. Maggi E, Chiesa R, Melissano G, et al. LDL oxidation in patients with severe carotid atherosclerosis-a study of in vitro and in vivo oxidation markers. Arterioscler Thromb 1994;14:1892–1899.

29. Wu R, Nityanand S, Berglund L, et al. Antibodies against cardiolipin and oxidatively modified LDL in 50-years-old men predict myocardial infarction. Arterioscler Thromb Vasc Biol 1997;17:3159–63.

30. George J, Harats D, Bakshi E, et al. Anti-oxidized low density lipoprotein antibody determination as a predictor of restenosis following percutaneous transluminal coronary angioplasty. Immunol Lett 1999;68:263–6.

31. Vaarala O, Alfthan G, Jauhiainen M, et al. Crossreaction between antibodies to oxidized low-density lipoprotein and to cardiolipin in systemic lupus erythematosus. Lancet 1993;341:923–5.

32. Wu R, Huang Y, Elinder LS, Frostegard J. Lysophosphatidylcholine is involved in the antigenicity of oxidized LDL. Arterioscler Thromb Vasc Biol 1998;18:626–30.

33. Itabe H, Yamamoto H, Suzuki M, et al. Oxidized phosphatidylcholines that modify proteins. J Biol Chem 1996;271:33208–17.

34. Horkko S, Miller E, Dudl E, et al. Antiphospholipid antibodies are directed against epitopes of oxidized phospholipids. J Clin Invest 1996;98:815–25.

35. Chang MK, Bergmark C, Laurila A, et al. Monoclonal antibodies against oxidized low-density lipoprotein bind to apoptotic cells and inhibit their phagocytosis by elicited macrophages: Evidence that oxidation-specific epitopes mediate macrophage recognition. Proc Natl Acad Sci USA 1999;96:6353–8.

36. Boyd HC, Gown G, Wolfbauer G, Chait A. Direct evidence for a protein recognized by a monoclonal antibody against oxidatively modified LDL in atherosclerotic lesions from a watanabe heritable hyperlipidemic rabbit. Am J Pathol 1989;135:815–26.

37. Palinski W, Ylä-Herttuala S, Rosenfeld ME, et al. Antisera and monoclonal antibodies specific for epitopes generated during oxidative modification of low density lipoprotein. Arteriosclerosis 1990;10:325–35.

38. Itabe H, Takeshima E, Iwasaki H, et al. A monoclonal antibody against oxidized lipoprotein recognizes foam cells in atherosclerotic lesions. Complex formation of oxidized phosphatidylcholines and polypeptides. J Biol

Chem 1994;269:15274–9.

39. Holvoet PG, Perez Z, Zhao E, et al. Malonaldehyde-modified low density lipoproteins in patients with atherosclerotic disease. J Clin Invest 1995;95:2611–9.

40. Hammer AG, Kager G, Dohr H, et al. Generation, characterization, and histochemical application of monoclonal antibodies selectively recognizing oxidatively modified apoB-containing serum lipoproteins. Arterioscler Thromb Vasc Biol 1995;15:704–13.

41. Lefvert AK. Heterogeneity of autoantibodies against cardiolipin and oxidatively modified LDLs revealed by human monoclonal antibodies. J Intern Med 2000;247:385–90.

42. Horkko S, Bird DA, Miller E, et al. Monoclonal autoantibodies specific for oxidized phospholipids or oxidized phospholipid-protein adducts inhibit macrophage uptake of oxidized low-density lipoproteins. J Clin Invest 1999;103:117–28.

43. Watson AD, Leitinger N, Navad M, et al. Structural identification by mass spectrometry of oxidized phospholipids in minimally oxidized low density lipoprotein that induce monocyte/endothelial interactions and evidence for their presence in vivo. J Biol Chem 1997;272:13597–607.

44. Palinski W, Horkko S, Miller E, et al. Cloning of monoclonal autoantibodies to epitopes of oxidized lipoproteins from apolipoprotein E-deficient mice. Demonstration of epitopes of oxidized low density lipoprotein in human plasma. J Clin Invest 1996;98:800–14.

45. Yagi K. A simple fluorometric assay for lipoperoxide in blood plasma. Biochem. Med. 1976;15:212–6.

46. Witztum JL, Steibrecher UP, Fisher M, Kesaniemi A. Nonenzymatic glucosylation of homologous LDL and albumin render them immunogenic in the guinea-pig. Proc Natl Acad Sci USA 1983;80:2757–61.

47. Haberland ME, Cheng L, Fong D. Malondialdehyde-altered protein occurs atheroma of waranabe heritable hyperlipidemic rabbits. Science 1988;241:215–7.

48. Rosenfeld ME, Palinski W, Ylä-Herttuala S, et al. Distribution of oxidation specific lipid-protein adducts and apolipoprotein B in atherosclerotic lesions of varying severity from WHHL rabbits. Arteriosclerosis 1990;10:336–49.

49. Knight JA. Free radicals: their presence in biological systems. In: Free Radicals, Antioxidants, Aging, and Disease. Washington DC: Amer Assn Clin Chem Press 1999:1–31.

50. Pratico D, Tangirala RK, Rader DJ, et al. Vitamin E suppresses isoprostane generation in vivo and reduces atherosclerosis in ApoE-deficient mice. Nat Med. 1998;4:1189–92.

51. Chisolm GM, Ma G, Irwin KC, et al. 7 beta-htdroperoxycholest-5-en-3 beta-ol, a component of human athero-

sclerotic lesions, is the primary cytotoxin of oxidized human low density lipoprotein. Proc Natl Acad Sci USA 1994;91:11452–6.

52. Esterbauer H, Jurgens G, Quehenberger O, Koller E. Autooxidation of human low density lipoprotein:loss of polyunsaturated fatty acids and vitamin E and generation of aldehydes. J Lipid Res 1987;28:495–509.

53. Jurgens G, Hoff HF, Chisolm GM, Esterbauer H. Modification of human serum low density lipoprotein by oxidation – characterization and pathophysiological implications. Chem Phys Lipids1987;45:315–36.

54. Parthasarathy S, Fong LG, Witztum JL, Steinberg D. Nonenzymatic oxidative cleavage of peptide bonds in apoprotein B 100. Proc Natl Acad Sci USA 1978;86:1046–50.

55. Quinn MT, Parthasarathy S, Steinberg D. Lysophosphatidylcholine: a chemotactic factor for human monocytes and its potential role in atherogenesis. Proc Natl Acad Sci USA 1988;85:2805–9.

56. Hansson GK, Jonasson L, Seifert PS, Stemme S. Immune mechanisms in atherosclerosis. Arteriosclerosis 1989;9:567–78.

57. Nilsson J, Regnstrom J, Frostegard J, Stiko A. Lipid oxidation and atherosclerosis. Herz 1992;17:263–9.

58. Esterbauer H, Waeg G, Puhl H, et al. Inhibition of LDL oxidation by antioxidants. Basel: Birkhäuser 1992;62:145–57.

59. Watson AD, Berliner JA, Hama SY, et al. Protective effect of high density lipoprotein associated paraoxonase-inhibition of the biological activity of minimally oxidized low density lipoprotein. J Clin Invest 1995;96:2882–91.

60. Cross CE, Traber M, Eiserich J, van der Vliet A. Micronutrient antioxidants and smoking. Br Med Bull 1999;55:691–704.

61. Freigang S, Horkko S, Miller E, et al. Immunization of LDL receptor-deficient mice with homologous malondialdehyde-modified and native LDL reduces progression of atherosclerosis by mechanisms other than induction of high titers of antibodies to oxidative neoepitopes. Arterioscler Thromb Vasc Biol 1998;18:1972–82.

62. Palinski W, Tangirala RK, Miller E, et al. Increased autoantibody titers against epitopes of oxidized low density lipoprotein in LDL-receptor-deficient mice with increased atherosclerosis. Arterioscler Thromb Vasc Biol 1995;15:1569–76.

63. Ohara Y, Peterson TE, Harrison DG. Hypercholesterolemia increases endothelial superoxide anion production. J Clin Invest 1993;91:2546–51.

64. Liao F, Andalibi A, deBeer FC, et al. Genetic control of inflammatory gene induction and NF-κ B-like transcription factor activation in response to an atherogenic diet in mice. J Clin Invest 1993;91:2572–9.

Atherosclerosis and Autoimmunity
Y. Shoenfeld, D. Harats and G. Wick, editors

Autoantibodies to Endothelial Cells and Oxidized LDL in Human Atherosclerosis and Hypertension

Johan Frostegård

Department of Medicine and CMM, Karolinska Hospital, Karolinska Institutet, Stockholm, Sweden

1. INTRODUCTION

According to the response to injury hypothesis, atherosclerosis starts as a damage to or dysfunction of the endothelium, leading to a low grade chronic inflammation present over many years, before acute ischemic events may occur as a result of plaque rupture and/or thrombosis. Atherosclerosis is a complex disease where risk factors as hypertension, hyperlipidemia, smoking and diabetes have been identified. Recently, inflammation as determined by circulating C-reactive protein has been demonstrated to enhance the risk of cardiovascular disease [1, 2]. Furthermore, patients with rheumatic autoimmune disases, especially SLE but also rheumatoid arthritis have an enhanced risk for cardiovascular disease [3]. Dyslipidemia, anti-phospholipid antibodies and systemic inflammation are features of SLE, which makes this disease interesting as a model for development of inflammation-related atherosclerosis [3, 4]. Also infectious agents have been implicated as risk factors for atherosclerosis, especially Chlamydia Pneumonia [5].

Relatively little is known about a putative role of immune reactions in hypertension, and in a majority of cases, the cause of this condition – essential hypertension – remains obscure. However, alterations of immunological factors such as decreased T cell responses and abnormalities in complement function as well as enhanced immunoglobulin levels have been reported in hypertension [6].

The atherosclerotic lesions start to develop early, while clinical symptoms come much later in life. The lesions are located just under the endothelium,

in the intima of large and middle sized arteries, and tend to accumulate in bifurcations. This is an interesting feature of the lesions not fully explained, though possibly related to the special characteristics of turbulent blood flow at these sites, leading to endothelial stress and/or damage [1].

Fatty streaks, the earliest lesions, are characterized by an infiltration of macrophages, and T cells into the intima and these inflammatory cells are then present in large amounts at all stages of disease development [7, 8] Many of the macrophages develop into lipid-filled foam cells, constituting a large part of the developing lesions, and a major lipid in foam cells is oxidized (ox) LDL [9]. Atherogenesis is also characterized by the migration and proliferation of smooth muscle cells from the media into the intima [1, 8]. Proinflammatory cytokines are produced in large amounts in the atherosclerotic lesions [10].

Epidemiological and immunopathological data thus indicate that atherosclerosis is an inflammatory disease [2, 8, 10].

Both the endothelium and oxLDL are thus clearly relevant in cardiovascular disease, and one focus of our studies has been the role of immune reactions and especially antibodies against oxLDL and endothelial cells (EC) in human atherosclerosis and hypertension.

2. IMMUNOLOGICAL MECHANISMS IN THE DEVELOPMENT OF ATHEROSCLEROSIS AND HYPERTENSION

Though it is clear that inflammation is a prominent feature of atherosclerosis, relatively little is known about how specific immune reactions influence disease development. In fact, animal experiments indicate that T and B cells are not necessary for the development of atherosclerotic lesions in the presence of severe hypercholesterolemia. However, they may play an important role in moderate degrees of hypercholesterolemia by modulating disease development [11, 12]. In general, the role of immune reactions in atherogenesis is likely to be very complex, and may depend both on antigen, animal model, and disease stage.

Cell-mediated immune reactions have been reported to be related both to an increase and a decrease in the development of atherosclerosis when different animal models were used. As much as a 42% decrease in atherosclerotic lesions was detected in apo E knock-out mice in the presence of moderate hypercholesterolemia and a combined immunodeficiency, as compared to apo E knock out controls [12]. In another study using apo E knock-out mice crossed into IFN-gamma-receptor knock-outs, atherosclerosis was greatly diminished [13]. Likewise, transfer of CD4+ aggravates atherosclerosis in immune-deficient mice [14]. Also transplantation atherosclerosis was aggravated by T cells [15]. Furthermore, in T cell ablated, immune deficient atherosclerosis prone C57BL/6J mice, atherosclerosis was inhibited [16]. On the other hand, other studies indicate that cell mediated immune reactions in rabbit models [17] and in atherosclerosis prone C57 BL/6J mice [18] suppress the development of atherosclerosis.

These apparently conflicting data indicate that studies of human atherosclerosis are necessary to settle this issue, though evidence is accumulating indicating that cell-mediated immunity indeed aggravates atherosclerosis in many disease settings. As will be discussed below, the nature of the immune reaction and antigen specificity is likely to be pivotal in determining outcome.

It is also possible that the role of the cell mediated immune system in atherogenesis may depend on the disease stage and on the presence of other risk factors, sex, and effects of hormonal and metabolic factors on cytokine profile in specific immune reactions. Furthermore, atherosclerosis may be the outcome of different disturbances – immunological, metabolic, infectious – and may in fact be more than one disease and available animal models may reflect only a proportion of human atherosclerosis.

3. ANTIBODIES AGAINST THE ENDOTHELIUM

According to the response to injury hypothesis, an early endothelial injury, or activation, is pivotal in atherogenesis. Since endothelial dysfunction is a feature also of early cardiovascular disease in general as hypertension, a possibility that we have been interested in is that antibodies to endothelial cells (aEC) or to antigens associated with EC may contribute to the development and/or pathogenesis of both hypertension and atherosclerosis, in addition to being markers of disease. We recently reported that aEC are associated not only with borderline hypertension, but also with early atherosclerosis [19]. Though this kind of studies must be followed up prospectively to give implications about causative factors, an intriguing finding was an association with endothelin in our study [19]. Since aEC in other systems induce endothelin [20], it is in principle possible that these antibodies may contribute to the pathogenesis of hypertension, a possibility presently under investigation in a prospective study. It is also possible that aEC may contribute to development of atherosclerosis by causing damage to and/or activation of EC. Clearly, further research both in humans prospectively and in animal models is needed to clarify this issue.

Enhanced aEC levels have been reported in systemic lupus erythematosus [21–23] and in other autoimmune diaseases, including rheumatoid arthritis with systemic manifestations, Wegener´s granulomatosis and vasculitis [21]. Enhanced aEC has been suggested to be disease activity marker in SLE [22], and in a previous study, aEC were also associated with advanced atherosclerosis [24].

An important question is which antigens related to or present on EC that are targets for aEC. Several studies indicate that factors in the protein component of cells may function as antigens under certain conditions [25–27]. Another non-mutually exclusive possibility that we have been interested in is that phospholipids in the cell membranes are targets for aEC and it has been demonstrated that antiphospholipid antibodies in patients with autoimmune disease cross react with EC [28]. We recently demonstrated that in high-titer sera, aEC cross react with oxLDL, and also with another phospholipid in oxLDL that is believed to be atherogenic, lysophosphatidylcholine [29; LPC]. Platelet activating factor (PAF) is an inflammatory phospholipid expressed by activated endothelial cells, and PAF-like phospholipids but not PAF itself are present in oxLDL [30]. We recently described a novel category of antibodies against PAF, which showed a strong association with early atherosclerosis, blood pressure and also metabolic factors [31]. Also PAF may be a target for aEC, and antibodies against PAF showed a stronger association with BHT than other factors tested, including blood lipids, metabolic factors, other autoantibodies, and endothelin. However, antibodies to PAF and oxLDL differ in subclass distribution, which supports the notion that they have a different origin and may play completely different roles in cardiovascular disease, (unpublished observation). Antibodies against PAF may therefore be a novel promising marker of early cardiovascular disease.

Both oxidized phospholipids and LPC are present in cells undergoing apoptosis [32], and an intriguing possibility presently under investigation in our laboratory is that aEC recognize apoptotic EC.

Recent data suggest that the immunological component to the development of atherosclerosis involve the expression of and reactivity to heat shock proteins (HSP). In addition to being constitutively expressed, heat shock proteins are induced in response to different biological and physicochemical agents [33]. They are important in repair processes and the intracellular assembly, folding and translocation of proteins [34]. HSP are highly conserved, which has led to the hypothesis that there is a link between immune responses to infection and the development of autoimmune reactions [35]. Further evidence indicating the importance of HSP in vascular disease comes from studies reporting elevated levels of Hsp65 antibodies in patients with carotid atherosclerosis [36], and borderline hypertension [37].

Although heat shock proteins are typically regarded as being intracellular, they can be expressed on the surface of stressed aortic endothelial cells and Hsp60 and Hsp70 has been identified in the serum of normal individuals [39]. We recently demonstrated that HSP60 is associated with borderline hypertension, early atherosclerosis and metabolic factors [39], and our previous data indicate that oxLDL can induce HSP from monocytes [40]. HSP on EC can thus be targets for some aEC, a notion supported by an association between aHSP and aEC [19]. Taken together, possible antigens on EC involve phospholipids and co-factors for phospholipids like ß2GPI, oxidized lipids and LPC, and also HSP´s. By recognizing these antigens on EC, aEC may contribute to endothelial activation and dysfunction, and thus contribute to development of both atherosclerosis and hypertension, in addition to being disease markers.

4. LDL-OXIDATION

LDL is a well established risk factor for atherosclerosis [9]. LDL is believed to become more atherogenic after modification, e.g.oxidation [9] but also other forms of modification as glycosylation [41], and enzymatic modification through hydrolysis, may render LDL atherogenic [42].

Oxidation of LDL results in the formation of a large amount of different compounds that may contribute to atherogenesis in different ways, though it is not clear which component of oxLDL is the most atherogenic. These compounds include fragmented apoB 100; reactive aldehydes that may form adducts with apoB; oxidized fatty acids, lipid peroxides, oxysterols and oxidized cholesterol; lysolipids including lysophosphatidylcholine (LPC) [43].

The LDL-oxidation hypothesis in atherosclerosis is based on several findings. Firstly, LDL from atherosclerotic lesions show signs of oxidation and biologically active oxLDL-epitopes are present even in human serum. Secondly, antioxidants retard atherogenesis in experimental antimal models. Thirdly, proatherogenic properties of LDL including uptake by macrophages and foam cell formation requires oxidation [44, 45].

LDL can become oxidized in vivo through several different mechanism, and it is not completelay clear which of these is the most important. LDL-oxidation can be induced by cupper or iron metal ions [43, 44]. Cells directly involved in atherogenesis oxidize LDL in vitro. Metal ions may be a prerequisite also for this type of modification, though superoxide and other free radicals from activated macrophages may contribute significantly. Another possibility is that nitric oxide (NO), released by endothelial or other cells, may oxidize LDL [44].

LDL can become oxidized through enzymes present in the atherosclerotic lesion as lipoxygenases and myeoloperoxidases. Lipoxygenases are intracellular enzymes inducing peroxidation of polyunsaturated fatty acids, generating biologically active oxygenated lipid products. Myeoloperoxidases are produced by macrophages, and promote lipid peroxidation [44].

Though animal experiments clearly indicate that antioxidants decrease atherogenesis, the situation in humans is less convincing [45]. It is possible that this reflects differences between experimental animal and human atherosclerosis and may also indicate that levels of antioxidants needed to induce decreased atherogenesis and/or cardiovascular disease in general, are too high in humans.

One of the active components of oxLDL is LPC, which is formed by oxidation of LDL [46] or phosphatidylcholine by enzymes with phospholipase A2-activity [47]. Recently we identified secretory phospholipase A2 type II (sPLA2-II, non-pancreatic type) expression and activity in both normal and atherosclerotic arterial wall [48]. This finding indicates that significant amounts of LPC may be generated in the arterial wall by hydrolysis of phospholipids in retained LDL. Furthermore, PLA2 may promote oxidation that is induced by lipoxygenase and metal ions [8]. PLA2 activity is enhanced in systemic inflammation as SLE and may be a link between inflammation, LDL-oxidation and atherosclerosis [49]. We also recently reported that LPC is involved in the antigenicity of oxLDL and it is thus possible that systemic inflammation promotes LPC production and renders LDL immunogenic partly through enzymatic modification [50].

5. IMMUNE-STIMULATORY, ATHEROGENIC AND PROHYPERTENSIVE PROPERTIES OF OXLDL

Earler studies demonstrate that oxLDL is inhibitory and toxic to endothelial and other cells [51, 52] and may thus cause endothelial injury to which atherosclerosis is a response. These toxic and/or inhibitory effects mainly occur when high doses of oxLDL are used.

However, when low doses are used, oxLDL is stimulatory to different cell types involved in atherogenesis indicating a dual role.

OxLDL induces chemotaxis in monocytes and T cells [53, 54], promotes differentiation of monocytes into macrophages [52], stimulates monocyte-endothelial interaction [52], and activate endothelial cells to enhanced adhesiveness and expression of adhesion molecules [55, 56]. Furthermore, oxLDL induces smooth muscle cell proliferation [57]. OxLDL stimulates production of monokines including IL-1ß [58], TNF [59, 60], IL-8 [61], IL-6 [62] and IL-12 [63].

By inducing immunogenic HSP 60/65 [40] and HSP 70 [64], oxLDL may promote immune reactions indirectly, and thus contribute to inflammatory reactions. HSP 60 was recently demonstrated in the circulation [65] and was shown to have proinflammatory properties [66]. We recently demonstrated that HSP60 is associated with early atherosclerosis and borderline hypertension [39].

To a large extent, these immune-stimulatory, proinflammatory and proatherogenic effects on endothelial cells and on cytokine production may be related to platelet activating factor (PAF)-like lipids formed in LDL during modification [60, 67–69].

We recently investigated the proinflammatory, cytokine-stimulatory properties of oxLDL by testing the effects of different compounds in the lipid moiety of oxLDL, including oxysterols, oxidized free fatty acid products, and LPC [69]. The only compound that could mimick oxLDL´s effects was LPC, possibly after modification by enzymes, since LPC itself is not likely to be a PAF-like lipid. It is still possible that other oxidized and/or hydrolysed compounds in oxLDL still may share these properties, and recently, a rare fragmented alkyl-phosphatidylcholine [70] was shown to be the major

PAF-like lipid in oxLDL. Further studies are needed to elucidate how these compounds interact with monocytes and T cells and how they are generated and transformed in the local environment of atherosclerotic lesions.

Proinflammatory Th1 cytokines dominate in advanced atherosclerotic lesions, where also monokines are abundand, especially IL-1ß and IL-6, but also TNF [10]. OxLDL and PAF-like lipids in oxLDL, including LPC, can induce production of these cytokines from inflammatory cells prepared directly from atherosclerotic lesions (unpublished observation).

Taken together, available evidence clearly indicate that oxLDL may be a major factor causing the inflammation in atherosclerotic lesions. Another important question is whether oxLDL is also a specific antigen for specific immune reactions. Available evidence indicate that this is indeed the case.

OxLDL activates T cells by a monocyte-dependent mechanism [58]. OxLDL mediated T cell activation occurs only at low levels of oxLDL, and we and others have reported that oxLDL instead tends to inhibit T cell activation at concentrations above 10–25 µg/ml [58, 71]. It is even possible that this oxLDL-mediated T cell inhibition is atherogenic, by inhibiting an adequate T cell response to other antigens, e g viral [71].

Antibodies of IgG type specific for oxLDL are present both in cardiovascular disease and in healthy controls [9]. This indicates that T helper cells are involved and these findings give further support to the notion that oxLDL can activate T cells. In line with this is also a study where 10% of a population of T cell cloned from human atherosclerotic lesions reacted specifically with oxLDL [72].

The mechanism behind oxLDL-promoted T cell activation remains to be elucidated. Several possibilities, not mutually exclusive, have been proposed.

OxLDL mediated T cell activation may be indirect, since oxLDL induces immunogenic HSP´s, which may be recognized by specific T-cells [40].

Anti-phospholipid antibodies cross react with oxLDL [73] and recently it has been demonstrated that plasma proteins like ß2 Glycoprotein I act as cofactors, potentiating the binding of antiphospholipid antibodies [74]. The antigen for aPL may be the co-factor itself, a complex betweeen lipids and peptide fragments, or an oxidized epitope on the lipid [75, 76]. Recently, aPL were demonstrated to be specific for oxidized forms of phospholipid [76]. The exact mechanisms and the nature of the antigenicity of phospholipids thus remains to be clarified, but one interesting possibility is that the phospholipid-cofactor complex is taken up by macrophages, which then present peptide fragments to T and B cells.

Yet another possibility is that lipids in oxLDL bind to CD1 receptors on monocytes [77].

The cross-reactivity between antiphospholipid antibodies and oxLDL indicates that an important part of the T-cell antigenicity of oxLDL is related to the lipid moiety, e.g. LPC, possibly in complex with plasma proteins or fragments thereof [50]. However, also apoB fragments may in principle contribute to T cell reactivity against oxLDL.

OxLDL is likely to promote T cell activation by inducing TNF [59, 60], IL-12 and other T cell stimulatory cytokines [63]. These may enhance the activity of T cell reacting to other antigens, possibly also break down products in the complicated atherosclerotic lesions. OxLDL may thus also promote T cell activation indirectly, functioning as an adjuvant. Whether this property of oxLDL could contribute to the T-cell help likely to be needed for anti-oxLDL antibody formation is not clear.

Little is known about a putative role of oxLDL in hypertension. However, oxLDL decreases vascular tonus by inhibiting nitric oxide release, an effect related to LPC [78]. By this mechanism, oxLDL and LPC may in principle increase blood pressure.

6. OXLDL AND ANTIBODY FORMATION

Antibodies to oxLDL of both IgG and IgM type are present in normal healthy individuals [8] and in in atherosclerotic plaques [79].

However, the role of humoral immune reactions in general in atherogenesis is not clear. It may be hypothesized that the physiological function of antibodies to OxLDL is to participate in the removal of these proinflammatory and proatherogenic compounds from the circulation and from the artery wall. This is an important role played by antibody reactions in general, e g in infections, where high levels of antibodies protect against disease. Low aOxLDL levels may therefore in principle predispose to progression of atherosclerosis. Recently, natural T15 antibodies, well known for their ability to provide protection from virulent pneumococcal infection, were demonstrated to be identical to IgM monoclonal antibodies against oxLDL [32]. AoXLDL could therefore be part of a defense system against different forms of modified or oxidized lipids occuring in bacteria, lipoproteins, and apoptotic or necrotic cells [32]. Accordingly recent reports indicate that immunization of experimental animals with OxLDL, leading to enhanced aOxLDL levels, inhibits atherosclerosis development [80, 81]. Furthermore, in early cardiovascular disease, as in borderline hypertension, aOxLDL levels were decreased [82] which was the case also with antibodies to a major compound in oxLDL, LPC [83].

On the other hand, several studies have demonstrated a positive association between the degree of atherosclerosis and antibody levels to OxLDL [84–86]. One possibility is that at a later stage of disease development, enhanced antibody levels reflect the chronic inflammation in the artery wall, aoxLDL thus being a marker of late but not early stage disease. In line with this are reports that in later stages of early vascular disease, as may occur in essential hypertension (as opposed to BHT), increased aOxLDL levels have been reported [87]. Thus, during the earliest stages of atherosclerosis, the humoral response may be low and the antibodies generated bound by antigens in tissue or in the circulation. Later, as lesions expand, a stronger humoral response may occur, and antibody levels rise as production of antibodies exceeds binding to tissues.

LPC in oxLDL has proinflammatory properties and is also toxic at higher concentrations and may thus play a role in atherogenesis [31]. Furthermore, LPC functions as a vasoconstrictor in experimental systems, inhibiting NO-mediated vasorelaxation [78]. An intriguing possibility is that anti-LPC and aOxLDL antibodies counteract these effects and aOxLDL and aLPC may thus play a role in the development of hypertension. In this scenario, antibodies related to oxLDL would thus play a different role in disease development than those generated as a response to endothelial antigens.

The decreased immune-reactivity to oxLDL and LPC in BHT individuals may also be due to a decreased production, either caused by a lower exposure to the antigen, or because this immune-response is down-regulated. In general, immunological tolerance may be induced by an oral intake of an antigen, as exemplified by collagen II in Rheumatoid arthritis-rat models [88]. Whether oral tolerance may also be present as a specific response against certain lipid-containing and even oxidized compounds in the food is not known, but this is a possibility that could be tested in animal models and in human epidemiological studies.

Antibodies to oxLDL most likely recognize several different epitopes generated by LDL-oxidation. Malondialdehydes are formed during oxidation of free fatty acid in LDL, and these form adducts with apoB 100 in LDL, that may function as antigenic epitopes present in atherosclerotic lesions [9]. As described, aOxLDL and anti-phospholipid antibodies (aPL) cross-react immunologically [73]. APL is an important factor behind arterial and venous thrombosis [89, 90]. The cross-reactivity implies that antibodies recognizing the phospholipids in oxLDL may be of importance in vascular disease. Interestingly, SLE is characterized by aggravated atherosclerosis and aPL is an important risk factor for cardiovascular disease in SLE patients as well as in the general population [91, 92]. However, antigens may recognize an array of other epitopes in oxLDL. The role of aOxLDL in regulating oxLDL uptake by scavenger receptors is not clear and aOxLDL may both enhance and decrease uptake, depending on experimental system [93, 94]. Another mechanism by which aoxLDL may interfere with atherogenesis and cause endothelial acitvation is through cross-reactivity between aOxLDL and endothelial cells [29]. However, differences between these antibody categories exist, since binding of aOxLDL and aLPC or a PAF in contrast to aPL, is not enhanced by a co-factor as ß2GPI [31, 95].

7. DISCUSSION AND CONCLUSIONS

Available data from both animal experiments and human studies clearly indicate that atherosclerosis is an inflammatory disease, and that the immune system may modulate the disease and both promote and decrease atherogenesis. The outcome of specific immune reactions may depend on which antigen is used, type of immune reaction and cytokine profile in the local milieu, and also stage of disease development.

For example, immunization with HSP leads to aggravated atherosclerosis [96], but when oxLDL is used as antigen, the disease decreases in experimental animals [79, 80]. Animal experiments testing effects of immunization with these (or other factors) on blood pressure have not been reported to my knowledge.

Taken together, it may be hypothesized that antibodies against antigens in oxLDL may protect against disease development, while those directed against the endothelium or factors related to it as ß2GPI, HSP, have an opposite effect. This notion is supported by data from animal experiments, where immunization with oxLDL decreased disease development. On the other hand, when HSP were used as antigen, atherosclerosis was aggravated.

In line with these reports from animal experiments are human studies implying that antibodies to HSP [36, 37] and also to EC [19] are enhanced both in established atherosclerosis and early cardiovascular disease as in borderline hypertension [19, 36, 37], while aOxLDL and aLPC are decreased [82, 83].

In another study, immunization with ß2GPI was shown to aggravate disease develoment [97], also this in line with human studies demonstrating enhanced antibody levels to this co-factor in early human cardiovascular disease [19]. Furthermore, ß2GPI may be an important antigen for endothelial cell antibodies, like PAF itself (unpublished observation), and both antibodies to PAF and endothelial cells were associated with early human atherosclerosis and also with endothelin [19, 31]. Indeed, among all factors tested including metabolic and lipid factors, aPAF showed the strongest association with BHT (unpublished observation).

If immunization procedures with some component of oxLDL and/or inhibitors of immune-stimulatory components of oxLDL using e.g. PAF-antagonistsm potent antioxidants and/or PLA2 inhibitors have a role in treatment of human atherosclerosis and hypertension clearly deserves further studies.

REFERENCES

1. Ross R. The pathogenesis of atherosclerosis – a perspective for the 1990s. Nature 1993;362:801.

2. Ridker PM, Cushman M, Stampfer MJ, Tracy RP, Hennekens CH. Inflammation, aspirin, and the risk of cardiovascular disease in apparently healthy men. N Engl J Med 1997;336:973.

3. Gladman DD. Prognosis of Systemic Lupus Erythematosus and factors that affect it. Curr Op Rheum 1990;2:694.

4. Lahita RG, Rivkin E, Cavanagh I, Romano P. Low levels of total cholesterol, high density lipoprotein and apolipoprotein A1 in association with anticardiolipin antibodies in patients with systemic lupus erythematosus. Arthr Rheum 1993;36:1566.

5. Cook PJ, Lip GY. Infectious agents and atherosclerotic vascular disease. Quarterly J Med 1996;89:427.

6. Fu ML. Do immune system changes have a role in hypertension? J Hypertension 1995;1259–65.

7. Jonasson L, Holm J, Skalli O, Bondjers G, Hansson GK. Regional accumulations of T cells, macrophages, and smooth muscle cells in the human atherosclerotic plaque. Arteriosclerosis 1986;6:131.

8. Ross R. Atherosclerosis – an inflammatory disease. N Engl J Med 1999;340:115.

9. Witztum JL. The oxidation hypothesis of atherosclerosis. Lancet 1994;344:793.

10. Frostegård J, Ulfgren AK, Nyberg P, Swedenborg, J, Hedin U, Andersson U, Wuttge D, Stemme S, Klareskog L and Hansson GK. Secretion of proinflammatory (Th1) cytokines in advanced human atherosclerotic plaques. Atherosclerosis 1999;145:33–43.

11. Fyfe AI, Qiao JH, Lusis AH. Immune-deficient mice develop typical atherosclerotic fatty streaks when fed an atherogenic diet. J Clin Invest 1994;94:2516–20.

12. Dansky HM, Charlton SA, McGee H, Harper M, Smith JD. T and B lymphocytes play a minor role in atherosclerotic plaque formation in the apolipoprotein E-deficient mouse. Proc Natl Acad Sci USA 1997;94:4642–46.

13. Gupta S, Pablo AM, Jiang Xc, Wang N, Tall AR and Schindler C. IFN-gamma potentiated atherosclerosis in ApoE knock-out mice. J Clin Invest 1997;99:2752–61.

14. Xinghua Zhou. Immune Mechanisms in Atherosclerosis. The role of T cells in murine models of atherosclerosis. Academic dissertation. Stockholm: Karolinska Institute 2000.

15. Nagano H, Lippy P, Taylor MK, Hasegawa S, Stinn JL, Becker G, Tilney NL and Mitchell RN. Coronary arteriosclerosis after T-cell-mediated injury in transplanted mouse hearts: role of interferon-gamma. Am J Pathol 1998;152:1187–97.

16. Emcson EE, Shen ML, Bell CG, Qureshi A. Inhibition

of atherosclerosis in CD4 T cell ablated and nude (nu/nu) C57BL/6 hyperlipidemic mice. Am J Pathol 1996;149:675–85.

17. Roselaar SE, Schonfeld G, Daugherty A. Enhanced development of atherosclerosis in cholesterol-fed rabbits by suppression of cell-mediated immunity. J Clin Inv 1995;96:1389–94.

18. Emeson EE, Shen ML. Accelerated atherosclerosis in hyperlipidemic C57BL/6 mice treated with cyclosporin A. Am J Pathol 1993;142:1906–15.

19. Frostegård J, Wu R, Haegerstrand C, Lemne C, de Faire U. Antibodies to endothelial cells in borderline hypertension. Circulation 1998;98:1092–1098.

20. Yoshio T, Masuyama J, Mimori A, Takeda A, Minota S, Kano S. Endothelin-1 release from cultured endothelial cells induced by sera from patients with systemic lupus erythematosus. Ann Rheum Dis 1995;54:361–365.

21. Navarro M, Cervera R, Font J, Reverter JC, Monteagudo J, Escolar G, Lopez-Soto A, Ordinas A, Ingelmo M. Anti-endothelial cell antibodies in systemic autoimmune diseases: prevalence and clinical significance. Lupus 1997;6:521–526.

22. Li JS, Liu MF, Lei HY. Characterization of anti-endothelial cell antibodies in the patients with systemic lupus erythematosus: a potential marker for disease activity. Clin Immunol and Immunopath 1996;79:211–216.

23. Hill MB, Phipps JL, Milford-Ward A, Greaves M, Hughes P. Further characterization of anti-endothelial cell antibodies in lupus erythematosus by controlled immunoblotting. Br J Rheum 1996;35:1231–1238.

24. Bergmark C, Wu R, de Faire U, Lefvert AK, Swedenborg J. Patients with early-onset peripheral vascular disease have increased levels of autoantibodies against oxidized LDL. Arterioscler Thromb Vasc Biol 1995;15:441–445.

25. Vazici ZA, Behrendt M, Cooper D, Goodfield M, Partridge L, Lindsey MJ. The identification of endothelial cell autoantigens. J Autoimmun 2000;15:41–49.

26. Ihn H, Sato S, Fujimoto M, Igarashi A, Yazawa N, Kubo M, Kikuchi K, Takehara and Tamaki K. Characterization of autoantibodies to endothelial cells in systemic sclerosis (SSc): association with pulmonary fibrosis. Clin Exp Immunol 2000;119:203–209.

27. Hill MB, Phipps JL, Hughes P, Greaves M. Anti-endothelial cell antibodies in primary antiphospholipid syndrome and SLE: patterns of reactivity with membrane antigens on microvascular and umbilical venous cell membranes. Br J Haematol 1998;103:416–21.

28. Del Papa N, Guidali L, Spatola L, Bonara B, Borghi MO, Tincani A, Balestriera G, Meroni PL. Relationship between anti-phospholipid and anti-endothelial cell antibodies III: beta 2 glycoprotein 1 mediates the antibody binding to endothelial membranes and induces the

expression of adhesion molecules. Clin Exp Rheumatol 1995;13:179–185.

29. Wu R, Svenungsson E, Gunnarsson I, Haegerstrand-Gillis C, Andersson B, Lundberg I, Schäfer-Elinder L, Frostegård J. Antibodies to adult human endothelial cells cross react with oxidized LDL and ß2-glycoprotein I. Clin Exp Immunol 1999;115:561–566.

30. Lehr HA, Seemuller J, Hubner C, Menger MD, Messmer K. Oxidized LDL-induced leukocyte/endothelium interaction in vivo involves the receptor for platelet-activating factor. Arterioscler Thromb 1993;13:1013–1017.

31. Wu R, Lemne C, de Faire U, Frostegård J. Antibodies to platelet activating factor in early cardiovascular disease. J Internal Med 1999;246:389–397.

32. Shaw PX, Hörkkö S, Chang MK, Curtiss LK, Palinski W, Silverman GJ, Witztum J. Natural antibodies with the T15 idiotype may act in atherosclerosis, apoptotic clearance and protective immunity. J Clin Invest 2000;105:1731–1740.

33. Wick G, Schett G, Amberger A, Kleindienst R, Xu Q. Is atherosclerosis an immunologically mediated disease? Immunol Today 1995;16:27–33.

34. Hightower LE. Heat shock, stress proteins, chaperones and proteotoxicity. Cell 1991;66:191–197.

35. Kiessling R, Grönberg A, Ivanyi J, Söderström K, Ferm M, Kleinau S, Nilsson E, Klareskog L. Role of Hsp60 during autoimmune and bacterial inflammation. Immunol Rev 1991;12:91–111.

36. Xu Q, Willeit J, Marosi M, Kleindienst R, Oberhollenzer F, Kiechl S, Stulnig T, Luef G, Wick G. Association of serum antibodies to heat shock protein 65 with carotid atherosclerosis. Lancet 1993;341:255–259.

37. Frostegård J, Lemne C, Andersson B, van der Zee R, Kiessling R, de Faire U. Association of serum antibodies to heat-shock protein 65 with borderline hypertension. Hypertension 1997;29:40–44.

38. Xu Q, Schett G, Seitz CS, Hu Y, Gupta RS, Wick G. Surface staining and cytotoxic activity of heat-shock protein 60 in stressed aortic endothelial cells. Circulation Res 1994;75:1078–1085.

39. Pockley G, de Faire U, Lemne C, Kiessling R, Frostegård J. Circulating Heat Shock Protein 60 is associated with Early Cardiovascular disease. Hypertension 2000;36:303–307.

40. Frostegård J, Kjellman B, Gidlund M, Jindal S, Kiessling R. Induction of heat shock protein in monocytic cells by oxidized low density lipoprotein. Atherosclerosis 1996;121:93–103.

41. Palinski W, Ylä-Herttuala S, Rosenfeld S, Butler SA, Socher S, Parthasarathy S, Curtiss LK, Witztum JL. Antisera and monoclonal antibodies specific for epitopes generated during the oxidative modification of low density lipoprotein. Arteriosclerosis 1990;10:325–335.

42. Kume N, Cybulsky MI, Gimbrone MA. Lysophosphatidylcholine, a component of atherogenic lipoproteins, induces mononuclear leukocyte adhesion molecules in cultured human and rabbit arterial endothelial cells. J Clin Inv 1992;90:1138–1144.

43. Esterbauer H, Gebicki J, Puhl H, Jürgens G. The role of lipid peroxidation and antioxidant in oxidative modification of LDL. Free Radic Biol Med 1992;13:241–290.

44. Heinecke JW. Oxidants and antioxidants in the pathogenesis of atherosclerosis: implications for the oxidized low density lipoprotein hypothesis. Atherosclerosis 1998;141:1–15.

45. Steinberg D. A critical look at the evidence for the oxidation of LDL in atherogenesis. Atherosclerosis Suppl 1997;131:S5–7.

46. Quinn MT, Parthasarathy S, Steinberg D. Lysophosphatidylcholine: a chemotactic factor for human monocytes and its potential role in atherogenesis. Proc Natl Acad Sci 1998;85:2805–09.

47. Liu M, Subbaiah PV. Hydrolysis and transesterification of platelet-activating factor by lecithin-cholesterol acyltransferase. Proc Natl Acad Sci USA 1994;91:6035–39.

48. Schäfer-Elinder L, Hedin U, Dumitrescu A, Larsson P, Frostegård J, Claesson HE. Presence of different isoforms of phospholipase A2 in tissue slices from atherosclerotic carotid plaque. Arteriosclerosis, Thrombosis and Vasc Biol 1997;17:2257–62.

49. Pruzanski W, Goulding N, Flower RJ, Gladman DD, Urowitz MB, Goodman PJ, Scott KF, Vadas P. Circulating Group II phospholipase A2 activity and antilipocortin antibodies in systemic lupus erythematosus. Correlative study with disease activity. J Rheum 1994;21:252–257.

50. Wu R, Huang YH, Schäfer-Elinder L, Frostegård J. Lysophosphatidylcholine is involved in the antigenicity of oxLDL. Arteriosclerosis, Thrombosis and Vasc Biol 1998;18:626–630.

51. Kosugi K, Morel DW, DiCorleto PE, Chisolm GM. Toxicity of oxidized low-density lipoprotein to cultured fibroblasts is selective for S phase of the cell cycle. J Cellular Physiol 1987;130:311.

52. Frostegård J, Nilsson J, Haegerstrand A, Hamsten A, Wigzell H, Gidlund M. Oxidized Low Density Lipoprotein induces differentiation and adhesion of human monocytes and the monocytic cell line U937. Proc Natl Acad Sci USA 1990;87:904–908.

53. Quinn MT, Parthasarathy S, Fong GL, Steinberg D: Oxidatively modified low density lipoprotein: a potential role in recruitment and retention of monocytes/macrophages during atherogenesis. Proc Natl Acad Sci USA 1987;84:2995–2998.

54. McMurray HF, Parthasarathy S, Steinberg D. Oxidatively modified low density lipoprotein is a chemoattractant for human T lymphocytes. J Clin Invest 1993;92(2):1004–8.

55. Berliner JA, Territo MC, Sevanian A, Ramin S, Kim JA, Bamshad B, Esterson M, Fogelman AM. Minimally modified low density lipoprotein stimulates monocyte endothelial interactions. J Clin Invest 1990;85:1260–1266.

56. Frostegård J, Haegerstrand A, Gidlund M, Nilsson J. Biologically modified low density lipoprotein increases the adhesive properties of vascular endothelial cells. Atherosclerosis 1991;90:119–126.

57. Chatterjee S. Role of oxidized human plasma low density lipoproteins in atherosclerosis: effects on smooth muscle cell proliferation. Mol Cell Biochem 1992;111:143–147.

58. Frostegård J, Wu R, Giscombe R, Holm G, Lefvert AK, Nilsson J. Induction of T cell activation by oxidized low density lipoprotein. Arteriosclerosis and Thrombosis 1992;12:461–467.

59. Jovinge S, Ares MP, Kallin B, Nilsson J. Human monocytes/macrophages release TNF-alpha in response to Ox-LDL. Arterioscler Thromb Vasc Biol 1996;16:1573–1579.

60. Frostegård J, Huang YH, Rönnelid J, Schäfer-Elinder L. PAF and oxidized LDL induce immune activation by a common mechanism. Arteriosclerosis, Thrombosis and Vasc Biol 1997;17:963–968.

61. Terkeltaub R, Banka BL, Solan J, Santoro D, Brand K, Curtiss LK. Oxidized LDL induces monocytic cell expression of interleukin-8, a chemokine with T-lymphocyte chemotactic activity. Arterioscler Thromb 1994;14:47–53.

62. Huang YH, Schäfer-Elinder L, Owman H, Lorentzen JC, Rönnelid J, Frostegård J. Induction of IL-4 by platelet activating factor. Clin Exp Immunol 1996;106:143–148.

63. Uyemura K, Demer LL, Castle SC, Jullien D, Berliner JA, Gately MK, Warrier RR, Pham N, Fogelman AM, Modlin RL. Cross-regulatory Roles of interleukin (IL)-12 and IL-10 in atherosclerosis. J Clin Invest 1996;97:2130–2138.

64. Zhu W, Roma P, Pellegatta F, Catapano AL. Oxidised-LDL induce the expression of heat shock protein 70 in human endothelial cells. Biochem Biophys Res Comm 1994;200:389–394.

65. Pockley AG, Bulmer J, Hanks BM, Wright BH. Identification of human heat shock protein 60 (Hsp60) and anti-Hsp60 antibodies in the peripheral circulation of normal individuals. Cell Stress & Chaperones 1999;4:29–35.

66. Kol A, Bourcier T, Lichtman A, Libby P. Chlamydial and human heat shock protein 60s activate human vascular endothelium, smooth muscle cells, and macro-

phages. J Clin Invest 1999;103:571–577.

67. Watson AD, Navab M, Hama SY, Sevanian A, Prescott, AM, Stafforini DM, McIntyre TM, La Du BN, Fogelman A, Berliner JA. Effect of platelet activating factoracetylhydrolase on the formation and action of minimally oxidized low density lipoprotein. J Clin Invest 1995;95:774–782.

68. Tokumura A. A family of phospholipid autacoids: occurrence, metabolism and bioactions. Prog Lipid Res 1995;34:151–184.

69. Huang YH, Schäfer-Elinder L, Wu R, Claesson HE, Frostegård J. Lysophosphatidylcholine induces proinflammatory cytokines by a PAF-receptor dependent mechanism. Clin Exp Immunol 1999;116:326–31.

70. Marathe GK, Davies SS, Harrison KA, Silva AR, Murphy RC, Castro-Faria-neto H, Prescott SM, Zimmermann GA, McIntyre TM. Inflammatory platelet-activating factor-like phospholipids in oxidized low density lipoproteins are fragmented alkyl phosphatidylcholines. J Biol Chem 1999;274:28395–404.

71. Caspar-Bauguil S, Tkaczuk J, Haure MJ, Durand M, Alcouffe J, Thomsen M, Salvayre R, Benoist H. Mildly oxidized low-density lipoproteins decrease early production of interleukin 2 and nuclear factor kB binding to DNA in acivated T-lymphocytes. Biochem J 1999;337:269–274.

72. Stemme S, Fager B, Holm J, Wiklund O, Witztum JL, Hansson GK. T lymphocytes from human atherosclerotic plaques recognize oxidized low density lipoprotein. Proc Natl Acad Sci USA 1995;92:3893–97.

73. Vaarala O, Alfthan G, Jauhiainen M, Leirisalo-Repo M, Aho K, Palosuo T. Crossreaction between antibodies to oxidised low-density lipoprotein and to cardiolipin in systemic lupus erythematosus. Lancet 1993;341:923–925.

74. McNeil HP, Simpson RJ, Chesterman CN, Krilis SA. Anti-phospholipid antibodies are directed against a complex antigen that includes a lipid-binding inhibitor of coagulation: beta 2-glycoprotein I (apolipoprotein H). Proc Natl Acad Sci 1990;87:4120–24.

75. Hörkkö S, Miller E, Branch DW, Palinski W, Witztum J. The epitopes for some antiphospholipid antibodies are adducts of oxidized phospholipid and ß2 glycoprotein 1 (and other proteins). Proc Natl Acad Sci 1997;94:10356–60.

76. Hörkkö S, Miller E, Dudl E, Reaven P, Curtiss LK, Zvaifler NJ, Terkeltaub R, Pierangeli SS, Branch W, Palinski W, Witztum J. Antiphospholipid antibodies are directed against epitopes of oxidized phospholipids. J Clin Inv 1996;98:815–825.

77. Beckman EM, Porcelli SA, Morita CT, Behar SM, Furlong ST, Brenner MB. Recognition of a lipid antigen by CD1 restricted AB+ T cells. Nature 1995;372:691–694.

78. Yokoyama M, Hirata K, Miyake R, Akita H, Ishikawa Y, Fukuzaki H. Lysophosphatidylcholine: essential role in the inhibition of endothelium-dependent vasorelaxation by oxidized low density lipoprotein. Biochem Biophys Res Commun 1990;168:301–308.

79. Ylä-Herttuala S, Palinski W, Butler S, Picard S, Steinberg D, Witztum J. Rabbit and human atherosclerotic lesions contain IgG that recognizes epitopes of oxidized low density lipoprotein. Arterioscl Thromb 1990;14:32–40.

80. Palinski W, Miller E, Witztum JL. Immunization of low density lipoprotein (LDL) receptor-deficient rabbits with homologous malondialdehyde modified LDL reduces atherogenesis. Proc Natl Acad Sci USA 1995;92:821–825.

81. Ameli S, Hultgårdh-Nilsson A, Regnström J, Calara F, Yano J, Cervek B, Shah PK, Nilsson J. Effect of immunization with homologous LDL and oxidized LDL on early atherosclerosis in hypercholesterolemic rabbits. Arterioscl Thromb Vasc Biol 1996;16:1074–9.

82. Wu R, de Faire U, Lemne C, Witztum J, Frostegård J. Serum antibodies to oxidized LDL are decreased in borderline hypertension. Hypertension 1999;33:53–59.

83. Wu R, Lemne C, de Faire U, Frostegård J. Antibodies to lysophosphatidylcholine – a novel factor in cardiovascular disease, negatively associated with borderline hypertension. Hypertension (in press).

84. Salonen JT, Yla-Herttuala S, Yamamoto R, Butler S, Korpela H, Salonen R, Nyssonen K, Palinski W, Witztum JL. Autoantibody against oxidized LDL and progression of carotid atherosclerosis. Lancet 1992;339:883–887.

85. Bergmark C, Wu R, de Faire U, Lefvert AK, Swedenborg J. Patients with early-onset peripheral vascular disease have increased levels of autoantibodies against oxidized LDL. Arterioscl Thromb and Vasc Biol 1995;15:441–445.

86. Maggi E, Chiesa R, Melissano G, Castellano R, Astore D, Grossi A, Finardi G, Bellomo G. LDL oxidation in patients with severe carotid atherosclerosis. A study of in vitro and in vivo oxidation markers. Arterioscl Thromb 14:1892–9.

87. Maggi E, Marchesi E, Ravetta V, Martignoni A, Finardi G, Bellomo G. Presence of autoantibodies against oxidatively modified low-density lipoprotein in essential hypertension: a biochemical signature of an enhanced in vivo low-density lipoprotein oxidation. J Hypertension 1995;13:129–38.

88. Thompson HS, Harper N, Bevan DJ, Staines NA. Suppression of collagen induced arthritis by oral administration of type II collagen: changes in immune and arthritic responses mediated by active peripheral suppression. Autoimmunity 1993;16:189–99.

89. Ginsburg KS., Liang MH, Newcomer L, Goldhaber SZ, Schur PH, Hennekens CH, Stampfer MJ. Anticardiolipin antibodies and the Risk for Ischemic Stroke and Venous Thrombosis. Ann Intern Med 1992;117:997–1002.

90. Vaarala O, Mänttäri M, Manninen V, Tenkanen L, Puurunen M, Aho K, Paluoso T. Anti-Cardiolipin Antibodies and Risk of Myocardial Infarction in a Prospecive Cohort of Middle-Aged Men. Circulation 1995;91:23–27.

91. Petri M, Perez-Gutthann S, Spence D, Hochberg MC. Risk Factors for coronary Artery Disease in Patients With Systemic Lupus Erythematosus. Am J Med 1992;93:513–519.

92. Drenkard C, Villa AR, Alarcón-Segovia D and Pérés-Vazquez ME. Influence of the Antiphospholipid Syndrome in the Survival of Patients with Systemic Lupus Erythematosus. J Rheumatol 1994;21:1067–1072.

93. Wu R, Lefvert AK. Autoantibodies against oxidized low density lipoprotein (oxLDL): characterization of antibody isotype, subclass, affinity and effect on the macrophage uptake of oxLDL. Clin Exp Immunol 1995;102:174–180.

94. Hörkkö S, Bird DA, Miller E, Itabe H, Leitinger N, Subbanagounder G, Berliner JA, Friedman P, Dennis EA, Curtiss LK, Palinski W, Witztum JL. Monoclonal autoantibodies specific for oxidized phospholipids or oxidized phospholipid-protein adducts inhibit macrophage uptake of oxidized low-density lipoproteins. J Clin Invest 1999;103:117–128.

95. Wu R, Svenungsson E, Gunnarsson I, Andersson B, Lundberg I, Schäfer-Elinder L, Frostegård J. Antibodies against lysophosphatidylcholine and oxidized LDL in patients with SLE. Lupus 1999;8:142–148.

96. Xu Q, Dietrich H, Steiner HJ, Gown AM, Schoel B, Mikuz G, Kaufmann SH, Wick G. Induction of arteriosclerosis in normocholesterolemic rabbits by immunisation with heat shock protein 65. Arteriosclerosis Thrombosis 1992;12:789–799.

97. George J, Arnon A, Gilburd B, Blank M, Levy Y, Aron-Maor A, Levkovitz H, Shaish A, Goldberg I, Kopolovic J, Harats D, Shoenfeld Y. Induction of early atherosclerosis in LDL-receptor Deficient mice mmunized with ß2-Glycoprotein I. Circulation 1998;98:1108–1115.

Atherosclerosis and Autoimmunity
Y. Shoenfeld, D. Harats and G. Wick, editors

Technical and Clinical Aspects about Autoantibody Assays for Oxidized Low Density Lipoprotein

Outi Närvänen, Jukka Luoma and Seppo Ylä-Herttuala

A.I.Virtanen Institute of Molecular Sciences, University of Kuopio, P.O.Box 1627, 70211 Kuopio, Finland

1. INTRODUCTION

Several studies have shown that oxidation of LDL plays an important role in the development of atherosclerosis [1]. A key finding is that macrophages do not take up native LDL (natLDL) but they rapidly take up oxidized LDL (oxLDL) which leads to formation of foam cells [2]. In addition, oxLDL is cytotoxic to various cell types [3] and chemotactic for blood monocytes [4]. The presence of oxLDL in vivo has been indicated in many studies [5]. It has been extracted from atherosclerotic lesions [6] but not from normal arteries [7], and epitopes of oxLDL have been detected in atherosclerotic lesions with immunological techniques [8–10]. Furthermore, antibodies against oxLDL have been demonstrated in atherosclerotic lesions of rabbits and humans [6,11], and in human serum [8,12].

2. LDL OXIDATION

LDL oxidation is a complex process which is not yet fully understood. Several mechanisms are present in atherosclerotic lesions which can lead to LDL oxidation in vivo, e.g. reactions with lipoxygenases, superoxide anion, hydroxyl radical, peroxynitrite, haem proteins, ceruloplasmin, myeloperoxidase and hypochlorite (reviewed in reference 5). OxLDL is not a homogenous particle but forms a complex structure. Apolipoprotein B-100 (apoB-100) is the major protein constituent in LDL. During oxidation of LDL both the protein and the lipid portion of the particle can be modified [13]. Malondialdehyde (MDA) and 4-hydroxynonenal (4-HNE) are the

main reactive aldehydes formed during LDL oxidation [14], which can further react with lysine residues of apoB-100. Thus, as a result of oxidation several new structures are formed on LDL and these oxidation-specific epitopes can be antigenic.

3. AUTOANTIBODIES AGAINST OXLDL IN CLINICAL STUDIES

To evaluate the relationship between LDL oxidation and the progression of atherosclerosis researchers have tried to measure the amount of oxLDL in circulation. It is, however, difficult because oxLDL is rapidly taken up by liver cells [15]. Some sensitive assays have been described [16,17] but most studies have focused on different indirect measurements to define the extent of LDL oxidation. Autoantibodies against oxLDL are found in human sera and measuring their levels is one way to evaluate the extent of LDL oxidation.

Autoantibodies against oxLDL react with oxidation specific epitopes, such as MDA-lysine and HNE-lysine and also with unknown epitopes present in copper-oxidized LDL [6,8,9,11,12]. Oxidized phospholipids can also form epitopes for autoantibodies [16,18]. Recent studies have shown that monoclonal IgM autoantibodies cloned from apoE-deficient mice recognize both the oxidized protein and the oxidized lipid moiety of oxLDL [18]. These antibodies were found to be structurally and functionally identical to natural T15 anti-phosphorylcholine antibodies [19]. In addition, it has been reported that healthy individuals produce antibodies against lysophosphatidylcholine, which is a major component of oxLDL [20].

Autoantibodies against oxLDL have been measured in many clinical studies (reviewed in reference 5) but the results are conflicting. Some follow-up studies have shown that increased titers of anti-oxLDL antibodies predict progression of carotid atherosclerosis [12] and myocardial infarction [22–23]. This finding is supported by the results of cross-sectional studies which show association between increased titers of anti-oxLDL antibodies and carotid atherosclerosis [21] or myocardial infarction [24]. Elevated levels of autoantibodies have also been associated to coronary artery disease [25,26], early peripheral atherosclerosis [27] and to a higher risk for coronary restenosis following percutaneous transluminal coronary angioplasty [28]. Other studies have not found any association between anti-oxLDL antibodies and carotid atherosclerosis [29,30], coronary heart disease [31,32] or restenosis [33]. Interestingly, Schumacher and coworkers found that patients with severe, acute myocardial infarction had transiently decreased levels of anti-oxLDL antibodies [34].

Most of the studies have evaluated the significance of autoantibodies in atherosclerosis-related diseases but also other relationships have been reported. Elevated titers of autoantibodies have been found in systemic lupus erythematosus (SLE) [35,36], pre-eclampsia [37] and chronic periaortitis [38]. It has been reported that hormone replacement therapy does not change anti-oxLDL antibody concentrations in healthy early postmenopausal women [39], but decreases the level of anti-oxLDL antibodies in postmenopausal women with coronary heart disease [40]. In addition, it has been found that cigarette smoking and hypercholesterolemia synergistically impair endothelial function and their combined presence is associated with increased levels of anti-oxLDL antibodies [41]. Furthermore, titers of anti-oxLDL antibodies were inversely associated with coronary flow reserve in normal subjects [42]. In another study it was found that oxLDL antibody titer and intima-media thickness of the carotid arteries correlated negatively in healthy population suggesting that immune response to oxLDL may have protective role at an early stage of atherosclerosis [43].

Results concerning anti-oxLDL antibodies in diabetes mellitus, which is a well-defined risk factor of atherosclerosis, are conflicting. It has been reported that the amount of anti-oxLDL antibodies is raised in patients suffering from either type 2 diabetes [44–46] or from type 1 diabetes [47] but in other studies no such association has been found [48,49]. However, Korpinen and coworkers showed that allthough patients with type 1 diabetes did not have higher antibody levels against oxLDL than healthy subjects, they had higher antibody levels against glycated LDL [49].

The above observations have raised the question whether anti-oxLDL antibodies are protective, proatherogenic or an epiphenomen. Some clinical studies have suggested that elevated levels of anti-oxLDL antibodies are a marker of advanced atherosclerosis [12,21–23] whereas other studies have found no such associations [29–33] or have reported decreased levels of anti-oxLDL antibodies in patients with myocardial infarction [30,34]. On the other hand, it has been shown that immunization of experimental animals with oxLDL reduces atherogenesis [50,51]. In addition, recent reports have demonstrated an inverse relationship between anti-oxLDL titer and carotid artery intima-media thickness [43] as well as between anti-oxLDL titer and plasma oxLDL concentration [52] in a healthy population, which suggests an antiatherogenic role of anti-oxLDL antibodies at an early stage of atherosclerosis. The significance of anti-oxLDL antibodies at different stages of atherosclerosis is not yet fully understood. Most of the clinical studies are cross-sectional, so there is a need for controlled follow-up studies utilizing standardized autoantibody assays.

4. AUTOANTIBODY ASSAYS

At present the amount of anti-oxLDL antibodies in humans has been measured using a variety of different EIA or RIA methods. Comparison of results between laboratories is difficult because no standard method exists. LDL used in the assays as antigen has been oxidized by incubation with copper ions [21,23–27,30,31,34,38,41,42,44] or by conjugation with MDA [12,22,32,35,44,49]. Interestingly, Salonen and coworkers showed that elevated levels of anti-oxLDL antibodies predicted progression of carotid atherosclerosis when MDA-modified LDL was used as antigen, but not with copper-oxidized

174

LDL [12], which may be due to the fact that oxLDL has fewer MDA-lysine residues per LDL particle than MDA-LDL. Thus, differences in antigen, even between different batches, may cause significant variation in results. The extent of LDL oxidation can be evaluated e. g. by measuring formation of thiobarbituric acid reactive substances (TBARS) [2], formation of conjugated dienes [53] or generation of fluorescent compounds during oxidation [54] before using oxLDL as antigen to ensure that the degree of oxidation is similar in different batches. Another way to evaluate antigen is to monitor apoB-100 breakdown products on Western blot with different antibodies [55].

In addition to antigen, test conditions also vary widely between laboratories. Incubation temperatures vary from +4°C [12,24,25,27,30–32,35] to room temperature [22] and 37°C [21,26,34] and sample dilutions from about 1:10 to 1:2500 [12,21,22,24,30,32,35,41]. Most commonly used blocking agents are bovine serum albumin (BSA) [12,26,31,34,41,42,48] and human serum albumin (HSA) [22,24,25,35] but fetal bovine serum [21], dry milk powder [30] and casein [32] have also been used. Furthermore, the expression of results varies between laboratories. Results are calculated as the antibody titer against oxLDL [23], the ratio of autoantibody binding to oxLDL and natLDL [12,21,24,25,32,35,41,48], the difference in absorbances between binding to oxLDL and natLDL [22,25,26,35,36], or the antibody titers are expressed as the ratio to a standard serum [30]. One study reported different results depending on the data expression and the blocking agent used [35]. Antibody concentrations expressed as the ratio or the difference between modified LDL and natLDL were higher in women with SLE than in controls, when HSA was used as the blocking agent. With two other blocking agents (BSA and Superblock) the antibodies were higher in SLE patients only when the results were presented as the difference. We have optimized our oxLDL ELISA and compared different ways to express the results [56]. We found that our results differed depending on the expression of results. Men with acute myocardial infarction (AMI) had higher anti-oxLDL titers when the results were expressed as a ratio between oxLDL and natLDL, as antibody titer against oxLDL or as difference between binding to oxLDL and natLDL, but not when the results were expressed as a ratio between antibody titer against oxLDL and a standard serum (oxLDL/stand) or as the oxLDL/natLDL ratio corrected with the standard serum (oxLDL/stand)/(natLDL/stand). On the contrary, in some other studies results have not differed when calculated in two different ways [27,30,32].

Recently, several groups have studied the specificity of autoantibodies against oxLDL. In SLE patients anti-oxLDL antibodies have correlated with titers against cardiolipin, which is an anionic phospholipid [36]. The correlation of these two antibodies was not confirmed in CHD patients [24]. It has been shown that antibodies against cardiolipin and oxLDL predict myocardial infarction in men [23] and that anti-cardiolipin antibodies were heterogenous in their binding to oxLDL indicating that these two antibodies may have different subspecificities [57]. Recent results suggest that anti-cardiolipin antibodies are directed against neoepitopes of oxidized phospholipids [58], which may be similar to the epitopes in oxLDL. However, oxLDL could also have epitopes which have formed after modification of the protein part of the particle and which are not common with cardiolipin. Furthermore, antibodies against lysophosphatidylcholine, a major component of oxLDL, have been detected in healthy individuals [20] and in patients with SLE [59].

5. CHARACTERIZATION OF AUTOANTIBODIES AGAINST OXIDIZED LDL AND STANDARDIZATION OF THE ASSAY

Anti-oxLDL antibodies have been analyzed by determining the antibody isotype and affinity. Antibodies, which were found both in patients with atherosclerosis and in controls, were mainly of IgG and IgM isotype and high affinities could be detected [11,60]. These results have been confirmed by another group, except that they determined affinities of purified antibodies to be from moderate-to-low [61]. In addition, they showed that the antibodies were primarily specific for oxLDL but had some cross-reactivity with MDA-LDL and natLDL, and two of the purified antibodies reacted also with cardiolipin. The results of Wu and coworkers [23] are interesting, because they found that antibodies, which predicted myocardial infarction in men, were of IgG and IgA isotype. In addition, one study reported that oxLDL antibodies contained immunoglobulins of the three major isotypes and were mainly of IgG isotype, subclasses 1 and 3 and these antibodies predominantly recognized MDA-derived epitopes [62].

Homogeneity of different batches of oxLDL used as ELISA antigen is of outmost importance. Koskinen and coworkers [63] have produced a reference human antibody standard for the assay of anti-oxLDL antibodies, which gives a more accurate calibration curve. Furthermore, they optimized a competitive immunoassay for oxLDL antibodies. Copper-oxidized LDL was used as antigen because it is very similar to the LDL found in atherosclerotic lesions [6]. In addition, they tested every sample unabsorbed and absorbed with oxLDL to assure the specificity of the results. It is clear that more precise and reproducible assays using standardized methods for the calculation of results are needed before the clinical significance of anti-oxLDL antibodies can be evaluated.

6. CONCLUSION

The role of anti-oxLDL autoantibodies in atherogenesis is not yet fully understood. The information provided by clinical studies has provided evidence that autoantibodies may be associated with the progression of atherosclerotic disease. However, further studies are needed to clarify whether autoantibodies are antiatherogenic, proatherogenic or just an unrelevant finding. There is a need for the development of standardized autoantibody assays to be used in well-controlled follow-up studies before the significance of anti-oxLDL autoantibodies as a risk factor for cardiovascular diseases can be fully evaluated.

7. ACKNOWLEDGEMENTS

This study was supported by grants from Kuopio University Hospital (EVO 5130) and by Quattrogene Ltd, Finland. Authors want to thank Ms Anne Martikainen and Ms Mervi Ovaskainen for skilful technical assistance.

REFERENCES

1. Steinberg D. Low density lipoprotein oxidation and its pathobiological significance. J Biol Chem 1997;272:20963–20966.
2. Steinbrecher UP, Parthasarathy S, Leake DS, Witztum JL, Steinberg D. Modification of low density lipoprotein by endothelial cells involves lipid peroxidation and degradation of low density lipoprotein phospholipids. Proc Natl Acad Sci USA 1984;81:3883–3887.
3. Chisolm GM. Cytotoxicity of oxidized lipoproteins. Curr Opin Lipidol 1991;2:311–316.
4. Quinn MT, Parthasarathy S, Fong LG, Steinberg D. Oxidatively modified low density lipoproteins: a potential role in recruitment and retention of monocyte/macrophages during atherogenesis. Proc Natl Acad Sci USA 1987;84:2995–2999.
5. Ylä-Herttuala S. Is oxidized low-density lipoprotein present in vivo? Curr Opin Lipidol 1998;9:337–344.
6. Ylä-Herttuala S, Palinski W, Rosenfeld ME, Parthasarathy S, Carew TE, Butler S, et al. Evidence for the presence of oxidatively modified low density lipoprotein in atherosclerotic lesions of rabbit and man. J Clin Invest 1989;84:1086–1095.
7. Ylä-Herttuala S, Jaakkola O, Ehnholm C, Tikkanen MJ, Solakivi T, Särkioja T, Nikkari T. Characterization of two lipoproteins containing apolipoproteins B and E from lesion-free human aortic intima. J Lipid Res 1988;29:563–572.
8. Palinski W, Rosenfeld ME, Ylä-Herttuala S, Gurtner GC, Socher SS, Butler SW, et al. Low density lipoprotein undergoes oxidative modification in vivo. Proc Natl Acad Sci USA 1989;86:1372–1376.
9. Haberland ME, Fong D, Cheng L. Malondialdehyde-altered protein occurs in atheroma of Watanabe heritable hyperlipidemic rabbits. Science 1988;24:215–218.
10. Rosenfeld ME, Palinski W, Ylä-Herttuala S, Butler S, Witztum JL. Distribution of oxidation specific lipid-protein adducts and apolipoprotein B in atherosclerotic lesions of varying severity from WHHL rabbits. Arteriosclerosis 1990;10:336–349.
11. Ylä-Herttuala S, Butler S, Picard S, Palinski W, Steinberg D, Witztum JL. Rabbit and human atherosclerotic lesions contain IgG that recognizes epitopes of oxidized LDL. Arterioscler Tromb 1994;14:32–40.
12. Salonen JT, Ylä-Herttuala S, Yamamoto R, Butler S, Korpela H, Salonen R, et al. Autoantibody against oxidised LDL and progression of carotid atherosclerosis. Lancet 1992;339:883–887.

13. Steinberg D, Parthasarathy S, Carew TE, Khoo JC, Witztum JL. Beyond cholesterol: Modification of low-density lipoprotein that increase its atherogenicity. N Engl J Med 1989;320: 915–924.

14. Esterbauer H, Gebicki J, Puhl H, Jürgens G. The role of lipid peroxidation and antioxidants in oxidative modification of LDL. Free Radical Biol Med 1992;13:341–390.

15. de Rijke YB, van Berkel TJC. Rat liver Kuppfer and endothelial cells express different binding proteins for modified low density lipoproteins. J Biol Chem 1994;14:824–827.

16. Palinski W, Hörkkö S, Miller E, Steinbrecher UP, Powell HC, Curtiss LK, et al. Cloning of monoclonal autoantibodies to epitopes of oxidized lipoproteins from apolipoprotein E-deficient mice. J Clin Invest 1996;98:800–814.

17. Holvoet P, Stassen J-M, Van Cleemput J, Collen D, Vanhaecke J. Oxidized low density lipoproteins in patients with transplant-associated coronary artery disease. Arterioscler Thromb Vasc Biol 1998;18:100–107.

18. Hörkkö S, Bird DA, Miller E, Itabe H, Leitinger N, Subbanagounder G, et al. Monoclonal autoantibodies specific for oxidized phospholipids or oxidized phospholipid-protein adducts inhibit macrophage uptake of oxidized low-density lipoproteins. J Clin Invest 1999;103:117–128.

19. Shaw PX, Hörkkö S, Chang M-K, Curtiss LK, Palinski W, Silverman GJ, et al. Natural antibodies with the T15 idiotype may act in atherosclerosis, apoptotic clearance, and protective immunity. J Clin Invest 2000;105:1731–1740.

20. Wu R, Huang YH, Elinder LS, Frostegård J. Lysophosphatidylcholine is involved in the antigenicity of oxidized LDL. Arterioscler Thromb Vasc Biol 1998;18:626–630.

21. Maggi E, Chiesa R, Melissano G, Castellano R, Astore D, Grossi A, et al. LDL oxidation in patients with severe carotid atherosclerosis. Arterioscler Thromb 1994;14:1892–1899.

22. Puurunen M, Mänttäri M, Manninen V, Tenkanen L, Alfthan G, Ehnholm C, et al. Antibody against oxidized low-density lipoprotein predicting myocardial infarction. Arch Intern Med 1994;154:2605–2609.

23. Wu R, Nityanand S, Berglund L, Lithell H, Holm G, Lefvert AK. Antibodies against cardiolipin and oxidatively modified LDL in 50-year-old men predict myocardial infarction. Arterioscler Thromb Vasc Biol 1997;17:3159–3163.

24. Erkkilä AT, Närvänen O, Lehto S, Uusitupa MIJ, Ylä-Herttuala S. Autoantibodies against oxidized low density lipoprotein and cardiolipin in patients with coronary heart disease. Arterioscler Thromb Vasc Biol

25. Lehtimäki T, Lehtinen S, Solakivi T, Nikkilä M, Jaakkola O, Jokela H, et al. Autoantibodies against oxidized low density lipoprotein in patients with angiographically verified coronary artery disease. Arterioscler Thromb Vasc Biol 1999;19:23–27.

26. Bui MN, Sack MN, Moutsatsos G, Lu DY, Katz P, McCown R, et al. Autoantibody titers to oxidized low-density lipoprotein in patients with coronary atherosclerosis. Am Heart J 1996;131:663–667.

27. Bergmark C, Wu R, de Faire U, Lefvert AK, Swedenborg J. Patients with early-onset peripheral vascular disease have increased levels of autoantibodies against oxidized LDL. Arterioscler Thromb Vasc Biol 1995;15:441–445.

28. George J, Harats D, Bakshi E, Adler Y, Levy Y, Gilburd B, et al. Anti-oxidized low density lipoprotein antibody determination as a predictor of restenosis following percutaneous transluminal coronary angioplasty. Immunol Lett 1999;68:263–266.

29. Iribarren C, Folsom AR, Jacobs DR Jr, Gross MD, Belcher JD, Eckfeldt JH. Association of serum vitamin levels, LDL, susceptibility to oxidation, and autoantibodies against MDA-LDL with carotid atherosclerosis. Arterioscler Thromb Vasc Biol 1997;17:1171–1177.

30. Hulthe J, Wikstrand J, Lidell A, Wendelhag I, Hansson GK, Wiklund O. Antibody titers against oxidized LDL are not elevated in patients with familial hypercholesterolemia. Arterioscler Thromb Vasc Biol 1998;18:1203–1211.

31. Virella G, Virella I, Leman RB, Pryor MB, Lopes-Virella MF. Anti-oxidized low-density lipoprotein antibodies in patients with coronary heart disease and normal healthy volunteers. Int J Clin Lab Res 1993;23:95–101.

32. van de Vijver LPL, Steyger R, van Poppel G, Boer JMA, Kruijssen DACM, Seidell JC, et al. Autoantibodies against MDA-LDL in subjects with severe and minor atherosclerosis and healthy population controls. Atherosclerosis 1996;122:245–253.

33. Eber B, Schumacher M, Tatzber F, Kaufmann P, Luha O, Esterbauer H, et al. Autoantibodies to oxidized low density lipoproteins in restenosis following coronary angioplasty. Cardiology 1994;84:310–315.

34. Schumacher M, Eber B, Tatzber F, Kaufmann P, Halwachs G, Fruhwald FM, et al. Transient reduction of autoantibodies against oxidized LDL in patients with acute myocardial infarction. Free Rad Biol Med 1995;18:1087–1091.

35. Craig WY, Poulin SE, Nelson CP, Ritchie RF. ELISA of IgG antibody to oxidized low-density lipoprotein: Effects of blocking buffer and method of data expression. Clin Chem 1994;40:882–888.

36. Vaarala O, Alfthan G, Jauhiainen M, Leirisalo-Repo

M, Aho K, Palosuo T. Crossreaction between antibodies to oxidized low-density lipoprotein and to cardiolipin in systemic lupus erythematosus. Lancet 1993;341:923–925.

37. Branch DW, Mitchell MD, Miller E, Palinski W, Witztum JL. Pre-eclampsia and serum antibodies to oxidized low-density lipoprotein. Lancet 1994;343:645–646.

38. Parums DV, Brown DL, Mitchinson MJ. Serum antibodies to oxidized low-density lipoprotein and ceroid in chronic periaortitis. Arch Pathol Lab Med 1990;114:383–387.

39. Heikkinen A-M, Niskanen L, Ylä-Herttuala S, Luoma J, Tuppurainen MT, Komulainen M, et al. Postmenopausal hormone replacement therapy and autoantibodies against oxidized LDL. Maturitas 1998;29:155–161.

40. Hoogerbrugge N, Zillikens MC, Jansen H, Meeter K, Deckers JW, Birkenhäger JC. Estrogen replacement decreases the level of antibodies against oxidized low-density lipoprotein in postmenopausal women with coronary heart disease. Metabolism 1998;47:675–680.

41. Heitzer T, Ylä-Herttuala S, Luoma J, Kurz S, Münzel T, Olschewski M, & al. Cigarette smoking potentiates endothelial dysfunction of forearm resistance vessels in patients with hypercholesterolemia: role of oxidized LDL. Circulation 1996;93:1346–1353.

42. Raitakari OT, Pitkänen O-P, Lehtimäki T, Lahdenperä S, Iida H, Ylä-Herttuala S, et al. In vivo low density lipoprotein oxidation relates to coronary reactivity in young men. J Am Coll Cardiol 1997;30:97–102.

43. Fukumoto M, Shoji T, Emoto M, Kawagishi T, Okuno Y, Nishizawa Y. Antibodies against oxidized LDL and carotid artery intima-media thickness in a healthy population. Arterioscler Thromb Vasc Biol 2000;20:703–707.

44. Bellomo G, Maggi E, Poli M, Agosta FG, Bollati P, Finardi G. Autoantibodies against oxidatively modified low-density lipoproteins in NIDDM. Diabetes 1995;44:60–66.

45. Griffin ME, McInerney D, Fraser A, Johnson AH, Collins PB, Owens D et al. Autoantibodies to oxidized low density lipoprotein: the relationship to low density lipoprotein fatty acid composition in diabetes. Diabet Med 1997;14:741–747.

46. Leinonen JS, Rantalaiho V, Laippala P, Wirta O, Pasternack A, Alho H, et al. The level of autoantibodies against oxidized LDL is not associated with the presence of coronary heart disease or diabetic kidney disease in patients with non-insulin-dependent diabetes mellitus. Free Rad Res 1998;29:137–141.

47. Mäkimattila S, Luoma JS, Ylä-Herttuala S, Bergholm R, Utriainen T, Virkamäki A, et al. Autoantibodies against oxidized LDL and endothelium-dependent vasodilation in insulin-dependent diabetes mellitus. Atherosclerosis 1999;147:115–122.

48. Uusitupa M, Niskanen L, Luoma J, Mercuri M, Rauramaa R, Vilja P, et al. Autoantibodies against oxidized LDL do not predict atherosclerotic vascular disease in non-insulin-dependent diabetes mellitus. Arterioscler Thromb Vasc Biol 1996;16:1236–1242.

49. Korpinen E, Groop P-H, Åkerblom HK, Vaarala O. Immune response to glycated and oxidized LDL in IDDM patients with and without renal disease. Diabetes Care 1997;20:1168–1171.

50. Palinski W, Miller E, Witztum JL. Immunization of low density lipoprotein (LDL) receptor-deficient rabbits with homologous malondialdehyde-modified LDL reduces atherogenesis. Proc Natl Acad Sci USA 1995;92:821–825.

51. Ameli S, Hultgårdh-Nilsson A, Regnström J, Calara F, Yano J, Cercek B, et al. Effect of immunization with homologous LDL and oxidized LDL on early atherosclerosis in hypercholesterolemic rabbits. Arterioscler Thromb Vasc Biol 1996;16:1074–1079.

52. Shoji T, Nishizawa Y, Fukumoto M, Shimamura K, Kimura J, Kanda H, et al. Inverse relationship between circulating oxidized low density lipoprotein (oxLDL) and anti-oxLDL antibody levels in healthy subjects. Atherosclerosis 2000;148:171–177.

53. Esterbauer H, Striegl G, Puhl H, Rotheneder M. Continuous monitoring of in vitro oxidation of human LDL. Free Radic Res Commun 1989;6:67–75.

54. Cominacini L, Garbin U, Davoli A, Micciolo R, Bosello O, Gaviraghi G, et al. A simple test for predisposition to LDL oxidation based on the fluorescence development during copper-catalyzed oxidative modification. J Lipid Res 1991;32:349–358.

55. Viita H, Närvänen O, Ylä-Herttuala S. Different apolipoprotein B breakdown patterns in models of oxidized low density lipoprotein. Life Sci 1999;65:783–793.

56. Närvänen O, Erkkilä A, Ylä-Herttuala S. Evaluation and characterization of ELISA measuring autoantibodies against oxidized low density lipoprotein. Atherosclerosis 2000;151:200.

57. Vaarala O, Puurunen M, Lukka M, Alfthan G, Leirisalo-Repo M, Aho K. Affinity-purified cardiolipin-binding antibodies show heterogeneity in their binding to oxidized low-density lipoprotein. Clin Exp Immunol 1996;104:269–274.

58. Hörkkö S, Miller E, Dudl E, Reaven P, Curtiss LK, Zvaifler NJ, et al. Antiphospholipid antibodies are directed against epitopes of oxidized phospholipids: recognition of cardiolipin by monoclonal antibodies to epitopes of oxidized low density lipoprotein. J Clin Invest 1996;98:815–825.

59. Wu R, Svenungsson E, Gunnarsson I, Andersson B, Lundberg I, Schafer Elinder L, et al. Antibodies against

lysophosphatidylcholine and oxidized LDL in patients with SLE. Lupus 1999;8:142–150.

60. Wu R, Lefvert AK. Autoantibodies against oxidized low density lipoproteins (oxLDL): characterization of antibody isotype, subclass, affinity and effect on the macrophage uptake of oxLDL. Clin Exp Immunol 1995;102:174–180.

61. Mironova M, Virella G, Lopes-Virella MF. Isolation and characterization of human antioxidized LDL autoantibodies. Arterioscler Thromb Vasc Biol 1996;16:222–229.

62. Virella G, Koskinen S, Krings G, Onorato JM, Thorpe SR, Lopes-Virella M. Immunochemical characterization of purified human oxidized low-density lipoprotein antibodies. Clin Immunol 2000;95:135–144.

63. Koskinen S, Enockson C, Lopes-Virella MF, Virella G. Preparation of a human standard for determination of the levels of antibodies to oxidatively modified low-density lipoproteins. Clin Diag Lab Immunol 1998;5:817–822.

179

Atherosclerosis and Autoimmunity
Y. Shoenfeld, D. Harats and G. Wick, editors

Is There a Role for Paraoxonase in Atherosclerosis and in Antiphospholipid Syndrome?

M. Lambert[1], P.-Y. Hatron[1], U. Michon-Pasturel[1], E. Hachulla[1], B. Devulder[1], J.-C. Fruchart[2] and P. Duriez[2]

[1]*Internal Medicine Department, University Hospital of Lille, France;* [2]*Research Laboratory on Lipids and Atherosclerosis, Inserm U 325, Pasteur Institute of Lille and University of Lille 2, Lille, France*

1. INTRODUCTION

Initial interest in paraoxonase (PON) was in the field of toxicology because its esterase activity in involved in the detoxification of organophosphate insecticides such as parathion and chlorpyrifos [1].

Recent findings have suggested that paraoxonase might be involved in vascular biology, and in lipid metabolism. Paraoxonase activity might reduce LDL oxidation which constitutes the initial step in atherogenesis.

2. HUMAN SERUM PARAOXONASE: STRUCTURE, SYNTHESIS, FUNCTIONS

Pesticides as organophosphorus, mainly parathion, are applied in agriculture. They are activated in vivo by cytochrome-P450-dependent, microsomal mono-oxygenases leading to the highly toxic oxygen analogue (oxon) by a process known as oxidative desulphuration.

In mammals, serum paraoxonase hydrolysed in the blood any oxon which escapes hepatic detoxification. Insects, birds, reptiles and fishes generally lack paraoxonase and this explain their susceptibility as target organisms for organophosphorus [2].

The human metabolism of organophosphorus is complexe but the molecular polymorphism of paraoxonase is probably a major determinant of the variable toxicity of organophosphorus among different persons and different populations.

Serum paraoxonase gene is located at q21-q22 on the long arm of chromosome 7. The cDNA for human paraoxonase predicts a 355 amino acid protein. There is a high degree of conservation between rabbit and human cDNA clones suggesting an important metabolic role for the enzyme and a large constraint on its evolution.

Serum paraoxonase is synthesized by liver but is also present in human lung, brain, pancreas and placenta.

Paraoxonase is associated with the HDL particles. This association was firstly described by electrophoresis of human precipitated HDL [3]. Paraoxonase is tightly associated with a specific HDL subspecies containing both apolipoprotein A-I and clusterin.

Serum paraoxonase is important in metabolizing different xenobiotics. Animal studies indicated an increase in HDL-paraoxonase activity after injection with bacterial endotoxin indicating the possibility that paraoxonase could hydrolyse the lipopolysaccharide that constitutes the endotoxin.

3. GENETICS OF HUMAN PARAOXONASE

European population displays a triphasic distribution of serum paraoxonase activity towards paraoxon, but not to some others substrates such as phenyl acetate. It is important to bear in mind that high-activity paraoxonase allozyme doesn't suggest a high hydrolyzing rate and so a high protective rate against lipid peroxidation. This triphasic distribution is evocative of a mendelian trait. But african and oriental paraoxonase activity distribution is unimodal, with a decrease in the frequency of the low-activity genotype.

Paraoxonase phenotyping depends on the differential response of the two isoenzymes to salt and pH. The hydrolysis of paraoxon by the high-activity isoenzyme is stimulated by 1 M NaCl, whereas the low-acivity isoenzyme is not. The ratio of salt-stimulated paraoxon hydrolysis to the hydrolysis of phenylacetate is therefore commonly used to assign a phenotype.

The molecular basis of the paraoxonase polymorphism has been shown to be an amino-acid substitution at position 192. The Q (low-activity) isoenzyme has Glutamine at position 192 while the R (high-activity) isoenzyme has Arginine at this position [4].

There is a second polymorphism on position 310 determining the second gene of paraoxonase (PON2) with a cysteine to serine substitution, which doesn't affect the ability of HDL to hydrolyse peroxides [5]. There is also a third gene, which doesn't affect lipid peroxidation.

4. PARAOXONASE AND LIPID METABOLISM

HDL can decrease lipid peroxide accumulation on LDL incubated under oxidizing conditions by an enzymatic mechanism. Studies indicated that paraoxonase was one of the components of HDL responsible for this activity [6]. HDL might inhibit atherosclerosis development through the so called "reverse cholesterol transport" but also by reducing LDL oxidation, which is responsible of foam cells formation and fatty streaks, the early signs of atherogenesis.

5. PARAOXONASE IN MICE

Those hypothesis have been confirmed in mice. Shih et al. [7] have produced paraoxonase knockout mice by targeted disruption of exon 1 affecting the PON1 gene. Homozygous mutant have no PON1 protein in plasma samples and no detectable enzymatic activity. HDLs isolated from those mice were unable to prevent LDL oxidation in a co-cultured cell model

of the artery wall. When fed on a high-fat, high cholesterol diet, PON1-null mice were more susceptible to atherosclerosis than their wild-type littermates [7].

6. PARAOXONASE IN HUMAN

In 1991, Mackness et al. have shown, in vitro, that human HDLs prevent the lipoperoxide formation in LDL. They demonstrated that purified paraoxonase from HDL had a similar effect and might be the HDL protective component [6].

Clinical studies were there performed to evaluate a putative relationship between paraoxonase and coronary artery disease. Some studies demonstrated that serum PON1 activity and concentration were significantly lower in patients with myocardial infarction [8].

The PON1–192 R polymorphism was positively associated with coronary heart disease in several case-controls studies [9, 10]. Nevertheless, Huibi Cao et al. showed that LDL protection against peroxidation is independent of paraoxonase esterase activity towards paraoxon and is unaffected by the Q-> R genetic polymorphism [11].

We have shown that the paraoxonase polymorphism might play a role in the regulation of coronary vasomotor tone in case of intra-coronary administration of serotonin [12].

7. PARAOXONASE AND ANTICARDIOLIPIN ANTIBODIES

It is largely demonstrated that anticardiolipin antibodies (aCL) are associated with antibodies against modified LDL, which are in vivo markers of LDL oxidation and of atherosclerosis [13]. aCL might be symptomatic of endothelial agression secondary to an oxidative stress.

We have confirmed that autoantibodies (IgG) directed against modified LDL were increased in patients positive for anticardiolipin antibodies. In a representative subgroup of these patients PON1 activity was dramatically decreased and the prevalence of the proatherogenic RR genotype of this enzyme was increased in patients who have developed arterial thrombosis. This study suggests that

PON1 abnormalities might play a role in the antiphospholipid syndrome and might constitute and aggravate pure arterial thrombosis in patients with antiphospholipid syndrome [14].

8. CONCLUSION

Paraoxonase polymorphism is involved in progression of atherosclerosis plaque, particularly in patients with the RR genotype. Moreover, a recent study suggest that anticardiolipin antibodies might be associated to the proatherogenic polymorphism of paraoxonase in patients presenting pure arterial thrombosis. A reduction in paraoxonase activity constitutes a decrease in anti-oxidative defense and might be associated with an increase in phospholipid oxidation of endothelial cell membrane. This phospholipid oxidation might resulted in antiphospholipid autoantibodies production. So, this genetical abnormality could explain one part of the clinical presentation of patients presenting antiphospholipid syndrome.

REFERENCES

1. Murphy SD in Toxicology: The basic Science of Poisons. Eds Doull J, Klassen C, Amdur M. New York: MacMillan 1980:357–408.
2. Brealey CJ, Walker CH, Baldwin BC. A-esterase activities in relation to the differential toxicity of pirimiphos-methyl to birds and mammals. Pesti Sci 1980;11:546–54.
3. Mackness MI, Hallam SD, Peard T, Warner S, Walker CH. The separation of sheep and human serum A-esterase activity into the lipoprotein fraction by ultracentrifugation. Comp Biochem Physiol 1985;83B:675–7.
4. Humbert R, Adler DA, Distecke CM, Hassett C, Omiecinski CJ, Furlong CE. The molecular basis of the human serum paraoxonase activity polymorphism. Nature Genet 1993;3:73–6.
5. Mackness B, Durrington PN, Mackness MI. Polymorphism of paraoxonase genes and low-density lipoprotein lipid peroxidation. Lancet 1999;353:468–9.
6. Mackness MI, Arrol S, Durrington PN. Paraoxonase prevents accumulation of lipoperoxides in low-density lipoprotein. FEBS 1991;286:152–4.
7. Shih DM, Gu L, Xia Y-R, Navab M, Li WF, Hama S et al. Mice lacking serum paraoxonase are susceptible to organophosphate toxicity and atherosclerosis. Nature 1998;394:284–7.
8. Ayub A, Mackness MI, Arrol S, Mackness B, Patel J, Durrington PN. Serum paraoxonase after myocardial infarction. Arterioscler Thromb Vasc Biol 1999;19:330–5.
9. Ruiz J, Blanché H, James RW, Blatter Garin MC, Vaisse C, Charpentier G et al. Gln-Arg 192 polymorphism of paraoxonase and coronary heart disease in type 2 diabetes. Lancet 1995;346:869–72.
10. Serrato M, Marian AJ. A variant of human paraoxonase / arylesterase (HUMPONA) gene is a risk factor for coronary artery disease. J Clin Invest 1995;96:3005–8.
11. Cao H, Girard-Globa A, Berthezene F, Moulin P. Paraoxonase protection of LDL against peroxidation is independent of its esterase activity towards paraoxon and is unaffected by the Q-> R genetic polymorphism. J Lipid Res 1999;40:133–9.
12. Bauters C, Amant C, Boulier A et al. Paraoxonase polymorphism (Gln192Arg) as a determinant of the response of human coronary arteries to serotonin. Circulation 2000;101:740–3.
13. Amengual O, Atsumi T, Khamashta MA, Tinahones F, Hughes GR. Autoantibodies against oxidized low-density lipoprotein in antiphospholipid syndrome. Br J Rheumatol 1997;36(9):964–8.
14. Lambert M, Boullier A, Hachulla E et al. Paraoxonase activity is dramatically decreased in patients positive for anticardiolipin antibodies. Lupus 2000;9(4):299–300.

Atherosclerosis and Autoimmunity
Y. Shoenfeld, D. Harats and G. Wick, editors

Anti-Prothrombin Antibodies in Thrombosis and Atherosclerosis

Yaniv Sherer[1], Miri Blank[1], O. Vaarala[2], Aviv Shaish[3], Yehuda Shoenfeld[1] and Dror Harats[3]

[1]*Department of Medicine B & Research Unit of Autoimmune Diseases, Sheba Medical Center, Tel-Hashomer, and Sackler Faculty of Medicine, Tel-Aviv University, Israel;* [2]*Department of Immunobiology, National Public Health Institute, Helsinki, Finland;* [3]*Institute of Lipid and Atherosclerosis Research, Sheba Medical Center, Tel-Hashomer, and Sackler Faculty of Medicine, Tel-Aviv University, Israel*

1. INTRODUCTION

Human factor II, or prothrombin, is a plasma zymogen that assembles with the activated forms of factor V, factor X and phospholipids to form the pro-thrombinase complex, which, in the presence of calcium ions, cleaves prothrombin into thrombin [1]. The antiphospholipid syndrome (APS) is composed of both clinical and laboratory criteria. In order to diagnose APS a patient should have at least one clinical manifestation (vascular thrombosis, pregnancy morbidity) and one typical serologic finding (medium to high titers of anti-cardiolipin antibodies (aCL) or positive lupus anti-coagulant (LAC) test on 2 or more occasions at least 6 weeks apart) [2]. However, it has been reported that antibodies that cause LAC activity require the presence of plasma proteins. Hence, it was found that anti-prothrombin antibodies (aPT) are often present in plasmas of patients with APS. Not all aPT detected by ELISA have LAC activity, and hence LAC assay would reveal only antibodies that inhibit coagulation. Therefore, as found by Rao et al. [3], aPT comprise a heterogeneous group of antibodies as IgG from LAC-positive samples recognize more than one epitope on prothrombin.

2. ANTI-PROTHROMBIN ANTIBODIES AND THROMBOSIS

Several reports support the association of aPT and thrombotic events in patients with and without APS

Table 1. Association of anti-prothrombin antibodies and thrombosis [6–10]

- APT levels were significantly higher in patients who experienced myocardial infarction/cardiac death than controls
- APT was related to increased risk of deep venous thrombosis of the lower extremity or pulmonary embolism
- APT was more prevalent in patients with Sneddon's syndrome
- APT was associated with thrombosis in patients with systemic autoimmune diseases
- Thrombotic events were more prevalent in APS and SLE patients positive to aPT

(Table 1). Horbach et al. [4] found that the presence of aPT correlates with a history of venous thrombosis, but not with arterial thrombosis. In a small study, the association between aPT and LAC was examined. It has been demonstrated that antibodies to prothrombin or to a complex of prothrombin and phosphatidylserine were found only in patients with LAC, whereas in the absence of LAC (even when aCL were present) these antibodies were absent [5].

IgG aPT and anti-β2GPI antibodies were measured at entry to a 5-year coronary prevention trial, and compared between 106 patients who experienced non-fatal myocardial infarction or cardiac death and 106 subjects without coronary episodes during the follow-up [6]. aPT levels were significantly higher in patients than in controls. Furthermore, level of aPT in the highest third of distribution, predicted a 2.5-fold increase in the risk of cardiac events. However, the distribution of β2GPI antibodies did not differ significantly between cases and controls [6]. In a similar study, the levels of anti-β2GPI, aPT, aCL and anti-oxidized LDL antibodies were compared between middle-aged men participating in a cancer prevention trial who had a follow-up of about 7 years. In a comparison of 265 individuals who had deep venous thrombosis of the lower extremity or pulmonary embolism and 265 controls, the risk of thrombosis was significantly increased only in relation to aPT, whereas no relation could be demonstrated to the other antibodies [7].

The presence of aPT was also evaluated in Sneddon's syndrome (cerebral ischemia associated with livedo reticularis), which is considered a form of APS. It has been found that aPT were elevated in 26 of 46 (57%) patients and in none of the controls [8]. This finding also increased the proportion of Sneddon's syndrome patients with at least one marker of APS from 65% to 78%. In another study, the presence and levels of IgG aPT, anti-β2GPI, aCL, and anti-annexin V antibodies were evaluated in patients with systemic autoimmune diseases [9]. Among patients, those with APS had higher frequency of aPT and anti-annexin V antibodies than patients with other autoimmune diseases. Moreover, both antibodies were significantly associated with thrombotic events [9]. In a series of 177 patients with autoimmune diseases, aPT was found in 47% of all patients, in 57% of patients with primary APS, and in 40% of SLE patients compared with only 5% in the controls [10]. Thrombotic events were more prevalent in patients positive to aPT, and the presence of aPT was found to be an independent risk factor for arterial thrombosis. However, whereas aPT were associated with both arterial and venous thrombosis in SLE patients, no such association was found in patients with primary APS [10]. Nevertheless, in APS patients aPT were associated with thrombocytopenia.

As opposed to these studies, fewer papers emphasize lack of association between aPT and thrombosis. The presence of aPT and anti-β2GPI antibodies were evaluated in patients with LAC and/or aCL. Both antibodies were more prevalent in APS and SLE patients, than in the miscellaneous group [11]. Even though aPT were related to venous thrombosis, multivariate analysis showed that only anti-β2GPI were independent risk factor for venous thrombosis. Similarly, the presence of several antibodies was evaluated in patients with SLE, lupus-like disease and healthy volunteers. Whereas aCL, anti-β2GPI and LAC had some sensitivity and specificity for thrombosis, there was no significant association between aPT and thrombosis [12].

In summary, most studies suggest that aPT might be associated with venous thrombosis, whereas the correlation with arterial thrombosis is still questionable.

3. MECHANISMS OF ACTION OF ANTI-PROTHROMBIN ANTIBODIES

When discussing mechanisms of action of aPT in APS or in thrombosis, it should be noted that as aPT represent a heterogeneous group of antibodies, different mechanisms are possible in different cases. For example, apart from thrombosis the presence of aPT might lead to hypoprothrombinemia and bleeding. That was the case in a patient with LAC who had aPT which formed an immune complex with prothrombin, rather than neutralized it [13]. Hypoprothrombinemia and consequently bleeding occurred due to rapid clearance of the prothrombin-antibody complex. Alternatively, in another case neutralization of prothrombin has been suggested as the mechanism of hypoprothrombinemia [14]. The antibody reacted with the fragment 2-A region of prothrombin, and the authors suggested that the neutralizing action of the antibody is impairment of prothrombin activation by prothrombinase complex, either by steric hindrance of the hydrolysis of prothrombin by factor Xa or by interference of the interaction of prothrombin with factor Va [14].

Regarding aPT-associated thrombosis, monoclonal aPT was isolated from a patient with APS, and it reacted with 3 phospholipids and showed LAC activity [15]. Since this aPT enhanced the binding of prothrombin to damaged endothelial cells, and shortened the endothelial cell-based plasma coagulation time, it has been suggested that aPT may promote coagulation in areas of damaged endothelial cells and hence be pro-thrombogenic in the host [15]. Field et al. [16] have demonstrated that enhanced binding of prothrombin to phospholipids in the presence of aPT/LAC increased thrombin production. Therefore, aPT/LAC might propagate coagulation by facilitating prothrombin interaction with damaged blood vessel wall.

It has been shown that aPT inhibited both the prothrombinase complex in a prothrombin- and phospholipid-dependent way, and the tenase complex and the inactivation of factor Va by activated protein C. Therefore, aPT increase the affinity of prothrombin to negatively charged phospholipids to such an extent that the aPT-prothrombin complex compete with the binding of other coagulation factors for the available negatively charged phospholipids. This results in prolongation of the clotting times in coagulation assays that are dependent on phospholipid concentrations in the system [17]. With respect to the pro-thrombogenic effects of aPT, it should be noted that the generated thrombin has also anti-thrombotic properties, for example the activation of the protein C pathway. Therefore, possible inhibition of thrombin generation by aPT could lead also to decreased activation of protein C and consequently decreased anti-coagulation. In addition, Puurunen et al. [18] showed that aPT cross-react with plasminogen. Hence, it is possible that aPT which cross-react with plasminogen create a risk factor for thrombosis also by interference with the fibrinolytic system.

4. ANTI-PROTHROMBIN ANTIBODIES AND ATHEROSCLEROSIS

Atherosclerosis is a histologic process in which the immune system has a major role. The presence of advanced atherosclerosis in patients with some autoimmune diseases (e.g. SLE) and the evidence of association between aCL, β2GPI and other autoantibodies with atherosclerosis [19–21] prompted us to test whether atherosclerosis is also associated with aPT. As to the best of our knowledge there is currently no data regarding this association in the literature, we used an animal model of atherosclerosis to test whether aPT are associated with one of the underlying causes of thrombosis, namely atherosclerosis.

5. METHODS

Mice and diets: LDL-receptor deficient mice were bred in the local animal house of the Institute of Lipid and Atherosclerosis Research (Sheba Medical Center, Tel-Hashomer, Israel). The mice were on 12-h dark/light cycles and were allowed access to food and water ad libitum. The study lasted 8 weeks in which the mice were fed a high-cholesterol Western-type diet containing 0.15-% cholesterol, 21% anhydrous milk fat, and 19.5% casein. The study group (10 mice) was injected once intra-dermal with prothrombin at a dose of 10μg while the control group (10 mice) was injected with PBS. Body weights were measured at the beginning of the study, and at 4 and 8 weeks. aPT levels were measured using ELISA at both groups at the end of the study.

Determination of lipid profile: At the beginning and at the end of the study blood was collected from the retroorbital plexus after 12 hrs of fasting. One mg of EDTA per ml blood was added to each sample. Total plasma cholesterol and triglycerides levels were determined by using an automated enzymatic technique (Boehringer Mannheim, Germany).

Assessment of the extent of atherosclerosis at the aortic sinus: Quantification of atherosclerotic fatty streak lesions was carried out by calculating the lesion size in the aortic sinus. Briefly, the heart and upper section of the aorta were removed from the animals and the peripheral fat cleaned carefully. The upper section was embedded in OCT medium and frozen. Every other section (5 μm thick) throughout the aortic sinus (400 μm) was taken for analysis. The distal portion of the aortic sinus is recognized by the 3 valve cusps, which are the junctions of the aorta to the heart. Sections were evaluated for fatty streak lesions after staining with oil red O. Lesion areas per sections were counted using a grid by an observer unfamiliar with the tested specimen.

Statistical analysis: Statistical analysis was carried out using the Students' t-test. P < 0.05 was accepted as statistical significant.

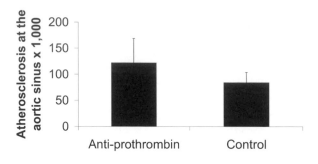

Figure 1. Mean levels of atherosclerosis (μm²) at the aortic sinus in the control and the aPT groups.

6. RESULTS

Both groups had similar weights when the study began, but at 4 weeks the control group weighted more than the aPT group (26.1±2.3 versus 23.6±1.7, P=0.03). Nevertheless, at the end of the study these weight gaps disappeared.

Regarding plasma lipid levels, there was no difference between the groups when the study began, but at the end of the study the aPT group had significantly lower levels of triglycerides and cholesterol than the control group (94±40 versus 187±66 and 783±355 versus 1363±582 mg/dl; P=0.005 and 0.04, respectively). The mean level of atherosclerosis extent in the aortic sinus was higher in the aPT group than in the controls (122,000±47,000 versus 84,000±20,000 μm²; Fig. 1), but the difference was not statistically significant. However, this non-significant more advanced atherosclerosis in the aPT group was in the presence of significantly decreased cholesterol levels compared with the control group.

The group that was injected with prothrombin developed elevated levels of aPT compared with practically no antibodies to prothrombin in the control group (1398±94 versus 0.07±0.03 IU/ml; P=0.001). There was no significant correlation between aPT levels and the extent of atherosclerosis in the aPT or control groups. However, in the aPT group higher cholesterol levels were significantly associated with smaller extent of atherosclerosis in the aortic sinus (Pearson correlation –0.84; P=0.02; Fig. 2). No such association was found in the control group.

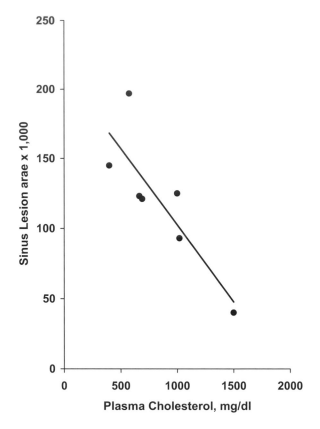

Figure 2. Inverse correlation between cholesterol levels and the extent of atherosclerosis in the aortic sinus (Pearson correlation –0.84; P=0.02) in the aPT group.

7. INTERPRETATION AND CONCLUSIONS

Literature reports on the association between aPT and thrombotic events suggest that these antibodies might be associated with thrombotic events in APS patients as well as in population at risk for thrombosis. Nonetheless, this association should be better clarified. As aCL and β2GPI are also markers of APS and were found to be associated with atherosclerosis, and as the aortic intima contains prothrombin and its related antigens [22], it was of an interest to test whether aPT are also related to atherosclerosis. Furthermore, the demonstration of thrombosis in mice is complicated [23]. In the presented animal model we demonstrate a trend of enhanced atherosclerosis caused by aPT injection. It seems that aPT was somehow toxic to the mice as it resulted in less weight gain and lower levels of triglycerides and cholesterol, the latter might have a beneficial effect on lipid profile. Nevertheless, in these conditions there was more atherosclerosis in the aPT group. Taking it together with the fact that higher cholesterol levels were significantly associated with smaller extent of atherosclerosis in the aPT group, it seems that aPT might be an independent risk factor for atherogenesis that could be more important than conventional risk factors such as hypercholesterolemia. More research in this field is obviously required to clarify the nature of association between aPT and atherosclerosis. This would be done using different animal models with various experimental protocols as wells as studies of association with human atherosclerosis.

REFERENCES

1. Furie B, Furie BC. The molecular basis of blood coagulation. Cell 1988;53:505–518.
2. Wilson WA, Gharavi AE, Koike T, Lockshin MD, Branch DW, Piette JC, Brey R, Derksen R, Harris EN, Hughes GR, Triplett DA, Khamashta MA. International consensus statement on preliminary classification criteria for definite antiphospholipid syndrome. Arthritis Rheum 1999;42:1309–1311.
3. Rao LVM, Hoang AD, Rapaport SL. Mechanism and effects of the binding of lupus anticoagulant IgG and prothrombin to surface phospholipids. Blood 1996;88:4173–4178.
4. Horbach DA, van Oort E, Donders RC, Derksen RH, de Groot PG. Lupus anticoagulant is the strongest risk factor for both venous and arterial thrombosis in patients with systemic lupus erythematosus. Comparison between different assays for the detection of anti-phospholipid antibodies. Thromb Haemost 1996;76:916–924.
5. Matsuda J, Saitoh N, Gotoh M, Kawasugi K, Gohchi K, Tsukamoto M. Phosphatidyl-serine dependent antiprothrombin antibody is exclusive to patients with lupus anticoagulant. Br J Rheumatol 1996;35:589–591.
6. Vaarala O, Puurunen M, Manttari M, Manninen V, Aho K, Palosuo T. Antibodies to prothrombin imply a risk of myocardial infarction in middle-aged men. Thromb Haemost 1996;75:456–459.
7. Palosuo T, Virtamo J, Haukka J, Taylor PR, Aho K, Puurunen M, Vaarala O. High antibody levels to prothrombin imply a risk of deep venous thrombosis and pulmonary embolism in middle-aged men – a nested case-control study. Thromb Haemost 1997;78:1178–1182.
8. Kalashnikova LA, Korczyn AD, Shavit S, Rebrova O, Reshetnyak T, Chapman J. Antibodies to prothrombin in patients with Sneddon's syndrome. Neurology 1999;53:223–225.
9. Lakos G, Kiss E, Regeczy N, Tarjan P, Soltesz P, Zeher M, Bodolay E, Szucs G, Szakony S, Sipka S, Szegedi G. Antiprothrombin and antiannexin V antibodies imply risk of thrombosis in patients with systemic autoimmune diseases. J Rheumatol 2000;27:924–929.
10. Munoz-Rodriguez FJ, Reverter JC, Font J, Tassies D, Cervera R, Espinosa G, Carmona F, Balasch J, Ordinas A, Ingelmo M. Prevalence and clinical significance of antiprothrombin antibodies in patients with systemic lupus erythematosus or with primary antiphospholipid syndrome. Haematologica 2000;85:632–637.
11. Forastiero RR, Martinuzzo ME, Cerrato GS, Kordich LC, Carreras LO. Relationship of anti β2-glycoprotein I and anti prothrombin antibodies to thrombosis and pregnancy loss in patients with antiphospholipid antibodies. Thromb Haemost 1997;78:1008–1014.
12. Swadzba J, De Clerck LS, Stevens WJ, Bridts CH, van Cotthem KA, Musial J, Jankowski M, Szczeklik A. Anticardiolipin, anti-β2-glycoprotein-I, antiprothrombin antibodies, and lupus anticoagulant in patients with systemic lupus erythematosus with a history of thrombosis. J Rheumatol 1997;24:1710–1715.
13. Baudo F, Redaelli R, Pezzetti L, Caimi TM, Busnach G, Perrino L, deCataldo F. Prothrombin-antibody coexistent with lupus anticoagulant (LA): clinical study and immunological characterization. Thromb Res 1990;57:279–287.
14. Cote HC, Huntsman DG, Wu J, Wadsworth LD, MacGillivray RT. A new method for characterization and epitope determination of a lupus anticoagulant-associated neutralizing antiprothrombin antibody. Am J Clin Pathol 1997;107:197–205.
15. Zhao Y, Rumold R, Zhu M, Zhou D, Ahmed AE, Le DT, Hahn B, Woods VL Jr, Chen PP. An IgG antiprothrombin antibody enhances prothrombin binding to damaged endothelial cells and shortens plasma coagulation times. Arthritis Rheum 1999;42:2132–2138.
16. Field SL, Hogg PJ, Daly EB, Dai YP, Murray B, Owens D, Chesterman CN. Lupus anticoagulants form immune complexes with prothrombin and phospholipid that can augment thrombin production in flow. Blood 1999;94:3421–3431.
17. de Groot PG, Horbach DA, Simmelink MJA, van Oort E, Derksen RHWM. Anti-prothrombin antibodies and their relation with thrombosis and lupus anticoagulant. Lupus 1998;7(Suppl 2):32–36.
18. Puurunen M, Manttari M, Manninen V, Palosuo T, Vaarala O. Antibodies to prothrombin crossreact with plasminogen in patients developing myocardial infarction. Br J Haematol 1998;100:374–379.
19. George J, Afek A, Gilburd B, Levy Y, Blank M,

Kopolovic J, Harats D, Shoenfeld Y. Atherosclerosis in LDL-receptor knockout mice is accelerated by immunization with anticardiolipin antibodies. Lupus 1997;6:723–729.

20. George J, Afek A, Gilburd B, Blank M, Levy Y, Aron-Maor A, Levkovitz H, Shaish A, Goldberg I, Kopolovic J, Harats D, Shoenfeld Y. Induction of early atherosclerosis in LDL-receptor-deficient mice immunized with beta2-glycoprotein I. Circulation 1998;98:1108–1115.

21. Sherer Y, Shemesh J, Tenenbaum A, Blank M, Harats D, Fisman EZ, Praprotnik S, Motro M, Shoenfeld Y. Coro-nary calcium and anti-cardiolipin antibody are elevated in patients with typical chest pain. Am J Cardiol 2000 (in press).

22. Smith EB, Crosbie L, Carey S. Prothrombin-related antigens in human aortic intima. Semin Thromb Haemost 1996;22:347–350.

23. Blank M, Eldor A, Tavor S, Ziporen L, Cines DB, Arepally G, Afek A, Shoenfeld Y. A mouse model for heparin-induced thrombocytopenia. Semin Hematol 1999;36(Suppl 1):12–16.

Atherosclerosis and Autoimmunity
Y. Shoenfeld, D. Harats and G. Wick, editors

Detection of Cellular Activity in Atherosclerosis by the Novel Cellscan System

Naomi Zurgil[1], Yair Levy[2], Boris Gilburd[2], Ella Trubiankov[3], Mordechai Deutsch[1], Yana Shafran[1] and Yehuda Shoenfeld[2]

[1]*The Jerome Schottenstein Cellscan Center, Department of Physics, Bar-Ian University, Ramat Gan, Israel;*
[2]*Department of Medicine B and the Research Unit of Autoimmune Diseases, Sheba Medical Center and Sackler Faculty of Medicine, Tel-Aviv University, Tel-Hashomer, Israel;* [3]*Medis-El Ltd, Yehud, Israel*

1. INTRODUCTION

In recent years considerable data have been accumulated regarding the involvement of immune system in atherogenesis [1, 2]. The previously neglected area was suggested by the presence of immunocompetent cells and immunoglobulin deposition in the vicinty of plagues, and by successful immunomodulation of the atherosclerotic process [3, 4]. A logical consequence of the results was a search for a putative (auto) antigen(s) that presumably triggers the 'ongoing' local inflammatory reaction [5–9].

Oxidized low-density lipoprotein (oxLDL) has been considered by many authorities to be an acceptable immunogen by virtue of numerous in vitro effects on the cellular constituents and by isolation of lesion T cells reactive with this antigen [10–16].

Lysophosphatidylcholine (LPC) is well known as an intermediate compound of the metabolism of phosphatidylcholine (PC), the main phospholipid component in all eukaryotic cells. LPC, which may be formed during oxidation of low density lipoprotein (LDL) [17], is a major component of oxidized LDL (oxLDL), accumulated in inflammatory and atherosclerotic lesions and is involved in the pathogenesis of inflammatory vascular disorders and in atherosclerosis.

LPC involvement in atherosclerosis is mainly associated with modulations of cell functions in the vessel wall. A variety of actions have been reported in response to LPC: induction of irreversible cell damage in cardiomyocytes [18], decrease in sensitivity of myocardial and aortic endothelium [19] to cholinergic stimulation, impairment contractility of arterial smooth muscle [20], modulation of platelet aggregation [21] and induction of apoptosis in endothelial cells [22].

The pro-inflammatory effects of LPC include induction of mitogenic effects on macrophages [23], activation of human T lymphocytes [24–26], induction of pro-inflammatory cytokine secretion [27], and initiation of monocyte and T lymphocyte chemotaxis [28, 29]. LPC was shown to upregulate adhesion molecules for monocytes and T lymphocytes as well as growth factors [30] and to stimulate adhesion and differentiation of lymphoid cells [31].

Recent studies suggested a role for inflammation in the pathophysiology of unstable angina. An increase in the percentage of IL-2 R positive T lymphocytes was evident in coronary lesions of patients with acute coronary syndromes, which indicated recent activation, and amplification of the immune response within the plaques [32]. Moreover, circulating lymphocytes are probably involved in the inflammatory reaction since they were shown to be activated in-patients with unstable angina [33, 34]. Circulating monocytes, which are constitutively activated in unstable angina, express numerous proatherogenic cytokines and upregulate acute phase proteins [35].

The fact that activated T cells are directly involved

in the pathogenesis of vascular disorders is reinforced by experimental studies in animal models. Thus, CD4+ T cell depletion degrades post-angioplastic atherosclerosis in rats [36] and reduce the incidence of spontaneous atherosclerosis in hyperlipidemic mice [37]. Similarly, T cell stimulation blockage in a post transplantation atherosclerosis model, resulted in reduced frequency and severity of the diseases [38].

An accumulation of LPC in the atherosclerotic lesions and an increase in its blood serum level was demonstrated in coronary heart disease patients [23, 39–53]. However, the way in which the increase of this modified lipid affects lymphocyte activation of atherosclerotic patients, remains unknown.

In vitro lymphocyte activation has been a standard approach for evaluating cell-mediated responses. Activation of T lymphocytes upon mitogenic or antigenic stimulation is typically measured either by the proliferative responses as a function of tritiated thymidine incorporation, or by induction of the production of IL-2 or its receptor [54]. These methods suffer from being time-consuming assays and, in addition, fail to provide information about functional responses of lymphocytes subpopulation or individual cells.

2. THE CELLSCAN APPARATUS

When polarized illumination is used to excite a fluorochrome-labeled cell, some of the fluorescence is emitted as depolarized light. The extent of depolarization reflects the molecular fluidity or mobility of the dye-bound molecule. Fluorescence polarization measurements have been used to characterize various physical parameters of cells [55].

The Cellscan apparatus is a laser scanning cytometer incorporating a unique cell carrier containing 10,000 wells, each of which can accommodate a single cell that allows repeated, high-precision fluorescence intensity (FI) and polarization (FP) measurements to be made on intact living cells under physiologic conditions [56]. The Cellscan is unique in its capability for repetitive measurement of individual cells in a population. It has been used to detect activation of lymphocytes, fibroblasts, and other responsive cells by mitogens, antigens, and growth factors, which is accompanied by detectable depolarization of intracellular fluorescence [57–60].

3. REACTIVITY OF PERIPHERAL BLOOD LYMPHOCYTES FROM PATIENTS WITH ATHEROSCLEROSIS TO OXLDL

In a previous work [61] we have shown that fluorescence intensity of fluorescein-labeled peripheral blood lymphocytes (PBL) was markedly decreased upon exposure to high doses (>25 µg/ml) of oxLDL concurrently with an increase in fluorescence polarization (FP). A specific and dose-dependent reduction in FP of the high-intensity cell subpopulations, accompanied by higher FI was evident in patients with ischemic heart disease upon exposure to low doses of oxLDL (up to 25 µg/ml). Maximal depolarization was shown upon triggering with 2 µg/ml of oxLDL. The polarization ratio (the mean polarization value of the specific cell population with and without activation) obtained for patients' lymphocytes was significantly lover (p< 0.01) than that of the control group (0.936 ±0.05 and 1.028 ± 0.055 respectively). These data suggest that PBL from patients with active ischemic heart disease show an increased reactivity to oxLDL. A 73% positivity rate was found for 22 ischemic heart disease patient compared with 5% in 22 control subjects.

The Cellscan system was used by us to monitor the effect of LPC on resting and activated peripheral blood lymphocyte (PBL) isolated from patients with IHD and from control subjects. Evidence is shown that LPC may exert stimulatory and inhibitory actions depending on the clinical status of the patients and the activation state of the cells.

4. INHIBITORY EFFECT OF LPC ON PHA ACTIVATED NORMAL PBL

In order to study the effect of LPC on PHA activated lymphocytes, PBL were incubated in the presence of PHA and 10µM LPC, three cytofluorometric markers for early lymphocyte activation were then measured in individual cells by the Cellscan cytometer: expression of CD25, RH123 uptake which reflect mitochondrial activity and mass, and fluorescein FP expressing intracellular matrix

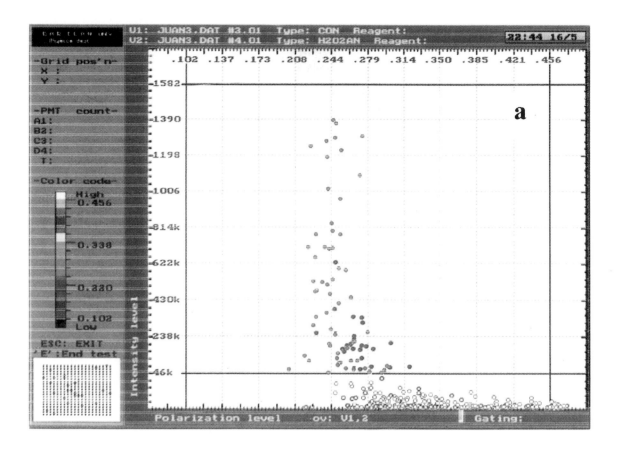

Figure 1a. Early lymphocyte activation in individual cells as estimated by the Cellscan cytometer: Scatter diagram of FI (ordinate) vs. FP (abscissa) of PBL population before (blue dots) and after (red dots) incubation in the presence of PHA. Fig. 1a: Cells were probed with FITC conjugated anti-CD25 for the expression of CD25.

organization.

Under the experimental conditions used here, the IL-2 receptor was detectable on surface of activated cells as early as 2–3h following stimulation (Fig. 1a). Concomitantly, a significant increase in uptake of RH123, a cationic fluorochrome that stains the mitochondria, was evident upon PHA stimulation (Fig. 1b). The use of FP measurement enables the discrimination between the specific fluorescence signals of anti CD25 and RH123, which exhibited discrete FP values, and the non-specific background signals.

The presence of LPC during PHA activation decreased the level of CD25 expression at the cell surface and inhibited the increase in mitochondrial membrane potential as measured by RH123 (Fig. 1c). The percentage of CD25 positive cells and FI of RH123 were lower by 40% and 30% respec-

tively.

We have previously shown that FP changes of fluorescein labeled lymphocytes reflect an early measure of lymphocyte stimulation [19, 23, 24, 27]. Fig. 2 depicts a three-dimensional histogram of FP vs. FI values of lymphocyte populations derived from a normal donor, triggered with PHA in the presence and absence of LPC. PHA activation resulted in a significant decrease in FP values of stimulated lymphocytes. The mean FP value of the cell population decreased from 0.204±0.024 to 0.191±0.023 (7.3% depolarization). Inhibition of mitogen-induced depolarization was evident when lymphocytes were treated with LPC (mean FP value 0.196±0.026, 4% depolarization – Fig. 2c).

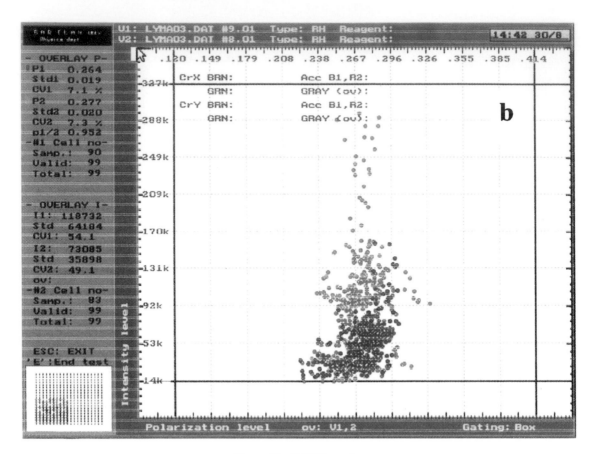

Figure 1b. RH123 uptake.

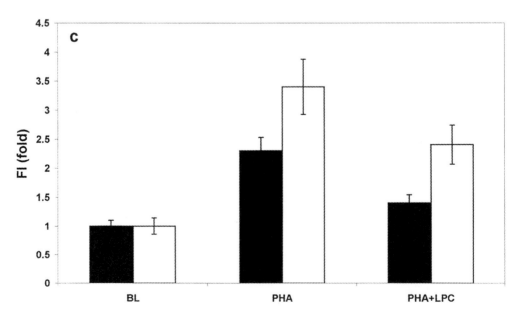

Figure 1c. Mean FI values of PBL probed with anti CD25 (■) or RH123 (□) before (BL) and after incubation in the presence of PHA (PHA) and PHA+10μM LPC (PHA+LPC). Values are averages with standard deviations.

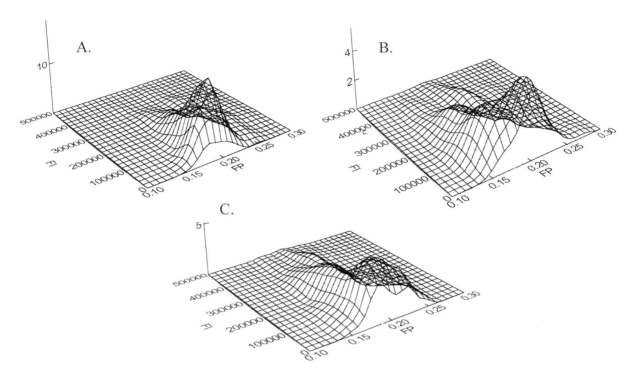

Figure 2. Effect of LPC on fluorescence polarization of activated lymphocytes. Three-dimensional distribution histogram of FP vs. FI values of lymphocyte population derived from a normal donor, before (A) and after PHA induced stimulation in the absence (B) and in the presence of LPC (C).

5. MODULATORY EFFECT OF LPC ON RESTING AND PHA ACTIVATED PBL FROM PATIENTS WITH ATHEROSCLEROSIS.

Intracellular FP of PHA activated peripheral lymphocytes from patients with advanced atherosclerosis and control subjects was monitored before and following exposure to LPC. Comparison of baseline FP values showed no significant difference between cells derived from atherosclerotic patients and healthy individuals (Fig. 3). The mean FP value of non-stimulated lymphocytes derived from 45 control subjects was 0.216±0.012, (Coefficient of variance (CV) of the average mean value between cell preparations of 45 individuals was 5.6%) while that of the 41 atherosclerotic patients was 0.211±0.012 (CV between individual patients was 7.1%). Following PHA stimulation the mean FP value decreased to 0.204±0.012 and 0.203±0.015 for healthy and diseased subjects respectively (Fig. 3).

The mean percent of depolarization upon expo-

sure of PHA activated peripheral lymphocytes to 10 uM LPC is shown in Fig. 5. As can be seen, LPC inhibited PHA induced depolarization by 71% in the control group (mean percentage of depolarization was 5.44±2.2%, and dropped to 1.57±1.2%), whereas inhibition of FP decreased by LPC was only 29% in IHD patients (4.04±2.3 and 2.87±1.82% depolarization without or with LPC respectively). Moreover, in resting lymphocytes, 10uM LPC alone induced a significant fluorescence depolarization in patients with atherosclerosis but not in the control group (Fig. 4). The mean decrease in FP of patients was found to be dose dependent, whereas in healthy subjects, no significant depolarization was evident in any of the LPC concentrations used (Fig. 5). In control measurements using 10 healthy subjects and 10 IHD patients, phosphatidylcholine (PC) did not show the activation response shown by LPC.

The effect of clinical status on intracellular FP induced by LPC is shown in Fig. 6. In non-stimulated lymphocytes, unstable angina patients exhibited higher reactivity to LPC than the group of

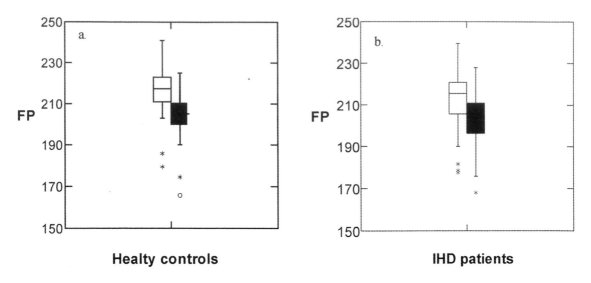

Figure 3. Distribution of baseline FP values in healthy controls and IHD patient populations. Box plots displaying medians and quartiles of mean FP values obtained from untreated (□) and PHA activated PBL (■) derived from 45 control subjects (a) and 40 atherosclerotic patients (b).

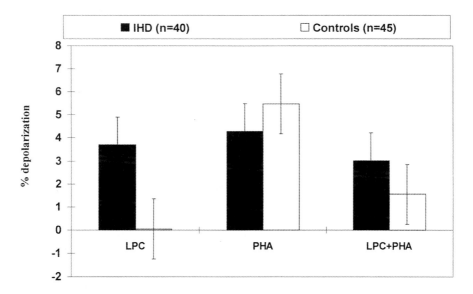

Figure 4. Effect of LPC on PBL's fluorescence depolarization. PBL from 45 control subjects (□) and 40 atherosclerotic patients (■) were activated by PHA in the presence or absence of 10M LPC. Mean percentage of depolarization and standard deviations are shown.

stable angina subjects. When PHA activated cells were exposed to LPC, a significant lower inhibition was evident both in stable and non-stable angina patients, with respect to the control group. In both groups of patients, no significant correlation was found between the degree of depolarization induced by LPC in resting lymphocytes and the percentage of inhibition shown in mitogen stimulated cells (Pearson coefficient = 0.002 and –0.03 for stable and non-stable angina respectively). It might therefore be concluded that LPC induced stimulatory or inhibitory effect on different populations of lymphocytes.

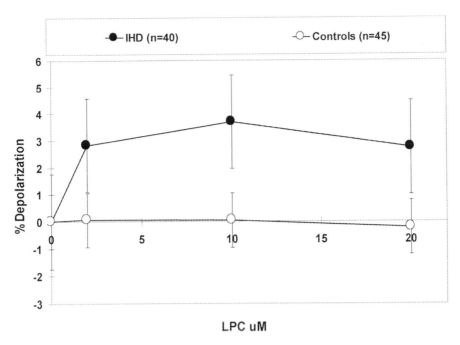

Figure 5. Activation of lymphocytes by LPC in healthy and atherosclerotic patients. Titration curves of LPC concentration vs. percent stimulation (% depolarization). Each dot represents mean values obtained from PBL of 45 control subjects (■) and 41 IHD (●) patients. The results are averages, and standard deviations are shown.

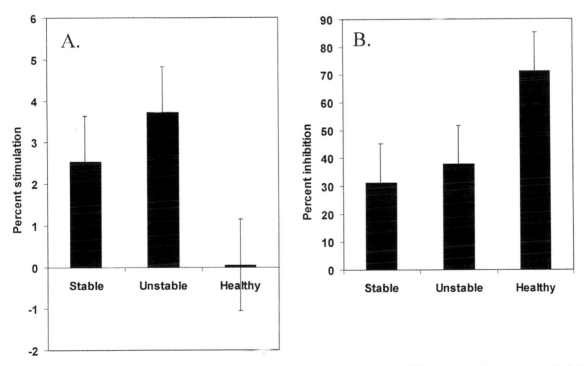

Figure 6. Effect of the clinical status on LPC induced changes in FP. Resting (A) or PHA stimulated lymphocytes (B) derived from 29 control subjects, 19 stable angina patients and 14 unstable angina patients were exposed to 10μM LPC. Mean percent of stimulation (A) and mean percent of inhibition of depolarization (B) in each subject group is presented. Standard deviations are shown.

6. CONCLUSIONS

One of the future prospects of these studies might be the advent of a simple and rapid noninvasive test that could assess the extent of atherosclerosis and possibly even the response to therapy, by monitoring the reactivity of PBL to oxLDL and LPC.

REFERENCES

1. Libby P, Hansson GK. Involvement of the immune system in human atherosclerosis: Current knowledge and unanswered questions. Lub Invest 1991;64:5–15.
2. Palinski W, Miller E, Wiztum JL. Immunization of low-density lipoprotein (LDL) deficient rabbits with homologous malondialdehyde-modified LDL reduces atherosclerosis. Proc Natl Acad Sci USA 1995;92:821–825.
3. Ameli S, Hultrgardh-Nilsson A, Regenstrom J, Calara F, Yana J, Cercek B, Shah PK, Nillson J. Effect of immunization with homologous LDL and oxidized LDL on early atherosclerosis in hypercholesterolemic rabbits. Arterioscler Thromb Vasc Biol 1996;16:1074–1079.
4. George J, Afek A, Gilburd B, Levkovitz H, Shaish A, Goldberg I, Kopolovic J, Wick G, Shoenfeld Y, Harats D. Hyperimmunization of apoE deficient mice with homologous MDA-low density lipoprotein suppresses early atherogenesis. Atherosclerosis 1998;138:147–152.
5. Xu Q, Dietrich H, Steiner HJ, Gown AM, Schoel B, Mikuz G, Kaufman SHE, Wick G. induction of arteriosclerosis in normocholesterolemic rabbits by immunization with heat shock protein 65. Arterioscler Thromb 1992;12:789–799.
6. George J, Shoenfeld Y, Afek A, Gilburd B, Keren P, Shaish A, Kopolovic Y, Wick G, Harats D. Enhanced fatty streak formation in C57BL/6J mice by immunization with heat shock protein 65. Arterioscler Thromb Vasc Biol 1999;19:505–510.
7. George J, Afek A. Gilburd B, Aron-Maor A, Shaish A, Levkovitz H, Blank M, Harats D, Shoenfeld Y. Induction of early atherosclerosis in LDL receptor deficient mice immunized with beta 2 glycoprotein 1. Circulation 1998;15:1108–1115.
8. George J, Harats D, Gilburd B, Afek A, Levy Y, Schneiderman J, Barshack I, Kopolovic J, Shoenfeld Y. Immunolocalization of β2-glycoprotein 1 (apolipoprotein H) to human atherosclerotic plaques: potential implications for lesion progression. Circulation 1999;99:2227–2230.
9. George J, Harats D, Gilburd B, Afek A, Shaish A, Levy Y, Kopolovic J, Shoenfeld Y. Adoptive transfer of beta-2-clycoprotein 1-reactive lymphocytes enhances athero-

sclerosis in LDL receptor deficient mice. Circulation 2000 (in press).
10. Yla-Hemuale SW, Palinski SW, Bulter S, Picard D, Steinberg D, Wiztum JL. Rabbit and human atherosclerotic lesion contain IgG that recognized epitopes of oxidized LDL. Arterioscler Thromb 1994;14:32–40.
11. Grundy SM. Role of low-density lipoproteins in atherosclerosis and development of coronary heart disease. Clin Chem 1995;41:139–146.
12. Holvoet P, Collen D. Oxidized lipoproteins in atherosclerosis and thrombosis. FASEB J 1994;8:1279–1284.
13. Steinberg DS, Parathasarathy TE, Carew JC, Khoo, Wiztum JL. Beyond cholesterol: Modification of low density lipoprotein that increases its atherogenicity. N Engl J Med 1989;320:915–924.
14. Wiztum J. The oxidation hypothesis of atherosclerosis. Lancet 1994;344:793–795.
15. Mironova M, Virella G, Lopes-Virella MF. Isolation and characterization of human antioxidized LDL autoantibodies. Arterioscler Thromb Vasc Biol. 1996;16:222–229.
16. Stemme S, Faber B, Holm J. T lymphocytes from human atherosclerotic plaques recognize oxidized low-density lipoprotein. Proc Natl Acad Sci USA 1995;92:3893–3897.
17. Hurt-Camejo E, Camejo G. Potential involvement of type II phospholipase A2 in atherosclerosis. Atherosclerosis 1997;132:1–8.
18. Chen M, Xiao CY, Hashizume H, Abiko Y. Phospholipase A2 is not responsible for lysophosphatidylcholine-induced damage in cardiomyocytes. Am J Physiol 1998;275:H1782–7.
19. Kamata K, Nakajima M. Ca2+ mobilization in the aortic endothelium in streptozotocin-induced diabetic and cholesterol-fed mice. Br J Pharmacol 1998;123:1509–16.
20. Leung YM, Xion Y, Ou YJ, Kwan CY. Perturbation by lysophosphatidylcholine of membrane permeability in cultured vascular smooth muscle and endothelial cells. Life Sci 1998;63:965–73.
21. Yuan Y, Schoenwaelder SM, Salem HH, Jackson SP. The bioactive phospholipid, lysophosphatidylcholine, induces cellular effects via G-protein-dependent activation of adenylyl cyclase. J Biol Chem 1996;271:27090–8.
22. Sata M, Walsh K. Endothelial cell apoptosis induced by oxidized LDL is associated with the down-regulation of the cellular caspase inhibitor FLIP. J Biol Chem 1998;273:33103–6.
23. Sakai M, Miyazaki A, Hakamata H, et al. Lysophosphatidylcholine plays an essential role in the mitogenic effect of oxidized low-density lipoprotein on murine macrophages. J Biol Chem 1994;269:31430–5.
24. Asaoka Y, Oka M, Yoshida K, Sasaki Y, Nishizuka

Y. Role of lysophosphatidyl-choline in T-lymphocyte activation: involvement of phospholipase A2 in signal transduction through protein kinase C. Proc Natl Acad Sci USA 1992;89:6447–551.

25. Asaoka Y, Yoshida K, Sasaki Y, et al. Possible role of mammalian secretory group II phospholipase A2 in T-lymphocyte activation: implication in propagation of inflammatory reaction. Proc Natl Acad Sci USA 1993;90:716–9.

26. Sakata-Kaneko S, Wakatsuki Y, Usui T, et al. Lysophosphatidylcholine upregulates CD40 ligand expression in newly activated human CD4+ T cells. FEBS Lett 1998;433:161–5.

27. Huang YH, Schafer-Elinder L, Wu R, Claesson H-E, Frostegard J. Lysophospha-tidylcholine (LPC) induces proinflammatory cytokines by a platelet-activating factor (PAF) receptor-dependent mechanism. Clin Exp Immunol 1999;116:326–31.

28. Quinn MT, Kondratenko N, Parthasarathy S. Analysis of the monocyte chemotactic response to lysophosphatidylcholine: role of lysophospholipase C. Biochim Biophys Acta 1991;1082:293–302.

29. Ryborg AK, Deleuran B, Thestrup-Pedersen K, Kragballe K. Lysophosphatidyl-choline: a chemoattractant to human T lymphocytes. Arch Dermatol Res 1994;286:462–5.

30. Kita T, Kume N, Ishii K, Horiuchi H, Arai H, Yokode M. Oxidized LDL and expression of monocyte adhesion molecules. Diabetes Res Clin Pract 1999;45:123–6.

31. Kume N, Cybulsky MI, Gimbrone MA. Lysophosphatidylcholine, a component of atherogenic lipoproteins, induces mononuclear leukocyte adhesion molecules in cultured human and rabbit arterial endothelial cells. J Clin Invest 1992;90:1138–44.

32. van der Wal AC, Piek JJ, de Boer OJ, et al. Recent activation of the plaque immune response in coronary lesions undergoing acute coronary syndromes. Heart 1998;80:14–8.

33. Neri Serneri GG, Prisco D, Martini F, et al. Acute T-cell activation is detectable in unstable angina. Circulation 1997;95:1806–12.

34. Kassirer M, Zeltser D, Prochorov V, et al. Increased expression of the CD11b/CD18 antigen on the surface of peripheral white blood cells in patients with ischemic heart disease further evidence for smoldering inflammation in patients with atherosclerosis. Am Heart J 1999;138:555–9.

35. Lee WH, Lee Y, Kim JR, et al. Activation of monocytes, T-lymphocytes and plasma inflammatory markers in angina patients. Exp Mol Med 1999;31:159–64.

36. Hancock WW, Adams DH, Wyner LR, Sayegh MH, Karnovsky MJ. CD4+ mononuclear cells induce cytokine expression, vascular smooth muscle cell proliferation, and arterial occlusion after endothelial injury. Am J Pathol 1994;145:1008–14.

37. Emeson EE, Shen ML, Bell CG, Qureshi A. Inhibition of atherosclerosis in CD4 T-cell-ablated and nude (nu/nu) C57BL/6 hyperlipidemic mice. Am J Pathol 1996;149:675–85.

38. Russell ME, Hancock WW, Akalin E, et al. Chronic cardiac rejection in the LEW to F344 rat model. Blockade of CD28-B7 costimulation by CTLA4Ig modulates T cell and macrophage activation and attenuates arteriosclerosis. J Clin Invest 1996;97:833–8.

39. Nishizuka Y. Intracellular signaling by hydrolysis of phospholipids and activation protein kinase C. Science 1992;258:607–14.

40. Ohara Y, Peterson TE, Zheng B, Kuo JF, Harrison DG. Lysophosphatidylcholine increases vascular superoxide anion production via protein kinase C activation. Arterioscler Thromb 1994;14:1007–13.

41. Inoue N, Hirata K, Yamada M, et al. Lysophosphatidylcholine inhibits bradykinin-induced phosphoinositide hydrolysis and calcium transients in cultured bovine aortic endothelial cells. Circ Res 1992;71:1410–21.

42. Kugiyama K, Ohgusi M, Sugiyama S, et al. Lysophosphatidylcholine inhibits surface receptor-mediated intracellular signals in endothelial cells by a pathway involving protein kinase C activation. Circ Res 1992;71:1422–8.

43. Shaikh NA, Downar E. Time course of changes in porcine myocardial phospholipid levels during ischemia. A reassessment of the lysolipid hypothesis. Circ Res 1981;49:316–25.

44. Pogowizd SM, Onufer JR, Kramer JB, Sobel BE, Corr PB. Induction of delayed after depolarizations and triggered activity in canine Purkinje fibers by lysophosphoglycerides. Circ Res 1986;59:416–26.

45. Mock T, Man RY. Mechanism of lysophosphatidylcholine accumulation in the ischemic canine heart. Lipids 1990;25:357–62.

46. Tanaka H, Ikeda U, Shigenobu K. Positive chronotropic and inotropic responses to lysophosphatidylcholine are mediated by norepinephrine released from myocardial sympathetic nerve terminals. Gen Pharmacol 1993;24:239–41.

47. Sato T, Ishida H, Nakazawa H, Arita M. Hydrocarbon chain length-dependent antagonism of acylcarnitines to the depressant effect of lysophosphatidylcholine on cardiac sodium current. J Mol Cell Cardiol 1996;28:2183–94.

48. Chen M, Hashizume H, Abiko Y. Effects of beta-adrenoceptor antagonists on Ca (2+)-overload induced by lysophosphatidylcholine in rat isolated cardiomyocytes. Br J Pharmacol 1996;118:865–70.

49. Chen M, Hashizume H, Xiao CY, Hara A, Abiko Y. Lysophosphatidylcholine induces Ca2+-independent cellular injury attenuated by d-propranolol in rat cardiomyocytes. Life Sci 1997;60:PL57–62.

50. Kang JX, Leaf A. Protective effects of free polyunsaturated fatty acids on arrhythmias induced by lysophosphatidylcholine or palmitoylcarnitine in neonatal rat cardiac muscles. Eur J Pharmacol 1996;297:97–106.

51. Undrovinas AI, Fleidervish IA, Makielski JC. Inward sodium current at resting potentials in single cardiac myocytes induced by the ischemic metabolite lysophosphatidylcholine. Circ Res 1992;71:1231–41.

52. Suslova IV, Korotaeva AA, Prokazova NV. Change in the equilibrium binding parameters of (3H)-quinuclidinylbenzilate in rabbit atrial membranes exposed to lysophosphatidylcholine (in Russian). Dokl Akad Nauk 1995;342:273–6.

53. Steinberg D, Parthasarathy S, Carew TE, Khoo JC, Witztum JM. Beyond cholesterol. Modifications of low-density lipoprotein that increase its atherogenicity. N Engl J Med 1989;320:915–24.

54. Hudson L, Hay FC. Mitogenic response. In: Practical Immunology, 3rd ed. Oxford: Blackwell 1989;154.

55. Zurgil N, Kaufman M, Deutsch M. Determination of cellular thiol levels in individual live lymphocytes utilizing fluorescence intensity and polarization measurements. J Immunol Methods 16:214–26.

56. Deutsch M, Weinreb A. Apparatus of high precision repetitive sequential optical measurement of living cells. Cytometry 1994;16:214–226.

57. Kaplan MR, Trubniykov E, Berke G. Fluorescence depolarization as an early measure of lymphocyte stimulation. J Immunol Methods 1997;201:15–24.

58. Zurgil N, Gerbat S, Langevitz P, Tishler M, Ehrenfeld M, Shoenfeld Y. Intracellular fluorescence polarization measurements by the Cellscan system: Detection of cellular activity in autoimmune disorders. Isr J Med Sci 1997;33:51–57.

59. Marder O, Shoval S, Eisenthal A, Fireman E, Skornic Y, Lifshitz-Mercer B, Deutsch M, Tirosh R, Weinreb A. Effect of interleukin (IL)-1α, IL-1β and tumor necrosis factor (TNF)-α on the intracellular fluorescein fluorescence polarization (IFFP) of human lung fibroblasts. Pathobiology 1996;321:1015–2008.

60. Eisenthal A, Marder O, Dotan D, Baron S, Lifschitz-Mercer B, Chaitchik S, Tirosh R, Weinreb A, Deutsch M. Decrease of intracellularfluorescein fluorescence polarization in human peripheral blood lymphocytes undergoing stimulation with phytohemagglutinin (PHA) concanavalin A (Con A), Pokeweed mitogen (PWM) and anti CD3. Biol Cell 1996;86:145–150.

61. Zurgil N, Levy Y, Deutsch M. Gilburd B, George J, Harats D, Kaufman M, Shoenfeld Y. Reactivity of peripheral blood lymphocytes (PBL) to oxLDL. A novel system to estimate atherosclerosis employing the Cellscan. Clin Cardiol 1999;22:526–532.

ANTI-ENDOTHELIAL CELL ANTIBODIES (AECA) AND ATHEROSCLEROSIS

Atherosclerosis and Autoimmunity
Y. Shoenfeld, D. Harats and G. Wick, editors

Pathogenicity of Antiendothelial Cell Autoantibodies

Anne Bordron[1], Ronan Révélen[1], Maryvonne Dueymes and Pierre Youinou

Laboratory of Immunology, Institut de Synergie des Sciences et de la Santé, Brest University Medical School, France

1. INTRODUCTION

Owing to their permanent contact with circulating immune effectors, endothelial cells (EC) have long been suspected of being a potential target for immune-mediated assault [1]. In spite of wide variations in the results [2], it is therefore not surprising that anti-EC antibodies (AECA) have been claimed to exist. Furthermore, these have been detected in a variety of clinical conditions [3], including systemic lupus erythematosis (SLE), rheumatoid arthritis (RA), Wegener granulomatosis (WG), systemic sclerosis (SSc), and Kawasaki syndrome (KS). Noteworthy is that all these disorders are characterized by vascular changes, leading to EC injury. AECAs have first been described by Lindqvist and Osterland [4], and then confirmed by Tan and Pearson [5], through immunofluorescence analysis. The reliability of staining with AECAs was subsequently established using purified IgG and F(ab')$_2$ fragments [6].

In view of the impressive diversity of conditions associated with AECAs, these certainly represent an extremely diverse family of autoantibodies [7]. However, in the light of this established fact, their presence in vasculitic diseases does not necessarily imply causation. In fact, the production of AECAs may follow, being merely a marker of vasculitis, rather than precede EC damage.

Evidence has indeed long been lacking that AECAs are pathogenic. Recent studies have, however, kindled a new debate on the pathogenicity of these intriguing autoantibodies [8]. Right now, it has

Table 1. Clues to the pathogenicity of AECAs

- Autoantibody levels fluctuate with disease activity
- The AECA test can identify disease subsets
- AECAs are associated with specific complications
- Circulating endothelial cells
- Enhanced level of serum thrombomodulin and E-selectin

to be highlighted that one of the most substantial pieces of evidence for the pathogenicity of at least some AECA subsets is the induction of experimental vasculitis in mice following passive transfer or active immunization with human autoantibodies [9]. Several effects of AECAs are indeed emerging, such as EC lysis, activation of the cells, enhanced expression of adhesion molecules along with the production of cytokines, or EC programmed cell death which has been shown to be a pivotal participant in the pathophysiology of vascular injury [10].

2. CLUES TO THE PATHOGENICITY OF AECAS

Although the pathogenicity of AECAs remains uncertain, the likelihood of such effects was first denoted by the observation that the autoantibody levels fluctuate with disease activity in patients with SLE, WG and KS (Table 1). Moreover, the pattern of AECA reactivity in a given SLE patient has been reported to change as the disease entered dif-

[1]Anne Bordron and Ronan Révélen were recipients of scholarships from the "Communauté Urbaine de Brest".

ferent phases [11]. AECAs have also been commonly detected in patients with systemic vasculitis, and their levels reported to parallel disease activity in WG [12], even more tightly than anti-neutrophil cytoplasm antibodies (ANCA). In keeping with these preliminary clinical observations, the time of sample collection might be important in the detection of AECAs in KS as suggested by Kaneko et al. [13]. Furthermore, the AECA test can identify particular subsets of SSc [14], vasculitides [15] or inflammatory myopathies [16] with related evolution. For example, the detection of AECAs in patients with primary Raynaud's phenomenon, limited SSc or diffuse SSc may help to determine the long-term prognosis of the disease. A significant trend for AECAs to increase with disease severity across these three groups of patients indicates that the AECA test can identify subsets of SSc with differing prognoses [14].

In this respect it is also of interest that the production of AECA is complicated by renal failure in SLE, vasculitis in RA and lung fibrosis in SSc and polymyositis/dermatomyositis. In practice, D'Cruz et al. calculated that the presence of AECAs conferred a positive value of 0.68 for the presence of nephritis in SLE [17], Heurkens et al. noticed that those RA patients with AECAs presented with vasculitis [18], while Cervera et al. [19] and Ihn et al. [20] showed that polymyositis/dermatomyositis and SSc, respectively, were associated with pulmonary fibrosis in the presence of AECAs.

Also consistent with the pathogenicity of AECAs is the detachment of ECs from affected vessels in thrombotic thrombocytopenic purpura which is a syndrome characterized by microvascular thrombosis and end-organ damage. Their appearance in the periphery related to disease activity, without the clear absence of inflammatory changes, suggests a possible role of AECAs in mediating microvascular injury in TPP, though this has recently been denied [21]. Finally, the finding that thrombomodulin, an EC-specific glycoprotein, and E-selectin, an EC adhesion molecule, are released by damage to these cells in WG and other vasculitis [22], is most probably relevant to this problem.

Table 2. Candidate target antigens for AECAs

Membrane components
- 11 proteins: 56–133 kDa
- 2 bands: 60 and 62 kDa
- 12 proteins: 16–88 kDa
- Heparan sulfate proteoglycans

"Planted antigens"
- Platelet factor 4 bound to sulfate proteoglycans
- DNA, histones, DNA/histone complexes
- Proteinase 3
- β2-glycoprotein I

3. AUTOANTIGENS RECOGNIZED BY AECAS

One of the prerequisites to delineate the mechanisms leading to AECA-mediated cell injury is to identify the target antigens of these autoantibodies. ECs from various tissues are heterogeneous with respect to their surface phenotype. Even in the same organ, the endothelium of large and small vessels, veins and arteries, exhibits significant heterogeneity, as a consequence of genetic diversity and their specialized microenvironment (reviewed in [7, 8, 23]). Yet, the fine identity of the autoantigens recognized by AECAs remains elusive, such that a vast array of EC surface components have proven to be candidate targets, even in individual patients. Indeed, immunoblotting techniques have revealed considerable discrepancies (Table 2). Just as examples, one group identified 11 proteins ranging in molecular weight from 56 to 133 kiloDaltons (kDa), a second group reported two bands of 60 and 62 kDa, and a third described 12 proteins ranging from 16 to 88 kDa (reviewed in [2, 7, 8]).

Specific target antigens of AECAs would also include vascular heparan sulfate proteoglycans or heparin-like molecules [24, 25]. Interestingly, the antibodies from patients with heparin-induced thrombocytopenia recognize platelet factor 4 complexed with heparin or bound to EC-heparan sulfate proteoglycans, thereby stimulating EC to express tissue factor and to bind platelets [21, 26, 27]. This is reminiscent of the observation that a subgroup of AECAs recognize heparan sulfate [24, 25]. It is certainly of note that certain autoantibodies referred to as AECAs are actually directed towards extracellular matrix and human collagen type IV in patients with systemic vasculitis [28]. Additionally, EC may up-regulate or express new antigenic determinants, upon activation or even in culture.

The majority of the AECA targets appear to be constitutive EC membrane proteins. If so, it is intriguing that EC preparations loose part of their reactivity following extensive washes with high molar buffers. This raises the possibility that some of the related autoantibodies are directed to proteins adherent to the membrane [29]. Three such proteins (so-called "planted antigens") are credible candidates: DNA, histones and DNA/histone complexes constitute the first set among these candidates [30]. Proteinase 3 which is the main target antigen of ANCA in WG, and most notably β_2-glycoprotein I (β_2GPI) are the other likely AECA-generating determinants. With regard to proteinase 3 in WG, this enzyme from degranulated polymorphonuclear neutrophils may produce EC injury through the binding to the EC surface and engagement of specific antibodies, even though some investigators advocate production of proteinase 3 by EC and, upon cytokine stimulation, surface expression of this enzyme [31]. β_2GPI appears to be the third and most noticeable adherent target antigen, and Del Papa et al. have indeed established that it binds to EC [32]. Concomitanlty, based on 3-dimensional modeling, binding studies with synthetic peptides and site-directed mutagenesis, the highly positively-charged motif Cys 281-Cys 288, located in the fifth domain of β_2GPI, has been identified as the major phospholipid (PL)-binding site [33]. This association is primarily electrostatic, as deduced from the inhibitory effect of increasing ionic strength and calcium ions. Importantly, β_2GPI binds to EC through the same amino acid sequence that is involved in binding to anionic PLs.

4. CYTOTOXIC ACTIVITY

The presence of complement-activating AECAs has been described in active SLE [6], possibly initiating EC lysis in nonorgan-specific autoimmune diseases. This phenomenon has not, however, been confirmed in such conditions by other investigators (reviewed in [7]). In this respect, KS has to be set apart. In their seminal study, Leung et al. established that inter-

leukin (IL)-1 and tumor necrosis factor (TNF) α rendered cultured EC susceptible to lysis by AECA [34]. The same holds true for nephropathia epidemica and other viral diseases [35]. These early findings are at variance with a recent study where AECAs were shown to be cytotoxic to ECs without cytokine pre-stimulation [14]. In contrast, sera from children with hemolytic-uremic syndrome were reported to contain complement-fixing IgG and IgM AECAs that lysed cultured ECs [36], and curiously to loose this activity after treatment of the cells with γ interferon. These data suggest that a unique class of AECAs is produced in this particular disease that may take part in the pathogenesis of vascular injury. Unfortunately, such an important observation has never been reproduced since then in KS or any other AECA-related disorder.

Other mechanisms, such as antibody-dependent cellular cytotoxicity (ADCC), might operate in some of them. These have been reported to mediate *in vitro* EC cytotoxicity in the presence of normal peripheral blood mononuclear cells. The specificity of ADCC was thus claimed to be supported by the absence of such a phenomenon in AECA-negative sera from patients with WG [37]. However, given the abnormally high ratio of effector cells to target cells, it is hard to believe that AECA-triggered ADCC represents one of the main *in vivo* mechanisms responsible for vascular damage. Likewise, polymorphonuclear neutrophils generate a significantly elevated cytotoxicity to ECs in SLE, but gel fractionation of these sera has demonstrated that other as yet unknown cytotoxic factors should be involved in the lysis. Despite previous positive results [38], it is also acknowledged now that ADCC is not influential in SSc.

5. ACTIVATION OF ECS

In addition, speculation about the mechanism of vascular conditions associated with AECAs has focused on enhanced expression of adhesion molecules, such as E-selectin, intercellular adhesion molecule 1 and vascular cell adhesion molecule 1, by ECs [39]. This enhanced expression, together with the production of chemotactic cytokines, e.g., IL-1β, IL-6, IL-8 and monocyte chemotatic protein 1, would facilitate adhesion of polymorphonuclear neutrophils and monocytes to the inflamed vessel walls, followed by their extravascular migration and granuloma formation [40]. The expression of tissue factor, which is a potent activator of coagulation, has also been recently shown (Renaudineau et al., unpublished results) to be augmented by AECAs.

Similar results have been obtained in WG [39], SSc [40] and SLE [41]. IgG AECAs from such patients would stimulate the release of cytokines, which might enhance adhesion molecule expression and leukocyte adhesion in an autocrine manner. Concomitantly, Blank et al. [42] have elegantly demonstrated that monoclonal AECAs generated from a patient with Takayasu arteritis activate ECs from large vessels. AECAs could thus play a pathogenetic role by activating ECs, rather than displaying a cytotoxic activity.

Since activation results in the loss of membrane thrombomodulin, we have evaluated its expression in ECs following incubation with AECAs (Bordron et al., unpublished results), and shown by flow cytometry that the mean fluorescence intensity of this surface molecule was reduced by 9 to 65%. In addition, to clarify the pathophysiological role of endothelin-1, the effect of sera from patients with SLE has been investigated [43]. IgM-AECAs may stimulate the release of endothelin-1 from ECs. This molecule may play an active role in the initiation and development of vascular injury.

6. APOPTOSIS-INDUCING AECAS

Apoptosis is a cell disruption, also designated as apoptosis, occurs with characteristic changes, e.g., ruffling and blebbing of the plasma membrane, (referred to as zeiosis), DNA fragmentation and nuclear condensation [44].

Plasma from patients with thrombotic thrombocytopenic purpura and sporadic hemolytic-uremic syndrome induces apoptosis in restricted lineages of human microvascular ECs, although the agents responsible for initiating ECs injury and the exact role played by AECAs remain unclear [45]. Pathogenic AECAs can thus be envisioned as a clinically relevant apoptotic stimulus, which may provide unique reservoirs of autoantigens in selected areas, just as viral infection or ultraviolet light do. The recent finding that one of the earliest events of a

chicken model of SSc is EC apoptosis [46] may also be highly relevant to this problem. Similar endothelial changes are also found in the initial phase of human generalized and local scleroderma. The role of associated AECAs in this process deserves to be discussed.

In view of the tight association [47–49] of AECAs with anti-PL antibodies (aPL), apoptosis may be suspected, inasmuch as it is widely acknowledged that early redistribution of plasma membrane anionic PL, most notably phosphatidylserine, is a general feature of the cellular commitment to apoptosis, regardless of the initiating stimulus. This phosphatidylserine translocation precedes DNA degradation and cell lysis in the apoptotic pathway, and presumably involves the combined actions of an activated scramblase and inhibited translocase.

The above observations prompted us to test the hypothesis that EC apoptosis is initiated by AECAs. In this study, incubation of EC with AECA derived from patients with vasculitis (particularly SSc) or mouse monoclonal AECAs resulted in the expression of phosphatidylserine on the surface of the cells, as established through the binding of fluorescein isothiocyanate-conjugated cationic annexin V [50]. Hypoploid cell enumeration, DNA fragmentation study and optical, immunofluorescence, confocal and electron microscopy analyses confirmed apoptosis of ECs. In some, but not all sera, a subgroup of AECAs may thus be pathogenic by inducing apoptosis and, thereby, encouraging autoimmune responses. Again, the identification of specific proteins and epitopes recognized by those apoptosis-inducing AECAs and clarification of the function of targets antigens is required to achieve a better understanding of the effects of AECAs on associated diseases. A minor family of membrane determinants might be involved in apoptosis, following stimulation with AECAs.

We have since extended these studies and found that AECA binding to ECs makes anionic PL accessible to anti-β_2GPI antibodies [51]. A mechanism by which some aPL bind to EC is proposed. Should phosphatidylserine become available, following the binding of AECA, circulating β_2GPI would attach to EC and, thereby, allow the recognition of the β_2GPI/PL complex by autoimmune aPL. Thus far, it has never been clearly established that anti-β_2GPI antibodies from patients with primary aPL syndrome recognize new epitopes formed after binding of the molecule to anionic structures or epitopes displayed by native β_2GPI when available at increased density (as one would expect for low-affinity antibodies). However, in line with the first interpretation is the recent report by Pittoni et al. that a monoclonal antibody from an SLE patient reacts with a cryptic epitope on β_2GPI, following binding to apoptotic cells [52].

Phosphatidylserine is a potent surface procoagulant, and surface blebs on apoptotic cells have been claimed to be sites of enhanced procoagulant activity. Further pursuit of possible procoagulant features in our model of AECA-induced apoptosis is thus of interest in light of a recent report that, during apoptosis induced by staurosporin and serum deprivation, ECs become procoagulant by increased phosphatidylserine expression and the loss of anticoagulant membrane components [53]. As previously suggested [54], aPL may represent a physiological mechanism to "shield" exposed phosphatidylserine and thus counteract excessive thrombin formation. Intriguingly, IgG with anti-EC activity has also been shown to be present in the serum of some healthy individuals [55]. Given that the repertoire of these natural AECAs differs from that of disease-associated autoantibodies, it is tempting to assume that these natural AECAs represent a normal response to dispose of unwanted cells with procoagulant surface activity. We have recently identified (Bordron et al., unpublished results) several AECA functional profiles: sera triggering activation of ECs and apoptosis, referred to as act+/apo+, those act–/apo+ or act+/apo–, and the remainder act–/apo– (although binding to ECs). There was no relationship between these functional profiles and the disease.

7. CONCLUDING REMARKS

To conclude, various effects have thus been allocated to AECAs (Table 3). Others might be confirmed in the near future, such as pregnancy loss [56]. Recent data provide additional insight into conceptualization of the mechanisms by which AECAs influence EC function. Although several issues remain unresolved, the hypothesis proposed regarding EC apoptosis provides a mechanism to link the production of aPL with the presence of pathogenic

Table 3. Potential pathogenic effects of AECAs

- Complement-dependent cytotoxicity
- Antibody-dependent cellular cytotoxicity
- Activation of endothelial cells
- Apoptosis of endothelial cells
- Pregnancy loss?

AECA subsets. Stimulating predictions derive from this model. Whether AECA-induced opsonization of ECs by aPLs occurs in a time-frame compatible with their clearance can be assessed by a time-course study.

Given the availability of an idiotypic manipulation model [18], it is feasible to assay serially aPLs in mice injected with AECAs. One hypothesis implies that the production of aPLs would be delayed. In addition, this sequence needs to be validated prospectively in a large number of patients and serial determination of AECAs, as well as aPLs, should be made in those originally found to be AECA-positive/aPL-negative. Evaluating the effects of Fcγ receptor polymorphisms on the capacity of macrophages to engulf phosphatidylserine-exposing and IgG aPL-bound ECs would also allow the hypothesis to be tested. Should the apoptotic EC clearance mechanisms operating *in vivo* be better defined, the consequences of impaired removal of these cells would be more easily tested. Finally and most importantly, studies are in progress to identify the cell surface epitope(s) recognized by AECAs [57], which should be considered in the design of new treatments for diseases associated with vasculitis.

REFERENCES

[1] Petty RG, Pearson JD. Endothelium, the axis of vascular health and disease. J Roy Coll Phys London 1989;92–102.

[2] Youinou P, Meroni PL, Khamashta MA, Shoenfeld Y. A need for standardization of the anti-endothelial cell antibody test. Immunol Today 1995;16:363–364.

[3] Youinou P. Antiendothelial cell antibodies and disease.

Intern Med Clin Lab 1995;3:7–10.

[4] Lindqvist KJ, Osterland CK. Human antibodies to vascular endothelium. Clin Exp Immunol 1971;9:753–760.

[5] Tan EM, Pearson CM. Rheumatic disease sera reactive with capillaries in the mouse kidney. J Clin Invest 1972;15:23–28.

[6] Cines DB, Lyss AP, Reeber M, Bina M, DeHoratius RJ. Presence of complement-fixing anti-endothelial cell antibodies in systemic lupus erythematosus. J Clin Invest 1984;73:611–625.

[7] Meroni PL, Youinou P. Endothelial cell antibodies. In: Peter JB, Shoenfeld Y, editors. Autoantibodies. Amsterdam: Elsevier, 1996;245–252.

[8] Meroni PL. What is going to happen tomorrow in the field of anti-endothelial cell autoantibodies related to vasculitis. Ann Med Interne 1994;145:467–468.

[9] Damianovich M, Gilburd B, Georges J, Del Papa N, Afek A, Goldberg L, Kopolovic Y, Roth D, Barkai G, Meroni PL, Shoenfeld Y. Pathogenic role of antiendothelial cell antibodies in vasculitis: an idiotypic experimental model. J Immunol 1996;156:4946–4951.

[10] Thompson CB. Apoptosis in the pathogenesis and treatment of disease. Science 1995;267:1456–1462.

[11] Li JS, Liu MF, Lei HY. Characterization of anti-endothelial cell antibodies in the patients with systemic lupus erythematosus: a potential marker for disease activity. Clin Immunol Immunopathol 1996;79:211–216.

[12] Chan TM, Frampton G, Jayne DRW, Perry GJ, Lockwood CM, Cameron JS. Clinical significance of anti-endothelial cell antibodies in systemis vasculitis: a longitudinal study comparing anti-endothelial cell antibodies and anti-neutrophil cytoplasm antibodies. Am J Kidney Dis 1993;22:387–392.

[13] Kaneko K, Savage COS, Pottinger BE, Shah V, Pearson JD, Dillon MJ. Antiendothelial cell antibodies can be cytotoxic to endothelial cells without cytokine pre-stimulation and correlate with ELISA antibody measurement in Kawasaki disease. Clin Exp Immunol 1994;98:264–269.

[14] Salojin KV, Le Tonquèze M, Saraux A, Nassonov EL, Dueymes M, Piette JC, Youinou P. Antiendothelial cell antibodies: useful markers of systemic sclerosis. Am J Med 1997;102:178–185.

[15] Salojin KV, Le Tonquèze M, Nassonov EL, Blouch MT, Baranov AA, Saraux A, Guillevin L, Fiessinger JN, Piette JC, Youinou P. Anti-endothelial cell antibodies in patients with various forms of vasculitis. Clin Exp Rheumatol 1996;14:163–169.

[16] Salojin KV, Bordron A, Nassonov EL, Shtutman VZ, Guseva NG, Baranov AA, Targoff IN, Youinou P. Antiendothelial cell antibody, thrombomodulin, and von Willebrand factor in idiopathic inflammatory myopathies. Clin Diagn Lab Immunol 1997;4:519–521.

[17] D'Cruz DP, Houssiau FA, Ramirez G, Baguley E, McCutcheon J, Vianna J, Haga HJ, Swana GT, Khamashta MA, Taylor JC, Davies DR, Hughes GRV. Antibodies to endothelial cells in systemic lupus erythematosus: a potential marker for nephritis and vasculitis. Clin Exp Immunol 1991;85:254–261.

[18] Heurkens AHM, Hiemstra PS, Lafeber GJM, Daha MR, Breedveld FC. Anti-endothelial cell antibodies in patients with rheumatoid arthritis complicated by vasculitis. Clin Exp Immunol 1989;78:7–12.

[19] Cervera R, Ramirez G, Fernandez-Sola J, D'Cruz D, Casademont J, Grau JM, Asherson RA, Khamashta MA, Urbano-Marquez A, Hughes GRV. Antibodies to endothelial cells in dermatomyositis: association with interstitial lung disease. Br Med J 1991;302:880–881.

[20] Ihn H, Sato S, Fujimoto M, Igarashi A, Yazawa N, Kubo M, Kikuchi K, Takehara K, Tamaki K. Characterization of autoantibodies to endothelial cells in systemic sclerosis: association with pulmonary fibrosis. Clin Exp Immunol 2000;119:203–209.

[21] Raife TJ, Atkinson B, Aster RH, McFarland JG, Gottschall JL. Minimal evidence of platelet and endothelial cell reactive antibodies in thrombotic thrombocytopenic purpura. Am J Hematol 1999;62:82–87.

[22] Boehme MWJ, Schmitt WH, Youinou P, Stremmel WR, Gross WL. Clinical relevance of elevated serum thrombomodulin and soluble E-selectin in patients with Wegener's granulomatosis and other systemic vasculitides. Am J Med 1996;101:387–394.

[23] Cines DB, Pollak ES, Buck CA, Loscalzo J, Zimmerman GA, McEver RP Pober JS, Wick TM, Konkle BA, Schwartz BS, Barnathan ES, McGrae KR, Hug BA, Schmidt AM, Stern DM. Endothelial cells in physiology and in the pathophysiology of vascular disorders. Blood 1998;91:3527–3561.

[24] Shibata S, Harpel PC, Gharavi A, Rand J, Fillit H. Autoantibodies to heparin from patients with antiphospholipid antibody syndrome inhibit formation of antithrombin III-thrombin complexes. Blood 1994;83:2532–2540.

[25] Renaudineau Y, Révélen R, Bordron A, Mottier D, Youinou P, Le Corre R. Two populations of endothelial cell antibodies cross read with heparin. Lupus 1998;7:86–94.

[26] Cines DB, Tomaski A, Tannenbaum S. Immune endothelial-cell injury in heparin-associated thrombocytopenia. N Engl J Med 1987;316:581–589.

[27] Visentin GP, Ford SE, Scott JP, Aster RH: Antibodies from patients with heparin-induced thrombocytopenia/thrombosis are specific for platelet factor 4 complexed with heparin or bound to endothelial cells. J Clin Invest 1994;93:81–88.

[28] Direskenerli H, D'Cruz D, Khamashta MA, Hughes

GRV. Autoantibodies against endothelial cells, extracellular matrix and human collagen type IV in patients with systemic vasculitis. Clin Immunol Immunopathol 1994;70:206–210.

[29] Del Papa N, Conforti G, Gambini D, La Rosa L, Tincani A, D'Cruz D, Khamashta M, Hughes GRV, Balestrieri G, Meroni PL. Characterization of the endothelial surface proteins recognized by antiendothelial antibodies in primary and secondary autoimmune vasculitis. Clin Immunol Immunopathol 1994;70:211–216.

[30] Chan TM, Frampton G, Staines NA, Hobby P, Perry GJ, Cameron JS. Different mechanisms by which anti-DNA MoAbs bind to human endothelial cells and glomerular mesangial cells. Clin Exp Immunol 1992;88:68–74.

[31] Mayet WJ, Csernok E, Szymkowiak C, Gross WL, Meyer zum Büschenfelde KHM. Human endothelial cells express proteinase 3, the target antigen of anticytoplasmic antibodies in Wegener's granulomatosis. Blood 1993;82:1221–1229.

[32] Del Papa N, Guidali L, Sala A, Buccellati C, Khamashta MA, Ichikawa K, Koike T, Balestrieri G, Tincani A, Hughes GRV, Meroni PL. Endothelial cells as target for antiphospholipid antibodies. Human polyclonal and monoclonal anti-β_2-glycoprotein I antibodies react in vitro with endothelial cells through adherent β_2-glycoprotein and induce endothelial activation. Arthritis Rheum 1997;40:551–561.

[33] Hörkkö S, Miller E, Branch DW, Palinski W, Witztum JL. The epitopes for some antiphospholipid antibodies are adducts of oxidized phospholipid and β_2 glycoprotein 1 (and other proteins). Proc Natl Acad Sci USA, 1997;10356–10361.

[34] Leung DYM, Collins T, Lapierre LA, Geha RS, Pober JS. Immunoglobulin M antibodies present in the acute phase of Kawasaki syndrome lyse cultured vascular endothelial cells stimulated by gamma interferon. J Clin Invest 1986;77:1428–1435.

[35] Wangel AG, Temonen M, Brummer-Korvenkontio M, Vaheri A. Anti-endothelial cell antibodies in nephropathia epidemica and other viral diseases. Clin Exp Immunol 1992;90:13–17.

[36] Leung DYM, Moake JL, Havens PL, Kim M, Pober JS. Lytic anti-endothelial cell antibodies in haemolytic-uraemic syndrome. Lancet 1988;2:183–186.

[37] Del Papa N, Meroni PL, Barcellini W, Sinico A, Radice A, Tincani A, D'Cruz D, Nicoletti F, Borghi MO, Khamashta MA, Hughes GRV, Balestrieri G. Antibodies to endothelial cells in primary vasculitides mediate in vitro endothelial cytotoxicity in the presence of normal peripheral blood mononuclear cells. Clin Immunol Immunopathol 1992;63:267–274.

[38] Penning CA, Cunnigham J, French MAH, Harrison G, Rowel NR, Hughes P. Antibody-dependent cellular

cytotoxicity of human vascular endothelium in systemic sclerosis. Clin Exp Immunol 1984;58:548–556.

[39] Del Papa N, Guidali L, Sironi M, Shoenfeld Y, Mantovani A, Tincani A, Balestrieri G, Radice A, Sinico RA, Meroni PL. Anti-endothelial cell IgG antibodies form patients with Wegener's granulomatosis bind to human endothelial cells in vitro and induce adhesion molecule expression and cytokine secretion. Arthritis Rheum 1996;39:758–766.

[40] Carvalho D, Savage COS, Black CM, Pearson JD. IgG antiendothelial cell autoantibodies form scleroderma patients induce leukocyte adhesion to human vascular endothelial cells in vitro. J Clin Invest 1996;97:111–119.

[41] Carvalho D, Savage COS, Isenberg D, Pearson JD. IgG anti-endothelial cell autoantibodies from patients with systemic lupus erythematosus or systemic vasculitis stimulate the release of two endothelial cell-derived mediators, which enhance adhesion molecule expression and leukocyte adhesion in an autocrine manner. Arthritis Rheum 1999;42:631–640.

[42] Blank M, Krause I, Goldkorn T, Praprotnik S, Livneh A, Langevitz, Kaganovsky E, Morgenstern S, Cohen S, Barak V, Eldor A, Weksler B, Shoenfeld Y. Monoclonal anti-endothelial cell antibodies from a patient with Takayasu arteritis activate endothelial cells from large vessels. Arthritis Rheum 1999;42:1421–1432.

[43] Yoshio T, Masuyama J, Mimori A, Takeda A, Minota S, Kano S. Endothelin-1 release from cultured endothelial cells induced by sera from patients with systemic lupus erythematosus. Ann Rheum Dis 1995;54:361–365.

[44] Evan G, Littlewood T. A matter of life and cell death. Science 1998;281:1317–1322.

[45] Mitra D, Jaffe EA, Weksler B, Hajjar KA, Soderland C, Laurence J. Thrombotic thrombocytopenic purpura and sporadic hemolytic-uremic syndrome plasmas induce apoptosis in restricted lineages of human microvascular endothelial cells. Blood 1997;89:1224–1234.

[46] Sgonc R, Gruschwitz MS, Dietrich H, Rechcis H, Gershwin ME, Wick G. Endothelial cell apoptosis is a primary pathogenetic event underlying skin lesions in avian and human scleroderma. J Clin Invest 1996;98:785–792.

[47] McCrae KR, DeMichele A, Samuels P, Roth D, Kuo A, Meng QH, Rauch J, Cines DB. Detection of endothelial cell-reactive immunoglobulin in patients with anti-phospholipid antibodies. Br J Haematol 1991;79:595–605.

[48] Vismara A, Meroni PL, Tincani A, Harris EN, Barcellini W, Brucato A, Khamashta MA, Hughes GRV, Zanussi C, Balestrieri G. Relationship between anti-cardiolipin and anti-endothelial cell antibodies in systemic lupus erythematosus. Clin Exp Immunol 1988;74:247–253.

[49] Le Tonquèze M, Dueymes M, Giovangrandi Y, Beigbeder G, Jouquan J, Pennec YL, Mottier D, Le Goff

P, Youinou P. The relationship of anti-endothelial cell antibodies to anti-phospholipid antibodies in patients with giant cell arteritis and/or polymyalgia rheumatica. Autoimmunity 1995;20:59–66.

[50] Bordron A, Dueymes M, Levy Y, Jamin C, Leroy JP, Piette JC, Shoenfeld Y, Youinou P. The binding of some antiendothelial cell antibodies induces endothelial cell apoptosis. J Clin Invest 1998;101:2029–2035.

[51] Bordron A, Dueymes M, Levy Y, Jamin C, Ziporen L, Piette JC, Shoenfeld Y, Youinou P. Antiendothelial cell antibody binding makes negatively-charged phospholipids accessible to antiphospholipid antibodies. Arthritis Rheum 1998;41:1738–1747.

[52] Pittoni V, Ravirajan CT, Donohoe S, Machin SJ, Mackie IJ, Lydyard PM, Isenberg DA. Human monoclonal antiphospholipid antibodies bind to membrane phospholipid and a cryptic epitope of β_2-glycoprotein I on apoptotic cells [abstract]. Arthritis Rheum 1998;41 suppl 12:S166.

[53] Bombeli T, Karsan A, Tist JF, Harlan JM. Apoptotic vascular endothelial cells become procoagulant. Blood 1997;89:2429–2432.

[54] Bevers EM, Smeets EF, Comfurius P, Zwall RFA. Physiology of membrane lipid asymmetry. Lupus 1994;3:235–240.

[55] Ronda N, Haury M, Nobrega A, Kaveri SV, Coutinho A, Kazatchkine MD. Analysis of natural and disease-associated autoantibody repertoires: anti-endothelial cell IgG autoantibody activity in the serum of healthy individuals and patients with systemic lupus erythematosus. Int Immunol 1994;6:1651–1660.

[56] Roussev RG, Stern JJ, Kaider BD, Thaler CJ. Anti-endothelial cell antibodies: another cause for pregnancy loss? Am J Repr Immunol 1998;39:89–95.

[57] Levy Y, Gilburd B, George J, Del Papa N, Mallone R, Damianovich M, Blank M, Radice A, Renaudineau Y, Youinou P, Wiik A, Malasavi F, Meroni PL, Shoenfeld Y. Characterization of murine monoclonal anti-endothelial cell antibodies (AECA) produced by idiotypic manipulation with human AECA. Int Immunol 1998;10:861–868.

Atherosclerosis and Autoimmunity
Y. Shoenfeld, D. Harats and G. Wick, editors

Functional Heterogeneity of Pathogenic Anti-Endothelial Cell Antibodies

Pier Luigi Meroni[1], Elena Raschi[2], Cinzia Testoni[1], Monica Riboni[1], Sonja Praprotnik[3], Yehuda Shoenfeld[4]

[1]*Allergy & Clinical Immunology Unit, Dept. of Internal Medicine, University of Milan, IRCCS Istituto Auxologico Italiano;* [2]*IRCCS Policlinico, Milan, Italy;* [3]*Dept. of Rheumatology, University Medical Centre, Ljubljana, Sloveni;* [4]*Dept. Medicine B, Tel-Hashomer, IsraelSchool, France*

1. INTRODUCTION

The term anti-endothelial cell antibodies (AECA) rather than identifying a homogenous group of autoantibodies just defines immunoglobulins characterized by their ability to react with endothelial structures. Actually, it is now widely accepted that AECA do represent a quite heterogeneous family of autoantibodies [1, 2].

The AECA heterogeneity is linked to different aspects: a) the autoantibodies display an association with different and unrelated diseases, b) their antigen specificity is widespread from constitutive to adhered molecules and from cell membrane to cytoplasmic structures, c) their occurrence and titres are related to disease activity in some conditions only, and finally d) their binding to endothelial cells ends into different functional effects (reviewed in [3]).

2. AECA HETEROGENEITY AND DISEASE ASSOCIATION

The most striking evidence of the AECA heterogeneity comes from the review of the pathological disorders in which these antibodies have been described (reviewed in [3, 4]). Different and unrelated diseases have been shown to display an anti-endothelial cell activity; table 1 reports the main conditions in which there is a sound evidence for AECA occurrence.

The common denominator for most of these pathological conditions is the presence of an immune-mediated inflammation of the vessel walls, but such a relationship cannot be found in all the AECA-positive diseases reported in literature. The best example is represented by the anti-phospholipid syndrome (APS) in which AECA are detected in the majority of the sera in spite of the fact that the disorder is characterized by a vasculopathy without strong signs of inflammation [5–7].

Firstly AECA have been described in systemic autoimmune vasculitis, both primary [8–10] and secondary to systemic autoimmune diseases [11]. This finding was not surprising keeping in mind the clear vessel wall inflammation characteristic of these disorders and the potential role for AECA to contribute to the process. Interestingly, AECA have been also found in Systemic Sclerosis (SSc) in which endothelial damage and/or activation is thought to play a pivotal role in inducing the eventual fibroblast hyperactivation [12–14].

Other diseases with an autoimmune pathogenesis but without a clear systemic vasculitis have been also found to be positive for AECA such as autoimmune endocrinopathies [3, 15, 16] or multiple sclerosis [17].

Quite different is the occurrence of an anti-endothelial activity in APS, a syndrome characterized by a vasculopathy and by a hypercoagulable state at least in part atributable to an endothelial activation/ dysfunction. More recently, the demonstration that most of the AECA activity in APS is due to antibodies able to recognize the "phospholipid co-factor" beta 2 glycoprotein I (β2GPI) expressed on the endothelial cell membranes explained the high prevalence of AECA in this disorder [18].

In line with the ability of endothelial cells to express HLA Class II antigens after cytokine activation, several groups described AECA in allograft rejection [19–22]. Interestingly, the anti-endothelial cell activity was found to be sustained also by antibodies that do not react with HLA molecules, suggesting a wider panel of endothelial antigens involved in host response to the graft and the potential role for these antibodies in the rejection phenomenon. The importance of AECA in transplantation was further underlined by the association between these antibodies and the accelerated atherosclerotic lesions frequently found in the graft vessels [23–25].

Such an association raised the hypothesis of a possible role for AECA in atherosclerosis as a potential antibody able to induce the activation/damage of the endothelium that is generally thought to represent a preliminary step for the atherosclerotic plaque formation [26]. However, not conclusive data have been reported to support this hypothesis up to now [27].

Anti-endothelial cell antibodies have been also described in small series of patients with different infectious processes [3, 28, 29]. It is difficult to state whether the appearance of these antibodies is the result of a specific autoimmune response driven by the infectious agent or just the emergence of B cell clones secreting natural autoantibodies in the course of a polyclonal B cell activation triggered by the infection [30].

As mentioned above, the presence of AECA in unrelated pathological conditions suggests the possibility that different and heterogeneous processes are likely responsible for the induction of AECA synthesis.

It should be noted that a high variability of AECA prevalences is reported in literature. Such a variability is mainly linked to the lack of standardization of the procedures for detecting AECA [31] and to the fluctuation of the AECA titres with disease activity, at least in some cases.

3. AECA HETEROGENEITY AND DISEASE ACTIVITY RELATIONSHIP

Anti-endothelial cell antibody positivity and titres have been frequently associated with disease activity and organ involvement (Table 1). In Wegener's Granulomatosis (WG) AECA disappeared in therapy-induced remissions and their titres increased during and even before flares [8, 9, 32, 33]. In Systemic Lupus Erythematosus (SLE) the presence of AECA has been associated with kidney involvement [34] and in Rheumatoid Arthritis AECA have been reported in patients with systemic vasculitic manifestations only [35]. Moreover, SSc patients positive for AECA displayed more frequently peripheral vasculitic lesions as well as pulmonary involvement [12, 13].

The close association between AECA and disease activity and/or vessel involvement strongly suggests a cause-effect relationship further supporting a potential pathogenic role for these antibodies. On the other hand, the lack of an association in other diseases suggests that AECA might be not involved in the pathogenesis, being just an epiphenomenon or alternatively that larger series or longer follow-up studies are required (reviewed in [3]).

4. AECA HETEROGENEITY AND ANTIGEN SPECIFICITY

Sera positive for AECA have been shown to recognize antigens expressed in large arterial and venous vessels, or in small vessels, such as omental, renal, skin and brain microvasculature. Moreover, no species restriction was found since AECA can cross-react with endothelial cell lines or with primary endothelial cell cultures of different animal origin (reviewed in [2, 3]). The characteristics of the antigens recognized by AECA in different pathological conditions are reported in Table 2.

By definition AECA are antibodies reacting with endothelial cells, nevertheless several groups clearly demonstrated a cross-reactivity with human fibroblasts and, at least in part, also with platelets and peripheral blood mononuclear cells (reviewed in [3]). However, studies with immunoprecipitation techniques and cross-absorption experiments showed that some AECA are directed against endothelial

Table 1. AECA prevalence and correlation with disease activity

Disease	Prevalence (%)	Reference	Correlation with disease activity
Primary autoimmune vasculitis			
Wegener granulomatosis			
Microscopic poliangiitis	55–80	[3, 8, 10, 55]	Yes
Kawasaki disease	up to 72	[56–59]	Yes
Takayasu arteritis	9	[60]	No
Giant cell arteritis	up to 50	[3]	No
Idiopathic retinal vasculitis	35	[61]	No
Behçet's disease	up to 50	[45]	Yes
Thromboangiitis obliterans	25–36	[3, 62]	No
Churg Strauss disease	50	[3]	No
Systemic autoimmune diseases:			
Systemic lupus erythematosus	up to 80	[31, 55, 63, 64]	Yes
Antiphospholipid syndrome	64	[65]	No
Rheumatoid arthritis with vasculitis	up to 65	[35, 55, 66]	Yes
Rheumatoid arthritis without vasculitis	up to 30	[35, 55, 66]	Yes
Scleroderma	20–80	[11, 13]	Yes
Mixed connective tissue disease	45	[55]	No
Polymyositis/dermatomyositis	44	[67]	No
Transplantation			
Heart and kidney allografts	up to 71	[19–25]	TxCAD[1]
Miscellaneous			
Hemolytic uremic syndrome	93	[68]	
Thrombotic thrombocytopenic purpura	100	[46, 68]	
Heparin induced thrombocytopenia	100	[38, 49]	
Inflammatory bowel disease	up to 55	[3, 69]	
Multiple sclerosis	23–75	[3]	
IgA nephropathy	32	[70]	
Diabetes mellitus	26–75	[3, 15, 71]	
Hypo-parathyroidism (autoimmune)	100	[3]	
Acute pre-eclampsia	50	[72]	
Rocky mountain spotted fever	50	[28]	
Viral infection	up to 18	[3]	
Borderline hypertension	(no prevalence reported)	[73]	
Hepatitis C virus mixed cryoglobulinemia	41	[29]	

[1]TxCAD: transplant coronary artery disease

structures only, suggesting that a specific antibody response against endothelial antigens does exist (reviewed in [3]; Meroni manuscript in preparation).

It is clear from the table that the reactivity is due to a family of antibodies against several antigens, being the majority shared in common by sera from different pathological conditions and only some being specific for a given disease. The AECA activity has been shown to be directed against constitutive cell membrane structures, but antibodies against intracellular constituents as well as extra-cellular matrix have been also described (reviewed in [3]). Some antigens can be expressed and/or up-regulated after endothelial cell activation induced by pro-inflammatory stimuli (reviewed in [3]).

Unfortunately no definite data are now available on the precise nature of the endothelial cell antigens. However part of the whole AECA population at least in SLE sera is apparently constituted by antibodies against sulphate proteoglycan or heparin like molecules, constitutively expressed on endothelial

Table 2. Characteristics of AECA

Disease	Antigen(s)	Detection	Cross-reactivity	Potential pathogenicity
WG/MPA	EC Ags 120 kDa plus other molecules ranging from 25 to 200 kDa	Cell-ELISA, IB[1], IP[2]	Dermal fibroblasts (++), PBMC[3] (+/−), RBC[4] (+/−)	C'-cytotoxicity (+/−), ADCC (+), EC activation (++)
KS	Enhanced expression by IL-1, TNFα, IFNγ IFNγ-induced Ags different from those induced by IL-1, TNFα Ags not immunoprecipitated	C'-cytotoxicity, cell-ELISA	No cross-reactivity with dermal fibroblasts or VSMC[5]	C'-cytotoxicity
HUS	Identified a 43 kDa cytosolic and nuclear protein IFNγ down-regulates the expression	C'-cytotoxicity	No cross-reactivity with dermal fibroblasts or VSMC	C'-cytotoxicity
TTP	Identified a 43 kDa cytosolic and nuclear protein Micro-vascular EC	C'-cytotoxicity, IIF[6]		C'-cytotoxicity, in large part due to IC[7] deposition EC activation (+)
SLE	EC Ags ranging from 25 to 200 kDa EC heparin-like molecules Adhered DNA-histone complexes Extracellular matrix components	C'-cytotoxicity, cell-ELISA, IB, IP, cytofluorimetry	Dermal fibroblasts (++), PBMC (+/−), RBC (+/− −)	C'-cytotoxicity (+/−), ADCC (+), EC activation (++)
APS	EC Ags ranging from 25 to 200 kDa Adhered β2GPI	Cell-ELISA, IB, IP	Dermal fibroblasts (++)	EC activation (++), ET-1[8] release (+), TF[9] expression (+/−) Protein C system inhibition
RA (vasculitis)	EC Ags ranging from 16 to 68 kDa	Cell-ELISA, IB, cytofluorimetry	Fibroblasts (++), PBMC (+), RBC (+/−)	No data
Scleroderma	EC Ags ranging from 16 to 200 kDa	C'-cytotoxicity, cell-ELISA, IB, cytofluorimetry.	Dermal fibroblasts (++), T-lymphoma cell line (+)	C'-fixation (+/−), EC activation (+) and apoptosis (+)
Behçet's disease	Micro- > macro-vascular EC	Cell-ELISA		
Takayasu arteritis	Macrovascular EC	Cell-ELISA, IIF, cytofluorimetry, C'-cytotoxicity		EC activation (+) (hu mAbs), C'-fixation (+/−)
AECA in transplantation	EC Ags (54–60, 97–110 kDa)	Cell-ELISA, C'-cytotoxicity, IIF, IB, cytofluorimetry	Not HLA-associated, in part shared by monocytes (VEC Ag)	C'-fixation (+/−), ADCC (+), EC activation (+/−)

[1]IB: immunoblotting; [2]IP: immunoprecipitation; [3]PBMC: peripheral blood lymphocytes; [4]RBC: red blood cells; [5]VSMC: vascular smooth muscle cells; [6]IIF: indirect immunofluorescence; [7]IC: immune complexes; [8]ET-1: endothelin 1; [9]TF: tissue factor.

cells. On the other hand, it is generally accepted that in autoimmune diseases blood group antigens or HLA Class I or II molecules are not involved (reviewed in [3]).

Besides constitutive endothelial antigens, AECA have been shown to recognize also molecules that adhere to endothelial cells (*planted antigens*) such as DNA or DNA/histone complexes [36, 37]. Similarly, in APS sera antibodies specific for the anionic phospholipid binding plasma protein β2GPI react with the molecule adhered to endothelial cell membranes (reviewed in [18]). On the other hand, antibodies reacting with platelet factor 4 (PF4) complexed to glycosaminoglycan molecules on the surface of endothelial cells may be part of the AECA detectable in heparin-associated thrombocytopenia [38]. Because of the close association between AECA and anti-neutrophil cytoplasmic antigens (ANCA) in primary vasculitis such as WG, several groups investigated the possible relationship between these two families of autoantibodies. It is now widely accepted that they are two distinct populations without any cross-reactivity [39, 40]. However, the main target of the cytoplasmic ANCA, namely proteinase-3 (PR3), has been shown to be able to adhere to the endothelial cell surface owing to its cationic charge and to be recognized by anti-PR3 antibodies [40]. So, even PR3 could be included into the list of the planted antigens responsible for an anti-endothelial antibody activity. Recently, two groups reported that the AECA activity might be, at least in part, due to antibodies that recognize bovine serum proteins adhered to the endothelial cell membranes and supplied by the serum component of the culture medium (Refs. [41], Meroni personal communication). Such a reactivity is likely related to heterospecific natural antibodies and can be easily eliminated by diluting the serum samples in buffer containing bovine serum.

Table 3 reports all the techniques that have been used for detecting AECA. The undiscriminated utilization of assays that do not distinguish between antibodies bound to cell membrane or cytoplasmic antigens further explains the heterogeneity in defining the AECA characteristics. Actually, while several studies – especially in primary and secondary systemic vasculitis – employed unfixed endothelial monolayers as a substrate, in other conditions authors fixed the cells so allowing the detection of antibodies directed against cytoplasmic constituents rather than against cell membrane antigens only.

The AECA reactivity with endothelial antigens common to vessels of different anatomical origin is apparently in contrast with the well known phenotypic and functional heterogeneity of endothelia and with the clinical observation that different pathological conditions are characterized by a selective involvement of peculiar anatomical vascular districts (reviewed in [42]).

A possible explanation would be that antibodies with comparable specificity/activity could induce different effects depending on the characteristics of the endothelium. Actually, it has been suggested that endothelium integrates different extracellular signals and responds differently to the same endogenous or exogenous injurious agents in different regions of the vascular tree districts (reviewed in [42]).

However, there are data supporting a selective reactivity of AECA for specific endothelia suggesting that the clinical manifestations could be dependent, at least in part, on the involvement of specific tracts of the vascular tree. For example, studies on AECA positive sera from patients with multiple sclerosis were shown to react with cerebral endothelial cells (BEC), but not with endothelial cells from umbilical cord vein (HUVEC) [43]. Additionally, children with Landau-Kleffner syndrome variant and autistic spectrum disorders had antibodies to BEC [44] and whole AECA positive sera from Behçet's patients display higher reactivity with human omental microvascular than with HUVEC [45, 46]. A recent study on the AECA specificity in primary APS and SLE revealed different bands when sera were tested with membrane antigens from HUVEC and from human microvascular endothelial cells (HMEC) [47]. As already mentioned, the anti-endothelial reactivity in APS is primarily against adhered β2GPI. In a recent study Meroni et al. (unpublished data) showed that the reactivity of anti-β2GPI antibodies to human BEC was higher than to HUVEC. Primary skin endothelial cells as well as a microvascular dermal endothelial cell line displayed comparable behaviour. The AECA pattern of reactivity with both micro- and macro- endothelial cells in APS is in accordance with the pathological feature of the disease where large vessel thrombosis may occur in conjuction with micro-

Table 3. Methods for the detection of AECA

Assays	Specificity	Sensitivity	Comments
IIF	+++	+ (++ with confocal microscopy)	Possibility to visualize cell membrane or cytoplasmic staining. Less convenient for large screenings.
Microcytotoxicity	++	+	Lowest sensitivity. Not always C'-fixation induces EC lysis.
Cytofluorimetry	+++	+	The use of EC suspensions might alter the apical distribution or the antigen density of cell membrane antigens.
Cell solid phase	+++	+++	Mild or no fixation is required to avoid false positivities due to the binding of antibodies reacting with cytoplasmic antigens. Cell solid phase with unfixed EC allows to detect antibodies reacting with *physiological* endothelial monolayers. Quantitative assay.
Cell membrane solid phase	++	+++	It is difficult to completely rule out any contamination of cytoplasmic structures in the cell membrane preparations. Quantitative assay.
IB	++	++	It is difficult to completely rule out any (EC membranes) contamination of cytoplasmic structures in the cell membrane preparations. It also requires large EC membrane preparations. Semi-quantitative assay. It permits biochemical characterization of the recognized antigens.
IP	+++	+++	Time and cell consuming assay. Not (radiolabelled EC membranes) convenient for large screenings. Semi-quantitative assay. When selective apical cell membrane labelling is performed, the assay detects antibodies against cell surface antigens.

vascular involvement. On the contrary, SLE AECA positive sera bind HUVEC and BEC in a comparable manner; moreover 17 SLE patients with central nervous system (CNS) involvement (and without anti-phospholipid antibodies) did not display higher reactivity against BEC (Meroni personal communication). Altogether these findings suggest that in SLE AECA are directed against antigens shared in common between both macro- and micro-vascular endothelium.

In other studies, a selective reactivity has been described: a) human monoclonal AECA IgG from Takayasu's patients possessed high activity against macrovascular endothelial cells (HUVEC), but none against microvascular endothelial cells (human bone marrow endothelial cells: HBMEC) [48]. Moreover, immunohistochemistry analysis demonstrated anti-human-aortic endothelial cell activity in contrast with the lack of reactivity of anti-microvascular endothelial cell antibodies (from patients with heparin-induced thrombocytopenia) or normal human IgG [48]. Such a selectivity is in line with the path-

ological characteristics of TA, which affects large arteries exclusively.

Further, affinity purified AECA F(ab)2 from patients with thrombotic thrombocytopenic purpura (TTP) bound and activated HBMEC and not large vessel endothelial cells (HUVEC)[46]. It is worth noting that TTP is characterized by small vessels thrombosis only (brain, kidney, skin), without a large blood vessel involvement.

Heparin-induced thrombocytopenia (HIT) is a complex clinical syndrome in which individuals sensitized to heparin may develop thrombocytopenia that may be associated with severe thromboembolic events [49]. The clinical manifestations are associated to antibodies directed against epitope/s formed by complexes between heparin or other glycosaminoglycans and platelet factor 4 (PF4) that can be expressed also on the endothelial cell membranes [38]. Antibodies from patients with HIT activate microvascular endothelial cells, while interaction with macrovascular endothelium occurred only after the cells had been pre-activated with TNFα

[37].

It is likely that within the large family of antibodies reactive with common endothelial antigens, antibodies specific for much more differential structures do exist and probably contribute to the differential clinical manifestation.

5. AECA HETEROGENEITY AND FUNCTIONAL EFFECTS

Antibody binding to endothelial cells have biological effects that have been extensively investigated in *in vitro* studies and in some *in vivo* experimental models (reviewed in [3]). Again, a huge heterogeneity was reported regarding the final phenotypic and/or functional modifications of the cells.

Although debated, some reports showed that AECA are able to fix complement (C') in primary and secondary vasculitis. In Kawasaki disease (KD) and Hemolytic uremic syndrome (HUS) a C'-dependent cytotoxicity was found on cytokine-activated (IFNγ, IL-1α/β, and TNFα) endothelial cells only. This finding points out that even C' fixation is heterogeneous among AECA and that a modulation of the endothelial phenotype may be necessary in some cases (reviewed in [3]). On the other hand, Fcγ receptor positive mononuclear cells can lyse endothelial monolayers sensitized by SSc or WG AECA-positive sera or their IgG fractions in an antibody dependent cellular cytotoxicity (ADCC). However, not all the sera displayed such an activity and there was no correlation with the antibody titres. An ADCC phenomenon has also been found with AECA positive sera from patients who received allografts (reviewed in [3]). Interestingly, SSc whole sera or IgG were shown to induce endothelial apoptosis [50] even in the presence of NK cells potentially able to mediate an ADCC [51]. It is not clear what conditions are able to shift the AECA effect from a cytotoxicity towards an apoptosis, but, once again these data stressed the heterogeneity of the antibody-mediated effects.

In strong contrast with the induction of a cell death, several groups recently demonstrated that both polyclonal as well as monoclonal AECA induce an endothelial activation in *in vitro* studies. Endothelial activation has been evaluated as the induction of a pro-adhesive and a pro-inflammatory as well as a pro-coagulant phenotype (reviewed in [3]). Several unrelated pathological conditions have been shown to reproduce such an activation and recent data focused on the pivotal role of the NFkB but not of Junk system in sustaining the cell response (Refs. [48, 52], Meroni in preparation). It is still to be investigated whether additional or alternative signalling pathways are involved by AECA from different diseases. Moreover, a murine AECA monoclonal antibody (mAb) derived from animals with an experimentally induced autoimmune vasculitis gave comparable results [53]. In some cases, endothelial activation has been shown only after cytokine (TNFα) treatment further stressing the AECA heterogeneity [47, 51].

Finally, AECA from APS or KD sera have been shown to affect endothelial cell migration *in vitro*, providing an additional biological effect to the above list [54].

6. CONCLUSIONS

The family of anti-endothelial cell antibodies includes antibodies directed against different antigens and able to mediate different functional effects on the cells. The assays that detect the whole AECA activity probably weaken the final message in the clinical practice. A similar situation is well known for anti-nuclear antibodies detected by indirect immunofluorescence in comparison to the identification of the single anti-nuclear antigen/antibody systems by more specific techniques. A more detailed analysis of the AECA activity could offer much sounder information from both a diagnostic and a prognostic point of view in spite of their heterogeneity.

REFERENCES

1. Shan H, Goldman J, Cunto G, Manupello J, Chaiken I, Cines DB, Silberstein LE. Heterogeneity of anti-phospholipid and anti-endothelial cell antibodies. J Autoimmun. 1998;11:651–660.

2. Praprotnik S, Blank M, Meroni PL, Rozman B, Eldor A, Shoenfeld Y. Classification of antiendothelial cell antibodies to antibodies against micro and macrovascular endothelial cell: is it practical? (submitted).

3. Meroni PL. Endothelial cell antibodies (AECA) from a laboratory curiosity to another useful autoantibody. In: Y. Shoenfeld ed. The Decade of Autoimmunity. Amsterdam: Elsevier Science 1999;285–294.

4. Belzina C, Cohen Tervaert JW. Specificity, pathogenicity, and clinical value of antiendothelial cell antibodies. Semin Arthritis Rheum 1997;27:98–109.

5. Vismara A, Meroni PL, Tincani A, Harris EN, Barcellini W, Brucato A, Khamashta MA, Hughes GRV, Zanussi C, Balestrieri G. Antiphospholipid antibodies and endothelial cells. Clin Exp Immunol 1988;74:247–253.

6. Cervera R, Khamashta MA, Font J, Ramirez J, D'Cruz D, Montalban J, Lopez-Soto A, Asherson RA, Ingelmo M, Hughes GRV. Anti-endothelial cell antibodies in patients with the antiphospholipid syndrome. Autoimmunity 1991;11:1–6.

7. Lie JT. Vasculitis in the antiphospholipid syndrome: culprit or consort? J Rheumatol 1994;21:397–399.

8. Ferraro G, Meroni PL, Tincani A, Sinico A, Barcellini W, Radice A, Gregorini G, Froldi M, Borghi MO, Balestrieri G. Anti-endothelial cell antibodies in patients with Wegener's granulomatosis and micropolyarteritis. Clin Exp Immunol 1990;79:47–53.

9. Frampton G, Jayne DR, Perry GJ, Lockwood CM, Cameron JS. Autoantibodies to endothelial cells and neutrophil cytoplasmic antigens in systemic vasculitis. Clin Exp Immunol 1990;82:227–232.

10. Savage COS, Pottinger BE, Gaskin G, Lokwood CM, Pusey CD, Pearson JD. Vascular damage in Wegener's granulomatosis and microscopic polyarteritis. Presence of anti-endothelial cell antibodies and their relation to anti-neutrophil cytoplasmic antibodies. Clin Exp Immunol 1991;85:14–19.

11. Rosenbaum J, Pottinger BE, Woo P, Black CM, Louzou S, Byron MA, Pearson JD. Measurement and characterization of circulating anti-endothelial cell IgG in connective tissue diseases. Clin Exp Immunol 1988;72:450–456.

12. Pignone A, Scaletti C, Matucci-Cerinic M, Vasquez-Abad D, Meroni PL, Del Papa N, Falcini F, Generini S, Rothfield N, Cagnoni M. Anti-endothelial cell antibodies in systemic sclerosis: significant association with vascular involvement and alveolo-capillary impairment. Clin Exp Rheum 1998;16:527–532.

13. Salozhin KV, Le Tonqueze M, Saraux A, Nassonov EL, Dueymes M, Piette JC, Youinou P. Antiendothelial cell antibodies: useful markers of systemic sclerosis. Am J Med 1997;102:178–185.

14. Isenberg DA, Black C. ABC of rheumatology. Raynaud's phenomenon, scleroderma, and overlap syndromes. Br Med J 1995;310:795–798.

15. Triolo G, Accardo-Palumbo A, Carbone MC, Ferrante A, Casiglia D, Giardina E. IgG anti-endothelial cell antibodies (AECA) in type I diabetes mellitus; induction of adhesion molecule expression in cultured endothelial cells. Clin Exp Immunol 1998;111:491–496.

16. Wangel AG, Kontianen S, Scenini T, Schlenzka A, Wangel D, Maenpaa J. Anti-endothelial cell antibodies in insulin-dependent diabetes mellitus. Clin Exp Immunol 1992;88:410–413.

17. Trojano M, Defazio G, Ricchiuti F, De Salvia R, Livrea P. Serum IgG to brain microvascular endothelial cell in multiple sclerosis. J Neurol Sci 1996;143:107–113.

18. Meroni PL, Del Papa N, Raschi E, Panzeri P, Borghi MO, Tincani A, Balestrieri G, Khamashta MA, Hughes GR, Koike T, Krilis SA. Beta2-glycoprotein I as a 'cofactor' for anti-phospholipid reactivity with endothelial cells. Lupus (suppl 2)1998;7:44–47.

19. Miltenburg AM, Meijer-Paape ME, Weening JJ, Daha MR, van Es LA, van der Woude FJ. Induction of antibody-dependent cellular cytotoxicity against endothelial cells by renal transplantation. Transplantation 1989;48:681–688.

20. Perrey C, Brenchley PE, Johnson RW, Martin S. An association between antibodies specific for endothelial cells and renal transplant failure. Transpl Immunol 1998;6:101–106.

21. Ationu A, Collins A. Molecular cloning and expression of 56–58 KD antigen associated with transplant coronary artery disease. Biochem Biophys Res Commun 1997;236:716–718.

22. Collins AD, Ationu A. The role of anti-endothelial antibodies in the immunopathogenesis of transplant associated coronary artery disease. Int J Molec Medicine 1998;1:439–452.

23. Dunn MJ, Crisp SJ, Rose ML, Taylor PM, Yacoub MH. Anti-endothelial antibodies and coronary artery disease after cardiac transplantation. Lancet 1992;339:1566–1570.

24. Ferry BL, Welsh KI, Dunn MJ, Law D, Proctor J, Chapel H, Yacoub MH, Rose ML. Anti-cell surface endothelial antibodies in sera from cardiac and kidney transplant recipients: association with chronic rejection. Trans Immunol 1997;5:17–24.

25. Faulk WP, Rose M, Meroni PL, Del Papa N, Torry RJ, Labarrere CA, Busing K, Crisp SJ, Dunn MJ, Nelson DR. Antibodies to endothelial cells identify myocardial damage and predict development of coronary artery disease in patients with transplanted hearts. Hum Immunol 1999;60:826–832.

26. Ross R. The pathogenesis of atherosclerosis: a perspective for the 1990s. Nature 1993;362:801–809.

27. George J, Meroni PL, Gilburd B, Adler Y, Raschi E, Harats D, Shoenfeld Y. Antiendothelial cell antibodies in patients with coronary atherosclerosis. Immunology Letters in press.

28. Walkner TS, Triplett DA. Serologic characteristic of Rocky Mountain spotted fever. Appearance of antibodies reactive with endothelial cells and phospholipids, and factors that alter protein C activation and prostacyclin secretion. Clin Microbiol Infect Dis 1991;95:725–732.

29. Cacoub P, Ghillani P, Revelen R, Thibault V, Calvez V, Charlotte F, Musset L, Youinou P. Piette JC. Anti-endothelial cell auto-antibodies in hepatitis C virus mixed cryoglobulinemia. J Hepatol 1999;31:598–603.

30. Toyoda M, Petrosian A, Jordan SC. Immunological characterization of anti-endothelial cell antibodies induced by cytomegalovirus infection. Transplantation 1999;68:1311–1318.

31. Youinou P, Meroni PL, Khamashta MA, Shoenfeld Y. A need for standardization of the anti-endothelial cell antibody test. Immunology Today 1995;16:363–364.

32. Gobel U, Eichhorn J, Kettritz R, Briedigkeit L, Sima D, Lindshau C, Haller H, Luft FC. Disease activity and autoantibodies to endothelial cells in patients with Wegener's granulomatosis. Am J Kidney Dis 1996;28:186–194.

33. Chan TM, Frampton G, Jayne DR, Hoppy P, Perry GJ, Lockwood CM, Cameron JS. Clinical significance of anti-endothelial cell antibodies in systemic vasculitis: A longitudinal study comparing anti-endothelial cell antibodies and anti neutrophil cytoplasmic antibodies. Am J Kidney Dis 1993;22:387–392.

34. D'Cruz DP, Houssian FA, Ramirez G, Baguley E, McCutcheon J, Vianna J, Haga HJ, Swana GT, Khamashta MA, Taylor JC, Davies DR, Hughes GRV. Antibodies to endothelial cells in systemic lupus erythematosus: a potential marker for nephritis and vasculitis. Clin Exp Immunol 1991;85:254–261.

35. Heurkens AHM, Hiemstra PS, Lafeder GJM, Daha MR, Breedveld FC. Antiendothelial cell antibodies in patients with Rheumatoid Arthritis complicated by vasculitis. Clin Exp Immunol 1989;78:7–12.

36. Chan TM, Frampton G, Staines NA, Hobby P, Perry GJ, Cameron JS. Different mechanisms by which anti-DNA moabs bind to human endothelial cells and glomerular mesangial cells. Clin Exp Immunol 1992;88:68–74.

37. Chan TM, Yu PM, Tsang LC, Cheng IKP. Endothelial cell binding by human polyclonal anti-DNA antibodies: relationship to disease activity and endothelial functional alterations. Clin Exp Immunol 1995;100:506–513.

38. Blank M, Shoenfeld Y, Tavor S, Praprotnik S, Boffa MC, Weksler BB, Walenga JM, Amiral J, Eldor A. Anti-PF4/heparin antibodies from patients with heparin-induced thrombocytopenia cause direct activation of microvascular endothelial cell. Blood (in press).

39. Meroni PL, Raschi E, Testoni C, Borghi MO. Anti-endothelial antibodies (AECA): characterization and pathogenetic role. Clin Exp Immunol (suppl)2000;120:4–5.

40. Taekema-Roelvinik MEJ, Daha MR. P2: Proteinase 3 is not expressed by but interacts with endothelial cells; relevance for vasculitis. Clin Exp Immunol (suppl 1)2000;120:3–4.

41. Revelen R, Bordron A, Dueymes M, Youinou P, Arvieux J. False positivity in a cyto-ELISA for anti-endothelial cell antibodies caused by heterophile antibodies to bovine serum proteins. Clin Chemistry 2000;46:273–278.

42. Rosenberg RD, Aird WC. Vascular-Bed Specific hemostasis and hypercoagulable states. New Engl J Med 1999;340:1555–1564.

43. Tsukada N, Tanaka Y, Miyagi K, Yanagisawa N, Okano A. Autoantibodies to each protein fraction extracted from cerebral endothelial cell membrane in the sera of patients with multiple sclerosis. J Neurology 1989;24:41–46.

44. Connolly AM, Chez MG, Pestronk A, Arnold TS, Mehta S, Deuel PK. Serum autoantibodies to brain in Landau-Kleffner syndrome variant, autism, and other neurological disorders. J Pediatr 1999;134:607–613.

45. Cervera R, Navarro M, Lopez-Soto A, Cid MC, Font J, Esparza J, Reverter JC, Monteagudo J, Ingelmo M, Marquez AU. Antibodies to endothelial cell in Behçet's disease: cell- binding heterogeneity and association with clinical activity. Ann Rheum Dis 1994;53:265–267.

46. Praprotnik S, Blank M, Tavor S, Eldor A, Weksler B, Shoenfeld Y. Anti endothelial cell antibodies (AECA) from patients with thrombotic thrombocytopenic purpura activate small vessels endothelial cells 2000 Int Immunol (in press).

47. Hill MB, Phipps JL, Hughes P, Greaves M. Anti-endothelial cell antibodies in primary antiphospholipid syndrome and SLE: pattern of reactivity with membrane antigens on microvascular and umbilical venous cell membranes. Br J Haematol 1998;103:416–421.

48. Blank M, Krause I, Goldkorn T, Praprotnik S, Livneh A, Langevitz P, Kaganovsky E, Morgenstern S, Cohen S, Barak V, Eldor A, Wekdler B, Shoenfeld Y. Monoclonal anti-endothelial cell antibodies from a patient with Takayasu arteritis activate endothelial cells from large vessels. Arthritis Rheum 1999;42:1421–1432.

49. Cines DB, Tomaski A, Tannenbaum S. Immune endothelial-cell injury in heparin-associated thrombocytopenia. N Engl J Med. 1987;316:581–589.

50. Bordron A, Dueymes M, Levy Y, Jamin C, Leroy JP, Piette JC, Shoenfeld Y, Youinou P. The binding of some human antiendothelial cell antibodies induces endothelial cell apoptosis. J Clin Invest 1999;101:2029–2035.

51. Sgonc R, Gruschwitz MS, Boeck G, Sepp N, Gruber J, Wick G. Endothelial cell apoptosis in systemic sclerosis is induced by antiendothelial cell antibody-dependent cellular cytotoxicity via CD95. Abstract. 2nd Int. Workshop on endothelial cells. Innsbruck, April, 2000.

52. Yazici ZA, Raschi E, Patel A, Testoni C, Borghi MO, Graham AM, Meroni PL, Lindsey N. Human monoclonal anti-endothelial cell IgG derived from B lymphocytes of a patient suffering from Systemic Lupus Erythematosus binds to human endothelial cells and induces a pro-adhesive and a pro-inflammatory endothelial phenotype in vitro. Submitted.

53. Levy Y, Gilburd B, George J, Del Papa N, Mallone R, Damianovich M, Blank M, Radice A, Renaudineau Y, Youinou P, Wiik A, Malavasi F, Meroni PL, Shoenfeld Y. Characterization of murine monoclonal anti-endothelial cell antibodies (AECA) produced by idiotypic manipulation with human AECA. Int Immunol 1998;10:861–868.

54. Lanir N, Zilberman M, Yron I, Tennenbaum G, Shechter Y, Brenner B. Reactivity patterns of anti-phospholipid antibodies and endothelial cells: effect of antiendothelial antibodies on cell migration. J Lab Clin Med 1998;131:548–556.

55. Westphal JR, Boerbooms AT, Schalwijk CJM, Kwast H, De Weijert M, Jacob C, Vierwinden G, Ruiter DJ, Van de Putte LB, De Waal RM. Anti-endothelial cell antibodies in sera of patients with autoimmune diseases: Comparison between ELISA and FACS analysis. Clin Exp Immunol 1994;96:444–449.

56. Leung DYM. Kawasaki syndrome. Curr Opin Rheumatol 1993;5:41–50.

57. Tizard EJ, Baguley E, Hughes GR, Dillon MJ. Antiendothelial cell antibodies detected by a cellular based ELISA in Kawasaki disease Arch Dis Childhood 1991;66:189–192.

58. Kaneko K, Savage CO, Pottinger BE, Shah V, Pearson JD. Antiendothelial cell antibodies can be cytotoxic to endothelial cells without cytokine pre-stimulation and correlate with ELISA antibody measurement in Kawasaki disease. Clin Exp Immunol 1994;98:264–269.

59. Fujieda M, Oishi N, Kurashige T. Antibodies to endothelial cells in Kawasaki disease lyse endothelial cell without pre-treatment. Clin Exp Immunol 1997;107:120–126.

60. Eichhorn J, Sima D, Thiele B, Lindschau C, Turowski A, Schmidt H, Schneider W, Haller H, Luft FC. Antiendothelial cell antibodies in Takayasu arteritis. Circulation 1996;94:2396–2401.

61. Edelsten C, D'Cruz D, Hughes GRV, Grahm EM. Antiendothelial cell antibodies in retinal vasculitis. Curr Eye Res 1992;11:203–208.

62. Eichhorn J, Sima D, Lindschau C, Turowski A, Schmidt H, Schneider W, Haller H, Luft FC. Anti-endothelial cell antibodies in thromboangiitis obliterans. Am J Med Sci 1998;315:17–23.

63. Li SJ, Liu MF, Lei HY. Characterisation of antiendothelial cell antibodies in the patient with systemic lupus erythematosus: potential marker for disease activity. Clin Immunol Immunopath 1996;79:211–216.

64. Van der Zee JM, Miltenburgh AM, Siegert CE, Daha MR, Breedveld FC. Anti-endothelial cell antibodies in systemic lupus erythematosus: enhanced antibody binding to interleukin-1 stimulated endothelium. Int Arch Allergy Immunol 1994;104:131–136.

65. McGrae KR, De Michele A, Samuels P, Roth D, Kuo A, Meg QH, Rauch J, Cines DA. Detection of endothelial cell reactive immunoglobulin in patients with anti-phospholipid antibodies. Br J Haematol 1991;79:595–605.

66. Salih AM, Nixon NB, Dawes PT, Mattey DL. Soluble adhesion molecules and anti-endothelial cell antibodies in patients with rheumatoid arthritis complicated by peripheral neuropathy. J Rheumatol 1999;26:551–555.

67. Cervera R, Ramirez G, Fernandez-Sola G, D'Cruz D, Casademont J, Gran JM et al. Antibodies to endothelial cells in dermatomyositis associated with interstitial lung disease. Brit Med J 1991;302:880–881.

68. Leung DYM, Moake JL, Havens PL, Kim M, Pober JS. Lytic anti-endothelial cell antibodies in haemolytic uremic syndrome. Lancet 1988;2:183–186.

69. Stevens TRJ, Harley SL, Groom JS, Cambridge G, Leaker B, Blake DR, Rampton DS. Anti-endothelial cell antibodies in inflammatory bowel disease. Dig Dis Sci 1993;38:426–432.

70. Yap HK, Sakai RS, Bahn L, Rappaport V, Woo KT, Anathuraman V, Lim CH, Chiang GS, Jordan SC. Anti-vascular endothelial cell antibodies in patients with IgA nephropathy: Frequency and clinical significance. Clin Immunol Immunopathol 1988;49:450–462.

71. Jones DB, Wallace R, Frier BM. Vascular endothelial cell antibodies in diabetic patients: Association with diabetic retinopathy. Diabetes Care 1992;15:552–555.

72. Rappaport VJ, Hirata G, Yap KH, Giordan SC. Antivascular endothelial cell antibodies in severe preeclampsia. Am J Obstet Gynecol 1990;162:138–146.

73. Frostegård J, Wu R, Gillis-Haegerstrand C, Lemne C, de Faire U. Antibodies to endothelial cells in borderline hypertension. Circulation 1998;98:1092–1098.

Atherosclerosis and Autoimmunity
Y. Shoenfeld, D. Harats and G. Wick, editors

The Aspect of Anti-Proteinase 3 Antibodies as AECA

Werner-J. Mayet and Andreas Schwarting

First Medical Dept., University of Mainz, Germany

1. INTRODUCTION

A few years ago only sparse data regarding the complex physiology of endothelial cells were available. As endothelial cells are in permanent contact with circulating antibodies, immunocomplexes, complement and other effectors of cell-mediated immunity play a key-role in the immunopathogenesis, especially of vasculitides.

Since their first description by Lindqvist and Osterland [1] and Tan and Pearson [2] anti-endothelial cell antibodies (AECA) have been found in connective tissue diseases and vasculitides. Currently it is discussed that AECA may play an important role during vessel destruction.

The target antigens of AECA are not fully characterized yet. As different associations of AECA with different diseases like systemic lupus erythematosus, Kawasaki disease, haemolytic uremic syndrome and vasculitides have been described a heterogeneous specificity has been discussed.

In a review of Meroni et al. [3] the authors report that AECA bind to a variety of antigenic structures in the membranes of endothelial cells. Direct pathogenic effects of AECA in several inflammatory disorders, however, are still a matter of debate.

The discovery of anti-neutrophil cytoplasmic antibodies (ANCA) has caused a great impact on the diagnostic procedure and clinical observation of systemic necrotizing vasculitides like Wegener's granulomatosis (WG), microscopic polyangiitis, Churg-Strauss syndrome and necrotizing glomerulonephritis.

There is persuasive circumstantial evidence for a pathogenic role of ANCA in ANCA-related vasculitides involving both neutrophils and vascular endothelial cells. The major stepthrough in the pathogenesis of ANCA related diseases was the identification of proteinase-3 (PR-3) as the main target antigen of ANCA in Wegener's Granulomatosis.

PR-3 has been described as a constituent of the azurophil granules of neutrophils [4–6]. It is a lysosomal protein identical with myeloblastin and a differentiation factor for myeloid precursor cells. Other functions are cleavage of elastin and other proteins of microorganisms and generation of chemotactic activities by forming alpha 1-proteinase inhibitor complexes [7].

PR-3 is physiologically inhibited by alpha-1-antitrypsin [8]. After fusion of alpha-granules with the plasma membrane during activation of neutrophils the cells release PR-3 [9]. This process can be induced by TNF-alpha *in vitro* [10].

Genes encoding PR-3, azurocidin and neutrophil elastase are closely clustered in this sequence within 50 kb of genomic DNA and have the same transcriptional orientation. The genes show the same exon-intron organization as neutrophil cathepsin G, mast cell chymase 1 and the lymphocyte serine proteases, granzymes A, B and H. The AZU-PR-3-NE gene cluster was mapped to the telomeric region on the short arm of human chromosome 19 (19p13,3) [11].

2. EXPRESSION OF PR-3 IN HUMAN ENDOTHELIAL CELLS

Endothelial cells (EC) are considered a possible target of an immune-mediated aggression during vasculitis due to their functional characteristics and

Table 1. Effects of anti-PR-3 antibodies on human endothelial cells

- Upregulation of E-Selectin
- Upregulation of VCAM-1
- Upregulation of ICAM-1
- Induction of endothelial cytotoxicity
- Induction of leakage response
- Induction of endothelial IL-8
- Induction of phosphoinositide hydrolysis
- Induction of tissue factor activity

because they are in direct contact with circulating humoral and cellular immune effectors [12].

During the past years a body of data regarding interaction of anti-PR-3 antibodies, with human EC (i. e. AECA properties of ANCA) became available (see Table 1).

Abbott et al. showed that a monoclonal antibody against the C-ANCA antigen and IgG-fractions of patient's sera specifically bind to endothelial cells [13].

In another study 59% of 168 ANCA positive patients revealed AECA-activity [14]. Pretreatment of cells with TNF-alpha or IFN-gamma led to an enhanced binding of antibodies.

An important prerequisite of these interactions is the expression of PR-3 in EC.

Until now it is still a matter of debate whether there is endogenous expression of endothelial PR-3 or exogenous PR-3 attached to EC, subsequently being recognized by ANCA.

In 1993 we were able to identify PR-3 in human EC using polymerase chain reaction (PCR) and affinity-purified anti-PR-3 antibodies as probes. We were also able to show a time-dependent translocation of PR-3 from the perinuclear region into the cytoplasm of EC and a transient membrane expression triggered by cytokines like TNF-alpha and IL-1 [15].

Priming of human umbilical vein endothelial cells (HUVEC) with TNF-alpha induced endothelial upregulation of PR-3 message and surface expression of this antigen as measured by cyto-ELISA

with a maximum occurrence after 2 h [16].

Translocation of PR-3 in EC could be characterized as an active process depending on protein synthesis.

TNF-alpha-induced membrane expression of PR-3 could be blocked with the RNA synthesis inhibitor actinomycin D, the protein kinase C (PKC) and proteinase A (PKA) inhibitor staurosporine, the specific PKA inhibitor calphostin C, the c-AMP-dependent PKA inhibitor KT5720 and the tyrosine kinase inhibitor genistein in a dose dependent manner. The effect of calphostin C was the most significant.

Pretreatment of cells with PMA for 48 h led to a downregulation of PR-3 expression. This effect could be overridden by TNF-alpha stimulation, i.e. TNF-alpha-induced membrane expression of PR-3 was resistant to down-regulation of PKC [17].

Meanwhile other authors were not able to detect PR-3 expression in EC [18, 19] performing PCR-analysis. One reason of this discrepancy, however, could be the dependency on different culture conditions *in vitro*. For this reason we studied the regulation of PR-3 mRNA-expression in EC under various culture conditions (different matrices, cytokine stimulation and oxygen restriction) by RT-PCR-technique.

For sufficient detectable PR-3 message with RT-PCR or protein with ELISA two conditions proofed to be essential: stimulation with TNF-alpha and growing EC on most natural matrices i. e. ECM (physiological extracellular matrix) and Matrigel® (extracted from basal membranes of Engelbreth-Holm-Swarm mouse tumor). TNF-alpha primed cells grown on physiologically composed matrices yielded the strongest expression of PR-3 mRNA [20].

Recently another mechanism of interaction of PR-3 with EC has been proposed [21].

The authors postulated that PR-3 is not expressed endogenously but exogenous PR-3 would bind to EC. They were able to demonstrate binding of digoxigenin-labelled PR-3 to EC cultured on cover-slips.

Digoxigenin-labeled PR-3 binds to HUVEC. Saturation was reached at 40 mg/ml. Binding of PR-3 to HUVEC was only detectable following detachment of the cells with PBS and 20 mM EDTA and was strongly reduced after treatment

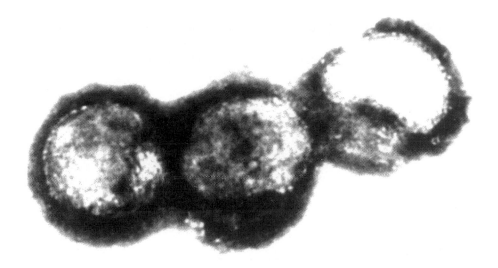

Figure 1. Cytospin of HUVEC and hybridization with PR-3 antisense probe (Digoxigenin-labelled). Specific PR-3 expression (× 1000).

with trypsin or dispase.

Affinity precipitation of HUVEC membrane proteins revealed a band of 111 kD under non-reducing conditions and bands at 55 and 63 kD under reducing conditions [21].

The authors reasoned that an endothelial membrane protein could be involved in the binding of PR-3. The nature of this putative receptor, however, remains to be elucidated.

3. ANTI-PR-3 ANTIBODIES AS AECA

When PR-3 at the surface of EC is accessible for ANCA after membrane translocation of endogenously expressed or attached exogenous PR-3, anti-PR-3 antibodies in patients with WG and other vasculitides can react as AECA. AECA could then exert specific effects on EC and modulate their state of activation via signal transduction events. During the last years, an increasing body of data became available regarding this issue.

Several authors have reported AECA in patients with WG. There are also target antigens different from ANCA [22, 23]. Performing immunoprecipitation of radiolabeled surface membrane proteins from HUVEC followed by Western blotting showed that WG patients displayed a constant precipitation pattern of 180, 155, 125, 68 and 25 kDa proteins

[24, 25].

In 1993 we were able to show that incubation of EC with affinity-purified anti-PR-3 antibodies led to a marked increase of neutrophil adhesion with a peak after 4 h and a rapid decrease after 8 h. Anti-PR-3 antibody induced adhesion occurred via the adhesion molecule E-selectin as confirmed by blocking experiments with specific antibodies to adhesion molecules. Anti-PR-3 antibodies induce E-selectin expression after binding to their target antigen [26].

Other experiments showed that incubation of HUVEC with anti-PR-3 antibodies led to a marked increase of endothelial VCAM-1 expression with a peak after 8 h. Increased adhesion of T-lymphocytes to HUVEC after binding of anti-PR-3 antibodies to their antigen could be confirmed by performing adherence assays. This effect could be inhibited by antibodies to VLA-4 [27].

It also has been shown that anti-PR-3 antibodies are able to induce expression of endothelial ICAM-1 [28].

Another important issue regarding a direct effect in immunopathogenesis of anti-PR3 antibodies in vasculitides is whether this subgroup of AECA could exert any direct effect on EC leading to apoptosis or cytolysis.

Purified antibodies to PR-3 display a lytic activity against EC with TNF-alpha with the help of

223

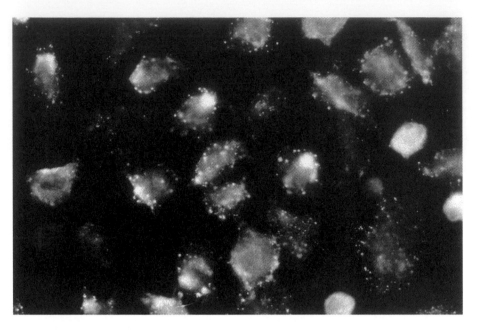

Figure 2. Indirect immunofluorescence of unfixed HUVEC treated with TNF-α (2 h). Reaction of affinity-purified anti-PR-3 antibodies with the target antigen translocated into the membrane.

cytokine-primed neutrophils as measured in a Cr-release assay.

PR-3 antibody-induced cytotoxicity required (i) expression of PR-3 on the surface of TNF-alpha-treated endothelial cells and (ii) co-cultivation of cytokine-primed neutrophils [29]. Therefore antibodies to PR-3 have cytotoxic effects on human EC.

About 100% specific cytotoxicity occurred after 4 h and was independent of complement. Cytotoxic effects were inhibited by coincubation with unprimed neutrophils or preincubation of PR-3 antibodies with purified antigen.

These data give a hint at a PR-3 antibody-mediated mechanism of endothelial injury via antibody-dependent cellular cytotoxicity in WG.

Meanwhile it is obvious that AECA with anti-PR-3 specificity can activate EC *in vitro*. Sibelius et al. were able to show that primed EC responded to low concentrations of anti-PR-3 antibodies (25 ng – 2.5 mg/ml), but not to control immunoglobulins, with pronounced and dose-dependent phosphoinositide hydrolysis, as assessed by accumulation of inositol phosphates. The signaling response peaked after 20 min in parallel with the appearance of marked prostacyclin and platelet-activating factor

synthesis. The $F(ab)^2$ fragment of anti-PR-3 antibodies was equally potent as anti-PR-3 antibodies themselves. Disrupture of the endothelial F-actin content by botulinum C2 toxin to avoid antigen-antibody internalization did not affect the response.

The authors conclude that anti-PR-3 antibodies are potent inductors of the preformed phosphoinositide hydrolysis-related signal transduction pathway in human endothelial cells [16].

De Bandt et al. report another effect of anti-PR-3 antibodies [30].

Tissue factor (TF) activity was generated in anti-PR-3-stimulated EC as shown by a chromogenic test. TF messenger RNA was found in anti-PR-3-stimulated cells as detected by reverse transcriptase-polymerase chain reaction. TF expression reached maximum levels 12 hours after exposure to the anti-PR-3 antibodies and did not require complement.

TF mRNA expression was inhibited by cycloheximide suggesting a requirement for protein synthesis. Thus, anti-PR-3 antibodies induce sequential expression of IL-1 alpha mRNA and TF mRNA, as well as their corresponding proteins.

In conclusion, anti-PR-3 antibodies can be considered as AECA. Although expression of the target antigen PR-3 in EC is still discussed controversially an increasing body of data regarding interaction of anti-PR-3 antibodies with EC became available. During this interaction EC can be activated indicating an important role of anti-PR-3 antibodies in the pathogenesis of ANCA related vasculitides.

As endothelial cells derived from large vessels differ from microvascular endothelium in terms of growing in cell culture or antigenic properties, further investigations involving various EC apart of HUVEC are required.

REFERENCES

1. Lindqvist KJ, Osterland CK. Human antibodies to vascular endothelium. Clin Exp Immunol 1971;9:753–760.
2. Tan EM, Pearson CM. Rheumatic disease sera reactive with capillaries in the mouse kidney. Arthritis Rheum 1972;15:23–28.
3. Meroni PL, Youinou P. Endothelial cell antibodies. In Peter J, Shoenfeld Y, eds. Amsterdam: Elsevier Science. Autoantibodies 1996;245–248.
4. Niles JL, McCluskey RT, Ahmad MF, Arnaout MA. Wegener's Granulomatosis autoantigen is a novel serine proteinase. Blood 1989;74:1888–1893.
5. Goldschmeding R., Van der Schoot CE, Ten Bokkel Huinink D, Hack CE, van den Ende ME, Kallenberg CGM, von dem Borne AEGKR. Wegener's Granulomatosis autoantibodies identify a novel diisopropylfluorophosphate-binding protein in the lysosomes of normal human neutrophils. J Clin Invest 1989;84:1577–1587.
6. Lüdemann J, Utecht B, Gross WL. Anti-neutrophil cytoplasm antibodies in Wegeners Granulomatosis recognize an elastinolytic enzyme. J Exp Med 1990;171:357–362.
7. Gross WL, Csernok E, Flesch BK. "Classic" anti-neutrophil cytoplasmic autoantibodies (cANCA). "Wegener's autoantigen" and their immunopathogenic role in Wegener's granulomatosis. J Autoimmun 1993;6:171–184.
8. Dolman KM, Van den Weil BA, Kam CM, Abbink JJ, Hack CE, Sonnenberg A, Powers JC, von dem Borne AEGKR, Goldschmeding R. Determination of proteinase 3/alpha1-antitrypsin complexes in inflammatory fluids. FEBS Lett 1992;314:117–121.
9. Calafat J, Goldschmeding R, Ringeling PL, Janssen H, van der Schoot CE. In situ localization by double-labeling immunoelectron microscopy of anti-neutrophil cytoplasmic autoantibodies in neutrophils and monocytes. Blood 1990;75:242–250.
10. Charles LA, Caldas MLR, Falk RJ, Terrell RS, Jennette JC. Antibodies against granule proteins activate neutrophils in vitro. J Leuk Biol 1991;50:539–546.
11. Jenne DE. Structure of the azurocidin, proteinase 3 and neutrophil elastase genes. Implication for inflammation and vasculitis. Am J Respir Crit Care Med 1994;150:147–154.
12. Cines DB, Lyss AP, Reeber M, Bina M, De Horatius RJ. Presence of complement-fixing anti-endothelial cell antibodies in systemic lupus erythematosus. J Clin Invest 1984;73:611–625.
13. Abbott F, Jones S, Lockwood CM, Rees AJ. Autoantibodies to glomerular antigens in patients with Wegener's granulomatosis. Nephrol Dialys Transplant 1989;4:1–8.
14. Savage CO, Pottinger BE, Gaskin G, Lockwood CM, Pusey CD, Pearson JD. Vascular damage in Wegener's granulomatosis and microscopic polyarteriitis. Presence of anti-endothelial cell antibodies and their relation to anti-neutrophil cytoplasm antibodies. Clin Exp Immunol 1991;85:14–19.
15. Mayet WJ, Csernok E, Szymkowiak C, Gross WL, Meyer zum Büschenfelde KH. Human endothelial cells express proteinase 3, the target antigen of anti-cytoplasmic antibodies in Wegener's Granulomatosis. Blood 1993;82:1221–1229.
16. Sibelius U, Hattar K, Schenkel A, Noll T, Csernok E, Gross WL, Mayet WJ, Piper HM, Seeger W, Grimminger F. Wegener's granulomatosis: anti-proteinase 3 antibodies are potent inductors of human endothelial cell signaling and leakage response. J Exp Med 1998;187:497–503.
17. Mayet WJ, Schwarting A, Orth T, Sibelius U Hattar K, Meyer zum Büschenfelde KH. Signal transduction pathways of membrane expression of proteinase 3 (PR-3) in human endothelial cells. Eur J Clin Invest 1997;27:893–899.
18. King WJ, Adu D, Daha MR, Brooks CJ, Radford DJ, Pall AA, Savage CO. Endothelial cells and renal epithelial cells do not express the Wegener's autoantigen proteinase 3. Clin Exp Immunol 1995;102:98–105.
19. Pendergraft WF, Alcorta DA, Segelmark M, Yang JJ, Tuttle R, Jennette JC, Falk RJ, Preston GA. ANCA antigens, proteinase 3 and myeloperoxidase, are not expressed in endothelial cells. Kidney Int 2000;57:1981–1990.
20. Mayet WJ. Expression of proteinase 3 by endothelial and other non-myeloid cells; relevance for vasculitis. Clin Exp Immunol 2000;120:2.
21. Taekema-Roelvink MEJ, Daha MR. Proteinase 3 is not expressed by but interacts with endothelial cells; relevance for vasculitis. Clin Exp. Immunol 2000;120:3–4.
22. Del Papa N, Gambini D, Meroni PL. Anti-endothelial antibodies and autoimmune diseases. Clin Rev Allergy 1994;12:275–286.

23. Youinou P, Meroni PL, Khamashta MA, Shoenfeld Y. A need for standardization of the anti-endothelial cell antibody test. Immunology Today 1995;16:363–364.

24. Del Papa N, Conforti G, Gambini D, La Rosa L, Tincani A, D'Cruz D, Khamashta M, Hughes GR, Balestrieri G, Meroni PL. Characterization of endothelial surface proteins recognized by anti-endothelial antibodies in primary and secondary autoimmune vasculitis. Clin Immunol Immunopathol 1994;70:211–216.

25. Ferraro G, Meroni PL, Tincani A, Sinicio A, Barcellini W, Radice A, Gregorini G, Froldi M., Borghi MO, Balestrieri G. Anti endothelial cell antibodies in patients with Wegener's granulomatosis and micropolyarteriitis. Clin Exp Immunol 1990;79:47–53.

26. Mayet WJ, Meyer zum Büschenfelde KH. Antibodies to proteinase 3 increase adhesion of neutrophils to human endothelial cells. Clin Exp Immunol 1993;94:440–446.

27. Mayet WJ, Schwarting A, Orth T, Duchmann R, Meyer zum Büschenfelde KH. Antibodies to proteianse 3 mediate expression of vascular cell adhesion molecule-1 (VCAM-1). Clin Exp Immunol 1996;103:259–267.

28. De Bandt M, Meyer O, Hakim J, Pasquier C. Antibodies to proteinase 3 mediate expression of intercellular adhesion molecule-1 (ICAM-1, CD 54). Br J Rheumatol 1997;36:839–846.

29. Mayet WJ, Schwarting A, Meyer zum Büschenfelde KH. Cytotoxic effects of antibodies to proteianse 3 (C-ANCA) on human endothelial cells. Clin Exp Immunol 1994;97:458–465.

30. De Bandt M, Ollivier V, Meyer O, Babin-Chevaye C, Khechai F, de Prost D, Hakim J, Pasquier C. Induction of interleukin-1 and subsequent tissue factor by anti-proteinase 3 antibodies in human umbilical vein endothelial cells. Arthritis Rheum 1997;40:2030–2038.

Atherosclerosis and Autoimmunity
Y. Shoenfeld, D. Harats and G. Wick, editors

Anti-Endothelial-Cell Antibodies (AECA) in Systemic Lupus Erythematosus: Clinical Relevance

Norbert Sepp and Gerlinde Obermoser

Department of Dermatology, University of Innsbruck, Austria

Antibodies to endothelial cells (AECA), first described by Lindqvist and Osterland [1] and Tan et al. [2] using kidney sections as substrates, are a heterogenous group of low
affinity autoantibodies directed against a variety of endothelial epitopes.

Since the last decade, there is a considerable renaissance in research on AECA [3]. Not surprisingly, consensus exists about the high prevalence of AECA in autoimmune disorders, in particular in systemic lupus erythematosus (SLE) [4].

AECA react with a variety of endothelial epitopes that have been partially characterized by immunoblotting techniques with whole endothelial cell extracts [5]. Analysis of the endothelial cell surface membrane antigens reacting with SLE sera indentified several constitutive endothelial proteins with a molecular weight ranging from 25 to 200 kDa [6–8]. Most of these proteins are also found in AECA from primary vasculits such as Wegener's granulomatosis and microscopic polyarteriitis [6], however some endothelial antigens are recognized by SLE sera only [6]. Anti-DNA and anti-ß2 glycoprotein I antibodies also show anti-endothelial activity due to their ability to recognize their counterpart molecules adhered on the endothelial cell surface [5, 9]. Using a human endothelial cell complementary DNA expression library it has been found that most of the AECA -positive SLE sera reacted with a ribosomal protein [3]. With regard to possible clinical associations it is interesting that Li et al. [10] found in patients suffering from lupus nephritis, vasculitis and hypocomplementemia IgG-AECAs

against a 66 kDa membrane antigen [10], those with thrombocytopenia had IgG-AECAs against a 55 kDa antigen, those with pleuritis had IgG-AECAs against a 18 kDa antigen [10].

Furthermore differences in both the pattern of antibody binding and band intensity have been demonstrated in endothelial cells deriving from human umbilical endothelial cells (HUVEC) and an immortalized human microvascular endothelial cell line (HMEC-1) [11, 38].

The prevalence of AECA in SLE reported in the literature varies from study to study. The IgG -AECA positivity ranged from 19–84% of SLE sera when determined by ELI SA and 72 to 88% by immunoblotting, suggestive of a higher sensitivity of immunoblotting techniques in the search for AECA antibodies [10, 12, 13]. The prevalence of AECA in SLE sera seems to be higher in those patients suffering from cutaneous vasculitis, the Raynaud phenomen, and lupus nephropathy [14, 15].

With regard to their clinical use, AECA levels parallel remission of lupus nephritis and sometimes become undetectable under immunosuppressive therapy. However no correlation was found between AECA and particular epitopes and certain disease manifestations [10].

AECAs may be a useful serological marker-independent on the presence of antibodies against native DNA and the Smith antigen (Sm), which is unaffected by therapy [16] to indicate a higher risk of lupus nephritis.

Sera obtained at the time of renal biopsy were positive for AECA in 81% of lupus nephritis patients versus 44% in SLE patients without renal involvement and in 10% of the healthy controls. The highest levels were detected in patients with diffuse proliferative glomerulonephritis, proteinuria/ the nephrotic syndrome [14] and also correlated with the Austin score activity index of glomerulonephritis [17]. This was independent on the detection of anti-double strand DNA antibodies, but correlated with elevated levels of circulating immune complexes. Similar results come from a study by Perry et al. [16].

In vitro, AECA-IgG from lupus sera was shown to induce upregulation of adhesion molecules and secretion of proinflammatory cytokines in endothelial cells. In accordance with these in vitro findings are in vivo reports of increased serum levels of soluble adhesion molecules in SLE patients [39, 40]. In fact, it is widely accepted that increased expression of cell surface adhesion molecules is followed by the release of their soluble forms into the circulation. These soluble forms of adhesion molecules are usually considered as an indirect evidence for the activation of different cell types including the endothelium. Increased interleukin 6 levels in active SLE may be related to an upregulated secretion of this cytokine following activation by AECA [18]. Therefore the binding of AECA to endothelial cell surfaces might transduce activation signals mediating both upregulation of adhesion molecules and cytokine secretion [19]. The specificity of AECA has been shown by the lack of endothelial modulation in the presence of IgG fractions from AECA-negative SLE sera.

Is there a relationship between anti-phospholipid antibodies and AECAs? These autoantibodies coexist in about one third of patients with non-organ specific autoimmune disorders [9]. They have in common the ability to activate human umbilical vein endothelial cells (HUVEC) as demonstrated by the increased expression of certain adhesion molecules (ICAM-1, VCAM-1, E-Selectin) [20].

The binding of AECA to endothelial cells was shown to be the first step leading to the transfer of anionic phopholipids such as phophatidylserine to the outer plasma membrane leaflet, as demonstrated by the binding of annexin V, and thereby initiating programmmed cell death [21, 22]. AECA induced apoptosis has in part replaced the previously predominating pathogenetic models of AECA by complement mediated or direct cytotoxic properties of

this class of autoantibodies. Using the anti-idiotype approach, Shoenfeld et al [23, 24] immunized mice with human IgG AECA, thereby generating murine AECA with the same binding and functional properties as their human counterpart in autoimmune diseases.

Over the past 40 years treatment of SLE has become more successful as reflected by a shift of the 5 years mortality rate approaching 50% in the 1950ies to a 10 years survival expectancy of SLE in the range of 90% today. However, prolonged survival of SLE patients has unmasked a number of formerly unknown complications; premature atherosclerotic cardiovascular disease. Rubin and coworkers [25] recognized the bimodal pattern of mortality in SLE: the early peak is associated with SLE activity whereas the second peak results, primarily, from complications of myocardial infarction and stroke. Although therapeutic regimens including corticosteroids may contribute to the pathogenesis of atherosclerosis in SLE patients , this is clearly not the only cause. Recent data suggests that stimulated arterial endothelium may play a role in the development of this late complication of SLE as well. By expressing adhesion molecules for monocytes (VCAM-1), arterial endothelium plays an active role in the cascade of events leading to atherosclerosis. Interaction of antiendothelial antibodies and stimulated T-cells with arterial endothelial cells, occupancy of the C1q receptors with immuncomplexes, may all contribute to the pathogenesis of atherosclerosis in patients with SLE [41–43].

Furthermore it has been recently appreciated that the enzyme sterol 27-hydroxylase plays a key role in the first line defense against atherosclerosis. This enzyme , highly expressed in arterial endothelium, catalyses the first step in the extrahepatic metabolism of cholesterol to 27-hydroxycholesterol: it is antiatherogenetic not only by suppression of smooth muscle proliferation, but also by diminishing foam cell formation by macrophages. Studies by Reis and coworkers [43] clearly demonstrate that immuncomplexes bound to the C1q receptor specifically downregulate the mRNA levels of sterol 27-hydroxylase both in arterial endothelial cells and in monocytes. However, an effect of antiendothelial cell antibodies on the expression of sterol-27 hydroxylase has not been tested. These studies show how immunological alterations common to SLE may have an influence on cholesterol metabolism and thereby leading to atherosclerosis.

The clinical spectrum of CNS affection by SLE encompasses a wide range from mild cognitive and affective dysfunction to more serious complications such as seizures, chorea, stroke, and myelopathy [26].

A number of – at present only for research purposes studied – antibodies and other serological markers have been investigated in this context. As for AECAs, they could be demonstrated in mice with neurological and behavioural defects after experimental induction of an anti-phospholipid syndrome [27]. A rise in AECA may be especially useful in suspected cerebral lupus since these patients can have completely normal C3 and anti-ds DNA levels [15].

Pulmonary hypertension is an increasingly recognized complication not only of scleroderma but also of SLE. Its association with the Raynaud phenomenon, anti-ribonucleoprotein and anti-cardiolipin antibodies is well established [18, 28]. Recently AECAs were demonstrated as an other serological marker in pulmonary hypertension, especially in association with digital vasculitis, Raynaud´s phenomenon or serositis suggesting that AECA may be involved in the pathogenesis of vascular injury leading to these manifestations. In vitro, AECA stimulate IL-6 release from EC, which has been associated with pulmonary hypertension in SLE [18, 29].

Correlation of skin changes in SLE with AECA is seen in digital vasculitis (causing nail fold or pulp infarcts, ulcers and/or splinter haemorrhages) and urticarial vasculitis [14, 36]. The Raynaud phenomenon was associated with high titres of AECA by several authors [10, 30].

Surprisingly arthritis – as the most common symptom of SLE and also an important clinical marker of disease activity – is not associated with the occurence of AECA [29].

There are only few reports on an association between serositis and AECA [10, 29].

The occurence of AECA is not limited to overt SLE, because antibodies reactive with endothelial cells have also been reported in women with hyperprolactinemia, a condition regarded as a predisposing condition to SLE [31].

SLE is largely a disease of women in their reproductive years; it may affect as many as 1 in 1000 young females [26].Consequently pregnancy in a lupus patient is of privotal interest to the clinican.

In principle, SLE can threat pregnancy in three different ways: (a) by a flare up in the mother, (b) by an increased risk of gestation-related disorders, and finally (c) by maternal autoantibodies translocated into the fetal circulation and thereby causing fetal endocarditis, hepatitis and thrombocytopenia [32, 33].

There has been much debate about autoantibodies as a cause of pregnancy loss. Anti-phospholipid antibodies were shown to promote thrombosis of placental vessels by lowering the level of annexin V on trophoblasts [34]. Both in idiopathic recurrent spontaneous abortion and lupus pregnancies increased levels of AECAs have been measured. Their pathogenetic role remains to be eluciated. Interestingly, some of the placentas studied carried histological features similar to allograft rejection (where AECAs have been already described in the 1980s).

Autoimmune thrombocytopenia occurs in as many as 25% of patients with SLE [32]. In contrast to leucopenia, an other ARA criterion [37], a low platelet count is of unfavorable prognostic significance. A pathogenetic overlap with idiopathic thrombocytopenic purpura (ITP) has been proposed earlier. There is some evidence that AECA may play a role in ITP via an ADCC.

An association of SLE with autoimmune endocrinopathies is well established. AECAs were demonstrated in hyperprolactinemia, hypothyroidism, and hypoparathyroidism [31].

In conclusion, anti endothelial cell antibodies may be a useful marker for vascular injury in systemic lupus erythematosus as demonstrated by a particularly high prevalence of AECA in the Raynaud phenomenon, cutaneous vasculitis, pulmonary hypertension and lupus nephritis. AECA brought new insights into the pathogenesis of SLE and once again demonstrated the pivotal role of the vascular endothelium.

It is generally accepted that lupus disease activity correlates with the prevalence of AECA especially in those patients with lupus nephritis. Therefore the occurence of AECA might be a serological marker of disease activity.

AECA may also explain long term complications of SLE due to accelaterated atherosclerosis similar to the phenomena seen in recipients of organ transplantation.

An association of the pattern and the binding properties of AECA in SLE with disease manifestaions has not yet been found. But above all, before AECAs can be introduced into routine clinical use, a standardized array of test systems for the detection of AECAs is mandatory [35].

REFERENCES

1. Lindqvist KJ, Osterland CK. Human antibodies to vascular endothelium. Clin Exp Immunol 1971;9(6):753–60.
2. Tan EM, Pearson CM. Rheumatic disease sera reactive with the capillaries in the mouse kidney. Arth Rheum 1972;15:23–8.
3. Shoenfeld Y, Alarcon-Segovia D, Buskila D et al. Frontiers of SLE: review of the 5th international congress of systemic lupus erythematosus, Cancun, Mexico, April 20–25, 1998. Semin Arthritis Rheum 1999;29(2):112–30.
4. Meroni PL, Del Papa N and Borghi M. Antiphospholipid and antiendothelial antibodies. Int Arch Allergy Immunol 1996;111(4):320–25.
5. Hill MB, Phipps JL, Milford-Ward A et al. Further characterization of anti-endothelial cell antibodies in systemic lupus erythematosus by controlled immunoblotting. Br J Rheumatol 1996;35(12):1231–38.
6. Del Papa N, Conforti G, Gambini D et al. Characterization of the endothelial surface proteins recognized by anti-endothelial cell antibodies in primary and secondary autoimmune vasculitis. Clin Immunol Immunopathol 1994;70(3):211–6.
7. van-der-Zee JM, Siegert CE, de-Vreede TA et al. Characterization of anti-endothelial cell antibodies in systemic lupus erythematosus (SLE). Clin Exp Immunol 1991;84(2):238–44.
8. Shan H, Goldman J, Cunto G et al. Heterogeneity of anti-phospholipid and anti-endothelial cell antibodies. J Autoimmun 1998;11(6):651–60.
9. Vismara A, Meroni PL, Tincani A et al. Relationship between anti-cardiolipin and anti-endothelial cell antibodies in systemic lupus erythematosus. Clin Exp Immunol 1988;74(2):247–53.
10. Li JS, Liu MF and Lei HY. Characterization of antiendothelial cell antibodies in the patients with systemic lupus erythematosus: a potential marker for disease activity. Clin Immunol Immunopathol 1996;79(3):211–16.
11. Lee KH, Bang D, Choi ES et al. Presence of circulating antibodies to a disease-specific antigen on cultured human dermal mirovascular endothelial cells in patients with Behcet's disease. Arch Dermatol Res 1999;291(7–9): 374–81.
12. Belizna C, Tervaert JW. Specifity, pathogenicity, and clinical value of antiendothelial cell antibodies. Semin Arthritis Rheum 1997;27(2):98–109.
13. Westphal JR, Boerbooms AM, Schalwijk JC et al. Anti-endothelial cell antibodies in sera of patients with autoimmune diseases: comparison between ELISA and FACS analysis. Clin Exp Immunol 1994;96(3):444–9.
14. D'Cruz DP, Houssiau FA, Ramirez G et al. Antibodies to endothelial cells in systemic lupus erythematosus: a potential marker for nephritis and vasculitis. Clin Exp Immunol 1991;85(2):254–61.
15. Chan TM, Cheng IKP. A prospective study on antiendothelial cell antibodies in patients with systemic lupus erythematosus. Clin Immunol Immunopathol 1996;78(1):41–6.
16. Perry GJ, Elston T, Khouri NA et al. Antiendothelial cell antibodies in systemic lupus erythematosus: correlations with renal injury and circulating markers of endothelial damage. Q J Med 1993;86(11):727–34.
17. Austin HA III, Muenz LR, Joyce KM et al. Prognostic factors in lupus nephritis. Contribution of renal histologic data. Am J Med 1983;75:382–91.
18. Yoshio T, Masuyama JI, Kohda N et al. Association of interleukin 6 release from endothelial cells and pulmonary hypertension in SLE. J Rheumatol 1997;24(3):489–95.
19. Carvalho D, Savage CO, Isenberg D. IgG anti-endothelial cell antibodies from patients with systemic lupus erythematosus or systemic vasculitis stimulate the release of two endothelial cell-derived mediators, which enhance adhesion molecule expression and leucocyte adhesion in an autocrine manner. Arthritis Rheum 1999;42(4):631–40.
20. George J, Blank M, Levy Y et al. Differential effects of anti-beta2-glycoprotein I antibodies on endothelial cells and on the manifestations of experimental antiphospholipid syndrome. Circulation 1998;97(9):900–6.
21. Bordron A, Dueymes M, Levy Y et al. The binding of some human antiendothelial cell antibodies induces endothelial cell apoptosis. J Clin Invest 1998;101(10):2029–35.
22. Bordron A, Dueymes M, Levy Y et al. Anti-endothelial cell antibody binding makes negatively charged phospholipids accessible to antiphospholipid antibodies. Arthritis Rheum 1998;41(10):1738–47.
23. Damianovich M, Gilburd B, George J et al. Pathogenic role of anti-endothelial cell antibodies in vasculitis. An idiotypic experimental model. J Immunol 1996;156(12):4946–51.
24. Levy Y, Gilburd B, George J et al. Characterization of murine monoclonal anti-endothelial cell antibodies

(AECA) produced by idiotypic manipulation with human AECA. Int Immunol 1998;10(7):861–8.

25. Rubin LA, Urowitz MB, Gladman DD et al. Mortality in systemic lupus erythematosus: the bimodal pattern revisited. Q J Med 1985;55:87–98.

26. Mills JA. Systemic lupus erythematosus. NEJM 1994;330(26):1871–9.

27. Ziporen L, Shoenfeld Y, Levy Y et al. Neurological dysfunction and hyperactive behavior associated with antiphospholipid antibodies. A mouse model. J Clin Invest 1997;100(3):613–9.

28. Ihn H, Sato S, Fujimoto M et al. Characterization of autoantibodies to endothelial cells in systemic sclerosis (SSc): association with pulmonary fibrosis. Clin Exp Immunol 2000;119(1):203–9.

29. Yoshio T, Masuyama J, Sumiya M et al. Antiendothelial cell antibodies and their relation to pulmonary hypertension in systemic lupus erythematosus. J Rheumatol 1994;21(11):2058–63.

30. Van-der-Zee JM, Miltenburg AM, Siegert CE et al. Antiendothelial cell antibodies in systemic lupus erythematosus: enhanced antibody binding to interleukin-1-stimulated endothelium. Int Arch Allergy Immunol 1994;104(2):131–6.

31. Fattorossi A, Aurbach GD, Sakaguchi K et al. Antiendothelial cell antibodies: detection and characterization in sera from patients with autoimmune hypoparathyroidism. Proc Natl Acad Sci USA 1988;85(11):4015–9.

32. Boumpas DT, Austin HA III, Fessler BJ. et al. Systemic lupus erythematosus: Emerging concepts. Ann Int Med 1995;122(12):940–50.

33. Boumpas DT, Austin HA III, Fessler BJ. et al. Systemic lupus erythematosus: Emerging concepts. Ann Int Med 1995;123(1):42–53.

34. Rand JH, Wu XX, Andree HA et al. Pregnancy loss in the antiphospholipid-antibody syndrome – a possible thrombogenic mechanism. N Engl J Med 1997;337(3):154–60.

35. Youinou P, Meroni PL, Khamashta MA et al. A need for standardization of the anti-endothelial-cell antibody test. Immunol Today 1995;16(8):363–4.

36. D'Cruz DP, Wisnieski JJ, Asherson RA et al. Autoantibodies in systemic lupus erythematosus and urticarial vasculitis. J Rheumatol 1995;22(9):1669–73.

37. Tan EM, Cohen AS, Fries JF et al. The 1982 revisited criteria for the classification of systemic lupus erythematosus. Arthritis Rheum 1982;25:1271–7.

38. Hill MB, Philipps JL, Hughes P et al. Anti-endothelial cell antibodies in primary antiphospholipid syndrome and SLE: patterns of reactivity with membrane antigens on microvascular endothelial and umbilical venous cell membranes. Br J Haematol 1998;103:416–421.

39. Carson CW, Beall LD, Hunder CG et al. Serum E-selectin is increased in vasculitis, scleroderma, and systemic lupus erythematosus. J Rheumatol 1993;20:809–814.

40. Gearing AJH, Hemingway I, Pigott R et al. Soluble forms of vascular adhesion molecules, E-selectin, ICAM-1 and VCAM-1: pathological significance. Ann N Y Acad Sci 1992;667:324–331.

41. Cybulsky MI, Gimbrone MA. Endothelial expression of a mononuclear leukocyte adhesion molecule during atherogenesis. Science 1991;251:788–791.

42. Javitt NB. Bile acid synthesis from cholesterol: regulatory and auxiliary pathways. FASEB J 1994;8(15):1308–1311.

43. Reiss AB, Malhotra S, Javitt NB et al. Occupancy of C1q receptors on endothelial cells (EC) by immune complexes downregulates mRNA for sterol 27-hydroxylase, the major mediator of extra-hepatic cholesterol metabolism. Arthritis Rheum 1998;41(suppl):579.

Atherosclerosis and Autoimmunity
Y. Shoenfeld, D. Harats and G. Wick, editors

Endothelial Cell Dysfunction in Atherosclerosis and Autoimmunity

Galina S. Marder[1] and H. Michael Belmont[2]

[1]Long Island Jewish Medical Center, NY, USA; [2]Hospital for Joint Diseases, NYU Medical Center, NY, USA

1. INTRODUCTION

Endothelial cells line the lumen of all blood vessels and form the interface between the blood and peripheral tissues. Traditionally, the role of endothelial cells was considered to be that of a gatekeeper. Passive deposition of cholesterol and its metabolites in the artery wall has been thought to be the key step in the pathophysiology of atherosclerosis. In recent years, however, attention has shifted to the role of primary vascular injury. Although many factors cause atherosclerosis, it has become clear now that endothelial cell perturbation and inflammation at the site of vascular injury plays an essential role in the initiation and progression of atherosclerotic disease.

In response to a diverse array of stimuli, activated endothelial cells exhibit a pro-inflammatory phenotype by up-regulation of adhesion molecules on their surface, leading to sequential steps in rolling, firm adhesion, and transmigration of leukocytes and monocytes to the site of injury. Formation and accumulation of foam cells in turn promotes neointimal proliferation and thinning of endothelium. These result in dysfunction of the endothelial cells, interaction with the platelets and stimulation of smooth muscle proliferation, leading to fibrous plaque and thrombus formation [1, 2].

The central role of endothelial cell-leukocyte interaction as an early response in the pathogenesis of atherosclerosis was demonstrated by experiments on C57BL/6 mice model with homozygous mutations for ICAM-1gene. This mutation, resulting in a deficiency of endothelial cell ICAM-1 expression, is associated with a protective role on the development of atherosclerosis in this animal model

Table 1. Reviewed factors stimulating endothelial cells and endothelial cells phenotypic responses that play an important role in pathogenesis of atherosclerosis and inflammatory vasculopathy

Stimuli	Response
Non-immunological	**Vascular tone**
mechanical forces: (transmural pressure, tension, hear stress) hypercholesterolemia, oxidized LDL, lysophosphatidilcholine	NO prostacyclin endothelin-1
Immunological	**Prothrombotic**
Cytokines: TNFα	Tissue factor
IL-1	vWF
γIFN	thrombomodulin
Activated complement products: C3a,C3b,C5a,MAC	
Autoantibodies: ACL	**Proadhesive**
AECA	
Anti-oxLDL	ICAM-1
Anti-dsDNA	VCAM-1
CD40/CD40L interaction	E-selectin
C1q receptors occupancy	

[3, 4]. Additionally, Systemic Lupus Erythematosus, a disease characterized by widespread vascular injury, has a high prevalence of premature atherosclerosis and represents an interesting model to study endothelial perturbation. This chapter will review the current literature on factors altering endothelial cell behavior and specific endothelial responses to these stimuli (Table 1).

2. ENDOTHELIAL PHENOTYPE

Endothelium plays a fundamental role in various physiologic functions, including vasoregulation, hemostasis, inflammation, and adhesion biology.

What determines the actual difference between the chronic lesion in atherosclerosis and the acute and subacute lesions of inflammatory vasculopathy? An understanding of the details of endothelial perturbation in response to stimuli may provide the explanation. Irrespective of the nature of the stimuli (immunogenic or direct mechanical forces), the endothelium responds by up-regulating adhesion molecules and recruiting leukocytes, shifting the phenotype to procoagulant by expressing tissue factor (TF), von Willebrand factor (vWF) and/or altering vascular tone.

2.1. Vascular Tone

In physiologic conditions equilibrium is maintained between relaxing and contracting factors. Prostacyclin (PGI2), which also inhibits the aggregation of platelets, and nitric oxide (NO), previously called endothelium-derived relaxing factor (EDRF), are the most potent mediators which endothellial cells contribute to the common pool of vasodilators. IL-1 and TNF-alpha were shown to be able to stimulate prostacyclin synthetase activity, therefore enhancing the production of prostacyclin by endothelial cells [5, 6]. Endothelin-1 is the most potent endothelium-derived contracting factor that modulates vascular smooth muscle tone. Endothelin-1 is not stored within the endothelial cell; it is synthesized in precursor form. Prepro-ET-1 mRNA was demonstrated within minutes of exposure to stimuli such as thrombin, cytokines, hypoxia, or shear stress [8, 9 in 7].

Endothelial perturbation due to various stimuli disrupts this fine balance. Specifically, subtle damage to the endothelium, as in hypertension or hyperlipidemia (via oxidized LDL) has a detrimental effect on nitric oxide production, leading to vasoconstriction [2]. In contrast, upregulation of iNOS expression leading to increased NO production was reported in the vascular lesions of temporal arteritis [10]. Similarly, Belmont and coworkers [11] reported increased serum NO level in patients with active SLE. Immunohistochemical analysis was performed on nonlesional skin of SLE patients and demonstrated colocalization of staining for iNOS and E-selectin, therefore pointing to endothelial cells as a source of excessive NO synthesis. It has been demonstrated that endothelial cells stimu-

lated by thrombin, acetylcholine, neurotransmitters, and serotonin, or the shear stress of flowing blood increase expression of iNOS leading to sustained production of high concentrations of NO, which promotes vasodilatation and increased permeability [5]. Conflicting results were published on the level of NO in vascular injury in scleroderma [12]. We speculate that the level of NO expression in different clinical settings depends on the duration and extent of endothelial injury and thereby shifts the balance to relaxation and permeability or to constriction and ischemia.

It is now recognized that the importance of endothelial NO is not limited to its role as a vasodilator. NO also is known to play a protective role by inhibiting platelet aggregation and reduction of platelet adherence to endothelial monolayer [11, 13].

Atsumi, Hughes et al. [7] hypothesized that induction of ET-1 by antiphospholipid antibodies contributes to the mechanism of vascular injury by increasing the arterial tone and, ultimately leading to arterial occlusion. They were able to demonstrate elevated plasma level of ET-1, that were significantly higher in APS patients with arterial stroke than in those with venous thrombosis, or in non-APS patients with stroke. In vitro experiments demonstrated that induction of prepro-ET-1 mRNA in cultured endothelial cells treated with human monoclonal aCL antibodies was significantly higher than in those primed with control monoclonal IgM. Similar results were obtained in earlier studies by incubating cultured endothelial cells with serum of patients with SLE compared to normal controls. ET-1 levels significantly correlated with the IgM AECA titer and immune complex concentration in sera from patients with SLE [14].

2.2. Prothrombotic Phenotype

By shifting the phenotype to procoagulant in response to stimulation, endothelial cells have a direct role in the mechanism of thrombosis, whether this is at a site of atherosclerotic plaque formation or focal vascular inflammation; or in circumstances characterized by diffuse endothelial activation, such as in SLE, catastrophic antiphospholipid syndrome (CAPS) or systemic inflammatory response syndrome (SIRS) [15, 16].

Von Willebrand factor (vWF) is a macromolecular protein complex, which plays a pivotal role in hemostasis. It functions as a carrier protein for plasma factor VIII, and mediates platelet adhesion to other platelets and to collagen exposed by damaged endothelium. Vascular endothelium is the major source of plasma vWF under physiologic and pathologic conditions. vWF is stored and released from endothelial cell secretory granules, along with its pro-peptide vWF:AgII. Elevated plasma von Willebrand factor was found in diabetes and other vasculopathies. Its level and the level of propeptide can serve as a marker of endothelial activation [17]. A group from Canada [18] demonstrated decreased peripheral dermal staining for endothelial vWF in systemic inflammatory response syndrome (SIRS) patients, as well as in healthy volunteers after TNF-alpha injection. This was associated with significantly greater plasma vWF levels, indicating degranulation in response to cytokine stimulation that predisposes to formation of platelet microthrombi, lodging in small capillaries, causing areas of local tissue ischemia.

Cultured endothelial cells in vitro express tissue factor (TF) in response to a great variety of stimuli [19]. The data in vivo are controversial; one group found an absence of expression of TF by endothelium overlying atherosclerotic plaques by in situ hybridization [20], but a later study reported endothelial expression of TF by using histochemical assessment [21]. Solovey and Hebbel demonstrated expression of TF by endothelial cells of sickle cell anemia patients during the acute vasooclusive episode, supported by concurence between TF antigen and mRNA expression [22].

2.3. Proadhesive Phenotype

Adhesion of leukocytes to vascular endothelium is one of the earliest events in acute immunogenic and nonimmunogenic inflammation [1].

The initial surface expression of adhesion molecules is the common endothelial response not only to a variety of atherogenic stimuli, but also to complement mediated vascular injury in SLE (immune complex mediated, as well as immune complex independent).

Many cells, including EC constitutively express ICAM-1, and its expression is upregulated by IL-1 or TNF-alpha. VCAM-1 is mainly present on endothelial cells activated by IL-1, TNF-alpha, interferon gamma or IL-4 [23]. Endothelial cells activated by IL-1, TNF alpha, or thrombin transiently express E-selectin, thereby mediating endothelial adhesion of neutrophils or memory lymphocytes [24]. Expression of these molecules promotes formation of vasoocclusive plaques, by interaction of endothelium with activated neutrophils, displaying up-regulation of beta2-integrin CD11b/CD18. The importance of this interaction was demonstrated in a recently studied model of vascular injury underlying thrombotic stroke [25]. Investigators used neutrophil-depleted or ICAM-1-deficient mice and demonstrated resistance of this model to focal cerebral ischemia and reperfusion injury provoked by experimental intraluminal occlusion of the cerebral artery. Elkon et al. [26] demonstrated in MRL/MpJ-FAS lpr mice that ICAM-1 deficiency results in a striking improvement in survival. Data from several groups analyzing the level of various adhesion molecules in SLE further support the notion that endothelial cells play a central role in systemic inflammatory response by exhibiting their adhesive properties. Immunohistological examination of non-sun exposed skin from SLE patients showed upregulation of the surface expression of all three adhesion molecules – E-selectin, ICAM-1, and VCAM-1 in patients with active SLE in otherwise histologically normal skin with no evidence of local immune complex deposition [27]. Elevation of soluble adhesion molecules (E-selectin, sICAM-1, sVCAM-1) also has been reported in active SLE [28]. A group from France [23] demonstrated increased level of sVCAM-1 in patients with primary APS, SLE-APS or systemic lupus erythematosus, compared to healthy controls or thrombosis controls.

3. STIMULI THAT ACTIVATE ENDOTHELIAL CELLS

Factors that alter the functional status of endothelium can be divided into two major categories: nonimmunological (such as direct mechanical forces, vasoactive mediators and products of oxidation) and immunological (cytokines, complement and autoantibodies).

3.1. Non-Immunological

The endothelium experiences three primary mechanical forces: transmural pressure, tension and shear stress. Sprague and others [29] have demonstrated flow-mediated modulation of endothelial activation markers, and Nagel et al. [30] reported up-regulation of ICAM expression in cultured human vascular cells in response to shear stress.

Recent studies have supported the view that hypercholesterolemia and oxidative stress are important inducers of atheroma formation. One of the actions of oxidized LDL is to induce endothelial dysfunction [31]. Erl and Weber demonstrated activation of endothelial cells by oxidized LDL (oxLDL) via distinct endothelial ligands, promoting adhesion of monocytes [32]. It is speculated that one of the mechanisms is a disruption of signal transduction [33]. Other mechanisms may be related to the liso-phosphatidyl-choline (LPC) moiety, one of the active components of oxLDL particle that induces superoxide endothelial cytotoxic effect via peroxinitrite production [33, 34]. Moreover, LPC is a major factor in the antigenicity of oxLDL [35, 36]. Antibodies against oxLDL were demonstrated both in normal, healthy individuals and in atherosclerotic plaques and were found to correlate with atherosclerosis progression [36]. The level of oxLDL antibodies has been correlated with titers for aCL in SLE patients [37, 34]. Several groups [37, 38] have demonstrated cross-reactivity of aPL and oxLDL underlying the link in development of atherosclerosis and immunological process.

3.2. Immunological

Cytokines are important mediators of endothelial cell activation. Specifically, TNFα, IL-1, and macrophage colony stimulating factor increase binding of LDL to endothelium and increase transcription of the LDL gene [31]. TNFα, IFN-γ and interleukin-1 stimulate adhesion molecule expression on endothelial cells. Few studies have reported increased levels of these cytokines in the circulation during vasculitis [39]. The Shwartzman phenomenon, originally described as a model of endotoxemia, currently is being used as a model of the widespread vasculopathy of SLE. It is recognized now that cytokines such as IL-1 and TNFα are the preparatory signals of the inflammatory process [27, 15]. These proinflammatry cytokines are capable of promoting atherosclerosis by stimulating the adhesive properties of endothelial cells. Accumulation of TNF-α [40] and IL-1 [41] was demonstrated in atheroscleroiic plaques of coronary arteries. It is also important to note that while endothelial cells are activated by cytokines, they also can produce IL-1, IL-6, IL-8 and TNF-α while stimulated [39, 46]. These cytokines can act as autocoids to up-regulate adhesion molecule expression. Kaplanski et al.[24] demonstrated induction of IL-8 production in a time and dose dependent fashion by thrombin-activated HUVEC; this effect was inhibited by the specific thrombin inhibitor hirudin.

Complement activation that can be either immune complex dependent or independent, plays an essential role in the mechanism of endothelial injury. This can explain the development of widespread vascular injury in SLE, an example of immune-mediated systemic inflammatory response, even without evidence of immune complex deposition in the tissue. Several products of the activated complement system (C3b, iC3b and C5a) are known to activate endothelial cells in vitro. More recently, Saadi and others [42] demonstrated that interaction of complement with endothelial cells and the assembly of membrane attack complex (MAC) leads to expression of P-selectin, activation of a protease that cleaves and releases heparan sulfate proteoglycan from the EC surface, and induces up-regulation of TF and COX-2. They concluded that activation of porcine aortic and microvascular endothelial cells upon MAC exposure involves the intermediate step of IL-1 release. By using endothelial cells transgenic for human decay-accelerating factor that inhibits complement convertase, these authors demonstrated that complement is required for endothelial activation. The presence of sCR1 prevented activation of aortic as well as microvascular endothelial cells [43].

Granular deposits of immunoglobulin and complement components were found within atherosclerotic lesion [44], suggesting that complement-dependent endothelial activation could play a role in pathogenesis of atherosclerosis.

Antibodies against endothelial cells and cardiolipin were found in a subset of patients with the clinical and angiographic diagnosis of severe premature atherosclerotic peripheral disease [45]. Recent research demonstrated that antibodies might contribute to the derangement of functional status of the endothelial cells, rather than simply displaying cell cytotoxicity. It has been reported that both polyclonal as well as monoclonal AECA induce EC activation in vitro. AECA have been shown to mediate release of vWF, arachidonic acid metabolites, ET-1 from endothelial cells and induce a pro-inflammatory and pro-coagulant phenotype of EC [46–49]. Statistically significant increase in expression of endothelial ICAM-1, VCAM-1, and E-selectin was demonstrated on human umbilical vein endothelial cells pretreated with AECA-positive sera from a scleroderma patient compared to cells pretreated with AECA-negative sera [49]. Neutralizing antibodies to IL-1, but not antibodies to TNF, substantially inhibited or blocked this activation, providing further evidence for the autocrine actions of IL-1. Del Papa and others [47] found that AECA IgG from Wegener's Granulomatosis patients up-regulate the expression of E-selectin, ICAM-1 and VCAM-1 and induce the secretion of IL-1, IL-6, IL-8, and MCP-1. Almost identical results were obtained from analysis of AECA-positive sera from Takayasu arteritis patients [48]. Another proposed mechanism is that binding of anti-endothelial cell antibody makes negatively charged phospholipids accessible to antiphospholipid antibodies [50], thereby further enhancing the activation of EC.

Crossreactivity between anti-ds DNA antibodies, cardiolipins and AECA has been observed in earlier studies [51, 52]. By using immunofluorescent staining, Smitanov and others were the first to demonstrate expression of cell adhesion molecules, including E-selectin, VCAM-1 and ICAM-1 by endothelial cells incubated with purified IgG from patients with high titers of anticardiolipin antibodies, even in the absence of clinical or serologic evidence of SLE [53]. They also established that this mechanism is β_2-glycoprotein–dependent.

A direct stimulatory effect of anti-dsDNA antibodies on endothelium, as indicated by the release of vWF, may have a pathogenic role on expression of adhesion molecules [54, 55]. These data can provide a link between SLE and premature atherosclerosis.

The interaction between CD40 and CD40L is another immune mediated interaction common to both SLE and atherosclerosis that leads to upregulation of adhesion molecules on endothelial cells [35]. CD-40 is a type 1 member of the TNF receptor superfamily of proteins, and is present on a wide variety of cells, including vascular endothelial cells. Ligation of this receptor on endothelial cells is known to increase expression of inflammatory adhesion molecules. Slupsky and others [56] demonstrated that platelets express the ligand of CD40 within seconds of exposure to agonist, and interact with endothelial cells to participate directly in the induction of an inflammatory response. The same authors also showed that activated platelets induce TF expression on endothelial cells in a CD40/CD40L-dependent manner. Moreover CD40 ligation on endothelial cells down-regulates the expression of thrombomodulin and adhesion molecule further implicating the procoagulant and proinflammatory phenotype of endothelial cells [57]. In a genetically modified murine model with hypercholesterolemia, blocking antibodies to CD40 reduced atherosclerotic lesion formation [58].

In SLE C1q immune complexes may be a source of arterial injury initiating atherogenesis. Lozada and others showed that immune complexes stimulate endothelial cells to express adhesion molecules E-selectin, ICAM and VCAM in the presence of a heat-labile complement component C1q. C1q depletion from serum or C1q protein synthesis inhibition on the surface of endothelial cells blocked the expression of adhesive proteins [59]. Moreover, Reiss et al. were able to demonstrate that occupancy of C1q receptors on endothelial cells by immune complexes down-regulated mRNA for sterol 27-hydroxylase, the enzyme that mediates peripheral cholesterol metabolism, interfering with the capacity of endothelium to convert cholesterol to anti-atherogenic metabolites and therefore enhancing atherogenesis [60].

In summary, we have described factors leading to endothelial perturbation and overlapping features of endothelial response in autoimmune disorders and atherosclerosis. The conversion of the endothelial phenotype to an adhesive and pro-thrombotic state, and interaction of inflammatory mediators with cholesterol metabolism driven by multiple immunological and non-immunological stimuli is the core of the pathophysiological link between mechanisms of inflammatory vasculopathy, thrombosis and atherosclerosis.

ACKNOWLEDGEMENT

Dr Robert Greenwald provided helpful advice and commentary.

REFERENCES

1. Price DT, Loscalzo J. Cellular adhesion molecules and atherogenesis. Am J Med 1999;107:85–97.
2. Vogel RA. Cholesterol lowering and endothelial function. Am J Med 1999;107:479–487.
3. Nageh MF, Sandberg ET, Marotti KR, Lin AH, Melchior EP, Bullard DC, Beaudet AL. Deficiency of inflammatory cell adhesion molecules protects against atherosclerosis in mice. Atheroscler Thromb Vasc Biol. 1997;7:1517–1520.
4. Walker G, Lanheinrich AC, Dennhauser E, Bohle RM, Dreyer T, et al. 3-Deazaadenosine prevents adhesion molecule expression and atherosclerotic lesion formation in the aortas of c57BL/6J mice. Atheroscler Thromb Vasc Biol. 1999;19(11):2673–2679.
5. Ramzi S. Cotran Endothelial cells, Textbook on Inflammation.
6. Zavoico GB, Ewenstein BM, Schafer AI, Pober JS. Interleukin-1 and related cytokines enhance thrombin-stimulated PGI_2 production in cultured endothelial cells without affecting thrombin-stimulated von Willebrand factor secretion or platelet activator factor biosynthesis. J Immunology 1989;1427:3993.
7. Atsumi T, Kamashta MA, Haworth RS, Brooks G, Amengual O, Ichikawa K, Koike T, Hughes G. Arterial disease and thrombosis in the antiphospholipid syndrome: a pathogenic role for Endothelin-1. Arthr Rheum 1998;41(5):800–807.
8. Marsen TA, Simonson MS, Dunn MJ. Thrombin induces the preproendothelin-1 gene in endothelial cells by a protein tyrosine kinase-linked mechanism. Circ Res 1995;76:987–995.
9. Kourembanas S, Marsden PA, McQuillan LP, Faller DV. Hypoxia induces endothelin gene expression and secretion in cultured human endothelium. J Clin Invest 1991;88:1054–1057.
10. Wagner AD, Bjornsson J, GoronzyJJ, Weyand CM. Potential role of TGF-β1 and nitric oxide in human vasculitis (abstract). Arthritis & Rheumatism 1996;39(suppl 9):S80.
11. Belmont HM, Levartovsky D, Goel A, Amin A, Giorno R, Rediske J, Skovorn ML, Abramson SB. Increased nitric oxide production accompanied by the up-regulation of inducible nitric oxide synthase in vascular endothelium from patients with systemic lupus erythematosus. Arthritis & Rheumatism 1997;40(10):1810–1816.
12. Andersen GN, Caidahl K, Kazza E, Petersson AS, Waldenstrom A, Mincheva-Nilson L, Rantapaa-Dahlqvist S. Correlation between increased nitric oxide production and markers of endothelial activation in Systemic sclerosis. Arthr Rheum 2000;43(5).
13. Radomski MW, Palmer RM, Moncada S. Endogenous nitric oxide inhibits human platelet adhesion to vascular endothelium. Lancet 1987;2:1057–1058.
14. Yoshio Y, Masuyama J, Mimori A, Takeda A, Minota S, Kano S. Endothelin-1 release from cultured endothelial cells induced by sera from patients with systemic lupus erythematosus. Ann Rheum Dis 1995;54(5):361–365.
15. Belmont HM, Abramson SB, Lie JT. Pathology and pathogenesis of vascular injury in systemic lupus erythematosus. Interactions of inflammatory cells and activated endothelium 1996;39(1):9–22.
16. Belmont HM, Abramson S. Systemic inflamatory response syndrome, systemic lupus erythematosus and thrombosis. Vascular manifextations of systemic autoimmune diseases. Ed. Cerveca and Asherson. In press.
17. Vischer UM, Emeis JJ, Bilo HJ, Stehouwer CD,Thomsen C, Rasmussen O, Hermansen K, Wollheim CB, Ingerslev J. vWillebrand factor as a plasma marker of endothelial activation in diabetes:improved reliability with parallel determination of the vWf propeptide. Thromb Haemost 1998;80(6):1002–1007.
18. McGill SN, Ahmed NA, Christou NV. Increased plasma von Willebrand factor in the systemic inflammatory response syndrome is derived from generalized endothelial cell activation. Crit Care Med 1998;26(2)296–300.
19. Edgington TS, Mackman N, Brand K, Ruf W. The structural biology of expression and function of tissue factor. Thromb Haemost 1991;66:67–79.
20. Wilcox JN, Smith KM, Schwartz SM, Gordon D. Localization of tissue factor in the normal vessel-wall and in the atherosclerotic plaque. Proc Natl Acad Sci 1989;86:2839–2843.
21. Thiruvikraman SV, Gudha A, Roboz J, Taubman MB, Nemerson Y, Falon JJ. In situ localization of tissue factor in human atherosclerotic plaques by binding of digoxigenin-labaled factors VIIa and X. Lab Invest 1996;75:451–461.
22. Solovey A, Gui L, Key NS, Hebbel RP. Tissue factor expression by endothelial cells in sickle cell anemia. J Clin Invest 1998;101(9):1899–1904.
23. Kaplanski G, Cacoub P, Farnarier C, Marin V, Gregoire R, Gatel A, Durand Jm, Harle JR, Bongrand P, Piette JC. Increased soluble vascular adhesion molecule-1 concen-

trations in patients with primary or systemic lupus erythematosus-related antiphospholipid syndrome. Arthritis Rheum 2000;43(1).

24. Kaplanski G, Fabrigoule M, Boulay V, Dinarello CA, Bongard P, Kaplanski S, et al. Thrombin induces endothelial type II activation in vitro: IL-1 and TNF-alpha-independent IL-8 secretion and E-selectin expression. J Immunol 1997;158(11):5435–5441.

25. Connolly ES Jr, Winfree CJ, Springer TA, Naka Y, Liao H, Yan SD, et al. Cerebral protection in homozygous null ICAM-1 mice after midddle artery occlusion: role of neutrophil adhesion in the pathogenesis of stroke. J Clin Invest 1996;97:209–216.

26. Bullard DC, King PD, Hicks MJ, Dupont B, Beaudet AL, Elkon KB. Intercellular adhesion molecule-1 deficiency protects MRL/MpJ-Fas (lpr) mice from early lethality. J Immunol 1997;159:2057–2067.

27. Belmont HM, Buyon J, Giorno R., Abramson SB. Upregulation of endothelial cel adhesion molecules characterizes disease activity in systemic lupus erythematosus: Schwartzman phenomenon revisited. Arthritis Rheum 1994;37:376–383.

28. Nyberg F, Acevedo F, Stephanson E. Different patterns of soluble adhesion molecules in systemic and cutaneous lupus eryhthematosus. J Immunol 1997;65:230–235.

29. Sprague EA, Cayatte AJ, Valente AJ, Shwartz CJ. Flow mediated modulation of selected biologic and molecular determinants related to vascular endothelial activation. J Vasc Surg 1992;15:919–921.

30. Nagel T, Resnick N, Atkinson WJ, Dewey CF, Gimbrone MA. Shear stress selectively upregulates intracellular adhesion molecule-1 expression in cultured human vascular endothelial cells. J Clin Invest. 1994;94:885–891.

31. Ross R. Atherosclerosis – an inflammatory disease. New Engl J Med 1999;340(2):115–123.

32. Erl W, Weber PC, Weber C. Monocytic cell adhesion to endothelial cells stimulated by oxidized low density lipoprotein is mediated by distinct endothelial ligands. Atherosclerosis 1998;136:297–303.

33. Crossman, DC. More problems with endothelium. QJM 1997;90(3):157–160.

34. Wu R, Huang YH, Elinder LS. Lysophosphatydylcholine is involved in the antigenicity of oxidized LDL. Atheroscler Thromb Vasc Biol 1998;18(4):626–630.

35. Manzi S, Chester M, Wasko M, Manzi S. Inflammation-mediated rheumatic diseases and atherosclerosis. Ann Rheum Dis 2000;50(5):321–325.

36. Bergmark C, Wu R, de Faire U, Lefvert AK, Swedenbort J. Patients with early onset peripheral vascular disease have increased levels of antibodies against oxidized LDL. Atheroscler Thromb Vasc Biol. 1995;15:441–445.

37. Vaarala O, Alfthan G, Jauhhiainen M, Lerisalo-Rpo M, Aho K, Palosuo T. Cross-reaction between antibodies to oxidized low-density lipoprotein and to cardiolipin in systemic lupus erythematosus. Lancet. 1993;341:923–925.

38. Hörkkö S, Miller E, Dudl E, Reaven P, Curtiss LK, Zvaifler NJ et al. Antiphospholipid antibodies are directed against epitopes of oxidized phospholipids: recognition of cardiolipin by monoclonal antibodies to epitopes of oxidized low density lipoprotein. J Clin Invest 1996;98:815–825.

39. Warner SJ, Auger KR, Libby P. Interleukin 1 induces interleukin 1. II. Recombinant human interleukin 1 induces interleukin 1 production by adult human vascular endothelial cells. J Immunol 1987;15;139(6):1911–1917. 40. Galea J, Armstrong J, Gadson P, Holden H, Francis SE, Holt CM. Interleukin-1 beta in coronary arteies of patients with ischemic heart disease. Arterioscler Thromb Vasc Biol 1996;16:1000–1006.

41. Barath P, Fishbein MC, Cao J, Berenson L, Helfant RH, Forrester JS. Detection and localization of tumor necrosis factor in human atheroma. Am J Cardiol 1990;65:297–302.

42. Saadi S, Holzknect RA, Patte CP, Stern DM, Platt JL. Complement-mediated regulation of tissue factor activity in endothelium. J Exp Med 1995; 182:1807–1814. Billiar TR. Nitric oxide: novel biology with clinical relevance. Ann Surg 1995;221:339–349.

43. Saadi S, Holzknecht RA, Patte CP, Platt JL. Endothelial cell activation by pore-forming structures:pivotal role for Interleukin-1. Circulation 2000;101(15):1867–1873.

44. Bruce IN, Gladman DD, Urowitz MB. Premature atherosclerosis in Systemic Lupus Erythematosus. Rheum Dis Clin North Am 2000;26(2).

45. Nityanand S, Bergmark C, deFaire U, Swedenborg J, Holm G, Lefvert AK. Antibodies against endothelial cells and cardiolipin in young patients with peripheral atherosclerotic disease. J Intern Med 1995;238(5):437–443.

46. Carvalho D, Savage COS, Isenberg D, Pearson JD. IgG anti-endothelial cell autoantibodies from patients with systemic lupus eythematosus or systemic vasculitis stimulate the release of two endothelial cell derived mediators which enhance adhesion molecule expression and leukocyte adhesion in an autocrine manner. Arthr Rheum 1999;42(4):631–639.

47. Del Papa N, Guidali L, Sironi M, Shoenfeld Y, Mantovani A, Tincani A, Baalestertrieri G, Radice A, Sinico RA, Meroni PL. Antiendothelial cell IgG antibodies from patients with Wegener's granulomatosis bind to human endothelial cells I vitro and induce adhesion molecule expression and cytokine secretion. Arthr Rheum 1996;39(5):758–767.

48. Blank M, Krause I, Goldkorn T, Praportnik S, A Livneh et al. Monoclonal antiendothelial cell anti-

bodies from a patient with Takayasu arteritis activate endothelial cells from large vessels. Arthr Rheum 1999;42(7):1421–1432.

49. Carvalho D, Savage C, Black CM, Pearson JD. IgG antiendothelial cell autoantibodies from scleroderma patients induce leukocyte adhesion to human vascular endothelial cells in vitro: induction of adhesion molecule expression and involvement of endothelium-derived cytokines. J Clin Invest 1996;97(1):111–119.

50. Bordon A, Dueymes M, Levy Y, Jamin C, Ziporen L, Piette JC, Schoefeld Y, Youinou P. Antiendothelial cell antibody binding makes negatively charged phospholipids accessible to antiphospholipid antibodies. Arthr Rheum 1998;41(10):1738–1747.

51. Koike T, Tomioka H, Kumagai A. Antibodies cross-reactive with DNA and cardiolipin in patients with systemic lupus erythematosus. Clin Exp Immunol 1983;59:449–456.

52. Hasselaar P, Deksen RHWM, Blokzijl L, PG de Groot. Crossreactivity of antibodies directed against cardiolipin, DNA, endothelial cells and blood platelets. Thromb Haemost 1990:63(2):169–173.

53. Simitanov R, LaSala JM, Lo SK, Gharavi AE, Sammaritano LR, Salmon JE, Silverstein RL. Activation of cultured endothelial cells by antiphospholipid antibodies. J Clin Invest. 1995;96(5):2211–2219.

54. Lai KN, Leung JCK, Lai KB, Lai FM, Wong KC. Increased release of von Willebrand factor antigen from endothelial cells by anti DNA autoantibodies. Ann Rheum Dis 1996;55(1):57–62.

55. Chan TM, Yu PM, Tsang KL, Cheng IK. Endothelial cell binding by human polyclonal anti-DNA antibodies: relationship to disease activity and endothelial functional alterations. Clin Exp Immunol 1995;100(3):506–513.

56. Slupsky Jr, Kalba M, Willuweit A, Henn V, Kroczek RA, Muller-Berhaus G. Activated platelets induce tissue factor expression on human umbilical vein endothelial cells by ligation of CD40. Thromb Haemost 1998 Dec:80(6):1008–1014.

57. Karnmann K, Hughes CC, Schechner J, Fanslow WC, Pober JS. CD40 on human endothelial cells: inducibility by cytokines and functional regulation of adhesion molecule expression. Proc Natl Acad Sci 1995;92:4342–4346.

58. Mach F, Schonbeck U, Sukhova GK, Atkinson E, Libby P. Reduction of atherosclerosis in mice by inhibition of CD40 signalling. Nature 1998;394:200–203.

59. Lozada C, Levin R, Huie M, Hirschhorn R, Naime D, Whitlow M, Recht PA, Golden B, Cronstein BN. Identification of C1q as the heat labile serum cofactor required for immune complexes to stimulate endothelial expression of the adhesion molecules E-selectin and intercellular and vascular cell adhesion molecules 1. Proc Nat Acad Sci 1995;92:8378–8382.

60. Reiss AB, Malhotra S, Javitt NB, Gross EA, Galloway AC, Montesinos MC, Cronstein BN. Occupancy of C1q receptors on endothelial cells by immune complexes downregulates mRNA for sterol 27-hydroxylase, the major mediator of extra-hepatic cholesterol metabolism. Arthr Rheum 1998;41(9)S:S79.

240

Atherosclerosis and Autoimmunity
Y. Shoenfeld, D. Harats and G. Wick, editors

Modulation of Endothelial Cell Function by Normal Polyspecific Human Immunoglobulins (IVIg)

Jean-Paul Duong Van Huyen[1,2], Jacques Chevalier[1], Michel D. Kazatchkine[1] and Srinivas Kaveri[1]

[1]INSERM U 430, Hôpital Broussais, Paris, France; [2]Laboratoire d'Anatomie Pathologique, Hôpital Européen Georges Pompidou, Paris, France

1. INTRODUCTION

Endothelium is not merely a barrier between the bloodstream and tissue, but, by virtue of their location, endothelial cells (EC) are continuously facing humoral factors and, in some circumstances, actively participate in inflammatory and immunomodulatory responses (for a review, see [1]). Thus, the endothelium plays a central role in the immunopathology of several vascular disorders in many inflammatory conditions such as Kawasaki disease, Wegener's granulomatosis, or vasculitides. It may act either as a target for injury or by encouraging the development of lesions because of its anatomical position and physiological function. Bound anti-endothelial cell antibodies (AECA) in kawasaki disease have the potential to mediate endothelial cell injury and lysis via either complement or by more subtle changes in endothelial cell functions. During inflammation, activated EC rapidly synthesize and release chemokines and cytokines, and express, in a few minutes or in a few hours, new adhesion molecules involved in the adhesion, rolling and diapedesis of leukocytes [1–3]. Among these newly synthesized molecules, monocyte chemoattractant protein 1 (MCP-1), granulocyte-colony stimulating factor (G-CSF), granulocyte-macrophage colony stimulating factor (GM-CSF), intercellular adhesion molecule-1 (ICAM-1) and vascular cell adhesion molecule-1 (VCAM-1), interleukins 1 and 6 (IL-1, IL-6), tumor necrosis factor alpha and beta (TNFα, TNFβ) play a key role and can be induced *in vitro* by numerous agents such as proinflammatory cytokines

IL-1β and TNF-α, [4–6] modified low density lipoproteins [7] and bacterial lipopolysaccharide [8].

Patients suffering from systemic inflammatory conditions such as dermatomyositis [9], and particularly, Kawasaki syndrome, are greatly benefitted from normal polyspecific human immunoglobulin (IVIg) treatment (for a review, see [10, 11]). IVIg has also been used in the treatment of anti-neutrophil cytoplasmic antigen (ANCA)-associated systemic vasculitis [12, 13]. The mechanisms of action of IVIg are, as yet, poorly understood although several mutually non-exclusive hypotheses have been proposed [14]. Our laboratory has recently undertaken several studies to address the potential role of IVIg on endothelial cell function by following both EC proliferation and EC expression of key adhesion molecules, chemokines and cytokines. Using HUVEC as target cells, we have shown that IVIg modulate the function of endothelial cells [15].

2. IVIG INHIBIT EC PROLIFERATION IN A DOSE- AND TIME-DEPENDENT MANNER

IVIg from different commercial sources including Sandoglobulin®, Gammagard® and Endobulin® inhibited HUVEC proliferation, as assessed by ³H-thymidine incorporation and cell enumeration, in a dose- and time-dependent manner (Fig 1 and data not shown). The inhibitory effect of IVIg was also reversible, in a dose- and time-dependent manner (Fig 2). At 48 hr of culture of EC, there was an

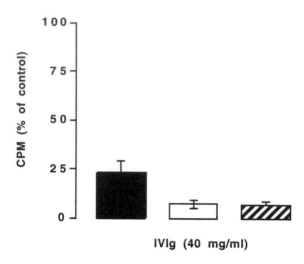

Figure 1. Comparative effect of different sources of IVIg on EC proliferation. Human umbilical vein endothelial cells (HUVEC) were obtained after a 4 min treatment of the umbilical vein with 0.15% collagenase I in phosphate buffer saline. The cells were cultured in medium M199 containing Earle's salts, L-glutamine, and 25 mM HEPES and supplemented with 20% fetal calf serum, 100 U/ml penicillin, 100 μg/ml streptomycin, and 0.25 μg/ml fungizone. In order to synchronize cells in a G_0/G_1 stage, FCS concentration was reduced to 1% for 24 hr. At the end of the depletion period, cells were replaced in M199/20% FCS and stimulated for various periods of time in the presence of 0.5 μCi ^{3}H-thymidine/well in the presence of 40 mg/ml of Sandoglobulin® (dark histogram), Gammagard® (open histogram) and Endobulin® (hatched histogram). At the end of incubation times, radioactivity was measured by liquid scintillation counter. Gammagard® and Endobulin® were more potent inhibitors than Sandoglobulin®.

abolition of the inhibitory effect of IVIg and the cell number progressively increased. Although the mechanisms underlying this escape of cells from the anti-proliferative action of IVIg after 48 hr is not clear, the phenomenon reflects the clinical picture following therapy with IVIg: a transient decrease of leukocyte count followed by a recovery in the count has been observed in volunteers infused with IVIg [16]. The drop in the number of live cells and the small increase in the number of dead cells, as assessed by FACS analysis (data not shown), clearly indicated that the inhibition of cell proliferation induced by IVIg is associated with an arrest of the cell cycle at the G_0/G_1 phase, rather than only due to a mortality of the cells. The observed inhibitory effect of IVIg on endothelial cell proliferation, was not merely due to a high concentration of protein since human albumin at 40mg/ml had no effect on the thymidine uptake by the cells (data not shown). Therefore, the changes in osmolarity provoked by the presence of sugar as stabilizing agent and the acidic pH used to prevent the precipitation of commercial IVIg preparations had little effect on HUVEC viability (data not shown). The mech-

anisms involved in the cell cycle arrest and mortality of cells remain unknown. We dissected the role of the variable region of Ig (F(ab')$_2$ fragments) and the constant Fc portion of Ig in the anti-proliferative effect of IVIg. We found that both F(ab')$_2$ and Fc were able to inhibit significantly, in a similar level, the proliferation of HUVEC (data not shown). Although the underlying mechanisms involved in the analogous effect observed with both F(ab')$_2$ and Fc portions of immunoglobulin are not clear as yet, a receptor-mediated mechanism cannot be ruled out. In vivo, it is most likely that both F(ab')$_2$ and Fc portions of immunoglobulins are involved in the immunomodulatory functions [17].

3. IVIG DOWN-REGULATE THE TNF-α- OR IL-1β-INDUCED EXPRESSION OF MESSENGER RNA ENCODING MAJOR PRO-INFLAMMATORY MOLECULES

Using semi-quantitative RT-PCR we have demonstrated that IVIg also down-regulated the TNF-α- or IL-1β-induced expression of messenger RNA

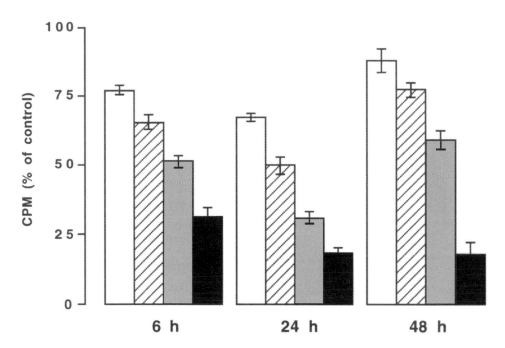

Figure 2. Kinetics of the inhibitory effect of IVIg on endothelial cell proliferation. HUVEC cells were maintained as described in the legend to Figure 1. Sandoglobulin was added at different concentrations (10mg/ml, open bars; 20 mg/ml, hatched bars; 30 mg/ml, grey bars and 40 mg/ml, dark bars) to the culture medium for various periods of time (6h, 24h and 48h) in the presence of 0.5 µCi ^{3}H-thymidine/well. At the end of incubation periods, radioactivity was measured by liquid scintillation counter. There was an inhibition of ^{3}H-thymidine incorporation by HUVEC cells in a dose- and time-dependent manner.

encoding major adhesion molecules, chemokines and pro-inflammatory cytokines in HUVEC. As the basal level of expression of adhesion molecules, chemokines and cytokines by HUVEC under our experimental conditions is low, we have induced the expression of the adhesion molecules ICAM-1 and VCAM-1, the chemokines MCP-1, M-CSF and GM-CSF and the proinflammatory cytokines TNF-α, IL-1β and IL-6 by two pro-inflammatory cytokines IL-1β and TNF-α, in order to evaluate the effect of IVIg on the expression of these molecules. IVIg significantly down-regulated the cytokine-induced expression of all these molecules involved in an inflammatory process, although IVIg alone, in concentrations ranging from 1 to 40 mg/ml, had no effect (Fig 3 and data not shown). One of the reasons for this blocking effect may be the anti-cytokine nature of IVIg, as IVIg contains antibodies directed against cytokines [18, 19]. However, we did not observe any difference in the proliferative responses of HUVEC either when IVIg was mixed with TNF-α or IL-1β before addition to the cells,

or when it was added after a preincubation of cells with the cytokines for 15 min (data not shown). We therefore believe that the inhibitory effect of IVIg on the cytokine-induced activation of HUVEC may not be exclusively due to neutralization of TNF-α or IL-1β by antibodies directed against these cytokines. Another possibility is that IVIg contains soluble receptors that "soak up" the TNF-α or IL-1β stimulators which abrogate the stimulatory effects of these cytokines. Further, it is also possible that in IVIg, anti-idiotypic antibodies bearing internal images of molecules that mimic such receptors may exist.

4. CONCLUSION

Our results suggest that some of the anti-inflammatory effects observed in patients treated with IVIg may be related to a decreased ability of endothelial cells to proliferate and to a down-regulation of the expression of molecules involved in the onset and

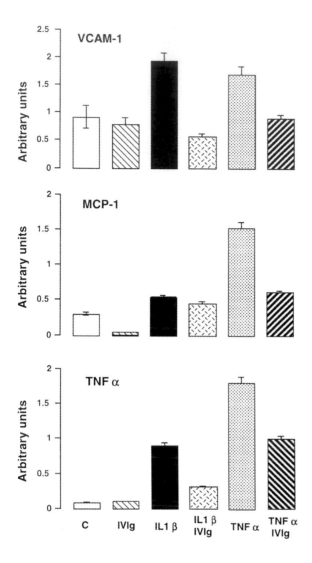

progression of inflammation. Although the relevance of these findings in *in vivo* situation needs further investigation, a possible beneficial effect of IVIg lies in the control of endothelial cell activation in the inflammatory conditions, since generation of microvessels is a salient feature of neoplasia and inflammation

REFERENCES

1. Carlos TM, Harlan JM. Leukocyte-endothelial adhesion molecules. Blood 1994;84:2068.
2. Matsushima KV, Oppenheim JJ. Interleukin-8 and MCAF: novel inflammatory cytokines induced by TNF and Il-1. Cytokines 1989;1:2.
3. Brady HR. Leukocyte adhesion molecules and kidney diseases. Kidney Int. 1994;45:1285.
4. Munro JM, Pober JS, Cotran RS. Tumor necrosis factor and interferon-g induce distinct patterns of endothelial activation and associated leukocyte accumulation in skin of Papio anubis. Am J Pathol 1989;135:121.
5. Osborn LR, Hession R, Tizard R, Vassala C, Luhowskyj S, Chi-Rosso G, Lobb R. Direct expression cloning of vascular cell adhesion molecule-1 and cytokine induced endothelial protein that binds lymphocytes. Cell 1989;248:415.
6. Scholz D, Devaux B, Hirche A, Potzsch B, Kropp B, Schaper W, Schaper J. Expression of adhesion molecules is specific and time-dependent in cytokine-stimulated endothelial cells in culture. Cell. Tissue Res. 1996;284:415.
7. Rajavashisth TB, Analibi A, Territo MC, Berliner JA, Navab M, Fogelman AM, Lusis AJ. Induction of endothelial cell expression of granulocyte and macrophage colony stimulating factors by modified low density lipoproteins. Nature 1990;344:254.
8. Jirik FR, Podor TJ, Hirano T, Kishimoto T, Loskutoff

Figure 3. Expression of messenger RNA encoding VCAM-1 adhesion molecules, MCP-1 chemokine and pro-inflammatory cytokine TNF-α. Endothelial cells were cultured in M199/20% FCS for 3–4 days to confluency and then incubated with IVIg (40 mg/ml), IL-1β (50 ng/ml), TNF-α (50 ng/ml), IL-1β (50 ng/ml) plus IVIg (40 mg/ml), TNF-α (50 ng/ml) plus IVIg (40 mg/ml). After 4 hours, mRNA were extracted and were reverse transcribed into cDNA with oligo(dT) and MMLV reverse transcriptase. The reverse transcription products were amplified with appropriate primers. The PCR fragments were analyzed by electrophoresis on 2% agarose gels and visualized by ethidium bromide staining. Polaroid photographs of ethidium bromide-stained gels were digitized into 512×512 pixel grey-scale images. The amount of nucleic acid, determined by densitometric analysis of the dots, was proportional to the logarithm of the optic density. Analysis was performed using the public domain NIH Image 1.51 program. The intensities of the cDNA bands for each protein were normalized to the GAPDH band intensities. IL-1β (50 ng/ml) and TNF-α (50 ng/ml) both induced an overexpression of mRNA encoding VCAM-1 (top panel), MCP-1 (midlle panel) and TNF-α (bottom panel) in a dose-dependent manner. While IVIg (40 mg/ml) alone had no significant effect on this synthesis, it down-regulated the mRNA expression induced by IL-1β or TNF-α. The intensities of the cDNA bands for each protein were normalized to the GAPDH band intensities. Experiments were run five times for each cell extract, coming from 3 to 5 different umbilical cords.

DJ, Carson DA, Lotz M. Bacterial lipopolysaccharide and inflammatory mediators augment IL-6 secretion by human endothelial cells. J. Immunol. 1989;142:144.

9. Dalakas M, Illa I, Dambrosia J, Soueidan S, Stein D, Otero C, Dinsmore S, McCrosky S. A controlled trial of high-dose intravenous immune globulin infusions as treatment for dermatomyositis. N. Engl. J. Med. 1993;329:1993.

10. Moller G. Immunoglobulin treatment: Mechanisms of action. Copenhagen: Munksgaard, 1994. Immunol. Rev.; vol 139).

11. Kazatchkine MD, Kaveri SV. Immunomodulation of autoimmune disease with intravenous immunoglobulin (IVIg). N. Engl. J. Med. 2000; in press.

12. Jayne DR, Lockwood CM. Pooled intravenous immunoglobulin in the management of systemic vasculitis. Adv Exp Med Biol 1993;336:469.

13. Lockwood CM. New treatment strategies for systemic vasculitis: the role of intravenous immune globulin therapy. Clin Exp Immunol 1996;1:77.

14. Kazatchkine MD, Dietrich G, Hurez V, Ronda N, Bellon B, Rossi F, Kaveri SV. V Region-mediated selection of autoreactive repertoires by intravenous immunoglobulin (IVIg). Immunol. Rev. 1994;139:79.

15. Xu C, Poirier B, Duong Van Huyen JP, Lucchiari N, Michel O, Chevalier J, Kaveri S. Modulation of endothelial cell function by normal polyspecific human intravenous immunoglobulins: a possible mechanism of action in vascular diseases. Am J Pathol 1998;153:1257.

16. Schnorf J, Arnet B, Burek-Kozlowska A, Gennari K, Rohner R, Spath PJ, Spycher MO. Laboratory parameters measured during infusion of immunoglobulin preparations for intravenous use and related tolerability. In: Kazatchkine MD, Morell A, eds. Intravenous immunoglobulin. Research and therapy. New York: Parthenon, 1996:312.

17. Fridman WH, Teillaud JL, Sautès C. Role of Fc receptors in immunomodulation by intravenous immunoglobulin. In: Kazatchkine MD, Morell A, eds. Intravenous immunogobulin. Research and therapy. New York: Parthenon, 1996:73.

18. Abe Y, Horiuchi A, Miyake M, Kimura S. Anti-cytokine nature of human immunoglobulin: one possible mechanism of the clinical effect of intravenous therapy. Immunol Rev 1994;139:5.

19. Svenson M, Hansen MB, Ross C, Diamant M, Rieneck K, Nielsen H, Bendtzen K. Antibody to granulocyte-macrophage colony-stimulating factor is a dominant anti-cytokine activity in Human IgG preparations. Blood 1998;91:2054.

ACCELERATED ATHEROSCLEROSIS IN DISEASE

Atherosclerosis and Autoimmunity
Y. Shoenfeld, D. Harats and G. Wick, editors

Cardiovascular Morbidity in the Hopkins Lupus Cohort[1]

Michelle Petri

Johns Hopkins University School of Medicine, Division of Rheumatology, Baltimore, MD 21205, USA

1. INTRODUCTION

In spite of multiple cohort studies emphasizing the increased survival in SLE [1, 2], the major cause of death in SLE in developed countries remains cardiovascular disease. Studies have shown varying prevalences of coronary artery disease, depending on whether it is defined clinically as angina/myocardial infarction/sudden death, or subclinically, using stress tests, echocardiograms, nuclear medicine scans, coronary catheterization or coronary calcification.

In the Hopkins Lupus Cohort, SLE patients are followed prospectively on a quarterly basis. The cohort includes a balance of African-American and Caucasian patients from the Baltimore community. Two types of cardiovascular damage – myocardial infarction and stroke – are tracked in this cohort, using the SLICC/ACR Damage Index [3, 4].

2. CORONARY ARTERY DISEASE

In 1992 we determined that coronary artery disease (CAD) (defined as angina, myocardial infarction, or sudden death) had occurred in 8.3% of the cohort. In a logistic regression model, duration of prednisone, hypertension, hypercholesterolemia, and morbid obesity were the best predictors [5] (Table 1).

In fact, the prevalence of CAD risk factors is astonishingly high in the Hopkins Lupus Cohort: African-Americans have on average 3.8 risk factors, and Caucasian patients have 3.6. The most common

risk factors are sedentary lifestyle, smoking, hypercholesterolemia, hypertension and obesity (Table 2). Sedentary lifestyle, current smoking, and obesity were more common in African-Americans than in Caucasians [6].

Our most recent analysis of factors predictive of CAD is shown in Table 3. As the cohort follow-up has lengthened, and the size of the cohort has grown, our ability to detect risk factors has increased. Of note, hypercholesterolemia is not included as a risk factor in this analysis. As part of the cohort protocol, only serum cholesterol is available. It is possible that LDL cholesterol, or other lipid parameters, would be a more informative risk factor.

Homocysteine is a major independent risk factor for both coronary artery disease and stroke in SLE [7]. Homocysteine predisposes to both atherosclerosis and thrombosis. In a clinical trial, we demonstrated that B-vitamin supplementation can reduce homocysteine in SLE [8].

We found that the lupus anticoagulant (but not anticardiolipin) was a risk factor for later CAD. This is reminiscent of previous work from our group [9] and others [10] that the lupus anticoagulant is a more specific predictor of thrombosis in SLE than is anticardiolipin antibody. The presence of antiphospholipid antibodies could predispose to CAD in several ways, by causing a thrombotic myocardial infarction [11], coronary vasculopathy [9] or atherosclerosis. Recent work has suggested that antiphospholipid antibodies may accelerate atherosclerosis by increasing uptake of oxidized LDL [12]. In addition, animal models have demonstrated that experimental antiphospholipid antibody syndrome is associated with atherosclerosis [13].

Many of the risk factors for CAD are a reflection

[1]The Hopkins Lupus Cohort is supported by AR 43727 and the Outpatient General Clinical Research Center RR 00052.

Table 1. Prediction of future coronary artery disease in the Hopkins Lupus Cohort: Multiple logistic regression model

	CAD	No CAD	t-test	p-value
Duration of prednisone (years)	14.3±11.3	7.2±7.2	2.85	0.005
Cholesterol – maximum mg/dL	271.2	214.9	3.9	0.0001
	CAD	No CAD	Odds ratio	95% CI
Hypertension, requiring treatment	79%	40%	5.5	1.8, 17.2
Obesity (NHANES definition)	58%	39%	2.1	0.8, 5.6

Table 2. Prevalence of CAD risk factors in the Hopkins Lupus Cohort

Characteristic	All females	White	Black
Number of patients	199	88	109
Sedentary life style	70%	53%	83%
Hypercholesterolemia (> 200 mg/dL)	55%	58%	52%
Hypertension, requiring treatment during cohort	39%	40%	39%
Obesity – NHANES definition	39%	30%	48%
Smoking – Current	37%	29%	44%
Hypercholesterolemia (> 240 mg/dL)	28%	24%	30%
Diabetes	6%	5%	7%
Mean number of risk factors (+ SD)	3.7±1.4	3.6±1.4	3.8±1.3

Table 3. Predictors of coronary artery disease in the Hopkins Lupus Cohort

Variable	OR (95% CI)	P-value
Age	1.08 (1.05–1.09)	0.001
Female sex	0.31 (0.19–0.55)	0.04
Homocysteine	1.05 (1.01–1.10)	0.02
Obesity	2.78 (1.61–4.76)	0.06
Hypertension	5.69 (3.53–9.18)	0.001
Diabetes mellitus	4.63 (2.75–7.82)	0.004
Higher creatinine	2.77 (1.79–4.27)	0.02
Lupus anticoagulant	3.79 (2.51–5.72)	0.002

of lupus-mediated organ damage. Hypertension and renal insufficiency are secondary to lupus nephritis, for example. Homocysteine levels are higher in SLE patients who have renal insufficiency or renal failure, as well. However, many of the risk factors are also aggravated by prednisone therapy, such as obesity, hyperlipidmia, and hypertension.

We have addressed the issue of the role of prednisone in accelerated atherosclerosis in two ways. First, in a prospective study analyzed using Generalized Estimated Equations (GEE), a regression technique appropriate for repeated measures, we showed that a 10 mg increase in prednisone led to significant increases in blood pressure, cholesterol, and weight [14]. Hydroxychloroquine use was able to reverse the effect on cholesterol (Table 4). Hydroxychlo-

Table 4. Multivariate analysis of factors affecting cholesterol in SLE patients: Longitudinal regression analysis

Variable	p value
Sex (women vs men)	0.001
Age	NS
Urine protein (3–4+)	< 0.001
Hydroxychloroquine (protective)	0.009
Diuretic use	0.04
Prednisone use	< 0.001

Table 5. Cox proportional hazards analysis of time to coronary artery disease

	RR (95% CI)	P-value
Cumulative corticosteroid	1.7 (1.2,2.4)	0.0024
High-dose corticosteroid	1.0 (0.3,3.0)	NS
Pulse methylprednisolone	1.1 (0.7,1.8)	NS

Table 6. Cox-proportional hazards analysis of time to stroke

	RR (95% CI)	P-value
Cumulative corticosteroid	1.0 (0.7,1.5)	NS
High-dose corticosteroid	3.4 (1.3,8.8)	0.01
Pulse methylprednisolone	0.9 (0.5,1.5)	NS

normal coronary arteries on catheterization, suggesting small vessel disease rather than atherosclerosis as the mechanism in some patients. Carotid duplex has been extensively studied by Manzi and colleagues [16], but it is not known if carotid atherosclerosis and coronary atherosclerosis are highly correlated in SLE. Secondly, the ideal interventions have not been studied. If the initial injury is lupus-mediated, traditional interventions may not be helpful. If progression is due to traditional risk factors, intervention may have to be multifactorial, because SLE patients have so many cardiovascular risk factors.

roquine is now used in about 50% of the Hopkins Lupus Cohort. It is interesting to speculate that the reason hypercholesterolemia is not found as a CAD risk factor in our most recent analyses is due to the widespread use of hydroxychloroquine in the cohort.

Our second approach to understanding the role of prednisone in cardiovascular disease has been a Cox-proportional hazards analysis. In this analysis corticosteroid exposure was examined in three ways: cumulative dose, high-dose exposure, and "pulse" intravenous methylprednisolone. Cumulative dose exposure was a significant risk factor in these analyses (Table 5) of the time to the cardiac event.

It is not clear that routine care of asymptomatic SLE patients should include screening tests for CAD, for two reasons. First, the best screening test has not been identified. The Toronto group has suggested that nuclear medicine technetium scans may identify SLE patients with subclinical coronary artery disease [15]. We share their interest in this area, but have found abnormal scans in patients with

3. STROKE

The most common cardiovascular event in the Hopkins Lupus Cohort is stroke (not myocardial infarction). Strokes are multifactorial, with risk factors including antiphospholipid antibodies, hypertension, and homocysteine [7]. Hypertension and homocysteine are both risk factors for atherosclerosis, but most strokes in our SLE patients are not ascribed to atherosclerosis.

Using Cox-proportional hazards analysis, we have examined the role corticosteroids play in the time to stroke (Table 6). Only the use of high-dose prednisone was associated with stroke. High-dose prednisone was also associated with an increase in hypertension (as we would have expected from our previous prospective analysis) that might explain the increase in stroke.

We have studied carotid duplex to screen for subclinical atherosclerosis in 433 SLE patients in the Hopkins Lupus Cohort. In this group of asymptomatic patients, 17% had an abnormal carotid duplex, with demonstration of atherosclerotic plaque.

Table 7. Risk factors for carotid atherosclerotic plaque in the Hopkins Lupus Cohort

Variable	OR	95% CI	P-value
A. Discrete variables			
Smoking	1.87	1.1–3.1	0.02
Renal insufficiency	2.21	1.1–4.5	0.04
Obesity	2.13	1.3–3.6	0.005
Hypertension	4.19	2.4–7.3	0.0001
Diabetes	3.44	1.6–7.4	0.002
Cholesterol	1.79	1.04–3.1	0.045
Aspirin use	0.54	0.3–0.96	0.04
Estrogen replacement therapy	2.48	1.4–4.5	0.004
B. Continuous variables			
Weight			0.0005
BP-systolic			0.0001
BP-diastolic			0.019
Age			0.0001
Years duration of Lupus			0.04
Highest Prednisone dose			0.04

Table 8. Risk factors for an abnormal transcranial Doppler in the Hopkins Lupus Cohort

Predictor	OR	95% CI	P-value
Cardiac valvular damage	7.69	1.71–34.3	0.02
Cardiac murmur	2.50	1.04–5.97	0.04
Muscle damage	5.44	1.30–22.5	0.04
Raynaud's	2.42	0.98–5.96	0.06
Anticardiolipin	3.86	1.52–9.80	0.005

Duplex carotid sonography was performed using commercially available high resolution linear transducers (5–10 MHz, Acuson 128XP, Hewlett Packard Image Point or ATL HDI 3000). Images were acquired of the distal common carotid arteries (CCA), carotid bulb and proximal internal carotid arteries (ICA) in the sagital plane. Intimal thickness was measured on the near and far walls of the distal CCA and Doppler spectrum tracings were taken in the first 2 cm of the proximal ICA. If atherosclerotic plaque was identified, transverse images and measurements of the plaque were also obtained.

Traditional cardiovascular risk factors are highly predictive of atherosclerotic plaque found on carotid duplex (Table 7). The highest dose of prednisone was associated with the presence of atherosclerotic plaque. Aspirin use appeared to be protective. Estrogen replacement therapy was associated with a higher frequency of atherosclerosis. Although this could reflect selection of higher-risk women for hormone replacement therapy, there are recent concerns that estrogen replacement may increase cardiovascular morbidity in normal women [17].

However, because we believe that the majority of strokes in SLE are not directly due to atherosclerosis, we have also examined a second screening test, transcranial Doppler (TCD), that detects microemboli.

In the general population, TCD is predictive of stroke in patients with high-grade carotid stenosis. It is also frequently abnormal in patients with antiphospholipid antibody syndrome [18]. We determined predictors of abnormal TCD in SLE patients, with no current symptoms of TIA or stroke, in a prospective study of 319 SLE patients.

A Pioneer TC 2020 model (Nicolet Biomedical Inc) TCD was used. The probe was placed on the temporal acoustic window superior and anterior to the external auditory meatus. Cerebral microemboli were counted for one hour, using a cut off of ≥ 9 dBs.

Eight percent of the TCDs were abnormal. There was no association with abnormal carotid duplex (only 4 patients had both an abnormal TCD AND an abnormal carotid duplex). Predictive variables were determined at cohort entry or during prospective follow-up before the TCD (Table 8). Low C3 (p=0.05) and low C4 (p=0.002) were also predictive of an abnormal TCD. Aspirin and hydroxychloroquine use were not protective against microemboli.

Abnormal TCDs in the Hopkins Lupus Cohort are associated with cardiac murmur and cardiac valvular damage. Because there is no association with abnormal carotid duplex, we believe the valvular damage is the source of the microemboli. Similarly,

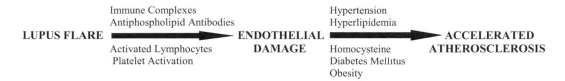

Figure 1. Model of accelerated atherosclerosis

anticardiolipin (aCL), a predictor of TCD, is also associated with Libman-Sacks, a known mechanism of valvular damage in SLE. This study strongly suggests that SLE patients with aCL should have screening cardiac echo (for valvular disease) and TCDs (to assess stroke risk). However, this study does not address treatment and cannot assess the actual risk of future stroke in SLE.

4. CONCLUSION

Cardiovascular morbidity is a major issue in SLE, both in terms of coronary artery disease and stroke. In the prospective Hopkins Lupus Cohort, the lupus anticoagulant has been a risk factor for CAD and anticardiolipin for stroke. The pathogenetic mechanisms leading to cardiovascular morbidity are complex, and involve not just atherosclerosis, but also thromboembolism and lupus-mediated vessel damage.

Atherosclerosis in SLE may be amenable to intervention, but it, too, is complicated in its pathogenesis. We have proposed a two-stage model, emphasizing that immune-mediated injury is likely primary, with traditional CAD risk factors then playing a secondary role in acceleration (Fig. 1). Prednisone is, therefore, a two-edged sword, being useful in dampening immune-mediated damage, but long-term being detrimental through aggravation of traditional CAD risk factors, including hyperlipidemia, hypertension and weight.

REFERENCES

1. Gladman DD, Urowitz MB. Morbidity in systemic lupus erythematosus. J Rheumatol 1987;14(suppl 13):223–226.
2. Wallace DJ, Podell T, Weiner J, Klinenberg JR, Forouzesh S, Dubois EL. Systemic lupus erythematosus – survival patterns: experience with 609 patients. J Am Med Assoc 1981;245:934–938.
3. Gladman D, Ginzler E, Goldsmith C, Fortin P, Liang M, Urowitz M, et al. Workshop Report. Systemic Lupus International Collaborative Clinics: development of a damage index in SLE. J Rheumatol 1992;19:1820–1821.
4. Gladman D, Ginzler E, Goldsmith C, Fortin P, Liang M, Urowitz M, et al. The development and initial validation of the Systemic Lupus International Collaborating Clinics/American College Rheumatology damage index for sytemic lupus erythematosus. Arthritis Rheum 1996;39:363–369.
5. Petri M, Perez-Gutthann S, Spence D, Hochberg MC. Risk factors for coronary artery disease in patients with systemic lupus erythematosus. Am J Med 1992;93:513–519.
6. Petri M, Spence D, Bone LR, Hochberg MC. Coronary artery disease risk factors in the Hopkins Lupus Cohort: prevalence, patient recognition, and preventive practices. Medicine 1992;71:291–302.
7. Petri M, Roubenoff R, Dallal GE, Nadeau MR, Selhub J, Rosenberg IH. Plasma homocysteine as a risk factor for atherothrombotic events in systemic lupus erythematosus. Lancet 1996;348:1120–1124.
8. Petri M, Vu D, Omura A, Yuen J, Selhub J, Rosenberg I, et al. Effectiveness of B-vitamin therapy in reducing plasma total homocysteine in patients with systemic lupus [abstract]. Arthritis Rheum 1998;41(9 (Suppl)):S241.
9. Petri M, Rheinschmidt M, Whiting-O'Keefe Q, Hellmann D, Corash L. The frequency of lupus anticoagulant in systemic lupus erythematosus: a study of 60 consecutive patients by activated partial thromboplastin time, Russell viper venom time, and anticardiolipin antibody. Ann Int Med 1987;106:524–531.
10. Derksen RHWM, Hasselaar P, Blokzijl L, Gmelig Meyling FHJ, de Groot PG. Coagulation screen is more specific than the anticardiolipin antibody ELISA in defining a thrombotic subset of lupus patients. Ann Rheum Dis 1988;47:364–371.
11. Hamsten A, Norberg R, Björkholm M, de Faire U, Holm G. Antibodies to cardiolipin in young survivors

of myocardial infarction: an association with recurrent cardiovascular events. Lancet 1986;1:113–116.

12. Hasunuma Y, Matsuura E, Makita Z, Nishi S, Koike T. Involvement of β_2-glycoprotein I and anticardiolipin antibodies in oxidatively modified low-density lipoprotein uptake by macrophages. Clin Exp Immunol 1997;107:569–573.

13. Shoenfeld Y. The significance of experimental models of systemic lupus erythematosus and antiphospholipid syndrome induced by idiotypic manipulation. Isr J Med Sci 1994;30:10–18.

14. Petri M, Lakatta C, Magder L, Goldman DW. Effect of prednisone and hydroxychloroquine on coronary artery disease risk factors in systemic lupus erythematosus: a longitudinal data analysis. Am J Med 1994;96:254–259.

15. Bruce IN, Burns RJ, Gladman DD, Urowitz MB. High prevalence of myocardial perfusion abnormalities in women with SLE [abstract]. Arthritis Rheum 1997;40(Suppl 9):S219.

16. Manzi S, Selzer F, Sutton-Tyrrell K, Fitzgerald SG, Rairie JE, Tracy RP, et al. Prevalence and risk factors of carotid plaque in women with systemic lupus erythematosus. Arthritis Rheum 1999;42:51–60.

17. Hulley S, Grady D, Bush T, Furberg C, Herrington D, Riggs B, et al. Randomized trial of estrogen plus progestin for secondary prevention of coronary heart disease in postmenopausal women. Heart and Estrogen/progestin Replacement Study (HERS) Research Group. JAMA 1998;280:605–613.

18. Brey RL, Carolin MK. Detection of cerebral microembolic signals by transcranial Doppler may be a useful part of the equation in determining stroke risk in patients with antiphospholipid antibody syndrome. Lupus 1997;6(8):621–624.

Atherosclerosis and Autoimmunity
Y. Shoenfeld, D. Harats and G. Wick, editors

Atherosclerosis in Systemic Lupus Erythematosus: Clinical Relevance

Sònia Jiménez, Manuel Ramos-Casals, Ricard Cervera, Josep Font and Miguel Ingelmo

Systemic Autoimmune Diseases Unit, Hospital Clínic, Barcelona, Catalonia, Spain

1. INTRODUCTION

The description of late-stage morbidity and mortality has been an important contribution to the understanding of systemic lupus erithematosus (SLE) in the past decade. In 1974, Urowitz et al. [1] described the bimodal pattern of mortality in SLE and found a second mortality peak in the long term outcome of SLE patients. Several epidemiological studies have analyzed this fact, suggesting the existence of a precocious and accelerated atherosclerosis in these patients. This condition has been recognized clinically with the diagnosis of coronary artery disease (CAD), namely myocardial infarction and angina, in young women with SLE. This accelerated atherosclerosis has also been recognized at postmortem examinations. In the largest series of SLE patients described since 1970, 6–20% of deaths were due to cardiovascular disease and 4–15% of deaths were due to cerebrovascular disease [2–7]. Many of these deaths were caused by atherosclerotic vascular disease occurring in premenopausal women. Thus, there is increasing evidence that traditional risk factors do not explain completely the atherosclerotic process in SLE, and recent studies have implicated new etiopathogenic factors.

2. ETIOLOGICAL FACTORS OF ATHEROSCLEROSIS IN SLE

2.1. Traditional Risk Factors

SLE patients have a high prevalence of "traditional" risk factors for atherosclerosis, related to clinical conditions and treatments received [8]. Nephritis may be associated with hypertension, nephrotic syndrome may cause hyperlipidemia, and arthritis and fatigue may reduce a patient's ability to exercise. These factors, along with smoking, obesity, diabetes mellitus and chronic renal failure may contribute to the increased prevalence of CAD in patients with SLE [9, 10]. In a 10-year prospective study in a cohort of 70 patients with lupus nephritis, the main causes of mortality were vascular complications (cardiovascular or cerebrovascular events) [11]. Additionally, the autopsy study of Bulkley and Roberts [12] showed that coronary atherosclerosis is a post-steroid era phenomenon. Petri et al. [13] have demonstrated that prednisone could indirectly accelerate atherosclerosis by increasing the levels of three traditional CAD risk factors, namely hypercholesterolemia, hypertension and obesity. Steroid therapy is associated with increased total cholesterol, very low density lipoproteins cholesterol (VLDL-C) and low density lipoproteins cholesterol (LDL-C) [14, 15], although only steroid doses greater than 10 mg/dL lead to significant changes in lipid levels [8, 16, 17]. Thus, corticosteroid treatment may accelerate atherosclerosis by worsening hypertension, hyperlipidemia, and diabetes mellitus, and by causing musculoskeletal morbidity that results in reduced physical activity [8, 12, 18, 19].

Other risk factors implicated in cardiovascular events in SLE patients include older age at SLE diagnosis [9, 20]. In a recent study, the incidence of stroke and myocardial infarction in SLE was estimated after controlling for expected events based on known population based risk models [21]. After adjustment for the classical risk factors, the risk for myocardial infarction and stroke was significantly increased, suggesting that the diagnosis of SLE or its treatment is the strongest known risk factor for cardiovascular disease in these patients.

To date, three large studies have assessed traditional risk factors for clinical CAD in patients with SLE [9, 20, 22], although the cohorts studied showed different ethnic characteristics. Older age at SLE diagnosis and hypercholesterolemia were found to be significantly associated with CAD in the three studies, and disease duration, duration of steroid therapy and hypertension were found to be associated in two [9, 20]. It might be argued that a cluster of CAD risk factors occurs in SLE, predisposing patients with SLE to CAD simply because they have more risk factors [23].

2.2. New Risk Factors

2.2.1. Metabolic risk factors

Several studies have shown that lipid abnormalities occur in untreated SLE [24]. This dyslipoproteinemia is characterized by elevated triglycerides and VLDL-C as well as reduced levels of high-density lipoprotein cholesterol (HDL-C) and apolipoprotein (Apo) A-1 [24, 25]. Some authors [26] have also found abnormalities in chylomicron (CM) clearance due to disturbances in their metabolism, characterized by decreased lipolysis and CM removal from the plasma [27]. These facts, as well as the basal pattern of lipid abnormalities of the untreated disease, suggest that SLE disease process directly influences the metabolism of VLDL-cholesterol. Addititionally, lipoprotein (a), an independent risk factor for CAD in the general population, has also been studied in SLE, and some studies [28] have found raised lipoprotein (a) levels and their association with myocardial infarction in patients with SLE [29].

Finally, elevation of serum homocysteine – that has both direct and indirect injurious effects on the endothelium – has recently been recognized as a risk factor for CAD in the general population. Some studies in SLE have found raised homocysteine levels [10] and their association with an increased risk for arterial thrombotic events in SLE [30]. Petri et al. [10] have disclosed several variables as predictive factors of elevated homocysteine levels in SLE, including male gender, diet, renal failure and prednisone intake.

2.2.2. Inflammatory factors

Currently, there is great interest in examining the role of inflammation in the pathogenesis of atherosclerosis [31–35]. Several studies have reported that modest elevations in C-reactive protein or serum amyloid A seems to identify a subset of patients with a worse prognosis from CAD [31, 32, 35, 37]. In SLE, Manzi et al. [36] have recently reported an association between atherosclerosis and inflammatory markers, such as C-reactive protein and fibrinogen.

2.2.3. Immunological factors

The pathogenesis of cardiovascular disease in SLE is likely multifactorial, involving an interaction between inflammation-induced and antiphospholipid antibody (aPL)-mediated vascular injury/thrombosis from the underlying disease as well as traditional risk factors. Many studies have shown the association of anticardiolipin antibodies (aCL) and the presence of CAD in SLE. Lahita et al. [38] suggested that aCL were associated with low total cholesterol, low HDL-cholesterol level and low apo A1 level. The presence of aCL may influence the lipid levels in patients with SLE and antiphospholipid syndrom (APS).

Matsura et al. [39] and Hasuma et al. [40] have postulated a possible pathogenetic mechanism: when aCL are not present, the "co-factor" (β-2-glycoprotein I or apolipoprotein H) acts as a natural protector against atherosclerosis, by inhibiting uptake of oxidized LDL. Antibodies to lipoproteins are consistently found in SLE, including antibodies to β-2-glycoprotein I – which is an HDL associated protein that have prognostic significance for the inflammatory process in SLE [41–44] – as well as antibodies to other HDL-associated proteins such as apoA-1 and apoA-2.

Finally, Vaarala et al. [45] described in 1993 the existence of a cross-reaction of antibodies to oxidized LDL as a possible mechanism involved in the development of accelerated atherosclerosis in SLE. It is conceivable that antibodies to oxidized LDL may enhance the accumulation of oxidized LDL in the endothelial cell walls [46].

Table 1. Epidemiological studies: Risk for CD in SLE

Study	Year	Design	Patients	Age of patients	Risk for MI	Risk for A	Risk for CVD
Jonsson et al. [47]	1989	prospective 1981–1986	86		9	–	–
Manzi et al. [20]	1997	prospective 1980–1993	498	25–34	∞	1.96	–
				35–44	50.43	2.35	–
				45–54	2.47	1.03	–
				55–64	4.21	2.33	–
Ward et al. [48]	1999	prospective 1991–1994	3851	18–44	8.5	–	8.7
			2754	45–64	2.8	–	2.5
			2137	≥ 65	0.7	–	0.7

CD: cardiovascular disease; MI: myocardial infarction; A: angor pectoris; CVD: cerebrovascular disease.

3. EPIDEMIOLOGY OF ATHEROSCLEROSIS IN SLE

3.1. Relative Risk

An increased risk for cardiovascular disease in SLE has been reported in various studies (Table 1). In 1989, Jonsson et al. [47] described a risk for CAD 9-fold greater in SLE patients compared with an age-matched general population. In another study [20], age-specific incidence rates of CAD from 498 SLE patients (SLE Cohort at Pittsburg) were contrasted with the age-specific rates in women (Framingham Offspring Study) followed during the same time period. This study reported that SLE women in the 35–44 age group were over 50 times more likely to have a myocardial infarction than controls (rate ratio=52.4%). In addition, a recent study performed in 8.742 SLE patients and age-matched controls demonstrated that the risk of hospitalization for myocardial infarction, cerebrovascular accident and congestive heart failure was respectively 2.27, 2.03 and 3.01, times greater for SLE patients between 18–44 years compared with controls [48]. Recently, analysis from the Canadian SLE population [21] revealed that the overall risk for myocardial infarction and stroke conferred by SLE, after controlling for the Framingham risk factors, was 8.3 and 6.7 fold, respectively.

3.2. Prevalence of Clinical Cardiovascular Disease

Epidemiologic studies have reported an increase in cardiovascular disease in SLE patients, with a prevalence that are strikingly high, given that most patients in these studies were young women.

Several studies have analyzed the prevalence of cardiovascular events in patients with SLE, such as myocardial infarction, angina, cerebrovascular accident or peripheral vascular disease (Table 2). These studies showed prevalences ranging between 2% and 20%. In 1987, Gladman and Urowitz [22] found a prevalence of 9% of CAD (angina or myocardial infarction) in a series of 507 SLE patients. In another study [9], cardiovascular disease (including angina, myocardial infarction and cardiac sudden death) was reported in 8% of 229 SLE patients from the Baltimore Lupus Cohort. Finally, the SUNY Heath Science Center at Brooklyn found a 15% prevalence of CAD in a series of 200 SLE patients [49]. In none of these studies, the previous treatment with steroids was related to cardiovascular events. Conversely, the traditional risk factors (hypertension, diabetes mellitus, high levels of cholesterol or triglycerides, postmenopausal status) were statistically related with cardiovascular manifestations. Although some authors [22] have found a relationship between previous cardiac features related to SLE (such as pericarditis or myocarditis) and atherosclerotic cardiovascular disease, most studies have found no association between cardiovascular

Table 2. Prevalence of cardiovascular disease (CD) in SLE

Study	Year	Patients	Design	Number of patients (%)		
				CAD	CVD	CD
Urowitz et al. [1]	1976	81	prospective	6 (7.4%)	–	–
Badui et al. [18]	1985	100	prospective	16 (16%)	3 (3%)	19 (19%)
Gladnan and Urowitz [22]	1987	507	prospective	45 (8.9%)	–	–
Jonsson et al. [47]	1989	86	prospective	17 (19.8%)	7 (8.1%)	29 (33.7%)
Shome et al. [101]	1989	65	retrospective	4 (1%)	–	–
Petri et al. [8]	1992	229	prospective	19 (8.3%)	–	–
Sultan et al. [49]	1994	200	prospective	30 (15%)	–	–
Heart-Holmes et al. [102]	1995	89	retrospective	5 (6%)	–	13 (13.4%)
Stahl-Hallengren et al. [100]	2000	85	prospective	12 (14.1%)	9 (11%)	21 (25%)
TOTAL				155/1442 (10.7%)	19/266 (7.1%)	72/360 (20%)

disease and SLE manifestations.

All these studies suggest that clinical atherosclerotic events are increased in prevalence and accelerated in their development in patients with SLE.

3.3. Mortality

Urowitz et al. [1] were among the first to recognize the significance of CAD in the late clinical course of patients with SLE. Analysis of the 11 deaths in their cohort at the University of Toronto revelated a bimodal distribution of mortality. Early deaths occurred within the first year after diagnosis and these patients died due to active SLE. The late deaths were attributed to myocardial infarctions. This led to the description of the phenomenon of a bimodal mortality pattern in SLE. Before this description, anecdotal reports of patients with SLE and myocardial infarctions were described [50–53]. Other cohorts [54–56] documented deaths from myocardial infarction during the 70s–80s, but these cohorts reported a mortality significantly lower than Urowitz et al. (3–4% vs 45% respectively) (Table 3). At that time, two autopsy studies [12, 57] confirmed the presence of CAD in women with SLE without overt clinical myocardial infarctions. Several other

investigators have attempted to estimate the prevalence of subclinical atherosclerosis in individuals with SLE using necropsy techniques. In an autopsy study of 22 young women with SLE, Haider and Roberts [57] found that 45% had at least one major coronary artery that was significantly narrowed by atherosclerotic plaques.

4. STUDY OF SUBCLINICAL CARDIOVASCULAR DISEASE IN SLE

The true prevalence of cardiovascular disease in living patients with SLE is unknown. Asymptomatic subclinical cardiovascular disease is an important concept because reflects more accurately the true prevalence of atherosclerosis. The diagnosis of the asymptomatic atherosclerotic disease in SLE may lead to an early and effective treatment of atherosclerosis with a preventive effect over their clinical complications. Several investigators have attempted to evaluate the frequency of subclinical CAD using electrocardiograms, echocardiograms, stress thallium scans, and dual-isotope myocardial perfusion imaging. In the 80s, some authors attempted an approach to study cardiovascular disease in SLE.

Table 3. Mortality studies from cardiovascular[a] disease (CD) on SLE

Study	Year	Period	No. patients	No. deaths	Deaths related to CD
Urowitz et al. [1]	1976	1970–1974	81	11	5 (45%)
Wallace et al. [92]	1981	1950–1980	609	128	26 (20%)
Rosner et al. [56]	1982	1965–1976	1103	222	12 (5.4%)
Rubin et al. [2]	1985	1970–1983	417	51	9 (17.6%)
Jonsson et al. [47]	1989	1979–1986	86	9	4 (44.5%)
Reveille et al. [4]	1990	1975–1984	389	89	8 (10.8%)
Petri et al. [8]	1992	1987–1992	229	10	2 (20%)
Abu-Shakra et al. [6]	1995	retrospective	665	124	31 (25%)
Ward et al. [7]	1995	1969–1983	408	144	32 (22%)
Aranow et al. [98]	1996	1966–1995 • 66–75 • 76–85 • 86–95	1080	270	 2% (CAD) / 0% (CVD) 3% (CAD) / 4% (CVD) 8% (CAD) / 4% (CVD)
Cervera et al. [99]	1999	1990–1995	1000	45	8 (17.7%)
Stahl-Hallengren et al. [100]	2000	1981–1986	121	17	13 (76%)

[a] Cardiovascular disease includes: coronary artery disease – CAD (myocardial infarction, angina or sudden death), cerebrovascular disease – CVD, and peripheral vascular disease – PVD

Badui et al. [18] analyzed 100 Mexican women with SLE by echocardiogram and electrocardiogram evaluation, and found evidence of ischemic heart disease in 16% of these women.

One of the main problems to detect subclinical cardiovascular disease is that most of the techniques have an invasive character. Because of this several studies have been started with the objective of optimizing several imaging techniques that though they do not present sensibility as high as arteriography, result bloodless and easy to accomplishing in patients tath in many ocasions present others complications.

By taking advantage of the growing use of vascular imaging techniques in cardiovascular research it is possible to increase our understanding of the prevalence and mechanisms of ischemic vascular disease in SLE and of the relative importance of associated factors. The ability to measure atherosclerosis in its subclinical stages will also allow better risk stratification.

4.1. B-mode Carotid Ultrasound

The carotid arteries are easily accessible to noninvasive study using ultrasound techniques. This technique provides no risk or discomfort to the patient and in trained hands can provide accurate and reliable measurements of atherosclerosis in its subclinical stages [58–61]. B-mode ultrasound allows detection and measurement of the intima-media wall tickness (IMT) and the degree of plaques in the carotid arteries. IMT may be the most sensitive marker for the earliest stages of atherosclerosis and is considered to be a marker of generalized atherosclerosis [62, 63]. B-mode ultrasound is widely used in epidemiologic studies that evaluate the prevalence and risk factors associated with atherosclerosis in large population-based samples [64–68]. Individuals with asymptomatic carotid disease are at increased risk for coronary heart disease, lower extremity arterial disease and death [69–75].

Recent studies have analyzed and measured the IMT and identified the existence of atherosclerotic plaques in patients with SLE. In 1997, atherosclerotic plaques were found in the 8% of 97 SLE patients from the Jonhs Hopkins cohort [76], and the variables significantly associated with focal plaque included race (black patients), hypertension, the number of years since SLE diagnosis and positive aPL. A high dose of prednisone, traditional cardiovascular risk factors such as hyperlipidemia or smoking, and the gender or age, were not related to the development of atherosclerosis. In another study, Roman et al. [77] analyzed 19 SLE patients with associated APS and 38 controls with a similar age and cardiovascular risk profile, and reported a similar carotid IMT in both groups, but a higher prevalence of discrete atherosclerotic plaque in SLE patients. In 1998, Merril et al. [78] found evidence of plaque by carotid ultrasound in 11 of 34 SLE patients with antibodies to apo A1. As compared with SLE patients without apoA1 antibodies and plaque, patients with these antibodies had strikingly lower cholesterol, lower levels of LDL and a low diastolic blood pressure. Manzi et al. [36] have also studied the prevalence of carotid atherosclerosis and associated risk factors in 175 women with SLE, measuring the carotid plaque and the IMT by B-mode ultrasound. In addition, traditional cardiovascular risk factors were determined at the time of the ultrasound scan. The independent variables related to plaque development were older age, higher systolic blood pressure, higher levels of LDL cholesterol, prolonged treatment with prednisone and a previous coronary event. Older age, a previous coronary event and elevated systolic blood pressure were also associated with an increased severity of plaque. However, the risk factors related to increased IMT were older age, elevated pulse pressure and higher Systemic Lupus International Collaborating Clinics (SLICC) disease damage score. Recently, Falaschi et al. [79] reported a serie of 26 juvenile-onset SLE patients, which showed an IMT significantly higher than a sex-age matched control group. The results of IMT measurements did not correlate with the age, disease duration, SLE Disease Activity Index (SLEDAI) score, SLICC/ACR score or cumulative prednisone dose. However, the patients with nephrotic range proteinuria had a significantly higher IMT than those without proteinuria.

We have recently performed carotid ultrasonographic study in 21 SLE patients (20 women and one man, mean age 38 years) and have observed focal plaque in 24% of patients, one of whom had known arterial disease (unpublished data).

4.2. Electron Beam Computed Tomography

Currently, new technology provides a noninvasive way to evaluate directly the coronary arteries. Coronary artery scanning by electron beam computed tomography (EBCT) has been shown to detect noninvasively and accurately calcified atherosclerotic plaque by both intravascular ultrasound and histologic criteria [80–83]. EBCT has also been used to detect progression over time of coronary calcification in a recent study by Maher et al. [84]. Since atherosclerosis may occur at an earlier age in the aorta than in the coronary arteries, EBCT can be used to detect aortic calcification, particularly in younger age groups. Preliminary reports indicated that, after intravenous injection of contrast agents, EBCT can accurately visualize the coronary artery lumen and detect stenoses noninvasively [85].

Thirteen SLE patients (age 33–48) with two or more risk factors (diabetes, hypertension, hypercholesterolemia, obesity and presence of aPL) were studied by EBCT [86]. The calcification score was compared to age and sex matched controls. Two of the SLE patients had calcification scores in the 70th percentile of age matched women without known CAD and three had scores in the 90th percentile.

4.3. Vascular Stiffness

Measures of vascular stiffness, such as aortic pulse wave velocity (PWV), are also showing promising results as an early marker of atherosclerosis . Stiffening of the aorta occurs with age due to fragmentation and degeneration of elastin, increases in collagen, and a thickening of the arterial wall [87]. A progressive dilation of the arteries accompanies this stiffening process. Aortic vascular stiffness has been analyzed by PWV in 165 women with SLE [88]. PWVwas significantly and positively associated with body mass index, systolic and diastolic blood oressure, tryglicerides, high fasting glucose levels, renal disease, C-reactive protein,fibrinogen, SLICC and focal carotid plaque detected by ultrasound.

4.4. Myocardial Perfusion Studies

Some studies have analyzed ischemia in SLE using coronary perfusion studies, such as thallium perfusion scan or dual-isotope myocardial perfusion imaging (DIMPI) [89]. These perfusion techniques rely on perfusion abnormalities, which could lead to a gross underestimation of the atherosclerotic burden and risk for future myocardial infarction.

Exercise thallium-201 cardiac scintigraphy was performed in 26 SLE patients from the Rheumatology Service of the Oregon Health Sciences University [90]. Segmental perfusion abnormalities were present in 10 (40%) patients: 5 had reversible defects suggesting ischemia, 4 had persistent defects consistent in scar and one patient had both reversible and persistent defects. There was no correlation between positive thallium results and duration of disease, amount of corticosteroid treatment, major organ system involvement or age. In other study, Dual-isotope myocardial perfusion abnormalities were seen in 40% of 60 SLE women at an early age (including six with a known history of CAD) at the University of Toronto [89]. Recently, Petri and Civclek [91] found abnormal myocardial SPECT in 33% (11 of 33) SLE patients. Age was the single variable associated to an abnormal myocardial SPECT scan. Myocardial SPECT scans are frequently abnormal in SLE patients with a normal carotid ultrasonography but are not associated with risk factors for atherosclerosis.

5. PREVENTION AND TREATMENT

5.1. Optimizing SLE Therapy

Physicians should perform an accurate evaluation of their SLE patients in order to an earlier detection and treatment of atherosclerotic lesions. A well-optimized control of SLE should include management of hypertension and dyslipemia, minimizing steroid dose and controlling other factors such as obesity or smoking. In addition, clinicians should routinely evaluate these patients for atherosclerotic risk factors and aggressively treat any that are present. One might speculate that more aggressive control of more traditional risk factors may be beneficial in reducing the risk of cardiovascular disease in these women.

There is a growing body of evidence that antimalarial agents may have beneficial effects on lipid profiles in SLE. Several studies have correlated the use of antimalarials with a reduction in cholesterol or triglicerid levels [13, 92–95]. Thus, antimalarials may have an additional therapeutic role in SLE to minimize the increase in lipid fractions in patients receiving steroid therapy. Petri et al. [13] found an association between hydroxychloroquine use and lower serum cholesterol, and it seems to be able to "balance" the hyperlipidemic effect of low doses of prednisone (10 mg). They also demonstrated the multifactorial effect of hydroxychloroquine on active SLE, hyperlipidemia, anti-platelet and "desludging" rheologic effect and a reduction in aPL titers [96].

5.2. Lipid Lowering Therapy

Large trials of aggressive LDL reduction in secondary prevention are now underway. Sub-studies of these groups of trials have shown additional benefits of statins in reducing events in the elderly, women, diabetics and reducing events of cardiac failure (30%), stroke or transient ischaemic attacks (30%) or peripheral vascular disease (28%). Similar benefits have been shown in patients without established coronary heart disease. Few data exist on the safety and efficacy of these drugs in patients with SLE apart from anecdotal reports. Further work is needed to investigate whether statins and fibrates can reduce cardiovascular disease in SLE.

Some authors suggest a more aggressive management of the lipid abnormalities in patients with SLE. Hallegua and Wallace [97] recommended that SLE patients should be started on lipid lowering agents earlier and the doses of these medications can be increased to maximal doses in order to keep the LDL levels at the recommended level of ≤ 130 mg/mL if patients do not have any symptoms of CAD. If CAD is present, then LDL levels should be reduced to ≤ 100 mg/ml, or to a level as low as possible.

5.3. Prevention

The marked increased mortality in SLE from accelerated atherosclerosis requires a higher state of vigilance in our SLE patients, and they must be monitored closely for symptoms and signs of CAD. Primary prevention of CAD is of paramount importance by cheking and treating hyperlipidemia, hyperglycemia and hypertension, counseling patients to stop smoking, exercise and help them lose weight. We should use the lowest dose of corticosteroids, adding other drugs, such as antimalarials or immunossuppresive agents. Finally, clinicians should be proactive in the use of non-invasive techniques in the screening for CAD.

REFERENCES

1. Urowitz MB, Bookman AM, Koehler BE, et al. The bimodal pattern of systemic lupus erythematosus. Am J Med 1976;60:221–225.
2. Rubin LA, Urowitz MB, Gladman DD. Mortality in systemic lupus erythematosus: the bimodal pattern revised. QJM 1985;55:87–98.
3. Helve T. Prevalence and mortality rates of systemic lupus erythematosus and causes of death in SLE patients in Finland. Scand J Rheumatol 1985;14:43–46.
4. Reveille JD, Bartolucci A, Alarcón GS. Prognosis in systemic lupus erythematosus: negative impact of increasing age at onset, black race, and thombocitopenia, as well as causes of death. Arthritis Rheum 1990;33:37–48.
5. Pistiner M, Wallace DJ, Nessim S, Metzger AL, Klinenberg JR. Lupus erythematosus in the 1980s: a survey of 570 patients. Semin Arthritis Rheum 1991;21:55–64.
6. Abu-Shakra M, Urowitz MB, Gladman DD, Gough J. Mortality studies in systemic lupus erythematosus. Results from a single center. I. Causes of death. J Rheumatol 1995;22:259–264.
7. Ward M, Pyun E, Studenski S. Causes of death in systemic lupus erythematosus: long-term followup of an inception cohort. Arthritis Rheum 1995;38:1492–1499.
8. Petri M, Spence D, Bone LR, Hochberg MC. Coronary artery disease risk factors in the Johns Hopkins Lupus Cohort: prevalence, recognition by patients, and preventive practices. Medicine (Baltimore) 1992;71:291–302.
9. Petri M, Perez-Gutthann S, Spence D, Hochberg MC. Risk factors for coronary artery disease in patients with systemic lupus erythematosus. Am J Med 1992;93:513–519.
10. Petri M, Roubenoff R, Dallal GE, Nadeau MR, Selhub J, Rosenberg IH. Plasma homocysteine as a risk factor for atherosclerotic events in systemic lupus erythematosus. Lancet 1996;348:1120–1124.
11. García-Carrasco M, Font J, Jiménez S, Ramos-Casals M, Cervera R, Nonell F, Sisó A, Torras A, Darnell

A, Ingelmo M. 10-year prospective study of morbidity and mortality in a cohort of 70 patients with lupus nephritis followed-up in a single center. Arthritis Rheum 1999;42(Suppl):S99.
12. Bulkley BH, Roberts WC. The heart in systemic lupus erythematosus and the changes induced in it by cortosteroid therapy: a study of 36 necropsy patients. Am J Med 1975;58:243–264.
13. Petri M, Lakatta C, MAgder L, Goldman DW. Effect of prednisone and hydroxycloroquine on coronary artery disease risk factors in systemic lupus erythematosus. Am J Med 1994;96:254–259.
14. Guba SC, Fink LM, Fonesca V. Hyperhomocystinemia: an emerging and important risk factor for thromboembolic and cardiovascular disease. Am J Clin Pathol 1996;105:709–722.
15. Selhub J, Jacques PF, Wilson PWF, at al. Vitamin status and intake as primary determinants of homocysteinemia in an elderly population. JAMA 1993;270:2693–2698.
16. MacGregor AJ, Dhillon VB, Binder A, et al. Fasting lipids and anticadiolipin antibodies as risk factors for vascular disease in systemic lupus erythematosus. Ann Rheum Dis 1992;1:152–155.
17. Leung KH, Koh ET, Feng PH et al. Lipid profiles in patients with systemic lupus erythematosus. J Rheumatol 1994;21:1264–1267.
18. Badui E, García-Rubi D, Robles E, Jiménez J, Juan L, Deleze M et al. Cardiovascular manifestations in systemic lupus erythematosus: prospective study of 100 patients. Angiology 1985;36:431–441.
19. Ettinger WH, Goldberg AP, Applebaum-Bowden D, Hazzard WR. dyslipoproteinemia in systemic lupus erythematosus: effect of corticosteriodis. Am J Med 1987;83:503–508.
20. Manzi S, Meilahn EN, Rairie JE, et al. Age-specific incidence rates of myocardial infarction and angina in women with systemic lupus erythematosus: comparision with the Framingham study. Am J epidemiol 1997;145:408.
21. Esdaile JM, Abrahamowitz M, Grodzicky T, Senecal JL, Panaritis T, Li Y et al. Myocardial infarction and stroke in SLE: markedly increased incidence after controlling for risk factors. Arthritis Rheum 1998;41(suppl 9):A629.
22. Gladman DD, Urowitz MB. Morbidity in systemic lupus erythematosus. J Rheumatol 1987;14:S13:223–226.
23. Urowitz MB, Gladman DD, Bruce I. Atherosclerosis and systemic lupus erythematosus. Curr Rheumatol Rep 2000;2:19–23.
24. Ilowite NT, Samuel P, Ginzler E et al. Dyslipoproteinemias in pediatric systemic lupus erythematosus. Arthritis Rheum 1988;31:859–863.
25. Borba EF, Bonfa E. Dyslipoproteinemias in systemic

lupus erythematosus: influence of disease, activity and anticardiolipin antibodies. Lupus 1997;6:533–539.

26. Borba EF, Bonfa E, Vinagre CG, et al. Imparied metabolism of artificial chylomicrons in systemic lupus erythematosus. Arthritis Rheum 1998;41 (supp l9):S79.

27. Borba EF, Bonfa E, Vinagre CG, Ramires JAF, Maranhao RC. Chylomicron metabolism is markedly altered in systemic lupus erythematosus. Arthritis Rheum 2000;43:1033–1040.

28. Rosengren A, Wilhelmsen L, Eriksson E, et al. Lipoprotein (a) and coronary heart disease: a prospective case-control study in a general poplulation sample of middle aged men. Br Med J 1990;301:1248–1251.

29. Petri m, Miller J, Ebert RF, et al. Lipoprotein (a) is predictive of myocardial infarction in SLE. Arthritis Rheum 1995;38(Suppl 9):S220.

30. Fijnheer R, Roest M, Haas FJ, et al. Homocysteine, methylenetetrahydrofolate reductase polymorfism, antiphospholipid antibodies and thromboembolic events in systemic lupus erythematosus: a retrospective cohort study. J Rheumatol 1998;25:1737–1742.

31. Ridker PM, Cushman M, Stampfer MJ, Tracy RP, Hennekens CH. Inflamation, aspirin, and the risk of cardiovascular disease in apparently healthy men. N Engl J Med 1997;336:973–979.

32. Maseri A. Inflamation, atherosclerosis and ischemic events-exploring the hidden side of the moon. N Engl J Med 1997;336:1014–1016.

33. Alexander RW. Inflamation and coronary artery disease. N Engl J Med 1994;331:468–469.

34. Tracy RP, Lemaitre RN, Psaty BM, Ives DG, Evans RW, Cushman M, et al. Relantionship of C-reactive protein to risk of cardiovascular disease in the elderly: results from the Cardiovascular Health Stydy and the rural health promotion project. Arterioscler Thromb 1997;17:1121–1127.

35. Kuller LH, Tracy RP, Shaten J, Meilahn EN. Relation of C-reactive protein and coronary heart disease in the MRFIT nested case-control study: multiple risk factor intervention trial. Am J Epidemiol 1996;144:537–547.

36. Manzi S, Selzer F, Sutton-Tyrrell K, Fitzgerald SG, Rairie JE, Tracy RP, Kuller LH. Prevalence and risk factors of carotid plaque in women with systemic lupus erythematosus. Arthritis Rheum 1999;42:51–60.

37. Levenson J, Giral P, Razavian M et al. Fibrinogen and silent atherosclerosis in subjects with cardiovascular risk factors. Atheroscler Thromb Vasc Biol 1995;15:1263–1268.

38. Lahita RG, Rivkin E, Cavanagh I, Romano P. Low levels of total cholesterol, high-density lipoprotein, and apolipoprotein A1 in association with anticardiolipin antibodies in patients with systemic lupus erythematosus. Arthritis Rheum 1993;36(11):1566–1574.

39. Matsura E, Katahira T, Igarashi Y, Koike T. β_2-Glycoprotein I bound to oxidatively modified lipoprotein could be targered by anticardiolipin antibodies. Lupus 1994;3:314 (abstract).

40. Hasuma Y, Matsura E, Makita Z et al. Involment of β_2-Glycoprotein I and anticardiolipin antibodies in oxidatively modified low-density lipoprotein uptake by macrophages. Clin Exp Immunol 1997;107:569–573.

41. George J, Gilburd B, Langewitz P et al. β_2-Glycoprotein I containing immune complexes in lupus patients: association with thrombocytopenia and lipoprotein (a) levels. Lupus 1999;8:116–120.

42. Shoenfeld Y, Harats D, George J. Atherosclerosis and the antiphosphplipid syndrome: a link unraveled? Lupus 1998;7(Suppl 1/2):S140–143.

43. Meroni PL, del Papa N, Raschi E et al. β_2-Glycoprotein I as a "cofactor" for antiphspholipid reactivity with endothelial cells. Lupus 1998;7(Suppl 1/2):S44–47.

44. Cuadrado MJ, Tinahones F, Camps MT, et al. Antiphospholipid anti-beta 2 glycoprotein I and anti-oxidised LDL antibodies in antiphospholipid syndrome. Q J Med 1998;91:619–626.

45. Vaarala O, Alfthan O, Jauhiainen M et al. Cross-reaction between antibodies to oxidised low-density lipoprotein and to cardiolipin in SLE. Lancet 1993;342:923–925.

46. Hughes GRV. Immunology, lupus and atheroma. Lupus 2000;9:159–160.

47. Jonsson H, Nived O, Sturfeit G. Outcome in systemic lupus erythematosus: a prospective study of patients from a defined population. Medicine (Baltimore) 1989;68:141–150.

48. Ward MM. Premature morbidity from cardiovascular and cerebrovascular diseases in women with systemic lupus erythematosus. Arthritis Rheum 1999;42:338–346

49. Sultan H, Benson J, Mirotznik J, Ginzler EM. Lack of evidence for corticosteroids as a risk factor for coronary artery disease in systemic lupus erythematosus. Presented at the Northeast Region American college of rheumatology Meeting, New York, June 1994.

50. Bonfiglio TA, Botti RE, Hagstrom JWC. coronary arteritis, occlusion and myocardial infarction due to lupus arythematosus. Am Heart J 1972;83:153–158.

51. Jensen G, Sigurd B. systemic lupus erythematosus and acute myocardial infarction. Chest 1973;64:653–654.

52. Tsakraklides VG, Blieden LC, Edwards JE. coronary atherosclerosis and myocardial infarction with systemic lupus erythematosus. Am Heart J 1974;87:637–641.

53. Meller J, Conde CA, Deppish LM et al. Myocardial infarction due to coronary atherosclerosis in three young adults with systemic lupus erythematosus. Am J Cardiol 1975;35:309–314.

54. Estes D, Christian C. The antural history of SLE by pro-

spective analysis. Medicine 1971;50:85–95.

55. Dubois EL, Wierzchowenscki M, Cox MB, Weiner JM. duration and death in systemic lupus erythematosus. An anlysis of 249 cases. JAMA 1974;227:1399–1402.

56. Rosner S, Ginzler EM, Diamond HS et al. A multicentes study of outcome in systemic lupus erythematosus. II. Causes of death. Arthritis Rheum 1982;25:612–617.

57. Haider YS, Roberts WC. Coronary arterial disease in systemic lupus erythematosus. Quantification of degrees of narrowinf in 22 necropsy patients (21 women) aged 16 to 37 years. Am J Med 1981;70:775–781.

58. Espeland MA, Craven TE, Riley WA, Corson J, Romont A, Furberg CD. Reliability of longitudinal ultrasonographic measurements of carotid intimal-medial thicknesses. Stroke 1996;5:343–344.

59. Li R, Cai J, Tegeler C, Sorlie P, Metcalf PA, Heiss G. Reproducibility of extracranial carotid atherosclerosis lesions assessed by B-mode ultrasound: the Atherosclerosis Risk in Communites Study. Ultrasound Med Biol 1996;22:791–799.

60. Persson J, Formgren J, Israelsson B, Berglund G. Ultrasound-determined intima media thickness and atherosclerosis. Direct and indirect validation. Atheroscler Thromb 1994;14:261–264.

61. Sutton-Tyrrell K, Wolfson SK, Thompson T, Kelsey SF. Measurement variability in duplex scan assessment of carotid atherosclerosis. Stroke 1992;23:215–220.

62. Salonen JT, Salonen R. Ultrasound B-mode imaging in observation studies of atherosclerotic progression. Circulation 1993;87Suppl II.II-56–57.

63. Pignoli P, Tremoli E, Poli A, Oreste P, Paoletti R. Intimal plus medial thickness of the arterial wall: a direct measurement with ultrasound imaging. circulation 1986;74:1399–1406.

64. The ARIC Investigators. The Atherosclerosis Risk in Communities (ARIC) Study: design and objectives. Am J epidemiol 1989;129:687–702.

65. Bots ML, Hofman A, DeJong PTVM, Grobbee DE. common carotid intima-media thickness as an indicator of atherosclerosis at other sites of the carotid artery: the Rotterdam Study. Ann Epidemiol 1996;6:147–153.

66. Heiss G, Sharett AR, Barnes R, Chambless LE, Szklo M, Alzola C, the ARIC Investigators. Carotid atherosclerosis measured by B-mode ultrasound in populations: associations with cardiovascular risk factors in the ARIC Study. Am J Epidemiol 1991;134:250–256.

67. O´Leary DH, Polak JF, Wolfson SK Jr, bond MG, Bommer W, Sheth S et al. on behalf of the CHS Collaborative Research Group. Use of sonography to evaluate carotid atherosclerosis in the elderly: the Cardiovascular Health Study. Stroke 1991;22:1155–1163.

68. The ACAPS Group. Rationale and desing for the Asymptomatic Carotid Artery Plaque Study (ACAPS).

Control CLin Trials 1992;13:293–314.

69. Salonen JT, Salonen R. Ultrasound B-mode imaging in obser vational studies of atherosclerotic progression. Circulation 1993;87Suppl II:II-56–65.

70. Burke GL, Evans GW, Riley WA, Sharrett AR, Howart G, Barnes RW, et al. for the ARIC Study Group. Arterial wall thickness is associated with prevalent cardiovascular disease in middle-aged adults: the Atherosclerosis Risk Communities (ARIC) Study. Atroke 1995;26:386–91.

71. Chambless LE, Heis G, Folsom AR, Rosamond W, Szklo M, Sharrett AR et al. Association of coronary heart disease incidence with carotid arterial wall thikcness and major risk factors: the Atherosclerosis Risk in Comunities (ARIC) Study, 1987–1993. Am J Epidemiol 1997;146:483–494.

72. Craven TE, Ryu JE, Espeland MA, Kahl FR, McKinney WM, Toole JF, et al. Evaluation of the associations between carotid artery atherosclerosis and coronary artery stenosis: a case control study. Circulation 1990;82:1230–1242.

73. Allan PL, Mowbray PI, Lee AJ, Fowkes GR. Relationship between carotid intima-media thickness ans symptomatic and asymptomatic peripheral arterial disease: the Edinburg Artery Study. Stroke 1997;28:348–353.

74. Sutton KC, Wolfson SK, Kuller LH. Carotid and lower extremity arterial disease in elderly adults with isolated systolic hypertension. Stroke 1987;18:348–353.

75. Durward QJ, Ferguson GG, Barr HWK. The natural history of asymptomatic carotid bifurcation plaques. Stroke 1982;25:1271–1277.

76. Petri M, Hamper U. Frequency of atherosclerosis detected by carotid duplex in systemic lupus srythematosus. Arthritis Rheum 1997;40:No.9(Suppl):S219.

77. Roman MJ, Salmon J, Sobel R et al. Premature athrosclerosis and myocardial hypertrophy in SLE and antiphospholipid antibogy syndrome. Arthritis Rheum 1997;40:S302.

78. Merril JT, Dinu AR, Sutton-Tyrrell K, Kuller L, Romano P, Lahita RG, Manzi S. Autoantibodies to apolipoprotein A1 (apo A1) in an SLE population: relation-ship to HDL levels and to carotid atherosclerosis by ultrasound assessment. Arthritis Rheum 1998;41:S139.

79. Falaschi F, Ravelli A, Martignoli A, Migliavacca D, Sartori M, Pistorio A, Perani G, Martini A. Nephrotic-range proteinuria, the major risk factor for early atheroscleosis in juvenile-onset systemic lupus erythematosus. Arthritis Rheum 2000;43:1405–1409.

80. Agatston AS, Janowitz WR, Kaplan G, Gasso J, Hildner F, Viamonte M, Jr. Ultrafast computed tomography-detected coronary calcium reflects the angiographic extents of coronary arterial atherosclerosis. Am J Cardiol 1994;74:1272–1274.

81. Kaufmann RB, Sheedy PF, Maher JE et al. Quantity of coronary artery calcium detected by electrom beam computed tomography in asymptomatic subjects and agiographically studied patients. Mayo Clin Proc 1995;70:223–232.

82. Rumberger JA, Simons DB, Fitzpatrick LA, Sheedy PF, Shwartz RS. coronary artery calcium area by electron-beam computed tomography and coronary atherosclerotic plaque area. A histopatologic correlative study. Circulation 1995;92:2157–2162.

83. Mintz GS, Pichard AD, Pompa JJ et al. Determinants and correlates of target lesion calcium in coronary artery disease: a clinical, angiographic and intravascular ultrasound study. J Am Coll Cardiol 1997;29:268–274.

84. Maheer JE, Bielak LF, Raz JA, Sheedy PF, Schwartz RS, Peyser PA. Progresion of coronary artery calcification: a pilot study. Mayo Clin Proc 1999;74:347–355.

85. Achenbach S, Moshage W, Ropers D, Nossen J, Daniel WG. Value Of electron-beam computed tomography for the noninvasive detection of haig-grade coronary-artery stenosis and occlusions. N Engl J Med 1998;339:1964–1971.

86. Von Feldt J. Coronary electron beam computed tomography (EBCT) in 13 SLE patients with 2 or more cardiovascular risk factors. Arthritis Rheum 1998;41:S139.

87. Lakatta EG, Mitchell JH, Promerance A, Rowe GG. human aging: changes in structure and function. J Am Coll Cardiol 1987;10:42A-47A.

88. Selzer F, Sutton-Tyrrel K, fitgeral S, Kuller L, Manzi S. Risk factors associated with arterial wall stiffness in women with SLE. Arthritis Rheum 1998;41:S139.

89. Bruce IN, Burns RJ, Gladman DD, Urowitz MB. High prevalence of myocardial perfusion abnormalities in women with SLE. Arthritis Rheum 1997;40:S219.

90. Hosenpud JD, Montanaro A, Hart MV, et al. Myocardial perfusion abnormalities in aymptomatic patinets with systemic lupus erythematosus. Am J Med 1984;77:286–292.

91. Petri M, Civelek C. Discordence of myocardial SPECT and carotid duplex in systemic lupus erythematosus (SLE). Arthritis Rheum 1998;41:S218.

92. Wallace DJ, Metzeger AL, Stecher VJ, et al. Cholesterol-lowering effect of hydroxychloroquine in patients with rheumatic disease: affects on lipid metabolism. Am J Med 1990;89:322–326.

93. Rahman P, Bruce I, Chung M et al. The cholesterol lowering effect of antimalarial drugs is enhanced in lupus patients on corticosteroids drugs. J Rheumatol 1999;26:325–330.

94. Hodis HN, Quismoro FP, Wickham E et al. The lipid, lipoprotein and apolipoprotein effects og hydroxichloroquine in patients with systemic lupus erythematosus. J Rheumatol 1993;20:661–665.

95. Tam LS, Gladman DD, Urowitz MB, Hallett D. correlation between fasting versus non fasting cholesterol and the effect of antimalarial agents on the fatinf lipid profile in systemic lupus erytjeamtosus (SLE. J Rheumatol 1999;26:1225.

96. Petri M. Hydroxychloroquine: past, present, future (editorial). Lupus 1998;7:65–67.

97. Hallegua DS, Wallace DJ. How accelerated atherosclerosis in SLE has changed our manegement of the disorder. Lupus 2000;9:228–231.

98. Arnow C, Soliman N, Ginzler E. Changing patterns of mortality in systemic lupus erythematosus (SLE) over three decades at an urban center. Arthritis Rheum 1996;39(Suppl):S213.

99. Cervera R, Khamashta M, Font J et al. Morbidity and mortality in systemic lupus erythematosus during 5-year period. A multicenter prospective study of 1000 patients. Medicine (Baltimore) 1999;78:167–175.

100. Stähl-Hallengren C, Jönsen A, Niven O, Sturfelt G. Incidence studies os systemic lupus erythematosus in Southern Sweden: increasinh age, deceasing frequency of renal manifestations and good prognosis. J Rheumatol 2000;3;685–691.

101. Shome GP, Sakauchi M, Yamane K et al. Ischemic heart diseaes In systemic lupus erythematosus. A retrospective study of 65 patients trated with prednisone. Japan J Med 1989;28:599–603.

102. Heart-Holmes M, Baethege BA, Broadwell L, Wolf RE. Dietary treatment of hyperlipidemia in patients with systemic lupus erythematosus. J Rheumatol 1995;22:450–454.

SLE as a Model of Autoimmune Atherosclerosis

Outi Vaarala

Department of Biochemistry, Helsinki, Finland

1. INTRODUCTION

The inflammatory reaction is a basic feature in the atherosclerotic vessel wall with lipid accumulation. The inflammatory cells, such as T-lymphocytes and macrophages, infiltrate the arterial intima and their role in the progression of atherosclerosis has been suggested to be crucial [1]. The risk of plaque rupture and formation of atherothrombosis depends more on the structural type of the plaque than on the size of the plaque (i.e. the degree of stenosis). Atherosclerotic plaques can be divided into "vulnerable" and "stable" plaques according to their risk for rupture and thrombosis. The "vulnerable" plaques may have a well-preserved lumen without angiographically evident flow-limiting stenosis but the arteries with "vulnerable" plaques seem to be the most infarct-prone arteries. Enhanced inflammation response in the "vulnerable" plaques, characterized by accumulation of macrophages and activated T lymphocytes, seems to be a crucial factor predisposing to plaque rupture and development of thrombosis. Recently, unspecific inflammatory markers such as elevated levels of serum C-reactive protein [2] and activation of peripheral blood lymphocytes [3] have been associated with the risk of coronary atherosclerosis. In the patients with coronary heart disease elevated concentration of C-reactive protein, ICAM-1 expressing CD8-lymphocytes, and the levels of antibodies to oxidized low-density lipoprotein showed an association with endothelial dysfunction, which is one of the earliest changes in atherosclerotic process [4].

Inflammatory changes may lead to the development of antigen-specific autoimmunity which

Table 1. Evidence for antiphospholipid autoimmunity in the pathogenesis of atherosclerosis

- Expression of autoantigens including modified LDL and β2-glycoprotein I in human atherosclerotic plaques [15, 22, 23]

- Antibodies to oxidised LDL, cardiolipin and prothrombin predict myocardial infarction [6–8, 24, 25]

- Antibodies to cardiolipin/β2-glycoprotein I increase the uptake of oxidised LDL by macrophages [14]

- Immunization with β2-glycoprotein I resulted in accelerated atherosclerosis in LDL-receptor deficient mice and apoE-knockout mice [16, 17]

- Antibodies crossreactive between cardiolipin and lysobiphosphatidic acid induced cholesterol accumulation into late endosomes [19]

occurs frequently in atherosclerosis. T lymphocyte clones derived from atherosclerotic plaques, the target tissue of autoimmune atherosclerosis, show autoreactivity against oxidatively modified low-density lipoprotein (LDL), the major autoantigen in atheroma [5]. Circulating autoantibodies to self-proteins, such as oxidised LDL, cardiolipin and prothrombin, occur in the patients with atherosclerosis [6–8]. In prospective studies the increased levels of antibodies to oxidised LDL, cardiolipin and prothrombin have been shown to predict the progression of atherosclerosis and myocardial infarction [6–8]. The autoantibodies associated with atherosclerosis may thus be involved with the development of atherothrombosis. These autoantibodies are frequently also found in the patients with systemic lupus erythematosus (SLE), an autoimmune disease accompanied with high mortality to coronary heart disease at early age [9].

2. AUTOIMMUNE ATHEROSCLEROSIS IN SLE

SLE is characterised by vascular inflammation with multiple immunological abnormalities. In the patients with SLE premature atherosclerosis is a clinical challenge [10–12]. The epidemiological studies by Susan Manzi and co-workers demonstrated that women with SLE in the 35- to 44-year age group had over 50 times higher rate ratio of cardiovascular events than healthy women of similar age [11]. According to the review by Bruce et al. subclinical coronary artery disease occurs at a frequency of about 35 to 40% in the patients with SLE [13]. Classical risk factors of atherosclerosis, such as the prolonged treatment with prednisone, high blood pressure and high levels of LDL cholesterol contribute to the atherosclerosis in SLE but SLE itself seems to be a risk factor for atherosclerotic complications beyond the classical risk factors. The autoimmune responses associated with SLE and antiphospholipid syndrome are suggested to be, at least parly, responsible for the enhanced atherogenesis. The studies on the atherogenic mechanisms of antiphospholipid antibodies have revealed the autoimmune mechanisms of common atherosclerosis, since the occurrence of these autoantibodies is not restricted to the patients with SLE or antiphosholipid syndrome but is associated also with common atherosclerosis.

3. ANTIBODIES BINDING TO β2-GLYCOPROTEIN I AND PHOSPHOLIPIDS

β2-glycoprotein I-binding antibodies represent the major population of antiphospholipid antibodies in the patients with antiphospholipid syndrome associated with SLE. These autoantibodies are associated with both arterial and venous thrombosis and are thus considered as prothrombotic autoantibodies. A role for antibodies to β2-glycoprotein I has

been suggested in atherogenesis based mainly on *in vitro* data and experimental studies in animal models of atherosclerosis.

In vitro studies suggest that antiphospholipid antibodies may contribute to the development of atherosclerotic process by enhancing of the lipid accumulation and inflammation in the arterial vessel wall. Antibodies to β2-glycoprotein I have been shown to enhance the accumulation of oxidised LDL into macrophages [14]. This effect was found when the antigen of these antibodies, β2-glycoprotein I, was added to the culture system. β2-glycoprotein I it self inhibited the accumulation of oxidised LDL into macrophages. The uptake of β2-glycoprotein I-LDL-autoantibody complexes by Fc-receptors may be the mechanism how these antibodies increase LDL uptake and contribute to the development of premature atherosclerosis in patients with antiphospholipid syndrome.

Studies by George et al. suggest that β2-glycoprotein I competes with oxidised LDL in the binding to endothelial cells and monocyte/macrophage cell line [15]. The same group also demonstrated that β2-glycoprotein I is found in the atherosclerotic plaques and shows colocalization with CD-4 positive lymphocytes. It is possible that β2-glycoprotein I is a target autoantigen in the atherosclerotic lesion. It must be emphasized, however, that β2-glycoprotein I is bound to LDL in circulation and thus it is accumulated into atheroma by the uptake of LDL.

Also animal studies indicate that immunity to β2-glycoprotein I contributes to the development of atherosclerosis. Immunization of LDL-receptor deficient or apolipoprotein E deficient mice with human β2-glycoprotein I led to the acceleration of early atherosclerosis [16, 17]. It is not known whether the acceleration of athersclerosis is mediated by antibodies to β2-glycoprotein I or by other mechanisms in the immunization experiments. Although the mechanisms are not known these studies suggest an involvement of β2-glycoprotein I in the atherosclerotic process.

The recent studies by Gruenberg's group have suggested that the target of antiphospholipid antibodies is lysobiphosphatidic acid (LBPA) which is an abundant lipid in the internal membranes of the multivesicular late endosomes [18]. This group has shown that antiphospholipid antibodies bind to late endosomes and that the presence of antiphosphol-

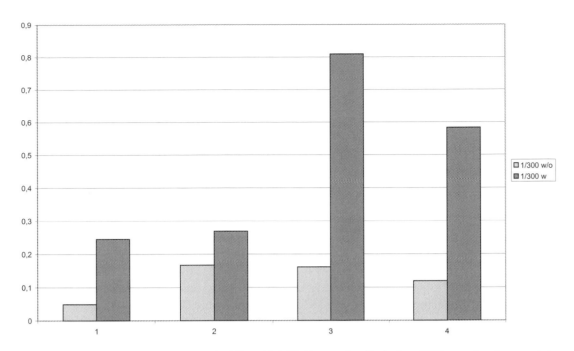

Figure 1. Binding of antibodies to lysophosphatidic acid (LBPA) coated wells in four SLE sera showing reactivity to late endosomes. The ELISA test was performed in β2-glycoprotein I-free conditions using gelatin as a blocking agent and serum dilution 1:300 in which the cofactor activity of serum β2-glycoprotein I for antiphospholipid antibodies is not detectable (1/300 w/o). When 10 μg/ml of β2-glycoprotein I was added to serum diluent, the binding of antibodies to LBPA enhanced remarkably suggesting that antibodies are directed to the complex of LBPA and β2-glycoprotein I (1/300w).

ipid antibodies in cell culture leads to cholesterol accumulation into late endosomes [19]. The changes in the cholesterol transport may be associated with the changes in the protein-sorting function of endosomes. Although the levels of antibodies to LBPA and to cardiolipin correlated, antiphospholipid antibodies showed binding only to the internal lipids of the late endosomes and not to mitochondrial cardiolipin [20]. The role of β2-glycoprotein I as the target antigen remained open in these studies.

In our preliminary studies we have confirmed the binding of antiphospholipid antibodies from patients with SLE to LBPA containing late endosomes (Vaarala et al. unpublished observations). However, in the SLE sera with reactivity to late endosomes, the binding of antibodies to solid-phase LBPA and cardiolipin was dependent on β2-glycoprotein I at serum dilutions in which serum derived endogenous β2-glycoprotein I is not functional (Fig. 1). This suggests that the primary antigenic target in late endosomes may be LBPA-β2-glycoprotein I complex. Accordingly, our findings emphasize the role

of β2-glycoprotein I as the target antigen for the antiphospholipid antibodies which may modify the intracellular traffic of cholesterol. These findings suggest that intracellular effects of antiphospholipid antibodies may play a role in the development of autoimmune atherosclerosis.

In a sero-epidemiological study, the antibodies to β2-glycoprotein I did not associate with myocardial infarction in dyslipidemic middle-aged men without autoimmune diseases[8]. In patients with SLE these antibodies are strongly associated with venous and arterial thrombosis. It remains to be elucidated whether the pathogenic mechanisms of these antibodies include other pathways beyond their contribution to blood coagulation.

4. ANTIBODIES TO OXIDISED LDL

The "oxidative-modification hypothesis" in the pathogenesis of atherosclerosis is based on the enhanced uptake of oxidised LDL by scavenger receptors of macrophages [21]. Inflammation in the atherosclerotic vessel wall leads to increased oxidative capacity which causes peroxidation of lipids. The end-products of lipid peroxidation further propagate changes in the proteins, such as production of malondialdehyde-conjugated LDL. The modifications of LDL by other mechanisms than oxidation may also potentiate its atherogenic nature. Generation of enzymatically modified LDL molecules may be important in the atherogenesis, especially hypochlorite conjugated LDL produced by myeloperoxidase [22].

Modified LDL molecules have been identified in the atherosclerotic vessels indicating their accumulation in the atherosclerotic plaques [22, 23]. The modified self-proteins induce autoimmune responses circulating autoantibodies to oxidised LDL have been reported patients with atherosclerosis [4, 5, 24, 25].

Elevated levels of autoantibodies to oxidised LDL have been reported to be markers or predictors of accelerated atherosclerotic process suggesting their importance in the pathogenesis of atherosclerosis. Two prospective studies in non-SLE subjects have shown that antibodies to oxidised LDL are predictive for myocardial infarction [24, 25] and progression of carotid atherosclerosis [6]. In addition, the levels of antibodies to oxidised LDL represented an independent determinant of impaired endothelium-dependent and endothelium-independent vasodilatation, which was detected in the forearm vasculature with a strain-gauge plethysmography in a series of patients with coronary heart disease [4]. These findings suggest that increased levels of antibodies to oxidised LDL in humans are closely associated with the atherosclerotic process in the vessel wall. However, it is not clear whether antibodies to oxidised LDL are markers of atherosclerotic process or contributors of this process.

Antibodies to oxidised LDL occur frequently also in the patients with SLE [26] and are associated with arterial thrombosis in these patients [27, 28]. Antibodies to oxidised LDL show heterogeneity in their antigenic-specificity. Since antibodies to oxidised LDL crossreact with antiphospholipid antibodies they are considered as members of the family of antiphospholipid antibodies [26, 29, 30]. A subpopulation of these antibodies binds to oxidised lipids in LDL molecule and are likely responsi-

ble for the crossreactivity with phospholipids such as cardiolipin [29, 30]. A major population of antibodies to oxidised LDL recognizes oxidised apolipoprotein B of LDL which is modified during oxidation [31]. Since small amount of plasma β2-glycoprotein I, an antigenic target of antiphospholipid antibodies, is bound to LDL molecule in circulation, antibodies to β2-glycoprotein I may also bind to oxidised LDL [32]. However, in some studies on SLE sera no crossreactivity between the antibodies to oxidised LDL and β2-glycoprotein I have been found [33, 34].

The frequent occurrence of antibodies to oxidised LDL and cardiolipin in SLE and antiphospholipid syndrome may be associated with enhanced oxidative stress and activate atherosclerotic process in SLE. The markers of enhanced lipid peroxidation are associated with antiphospholipid antibodies indicating increased oxidative stress in SLE [35, 36].

The pathogenic role of antibodies to oxidised LDL have been suggested by studies showing that *in vitro* these antibodies enhance the accumulation of LDL into macrophages [37]. However, immunization with oxidised LDL has been shown to protect from atherosclerosis in ApoE deficient mice [38] and in LDL-receptor deficient mice [39]. This protective effect was, however, not dependent on the generation of antibodies to oxidised LDL since immunization with native LDL was prevented atherosclerosis despite of the absence of antibodies to oxidised LDL in the mice. The authors suggested that the protection was related to T-cell dependent mechanisms [39]. The question of the pathogenic role of antibodies to oxidised LDL remains open. It is possible that the induced immune response to oxidised LDL in atherosclerosis is related to the housekeeping functions of the immune system, and serves as a marker of atherosclerotic process.

5. ANTIBODIES BINDING TO PROTHROMBIN

Prothrombin is an antigenic target of antiphospholipid antibodies in SLE. Some prothrombin-binding antibodies cause prolongation of in vitro clotting time which is called lupus anticoagulant activity [40]. Antibodies to prothrombin have been associated with the myocardial infarction in a prospective follow-up of healthy dyslipidemic men [8]. A two-fold risk of myocardial infarction was found in middle-aged men with antibody levels to prothrombin in the highest tertile when compared to the men with antibody levels in the lowest tertile. This risk was multiplied by an additive manner when the joint effect with other risk factors for myocardial infarction was accounted, such as high levels of antibodies to oxidised LDL, smoking and high Lp(a) levels. These findings suggest that autoimmunity to prothrombin may be associated with atherothrombosis. The mechanisms involved with the development of atherothrombosis may be related to the procoagulant activity of these antibodies *in vivo* as we have suggested [41]. However, it is possible that antibodies binding to prothrombin may be involved with atherosclerotic process as our preliminary studies in LDL-receptor knockout mice suggest [42].

REFERENCES

1. Libby P. Molecular bases of the acute coronary syndromes. Circulation 1995;91:2844–2850.
2. Mendall MA, Patel P, Ballam L, Strachan D, Northfield TC. C reactive protein and its relation to cardiovascular risk factors: a population based cross sectional study. BMJ 1996;312:1061–1065.
3. Neri Serneri GG, Prisco D, Martini F, Gori AM, Brunelli T, Poggesi L, Rostagno C, Gensini GF, Abbate R. Acute T-cell activation is detectable in unstable angina. Circulation 1997;95:1806–1812.
4. Sinisalo J, Paronen J, Mattila KJ, Syrjälä M, Alfthan G, Palosuo T, NieminenMS, Vaarala O. Relation of inflammation to vascular function in patients with coronary heart disease. Atherosclerosis 2000;149:403–411.
5. Stemme S, Faber B, Holm J, Wiklund O, Witztum JL, Hansson GK, T lymphocytes from human atherosclerotic plaques recognize oxidised low density lipoprotein. Proc. Natl. Acad. Sci. USA 1995;92:3893–3897.
6. Salonen JT, Ylä-Herttuala S, Yamamoto R, Butler S, Korpela H, Salonen R, Nyyssönen K, Palinski W, Witztum JL. Autoantibody against oxidized LDL and progression of carotid atherosclerosis. Lancet 1992;339:883–887.
7. Vaarala O, Mänttäri M, Manninen V, Tenkanen L, Puurunen M, Aho K, Palosuo T. Anti-cardiolipin antibodies and risk of myocardial infarction in a prospective cohort of middle-aged men. Circulation 1995;91:23–27.
8. Vaarala O, Puurunen M, Mänttäri M, Manninen V, Aho K, Palosuo T. Antibodies to prothrombin imply a risk of myocardial infarction in middle-aged men. Thromb Haemost 1996;75:456–459.
9. Vaarala O. Antiphospholipid antibodies and atherosclerosis. Lupus 1996;5:442–447.
10. Urowitz MB, Bookman AAM, Koehler BE, Gordon DA, Smythe HA, Ogryzlo MA.The bimodal mortality pattern of systemic lupus eryhtematosus. Am J Med 1976;69:221–225.
11. Manzi S, Meilahn EN, Rairie JE, Conte CG, Medsger TA, Jansen-McWilliams L, D'Agostino RB, Kuller LH. Age-specific incidence rates of myocardial infarction and angina in women with systemic lupus erythematosus: comparison with the Framingham Study. Am J Epidemiol 1997;145:408–415.
12. Ward MM. Premature morbidity from cardiovascular and cerebrovascular diseases in women with systemic lupus erythematosus. Arthritis Rheum 1999;42:338–346.
13. Bruce IN, Gladmann DD, Urowitz MB. Premature atherosclerosis in systemic lupus erythematosus. Rheum Dis Clin North America 2000;26:257–278.
14. Hasunuma Y, Matsuura E, Makita Z, Katahira T, Nishi S, Koike T. Involvement of β2-glycoprotein I and anticardiolipin antibodies in oxidatively modified low-density lipoprotein uptake by macrophages. Clin Exp Immunol 1997;107:569–573.
15. George J, Harats D, Gilburd B, Afek A, Levy Y, Schneiderman J, Barshak I, Kopolovic J, Shoenfeld Y. Immunolocalization of β2-glycoprotein I (Apolipoprotein H) to human atherosclerotic plaques. Potential implications for lesion progression. Circulation 1999;99:2227–2230.
16. George J, Afek A, Gilburd B, Blank M, Levy Y, Aron-Maor A, Levkovitz H, Shaish A, Goldberg I, Kopolovic J, Harats D, Shoenfeld Y. Induction of early atherosclerosis in LDL-receptor-deficient mice immunized with beta2-glycoprotein I. Circulation 1998;98:1108–1115.
17. Afek A, George J, Shoenfeld Y, Gilburd B, Levy Y, Shaish A, Keren P, Janackovic Z, Goldberg I, Kopolovic J, Harats D. Enhancement of atherosclerosis in beta-2-glycoprotein I-immunized apolipoprotein E-deficient mice. Pathobiology 1999;67:19–25.
18. Kobayashi T, Stang E, Fang KS, de Moerloose P, Parton RG, Gruenberg J. A lipid associated with the antiphospholipid syndrome regulates endosome structure and function. Nature 1998;392:193–197.
19. Kobayashi T, Beuchat MH, Lindsay M, Frias S, Palmiter RD, Sakuraba H, Parton RG, Gruenberg J. Late endosomal membranes rich in lysobisphosphatidic acid regulate cholesterol transport. Nature Cell Biology 1999;1:113–118.
20. Galve-de Rochemonteix B, Kobayashi T, Rosnoblet C, Lindsay M, Parton RG, Reber G, de Maistre E, Wahl D,

271

Kruithof EK, Gruenberg J, de Moerloose P. Interaction of anti-phospholipid antibodies with late endosomes of human endothelial cells. Arteriosclerosis Thromb Vasc Biology 2000;20:563–574.

21. Witztum JL. The oxidation hypothesis of atherosclerosis. Lancet 1994;344:793–795.

22. Hazell LJ, Arnold L, Flowers D, Waeg G, Malle E, Stocker R. Presence of hypochlorite-modified proteins in human atherosclerotic lesions. J Clin Invest 1996;97:1535–1544.

23. Yla-Herttuala S, Palinski W, Rosenfeld ME, Parthasarathy S, Carew TE, Butler S, Witztum JL, Steinberg D. Evidence for the presence of oxidatively modified low density lipoprotein in atherosclerotic lesions of rabbit and man. J Clin Invest 1989;84:1086–1095.

24. Puurunen M, Mänttäri M, Manninen V, Tenkanen L, Alfthan G, Ehnholm C, Vaarala O, Aho K, Palosuo T. Antibody against oxidized low-density lipoprotein predicting myocardial infarction. Arch Intern Med 1994;154:2605–2609.

25. Wu R, Nityanand S, Berglund L, Lithell H, Holm G, Lefvert AK. Antibodies against cardiolipin and oxidatively modified LDL in 50-year-old men predict myocardial infarction. Arterioscler Tromb Vasc Biol 1997;17:3159–3163.

26. Vaarala O, Alfthan G, Jauhiainen M, Leirisalo-Repo M, Aho K, Palosuo T. Crossreaction between antibodies to oxidised lipoprotein and to cardiolipin in systemic lupus erythematosus. Lancet 1993;341:923–925.

27. Amengual O, Atsumi T, Khamashta MA, Tinahones F, Hughes GR. Autoantibodies against oxidized low-density lipoprotein in antiphospholipid syndrome. Br J Rheumatol 1997;36:964–968.

28. Cuadrado MJ, Tinahones F, Camps MT, de Ramon E, Gomez-Zumaquero JM, Mujic F, Khamashta MA, Hughes GR. Antiphospholipid, anti-beta 2-glycoprotein I and anti-oxidized-low-density antibodies in antiphospholipid syndrome. Q J Med 1998;91:619–626.

29. Vaarala O, Puurunen M, Lukka M, Alfthan G, Leirisalo-Repo M, Aho K, Palosuo T. Affinity-purified cardiolipin-binding antibodies show heterogeneity in their binding to oxidised low-density lipoprotein. Clin Exp Immunol 1996;104:269–274.

30. Hörkkö S, Miller E, Dudl E, Reaven P, Curtiss LK, Zvaifler NJ, Terkeltaub R, Pierangeli SS, Branch DW, Palinski W, Witztum JL. Antiphospholipid antibodies are directed against epitopes of oxidized phospholipids. J Clin Invest 1996;98:815–825.

31. Palinski W, Yla-Herttuala S, Rosenfeld ME, Butler SW, Socher SA, Parthasarathy S, Curtiss LK, Witztum JL. Antisera and monoclonal antibodies specific for epitopes generated during oxidative modification of low

density lipoprotein. Arteriosclerosis 1990;10:325–335.

32. Matsuura E, Katahira T, Igarashi Y, Koike T. β2-glycoprotein I bound to oxidatively modified lipoproteins could be targeted by anticardiolipin antibodies. Lupus 1994;3:314.

33. Matsuda J, Gotoh M, Kawasugi K, Gohchi K, Tsukamoto M, Saitoh N. Negligible synergistic effect of beta2-glycoprotein I on the reactivity of antioxidized low-density lipoprotein antibody to oxidized low-density lipoprotein. Am J Hematol 1996;52:114–116.

34. Tinahones FJ, Cuadrado MJ, Khamashta MA, Mujic F, Gomez-Zumaquero JM, Collantes E, Hughes GR. Lack of cross-reaction between antibodies to beta2-glycoprotein-I and oxidized low-density lipoprotein in patients with antiphospholipid syndrome. Br J Rheumatol 1998;37:746–749.

35. Iuliano L, Pratico D, Ferro D, Pittoni V, Valesini G, Lawson J, FitzGerald GA, Violi F. Enhanced lipid peroxidation in patients positive for antiphospholipid antibodies. Blood 1997;90:3931–3935.

36. Ames PR, Nourooz-Zadeh J, Tommasino C, Alves J, Brancaccio V, Anggard EE. Oxidative stress in primary antiphospholipid syndrome. Thrombosis Haemostasis 1998;79:447–449.

37. Lopes-Virella MF, Binzafar N, Rackley S, Takei A, La Via M, Virella G. The uptake of LDL-IC by human macrophages: predominant involvement of the Fc gamma RI receptor. Atherosclerosis 1997;135:161–170.

38. George J, Afek A, Gilburd B, Levkovitz H, Shaish A, Goldberg I, Kopolovic Y, Wick G, Shoenfeld Y, Harats D.Hyperimmunization of apo-E-deficient mice with homologous malondialdehyde low-density lipoprotein suppresses early atherogenesis. Atherosclerosis 1998;138:147–152.

39. Freigang S, Horkko S, Miller E, Witztum JL, Palinski W.Immunization of LDL receptor-deficient mice with homologous malondialdehyde-modified and native LDL reduces progression of atherosclerosis by mechanisms other than induction of high titers of antibodies to oxidative neoepitopes. Arterioscler Thromb Vasc Biol 1998;18:1972–1982.

40. Galli M, Barbui T. Antiprothrombin antibodies: detection and clinical significance in the antiphospholipid syndrome. Blood 1999;93:2149–2157.

41. Puurunen M, Palosuo T, Lassila R, Anttila M, Vaarala O. Immunologic and hematologic properties of antibodies to prothrombin and plasminogen in a mouse model. Lupus (in press).

42. Sherer Y, Blank M, Vaarala O, Shaish A, Shoenfeld Y, Harats D. Antiprothrombin antibodies in thrombosis and atherosclerosis. Atherosclerosis and Autoimmunity 2001;187–192.

Oxidant Stress in SLE Patients: Relationship to Atherosclerosis

Francesco Violi, Fausta Micheletta and Luigi Iuliano

Institute of Clinical Medicine I, University La Sapienza, Rome, Italy

1. INTRODUCTION

Patients with systemic lupus erythematosus (SLE) have a natural history complicated by atherosclerosis and related vascular disease. Life expectancy of SLE is much less than that of general population and this is also a consequence of high rate of cardiovascular and cerebrovascular disease. In SLE patients 6–20% of deaths are due to cardiovascular disease and 4–15% of death are due to cerebrovascular disease [1–6]. Cardiovascular and cerebrovascular disease also causes a high rate of morbidity: 6–17% and 3–15% of SLE patients may in fact experience coronary heart disease or ischemic stroke respectively [7–12]. Ward [13] examined the reason for acute hospitalization in a large cohort of SLE patients and age-matched control group. He also stratified the two groups for 3 ages strata (18–44 years, 45–64 years and ≥ 65 years) and evaluated the rate of cardiovascular events in each stratified group. While in the middle age and elderly group the rate of cerebrovascular disease and coronary heart disease was not different, in young patients with SLE the rate of cardiovascular events was much higher than that of control population. In particular SLE patients were 2.27 times more likely to be hospitalized for myocardial infarction and 2.05 times more likely to be hospitalized for cerebrovascular disease than control population. The reason for such difference is still unclear. As the SLE patients are usually treated with corticosteroids, an attractive hypothesis was that metabolic disorders, related to this therapy, could account for accelerated atherosclerosis [14, 15]. This suggestion, however, has not been proved as a major prevalence of diabetes, dyslipidemia and hypertension has not been detected in SLE popula-

tion compared to general population. This lack of association was also reinforced by Ward's study, that did not find an increased of these above reported risk factors in SLE population showing a higher rate of cardiovascular events. Petri et al. [16] evaluated the relationship between vascular disease and homocysteine in 337 SLE patients. Homocysteine is a non-essential, sulphur-containing aminoacid produced as a result of methionine catabolism. Homocysteine has been reported to exert deleterious effect on vascular endothelium and several studies showed a direct correlation between plasma homocysteine and arterial thrombosis. Petri et al. [16] found raised concentration of homocysteine in 15% of SLE population. In multivariate analysis homocysteine was an independent predictor only of stroke, while arterial thrombosis was associated with homocysteine but not significantly. Even if these data are interesting, they do not help to clear-cut explain the increased risk for cardiovascular disease in SLE population.

2. ATHEROSCLEROSIS AND OXIDANT STRESS IN SLE PATIENTS

Atherosclerosis seems to be dependent on an inflammatory process occurring in the arterial wall as a consequence of enhanced oxidative stress [17, 18]. The hypothesized sequence of events assumes that LDL cross the endothelial layer, undergo oxidation trough still unclear mechanism, and are taken up by scavenger receptors on macrophages that became foam cells [19]. Several lines of evidence accumulated in the last two decades support this hypothesis. From these data the scavenger receptors, which recognize only oxidized LDL but not native LDL, are the pathway of cholesterol influx in macrophage, the main cell type of the atherosclerotic lesion. LDL oxidation has been produced in vitro by physiological plausible mechanisms, and antioxidants inhibit LDL oxidation and accumulation of cholesterol in macrophages [19, 20]. Several studies have shown inhibition of experimental atherosclerosis in animal models by natural and synthetic antioxidants [19, 21].

LDL extracted from human atherosclerotic plaque resulted similar to the LDL oxidized in vitro [20]. In addition, isoprostanes, specific markers of lipid peroxidation, have been isolated from the atherosclerotic lesions. Isoprostanes are enzyme-independent arachidonic acid peroxidation products: in this pathway arachidonic acid is converted by a free radical-mediated catalysis into prostaglandin-like substances named isoprostanes (IPFs) [22]. Sensitive and specific methods of assay have been made based on mass spectrometry negative ion chemical ionization [23]. Two isoprostane isomers, $IPF_{2\alpha}$-III and $IPF_{2\alpha}$-VI (8-iso-Prostaglandin-$F_{2\alpha}$ and isoprostane-$F_{2\alpha}$ I correspond with the new nomenclature to Isoprostane-$F_{2\alpha}$-III and Isoprostane-$F_{2\alpha}$-VI [24]), have been isolated from freshly excised human atherosclerotic lesions obtained at carotid endoarterectomy, and a monoclonal antibody against $IPF_{2\alpha}$-III stained macrophages in the lesions [25].

Isoprostanes have been isolated in plasma and urine of animals and humans in conditions of high oxidant stress [23]. The interest of isoprostanes, based in their use as markers of oxidant stress, has been increasingly relevant because most of them possess biological activity [22]. In particular, they are able to increase vascular tone and enhance platelet responsiveness to common agonists. We have recently shown that SLE patients have enhanced oxidative stress inasmuch as they showed increased urinary excretion of isoprostanes $IPF_{2\alpha}$-III and $IPF_{2\alpha}$-VI. These data have potential relevance for understanding the relationship between SLE and atherosclerosis because isoprostanes are formed upon LDL oxidation. Thus, the increase of isoprostanes could provide further support to the study of Hörkko [26] et al., who found enhanced title of antibodies against oxidized LDL in SLE patients. As a recent prospective study demonstrated that atherosclerosis extent correlated with the presence of anti-bodies against oxidized LDL [27], the increase of isoprostanes on one hand could explain the enhanced rate of atherosclerotic process in SLE patients and, on the other hand, may represent an interesting marker to assess atherosclerotic progression in this clinical setting.

3. OXIDANT STRESS AND ANTIPHOSPHOLIPID ANTIBODIES

SLE is an autoimmune disease of unknown cause [28], in which the presence of antiphospholipid antibodies (aPL) in plasma confers a striking risk of venous as well as arterial thrombotic events and fetal wastage [29–32]. It is unknown whether this represents a direct causative effect of aPL or the association with an unknown risk factor. Experimental evidence suggests that aPL may modify procoagulant proteins and/or interfere with the anticoagulant function of endothelium [30]. The nature of aPL is currently being explored with the objective of addressing its functional importance in thrombogenesis.

Hörkko et al. [26] have recently shown that aPL are directed against epitopes of oxidized phospholipids and suggested that aPL may result from phospholipid oxidation. To test this hypothesis in vivo, we measured the urinary excretion of IPFs in SLE patients with or without aPL positivity with the aim of assessing if there was a relationship between IPFs and aPL [33]: IPFs were used as a marker of lipid peroxidation because they are elevated in clinical settings associated with oxidant stress [34–36] and are generated during low density lipoproteins oxidation in vitro in temporal correlation with formation of lipid peroxides [37]. We found that urinary IPFs excretion was higher in patients with SLE than in age- and gender-matched controls. However, within the patients, those positive for aPL had higher levels of the isoprostanes. Indeed, whereas 82% of the SLE patients who were aPL-positive had levels of urinary IPFs above the upper bound of 95% confidence interval for its excretion in healthy individuals (154 pg/mg creatinine), only 16% of the aPL-negative SLE patients fell into this category. Urinary excretion of the compounds also correlated with the absolute levels of aCL. This observation, given the mechanism of formation of isoprostanes [38–40], is consistent with the hypothesis that aPL are directed against oxidized epitopes in phospholipids. However, a cause-effect relationship between oxidant stress and aPL has not yet demonstrated in humans.

4. OXIDANT STRESS, INFLAMMATION AND THROMBOSIS

Oxidant stress may characterize inflammatory episodes in autoimmune diseases such as SLE [41]. Accordingly, it has been shown that monocytes may generate IPFs in response to inflammatory stimuli in vitro [42], and have immunolocalized that IPF_{2a} in macrophage of human atherosclerotic plaque [25]. Thus, it is of interest that in SLE patients levels of IPFs excretion correlated with plasma TNFα, which is generated by activated monocytes and is elevated in the active phase of disease [43, 44]. These data arise the question as to whether inflammation may represent a *primum movens* of a sequence of events leading to the formation of antiphospholipid antibodies and to the induction of endothelial damage. As far as the first part is concerned, there is no evidence *in vivo* that inflammation and more in particular oxidative stress plays a causative role in the formation of aPL. As far as the relationship between inflammation and endothelial damage is concerned, there are many data *in vitro* and *in vivo* in support of this hypothesis. Among mechanisms linking immune-mediated inflammatory response and endothelial perturbation in SLE, in vitro experiments focused on the role of cytokines [45]. It was shown that TNFα is cytotoxic for endothelial cells *in vitro,* induces procoagulant activity in cultured endothelial cells [46, 47], and induces *in vitro* and *in vivo* von Willebrand factor (vWf) release from endothelial cells [48, 49]. All these data suggest that TNFα could mediate activation of the clotting system by interfering with the function of endothelial cells.

To further explore the relationship between inflammation and endothelial damage we measured aPL, anti-endothelial cell antibodies, circulating levels of prothrombin fragment F1+2, a marker of thrombin generation, TNFα, tissue-type plasminogen activator (tPA), and vWf in SLE patients and healthy subjects [50]. Patients positive for aPL had higher prevalence of anti-endothelial cell antibodies and higher levels of F1+2 than aPL negative ones. Endothelial perturbation, revealed by the elevated plasma levels of both t-PA and vWf, was significantly associated with aPL positivity. High circulating levels of F1+2 was detected in all but one patient in whom aPL positivity and endothelial perturbation coexisted, and in no aPL positive patients without endothelial perturbation; F1+2 was significantly correlated with vWf and t-PA only in aPL positive patients. Also endothelial perturbation was closely associated with high values of TNFα, antiphospholipid, and anti-endothelial cell antibodies. In 31 patients without a clinical history of thrombosis followed up for 3 years, aPL-positive patients with endothelial perturbation showed higher F1+2 and TNFα values than aPL-positive patients without endothelial dysfunction. This study showed that in SLE patients, aPL positivity is associated with an ongoing prothrombotic state only in the presence of endothelial perturbation, and also suggested that aPL and TNFα might cooperate in inducing endothelial perturbation.

The close relationship between TNFα and aPL may be also of interest for explaining the increased prothrombotic state observed in patients positive for antiphospholipid antibodies. Thus, TNFα promotes activation of the clotting system by enhancing expression of tissue factor, a glycoprotein of the extrinsic pathway that converts factor X to Xa [51]. This effect could be also mediated by prooxidant property of TNFα: thus several lines of evidence suggest that oxygen free radicals contribute to cell activation [52]. Actually, antioxidants have been reported to inhibit lipopolysaccharide-induced transcriptional and post-transcriptional expression of macrophage tissue factor [53, 54]. Furthermore, human monocytes exposed to copper-induced oxidant stress had an enhanced expression of tissue factor, which was again inhibited by antioxidants [55]. These data prompted us to hypothesize that the enhanced lipid peroxidation observed in aPL-positive patients could be an important mechanism leading to the activation of clotting system. To test this hypothesis we measured the urinary excretion of isoprostanes $IPF_{2\alpha}$-III and $IPF_{2\alpha}$-VI and the circulating levels of the prothrombin fragment F1+2 in antiphospholipid antibodies-positive patients, in antiphospholipid antibodies-negative patients with SLE, and in healthy subjects [56]. Furthermore,

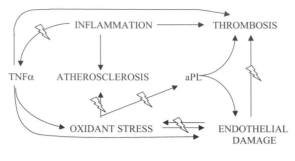

↯ denotes inhibition by antioxidants

Figure 1. Hypothetical mechanisms linking inflammation with vascular disease in SLE patients. Oxidant stress is induced by enhanced free radicals release by inflammation activated monocytes and altered endothelial cells. Activated monocytes generate TNFα that induces endothelial dysfunction and perpetuates inflammation. Oxidant stress may promote the formation of aPL which in turn are thrombogenic by direct altering procoagulant proteins, and by inducing endothelial dysfunction. Thrombosis is triggered by TNFα through expression of TF and activation of factors that promote endothelial damage. Inflammation and oxidant stress are the main determining factor of atherogenesis. Antioxidant could inhibit several steps of this process.

patients positive for antiphospholipid antibodies were treated with or without antioxidant vitamins (vitamin E at 900 IU/day and vitamin C at 2,000 mg/day) for four weeks. Compared with antiphospholipid antibodies-negative patients, antiphospholipid antibodies-positive patients had higher urinary excretion of isoprostane $IPF_{2\alpha}$-III, isoprostane $IPF_{2\alpha}$-VI, and plasma levels of the prothrombin fragment F1+2. In antiphospholipid-positive patients, F1+2 significantly correlated with isoprostanes $IPF_{2\alpha}$-III and $IPF_{2\alpha}$-VI. After four weeks of supplementation with antioxidant vitamins, we found a significant decrease in F1+2 levels concomitantly with a significant reduction of both isoprostanes $IPF_{2\alpha}$-III and $IPF_{2\alpha}$-VI. No change of these variables was observed in patients not receiving antioxidant treatment. This study suggested that lipid peroxidation might contribute to the activation of clotting system in patients positive for antiphospholipid antibodies because antioxidant treatment has been able to reduce the rate of thrombin generation in vivo.

5. CONCLUSION

On the basis of the above reported findings, it may be postulated that oxidative stress plays a pivotal role in inducing and perpetuating vascular damage in SLE patients and in so far contributing to the formation of atherosclerotic plaque (Fig.1). Thus, oxidative stress could facilitate the formation of aPL and induce vascular damage, so contributing to increase the risk for thrombotic episodes. Inflammation would represent a plausible mechanism leading to increased oxidant stress, therefore its modulation by appropriate therapy could result in inhibiting oxidative stress and eventually reducing atherosclerosis and its complications.

REFERENCES

1. Rubin LA, Urowitz MB, Gladman DD. Mortality in systemic lupus erythematosus: the bimodal pattern revisited. QJM 1985;55:87–98.
2. Helve T. Prevalence and mortality rates of systemic lupus erythematosus and causes of death in SLE patients in Finland. Scand J Rheumatol 1985;14:37–48.
3. Reveille JD, Bartolucci A, Alarcòn GS. Prognosis in systemic lupus erythematosus: negative impact of increasing age at onset, black race, and thrombocytopenia, as well as causes of death. Arthritis Rheum 1990;33:37–48.
4. Pistiner M, Wallace DJ, Nessim S, Metzger AL, Klinenberg JR. Lupus erythematosus in the 1980s: a survey of 570 patients. Semin Arthritis Rheum 1991;21:55–64.
5. Abu-Shakra M, Urowitz MB, Gladman DD, Gough J. Mortality studies in systemic lupus erythematosus: results from a single center. I. Causes of death. J Rheumatol 1995;22:1259–1264.
6. Ward MN, Pyun E, Studenski S. Causes of death in systemic lupus erythematosus: long-term followup of an inception cohort. Arthritis Rheum 1995;38:1492–1499.
7. Badui E, Garcia-Rubi D, Robles E, Jimenez J, Juan L, Deleze M et al. Cardiovascular manifestations in systemic lupus erythematosus: prospective study of 100 patients. Angiology 1985;36:431–441.
8. Gladman DD, Urowiz MB. Morbidity in systemic lupus erythematosus. J Rheumatol 1987;14,Suppl 13:223–226.
9. Petri M, Perez-Gutthann S, SpenceD, Hochberg MC. Risk factors for coronary artery disease in patients with systemic lupus erythematosus. Am J Med 1992;93:513–519.

10. Jonsson H, Nived O, Stuefelt G. Outcome in systemic lupus erythematosus: a prospective study of patients from a defined population. Medicine (Baltimore) 1989;68:141–150.

11. Sturfelt G, Eskilsson J, Nived O, Truedsson L, Valind S. Cardiovascular disease in systemic lupus erythematosus: a study of 75 patients from a defined population. Medicine (Baltimora) 1992;71:216–223.

12. Manzi S, Meilahn EN, Rairie JE, Conte CG, Medserg TA Jr, Jansen-McWilliams L et al. Age-specific incidence rates of myocardial infarction and angina in women with systemic lupus erythematosus: comparison with the farmingham study. Am J Epidemiol 1997;145:408–415.

13. Ward MN. Premature morbidity from cardiovascular and cerebovascular diseases in women with systemic lupus erythematosus. Artritis Rheum 1999;42:338–346.

14. Bulkley BH, Roberts WC. The heart in systemic lupus erythematosus and the changes induced in it by corticosteroid therapy. Am J Med 1975;58:243–264.

15. Ettinger WH, Golderg AP, Applebaum-Bowden D, Hazzard WR. Dyslipoproteinemia in systemic lupus erythematosus: effect of corticosteroids. Am J Med 1987;83:503–508.

16. Petri M, Roubenoff R, Dallal GE, Nadeau MR, Selhub J, Rosenberg IH. Plasma homocysteine as a risk factor for atherotrombotic events in systemic lupus erythematosus. Lancet 1996;348:1120–1124.

17. Ross R. Atherosclerosis – An inflammatory disease. New Engl J Med 340;114–126.

18. Steinberg D. Low Density Lipoprotein oxidation and its pathobiological significance. J Biol Chem 1997;272:20963–20966.

19. Steinberg D. Oxidative modification of LDL and atherosclerosis. Circulation 1997;95:1062–1071.

20. Esterbauer H, Gehicki J, Puhl H, Jurgens G. The role of lipid peroxidation and antioxidants in oxidative modification of LDL. Free Rad Biol Med 1992;13:341–390.

21. Praticò D, Tangirala RK, Rader D, Rokach J, Fitzgerald GA. Vitamin E suppresses isoprostane generation in vivo and reduces atherosclerosis in Apo E-deficient mice. Nature Med 1998;4:1189–1192.

22. Praticò D. F_2-isoprostanes: sensitive and specific noninvasive indices of lipid peroxidation in vivo. Atherosclerosis 1999;147:1–10.

23. Lawson JA, Rokach J, fitzgerald GA. Isoprostanes: formation, analysis and use indices of lipid peroxidation in vivo. J Biol Chem 1999;274:24441–24444.

24. Rocach J, Khanapure SP, Hwang SW, Adiyaman M, Lawson JA, FitzGerald GA. Nomenclature of isoprostanes: a proposal. Prostaglandins 1997;54:853–856.

25. Praticò D, Iuliano L, Mauriello A, Spagnoli L, Lawson JA, Maclouf J, Violi F, FitzGerald GA. Localization of distinct F_2-isoprostanes in human atherosclerotic lesions. J Clin Invest 1997;100:2028–2034

26. Hörkko S, Miller E, Dudl E, Reaven P, Curtis LK, Zvaifler NJ, Terkeltaub R, Pierangeli SS, Branch DW, Palinski W, Witztum JL. Antiphospholipid antibodies are directed against epitopes of oxidized phospholipids. Recognition of cardiolipin by monoclonal antibodies to epitopes of oxidized low density lipoprotein. J Clin Invest 1996;98:815–815.

27. Palinski WP, Tangirala E, Miller E, Young SG, Witztum JL. Increased autoantibody titers against epitopes of oxidized low density lipoproteins in LDL receptor-deficient with increased atherosclerosis. Arterioscler Thromb Vasc Biol. 1995;15:1569–1576.

28. Mohan C, Datta SK. Lupus: key pathogenic mechanism and contributing factors. Clin Immunol Immunopathol 1995;77:209–220.

29. Harris EN, Gharavi AE, Boey ML, Patel BM, Mackworth-Young CG, Loizou S, Hughes GRV. Anticardiolipin antibodies: detection by radioimmunoassay and association with thrombosis in systemic lupus erythematosus. Lancet 1983;2:1211–1214.

30. Hughes GRV. The antiphospholipid syndrome: ten years on. Lancet 1993;ii:341.

31. Ferro D, Saliola M, Quintarelli C, Valesini G, Basili S, Grandilli MA, Bonavita MS, Violi F. Methods for detecting lupus anticoagulant and their relation to thrombosis and miscarriage in patients with systemic lupus erythematosus. J Clin Pathol 1992;45:332–338.

32. Vaarala O, Mänttäri M, Manninem U, Tenkanen L, Puurunen M, Aho K, Palosuo T. Anticardiolipin antibodies and risk of myocardial infarction in prospective cohort of middle aged men. Circulation 1995;91:23–27.

33. Iuliano L, Praticò D, Ferro D, Pittoni V, Valesini G, Lawson J, FitzGerald GA, Violi F. Enhanced lipid peroxidation in patients positive for antiphospholipid antibodies. Blood 1997;90:3931–3935.

34. Delanty N, Reilly M, Praticò D, FitzGerald DJ, Lawson JA, FitzGerald GA. 8-epi-$PGF_{2\alpha}$ specific analysis of an isoeicosanoid as an index of oxidant stress in vivo. Br J Clin Pharmacol 1996;42:15–19.

35. Reilly M, Delanty N, Lawson JA, FitzGerald GA. Modulation of oxidant stress in vivo in chronic cigarette smokers. Circulation 1996;94:19–25.

36. Delanty N, Reilly M, Praticò D, Lawson JA, Onishi ST, FitzGerald DJ, FitzGerald GA. 8-epi-$PGF_{2\alpha}$ generation during coronary reperfusion: a potential quantitative marker of oxidative stress in vivo. Circulation 1997;95:2492–2499.

37. Lynch SM, Morrow JD, Roberts II JL, Frei B. Formation of non-cyclooxygenase-derived prostanoids (F2-isoprostanes) in plasma and low density lipoprotein exposed to oxidative stress in vivo. J Clin Invest

1994;93:998–1004.

38. Morrow JD, Hill KE, Burk RF, Nammour TM, Badr KF, Roberts LJ. A series of prostaglandin F2-like compounds are produced in vivo in humans by a non-cyclooxygenase, free radical-catalyzed mechanism. Proc Natl Acad Sci USA 1990;87:9383–9387.

39. Morrow JD, Awad JA, Boss HJ, Blair IA, Roberts LJ. Non-cyclooxigenase-derived prostanoids (F2 isoprostanes) are formed in situ on phospholipids. Proct Natl Acad Sci USA 1992;89:10721–10725.

40. O'Connor DE, Mihelich ED, Coleman MC. Stereochemical course of the autoxidative cyclization of lipid hydroperoxides to prostaglandin-like bicyclo endoperoxides. J Am Chem Soc 1984;106:3577–3581.

41. Halliwell B, Gutteridge GMC. Free radicals, ageing, and disease, in Halliwell B, Gutteridge GMC (eds): Free radicals in biology and medicine. New York, NY, Oxford University Press 1989, p 416.

42. Praticò D, FitzGerald GA. Generation of 8-epiprostaglandin F2alpha by human monocytes. Discriminate production by reactive oxygen species and prostaglandin endoperoxide synthase-2. J Biol Chem 1996;271:8919–8924

43. Beutler B, Cerami A. The biology of cachetin/TNF. A primary mediator of the host response. Ann Rev Immunol 1989;7:625–655.

44. Al-Janadi M, Al-Balla S, Al-Dalaan A, Raziuddin S. Cytokine profile in systemic lupus erythematosus, rheumatoid arthritis and other rheumatic disease. J Clin Immunol 1993;13:58–67.

45. Kahaleh MB. The role of vascular endothelium in the pathogenesis of connective tissue disease: endothelial injury, activation, participation and response. Clin Exp Rheumatol 1990;8:595–601.

46. Bevilacqua MP, Pober JS, Majeau GR, Fiers W, Cotran RS, Gimbrone MA Jr. Recombinant tumor necrosis factor induces procoagulant activity in cultured huamn vascular endothelium: characterization and comparison with the action of interleukin-1. Proc Natl Acad Sci USA 1986;83:4533–4537.

47. Mulder AB, Hegge-Paping KSM, Magielse CPE, Blom NR, Smit JW, Van der Meer J, Halie MR, Bom VJJ. Tumor necrosis factor alpha-induced endothelial tissue factor is located on the cell surface rather than in the subendothelial matrix. Blood 1994;84:1559–1566.

48. Kahaleh MB, Smith EA, Soma Y, LeRoy EC. Effect of lymphotoxin and tumor necrosis factor on endothelial and connective tissue cell growth and function. Clin Immunol Immunopathol 1988;49:261–272.

49. Van der Poll T, Van Deventer SJH, Pasterkamp G, Van Mowrik JA, Buller HR, Ten Cate JW. Tumor necrosis factor induces von Willebrand factor release in healthy humans. Thromb Heamost 1992;67:623–626.

50. Ferro D, Pittoni V, Quintarelli C, Basili S, Saliola M, Caroselli C, Valesini G, Violi F. Coexistence of antiphospholipid antibodies and endothelial perturbation in systemic lupus erythematosus patients with ongoing prothrombotic state. Circulation 1997;95:1425–32.

51. Mann KG, van 't Veer C, cawthern K, Butenas S. The role of tissue factor in initiation of coagulation. Blood Coagul Fibrinolysis 1998;Suppl 1:S3–7.

52. Irani K, Xia Y, Zweier JL, Solot SL, Der CJ, Fearon ER, Sundaresan M, Finkel T, Goldschidt-Clermont PJ. Mitogenic signaling mediated by oxidants in ras-transformed fibroblast. Science 1997;275:1649–1652.

53. Brisseau GF, Dackin APB, Cheung PY, Christie N, Rotstein OD. Posttranscriptional regulation of macrophages tissue factor expression by antioxidants. Blood 1995;85:1025–1035.

54. Oeth P, Mackman N. Salicylates inhibit lipopolysaccharyde-induced transcriptional activation of the tissue factor gene in human monocytic cells. Blood 1995;86:4144–4152.

55. Crutchley DJ, Que BG. Copper-induced tissue factor expression in human monocytic THP-1 cells and its inhibition by antioxidant. Circulation 1995;92:238–243.

56. Praticò D, Ferro D, Iuliano L, Rokach J, Conti F, Valesini G, FitzGerald GA, Violi F. Ongoing prothrombotic state in patients with antiphospholipid antibodies: a role for increased lipid peroxidation. Blood 1999;93:3401–7.

Atherosclerosis and Autoimmunity
Y. Shoenfeld, D. Harats and G. Wick, editors

Antiphospholipid Syndrome and Atherosclerosis

Olga Amengual[1], Tatsuya Atsumi[2], Munther A. Khamashta[1] and Graham R.V. Hughes[1]

[1]*Lupus Research Unit, The Rayne Institute, St. Thomas' Hospital, London, United Kingdom;* [2]*Department of Medicine II, Hokkaido University School of Medicine, Sapporo, Japan*

1. INTRODUCTION

Atherosclerosis is a systemic disease of multifactorial origin characterized by deposition of lipids in the vessel walls. The symptoms appear due to the flow-limiting stenosis in the atherosclerotic vessels or to the formation of atherothrombosis. Atherosclerosis has been recently viewed as a complicated interaction which involves T cells, macrophages, endothelial and smooth muscle cells and it has been suggested that immunity against modified/cryptic self-antigens can influence the fate of the atherosclerotic lesions [1]; candidates autoantigen are oxidized lipoproteins, particularly oxidized low density lipoproteins (ox-LDL) [2], heat shock proteins [3] and β2Glycoprotein I (β2GPI) [4]. It is thought that the oxidative modification of lipoproteins such as LDL or lipoprotein (a) (Lp(a)) play a major role in the pathogenesis of the atherosclerotic lesion [2, 5, 6]. An early event in atherosclerosis is the accumulation of cholesterol-laden foam cells which originate mainly from monocyte-macrophage [5]. Macrophages take up chemically modified LDL but not native LDL. These events lead to chemotaxis of monocytes and the production of endothelial cell adhesion molecules contributing to functional impairment of the vasomotor properties of involved arteries [7]. Furthermore oxidative phenomena are also implicated in the immunogenicity of lipoproteins. Oxidation of LDL induces a specific immune response and specific immunoglobulins against ox-LDL have been found in atherosclerotic lesions [8] and in human sera viewed as independent predictors of carotid atherosclerosis progression [9].

The antiphospholipid syndrome (APS) is charac-terized by recurrent thrombosis (both venous and arterial) and pregnancy loss in association with the presence of antiphospholipid antibodies (aPL) [10, 11]. APS is recognized as one of the most common prothrombotic disorders but also this syndrome has been described as "a crossroads of autoimmunity and atherosclerosis" [12]. Evidences have shown that aPL are a part of a large family of autoantibodies against phospholipid-binding plasma proteins [13]. One of the most characterized antigenic target for these antibodies is β2GPI, a highly glycosylated protein with normal plasma concentration of 200 μg/ml. It consists in a single chain polypeptide of 326 amino acids, with an approximate molecular weight of 50 KiloDalton [14] that avidly binds negatively charged surfaces and substances [15]. Recent evidence showed that immune response towards β2GPI may play an important role in atherogenesis, serving as a possible target for antigen specific therapies [16].

2. LIPOPROTEINS AND ATHEROSCLEROSIS

2.1. Low-Density Lipoprotein

Epidemiological studies have established that an elevated plasma level of LDL represents one of the most important risk factors for the development of atherosclerosis [17]. The LDL particle consists of a hydrophobic core of cholesteryl esters and triglycerides surrounded by phospholipids, cholesterol and apolipoprotein B 100 and represents one of the major cholesterol-carrier lipoproteins in plasma.

Oxidative modification of LDL is an important event in the pathogenesis of the atherosclerotic lesions [5, 18, 19]. There is a large body of evidence supporting the presence of ox-LDL particles in the early phase of the atherosclerotic plaque formation [20–22]. The oxidized molecule is greatly different from its native counterpart and is not longer recognized by specific monocyte/macrophage receptors, rather is taken up by the scavenger pathway [7] and may favour the recruitment and migration of monocytes and leukocytes within arterial vessels [23]. Ox-LDL has been shown to be cytotoxic to various cells such as endothelial cells, monocytes and macrophages [24]. In addition, ox-LDL is more immunogenic than its native form, eliciting specific antibodies against ox-LDL (anti ox-LDL) that have been found in atherosclerotic lesions [8]. These autoantibodies may promote the uptake of ox-LDL from monocytes [25] and have been related to the atherosclerotic process. Anti ox-LDL may bind to ox-LDL leading to the formation of immune complexes which are taken up at an enhanced rate by Fc receptors on macrophages by the scavenger pathway contributing to the atherogenic process [25, 26].

2.2. Lipoprotein (a)

Lp(a), first described by Berg in 1963 [27], is another lipoprotein that represent a major risk factor for premature atherosclerotic vascular disease [6]. Lp(a) consists of a core of cholesteryl-esters, a surface layer of phospholipids, free cholesterol and a molecule of apolipoprotein B 100. The structure of Lp(a) resembles that of LDL, except for the addition of a large glycoprotein, apolipoprotein (a) (apo(a)), bound to apolipoprotein B 100 by disulfide linkage [28, 29]. Apo(a) is a highly polymorphic protein whose size depends upon the number of Kringle IV type-2 repeats. The total number of reported Kringle IV repeats varies in individuals between 12 and 51, including 3–42 repeats of Kringle IV type-2 [30]. Plasma Lp(a) levels are inversely correlated to apo(a) isoform size [31, 32] and varies from almost zero to 1000 mg/l. Family studies have suggested that plasma Lp(a) levels are affected by hereditary, rather than environmental factors [33, 34] and that the apo(a) gene accounts for almost the entire heritability [35]. In addition to the Kringle IV repeat polymorphism effects, further variations in non-coding and/or coding regions of the apo(a) gene have been hypothesized since Lp(a) concentration may vary over 100-fold within the same size of apo(a) isoform [36]. A number of polymorphic sites have been investigated, such as (TTTTA) n repeat at position −1400 [32, 37, 38], G/A at −772, C/T at +93, G/A at +121 [39–41], Thr/Met at amino acid position 66 in Kringle IV type 10 [42].

Many studies have shown that Lp(a) is a major risk factor for atherosclerotic/thrombotic disease [43]. High plasma levels of Lp(a) have been noted in patients with autoimmune diseases, such as systemic lupus erythematosus (SLE) [44–46], rheumatoid arthritis [47] and Behçet disease [48], Our group have showed that APS patients have elevated plasma Lp(a) levels and a fibrinolysis impairment that might contribute to the thrombotic tendency in APS [49]. Yamazaki et al [50] and Kawai et al [46] claim an association between a history of arterial thrombosis and Lp(a) in patients with APS and lupus patients (including secondary APS). Lp(a) pathogenicity has been linked to its thrombogenic and atherogenic potential. Apo(a) shows a striking homology, approximately 80%, with plasminogen structure [51]. The presence of many homologous Kringle repeats in apo(a) may produce in vivo competition with plasminogen for binding to fibrin and to plasminogen receptors on endothelial cells. It could thus inhibit fibrinolysis on the vessel wall. The inverse relation between Lp(a) and activated transforming growth factor beta (TGF-β) levels is probably due to competitive inhibition of plasminogen conversion to plasmin, which is necessary for activation of TGF-β. Low levels of activated TGF-β in intimal plaques are likely to stimulate smooth muscle cell invasion and proliferation [52]. In vitro studies have also shown that Lp(a) activates endothelial cells, inducing plasminogen activator inhibitor-1 [53] and endothelin-1 [54], which may also relate to the thrombogenicity of Lp(a). On the other hand, the LDL-like properties of Lp(a) might mimic the LDL role in the atherogenesis. Lp(a) is oxidized after incubation with mononuclear cells [55]; oxidized Lp(a) in the form of malondialdehyde-modified (MDA)-Lp(a) is avidly taken up by human monocyte-macrophages via scavenger receptors [56] and is found in association with macrophages in the atheromatous plaque [57]. Lp(a) or apo(a) plays a role as an endothelial activator, inducing monocyte chemotactic activity [58]. The recruitment of monocytes/macrophages into the arterial subendothelium is an early event in the formation of the plaque.

3. ANTIBODIES AGAINST OXIDIZED PLASMA LIPOPROTEINS

The oxidative modification of lipoproteins have been reported to induce a humoral response. Different forms of oxidized LDL such as MDA-LDL or copper-oxidized LDL induce the production of a heterogeneous population of specific antibodies against oxidatively modified LDL (anti ox-LDL)[25]. Anti ox-LDL were initially reported in patients with chronic periaortitis [59] and subsequently detected in subjects with progressive carotid atherosclerosis [9], SLE [60, 61] and in other disease states [62–64]. These antibodies have been also found in patients with APS, both primary and secondary [65, 66]. Levels of antibodies against MDA-LDL were found to be higher in APS patients with a history of arterial thrombosis [65].

Recently, antibodies reacting against MDA-Lp(a) (anti MDA-Lp(a)) have been reported in patients with APS [67]. IgG anti MDA-Lp(a) was detected in 37% (38/104) of patients with APS but in only 6% of healthy controls (6/106) (p<0.0001). Levels of anti MDA-Lp(a) were also higher in patients that in healthy controls (p<0.0001). Anti MDA-Lp(a) strongly correlated with antibodies against MDA-LDL in this population. A significant cross-reactivity have been detected between both populations of antibodies suggesting the involvement of a common epitope in the reactivity of the majority of antibodies against oxidatively-modified lipoproteins and supporting the possible pathogenicity of Lp(a) in its oxidized moiety. However additional experiments to further characterize these antibodies and their specificities are required.

The pathogenic role of antibodies against oxidized-lipoproteins still remains uncertain. The presence of anti ox-LDL in serum may represent a marker of inappropriate ox-LDL generation [68]. However, there is several evidence supporting their involvement in the development of atherosclerosis including: a correlation between anti ox-LDL and disease progression in carotid atherosclerosis [9];

the predictive value of anti ox-LDL for myocardial infarction [68]; the presence of immune complexes consisting of ox-LDL and anti ox-LDL within atherosclerotic plaques [69]; and lastly in vitro radiolabelled ox-LDL is taken up faster by a monocyte/macrophage-like line in the presence of anti ox-LDL than in the presence of ox-LDL alone [25]. Furthermore cross-reactivity has been shown between anticardiolipin antibodies (aCL) and oxidized lipoproteins (MDA-LDL) a major autoantigen in the atherosclerotic plaques, in SLE patients [60, 70]. The cross-reactivity between aPL and ox-LDL has been extensively studied showing that monoclonal aCL established from NZW/BXSBF1 mice [71] and from apo E deficient mice bound to ox-LDL [72]. This interaction also increase the uptake of oxidized-lipoproteins by macrophages promoting its transformation into foam cells. The infusion of ox-LDL, but not LDL, aggravates the clinical manifestations of experimental APS [73]. In addition, studies using purified IgG containing aCL found that ox-LDL bind in some fractions, implying that some aCL may have binding activity to ox-LDL [74]. Antibodies binding to ox-LDL could be considered as part of the aPL family because LDL contains both phospholipids and lipid-binding protein, thus anti ox-LDL need to be assessed as a potential marker of APS, specially in those with arterial disease. Anti MDA-Lp(a) are closely related to anti MDA-LDL and may represent a different subset of autoantibodies in the APS. The presence of antibodies against oxidized-lipoproteins in those patients supports the hypothesis of the possible role of oxidative phenomena in the pathogenesis of vascular complications in the APS.

4. β2GPI, ANTIβ2GPI AND VASCULAR COMPLICATIONS

The APS is an acquired thrombophilia where both venous and arterial thrombosis may take place in the presence of aPL and it has been reported that a number of these patients also develop accelerated atheroma [75]. Intensive attention has recently been focused in the identification of the autoantigenic materials expressed within atherosclerotic plaques that may influence the fate of the lesions. One of the candidate proteins is β2GPI [4], a plasma pro-

Table 1. Inhibitory effect of β2Glycoprotein I in coagulation system

	Reference
Contact activation of intrinsic coagulation pathway	[84]
Factor XII activation	[85]
Factor Xa generating activity	[86]
Prothrombinase activity	[87]
ADP-induced platelet aggregation	[88]
Protein C pathway	[89]

tein composed of five homologous domains which are designated short consensus repeats/complement control protein repeats or sushi structures of some 60 amino acids each [76]. In 1990, three groups independently reported that aCL which were associated with APS, bound to cardiolipin (CL) in the presence of β2GPI [77–79]. The phospholipid binding site is present within the fifth domain of β2GPI [80], whereas the domain fourth is dominantly involved in expressing the possible epitope for aCL [81]. Matsuura et al [82] and Roubey et al [83] showed that aCL bound to β2GPI in the absence of CL if β2GPI was coated onto polystyrene irradiated plates where oxygen was introduced by radiation, implying that aCL can bind not only CL-β2GPI complex but also β2GPI alone. Thus aPL related with the clinical manifestations of APS recognize a cryptic epitope on β2GPI which appears when β2GPI interact with solid-phase negatively charged phospholipids [82]. In vitro data suggest that β2GPI may play a role in physiological homeostasis of the coagulation system [84–89] (Table 1). β2GPI has an immunomodulatoy effect in experimental APS which demonstrate the importance of β2GPI in the pathogenesis of APS [90]. The significance of this protein has recently been highlighted due to the fact that it possesses several properties of relevance to progression of human atherosclerotic plaques: a) its ability to bind negatively charged surfaces including activated cells and platelets or apoptotic cells, b) its role as an important target for binding autoimmune aPL in the in vitro activation of endothelial cells and c) its ability to scavenge modified cellular surfaces

and foreign particles from circulation [91]. In addition β2GPI has been found abundantly present in human atherosclerotic plaques from carotid arteries, more prominent in subendothelial regions and in the intimal-mediated border of the lesions, colocalized with CD4-positive lymphocytes. These findings suggest that β2GPI may serve as target for an immune-mediated reaction that can influence the acceleration of the ongoing local inflammatory reaction [92]. On the other hand studies using β2GPI showed that β2GPI directly bound to ox-LDL and that the uptake of ox-LDL to macrophages was inhibited in the presence of exogenous β2GPI. Conversely the simultaneous addition of human β2GPI and monoclonal aCL derived from NZW x BXSB-F1 mice, an animal model of APS or antiβ2GPI from BALB/C mice immunized with human β2GPI, enhances the binding of ox-LDL to macrophages [93]. Thus ox-LDL may be targeted not only by antibodies directed to negatively charged phospholipids, but also by antiβ2GPI via β2GPI adhesion [93]. Therefore, β2GPI may be an anti-atherogenic protein. In the absence of aCL, β2GPI has an anti-atherogenic function by inhibiting the uptake of ox-LDL by macrophages. Subsequently antibodies against β2GPI, frequently found in patients with APS [94] may have a role in atherogenesis in these patients.

Humoral and cellular mechanisms have been proposed to participate in the onset and/or progression of thrombosis/atherosclerosis in patients with APS. Inflammation mechanism induce oxidative modification on lipoproteins and the immune response may contribute to accelerated atherosclerosis plaque formation and thrombotic events in these patients. On the other hand plasma Lp(a) may play a role as an endothelial agonist inducing chemotactic activity and vascular complications. In Fig. 1 the proposed mechanisms that has been implicated in the pathogenesis of vascular complications in the APS are illustrated.

5. CONCLUSIONS

There are multifactorial determinants involved in the development of vascular complications in patients with aPL. APS represent a prothrombotic stage in which atherosclerosis changes may be associ-

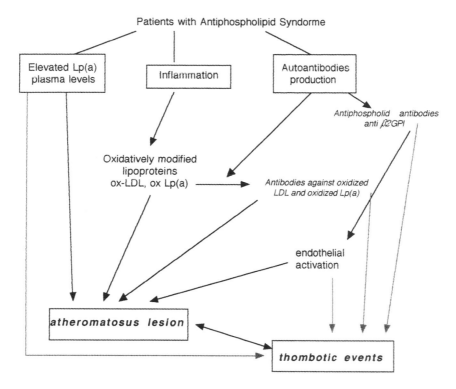

Figure 1. Pathogenesis of atherosclerosis and thrombosis in the APS.

aPL antiphospholipid antibodies, Lp(a) lipoprotein (a), LDL: low density lipoprotein, antiβ2GPI: anti β2Glycoprotein I.
The pathogenesis of the atherosclerotic lesions in patients with aPL is likely to be multifactorial. High plasma levels of Lp(a) are associated with atherosclerosis, playing a role as an endothelial activator. Elevated Lp(a) plasma levels inhibit fibrinolysis and thus might contribute to the thrombotic tendency in these patients. Inflammatory mechanism induce oxidative modification on lipoproteins (LDL or Lp(a)); oxidation enhances the uptake of lipoproteins by macrophages scavenger receptor and the development of atherosclerotic plaque. The humoral response against oxidized lipoproteins leads to the production of specific autoantibodies which contribute to the atherogenic process and to the development of arterial thrombosis in these patients. aPL (antiβ2GPI) leads to endothelial cell activation, which represent one of the early stages in the pathogenesis of atheroma.

ated with a high risk of atherothrombosis. Patients with this syndrome have increased levels of antibodies against oxidatively-modified lipoproteins, a subset of antibodies related to arterial thrombosis and accelerated atherosclerosis. The immuno-suppression may influence both thrombotic and atherosclerotic complications in affected patients. However additional studies are needed to determine the pathogenic role of these antibodies that will represent an important step in the understanding of the pathological events in APS.

ACKNOWLEDGEMENT

This work was supported by grants from Lupus UK. The authors thank Dr. Beverly Hunt for a critical review of the manuscript.

REFERENCES

1. Libby P, Hansson GK. Involvement of the immune system in human atherogenesis: current knowledge and unanswered questions. Lab Invest 1991;64:5–11.
2. Witztum JL. The oxidation hypothesis of atherosclerosis. Lancet 1994;344:793–795.
3. Wick G, Schett G, Amberger A, Kleindienst R, Xu Q. Is atherosclerosis an immunologically mediated disease?

Immunol Today 1995;16:27–33.

4. George J, Afek A, Gilburd B, Blank M, Levy Y, Aron-Maor A, et al. Induction of early atherosclerosis in LDL receptor deficient mice immunized with β2 glycoprotein I. Circulation 1998;15:1108–1115.

5. Steinberg D, Parthasarathy S, Carew TE, Khoo JD, Witztum JL. Beyond cholesterol: modifications of low-density lipoprotein that increase its atherogenicity. N Engl J Med 1989;320:915–924.

6. Dahlen G, Guyton JR, Attar M, Farmer JA, Kautz JA, Gotto AMJ. Association of plasma levels of lipoprotein (a), plasma lipids, and other lipoproteins with coronary artery disease documented by angiography. Circulation 1986;74:758–765.

7. Witztum JL, Steinberg D. Role of oxidized low density lipoprotein in atherogenesis. J Clin Invest 1991;88:1785–1792.

8. Ylä-Herttuala S, Butler SW, Picard S, Palinski W, Steinberg D, Witztum JL. Rabbit and human atherosclerotic lesions contain IgG that recognizes MDA-LDL and copper-oxidised LDL. Atherosclerosis 1991;11:1209–1222.

9. Salonen JK, Ylä-Herttuala S, Yamamoto R, Butler S, Korpela H, Salonen R, et al. Autoantibody against oxidised LDL and progression of carotid atherosclerosis. Lancet 1992;339:883–887.

10. Hughes GRV. The antiphospholipid syndrome: ten years on. Lancet 1993;342:341–344.

11. Wilson WA, Gharavi AZ, Koike T, Lockshin MD, Branch DW, Piette JC, et al. International consensus statement on preliminary classification criteria for definite antiphospholipid syndrome. Arthritis Rheum 1999;42:1309–1311.

12. Shoenfeld Y. The anti-phospholipid (Hughes) syndrome: a crossroads of autoinmmunity and atherosclerosis. Lupus 1997;6:559–560.

13. Roubey RAS. Autoantibodies to phospholipid-binding plasma proteins: a new view of lupus anticoagulants and other "antiphospholipid" autoantibodies. Blood 1994;84:2854–2867.

14. Kandiah D, Krilis SA. Beta2-Glycoprotein I. Lupus 1994;3:207–212.

15. Wurm H. beta2-glycoprotein (apolipoprotein H) interactions with phospholipid vesicles. Int J Biochem 1984;16:511–515.

16. George J, Shoenfeld Y, Harats D. The involvement of β2-Glycoprotein I (β2GPI) in human and murine atherosclerosis. J Autoimmunity 1999;13:57–60.

17. Ginsberg HN, Goldber IJ. Disorders of lipoprotein metabolism. In: Isselbacher KJ, ed. Harrison' Principles of Internal Medicine. 14th ed. United States of America: 1998: 2138–2149.

18. Palinski W, Rosenfeld ME, Ylä-Herttuala S, Gurtner GC, Socher SA, Butler SW, et al. Low-density lipoprotein undergoes oxidative modifications in vivo. Proc Natl Acad Sci USA 1989;86:1372–1376.

19. Steinberg D, Witztum JL. Lipoproteins and atherogenesis: current concepts. JAMA 1990;264:3047–3052.

20. Ylä-Herttuala S, Palinski W, Rosenfeld ME, Parthasarathy S, Carew TE, Butler SW, et al. Evidence for the presence of oxidatively modified low-density lipoprotein in atherosclerotic lesions of rabbit and man. J Clin Invest 1989;85:1086–1095.

21. O' Brien KD, Alpers CE, Hokanson JE, Wang S, Chait A. Oxidation-specific epitopes in human coronary atherosclerosis are not limited to oxidized low-density lipoprotein. Circulation 1996;94:1216–1225.

22. Steinberg D. Role of oxidized LDL and antioxidants in atherosclerosis. Adv Exp Med Biol 1995;369:39–48.

23. Berliner JA, Territo MC, Sevanian A, Ramin S, Kim JA, Bamshad B, et al. Minimally modified low-density lipoprotein stimulates monocyte endothelial interactions. J Clin Invest 1990;85:1260–1266.

24. Coffey MD, Cole RA, Colles SM, Chisolm GM. In vitro cell injury by oxidized low density lipoprotein involves lipid hydroperoxide-induced formation of alkoxyl, lipid and peroxyl radicals. J Clin Invest 1995;96:1866–1873.

25. Wu R, Lefvert AK. Autoantibodies against oxidized low density lipoproteins (oxLDL): characterization of antibody isotype, subclass, affinity and effect on the macrophage uptake of oxLDL. Clin Exp Immunol 1995;102:174–180.

26. Khoo JC, Miller E, Pio F, Steinberg D, Witztum JL. Monoclonal antibodies against LDL further enhance macrophage uptake of LDL aggregates. Arterioscler Thromb 1992;12:1258–1266.

27. Berg K. A new serum type system in man: The Lp(a) system. Acta Pathol Microbiol Scand 1963;59:369–382.

28. Scanu AM, Fless GM. Lipoprotein(a): heterogeneity and biological relevance. J Clin Invest 1990;85:1709–1715.

29. Gaubatz JW, Heldeman C, Gotto AMJ, Morrisett JD, Dahlén GH. Isolation and characterization of the two major apoproteins in human lipoprotein(a). J Biol Chem 1983;258:4582–4589.

30. Lackner C, Cohen JC, Hobbs HH. Molecular definition of the extreme size polymorphism in apolipoprotein (a). Hum Mol Genet 1993;2:933–940.

31. Utermann G, Menzel HJ, Kraft HG, Duba HC, Kemmler HG, Seitz C. Lp(a) glycoprotein phenotypes. Inheritance and relation to Lp(a)-lipoprotein concentrations in plasma. J Clin Invest 1987;80:458–465.

32. Brazier L, Tiret L, Luc G, Arveiler D, Ruidavets JB, Evans A, et al. Sequence polymorphisms in the apolipoprotein (a) gene and their association with lipoprotein (a) levels and myocardial infarction. The ECTIM Study.

Atherosclerosis 1999;144:323–333.

33. Austin MA, Sandholzer C, Selby JV, Newman B, Krauss RM, Utermann G. Lipoprotein (a) in women twins: heritability and relationship to apolipoprotein (a) pheno types. Am J Hum Genet 1992;51:829–840.

34. Boomsma DI, Kaptein A, Kempen HJ, Gevers Leuven JA, Princen HM. Lipoprotein(a): relation to other risk factors and genetic heritability. Results from Dutch parent-twin study. Atherosclerosis 1993;99:23–33.

35. DeMeester CA, Bu X, Gray RJ, Lusis AJ, Rotter JI. Genetic variation in lipoprotein(a) levels in families enriched for coronary artery disease is determined almost enterely by the apolipoprotein(a) gene locus. Am J Hum Genet 1995;56:287–293.

36. Cohen JC, Chiesa G, Hobbs HH. Sequence polymorphisms in the apolipoprotein(a) gene. Evidence for dissociation between apolipoprotein(a) size and plasma lipoprotein(a) levels. J Clin Invest 1993;91:1630–1636.

37. Trommsdorff M, Kochl S, Lingenhel A, Kronenberg F, Delport R, Vermaak H, et al. A pentanucleotide repeat polymorphism in the 5′ control region of the apolipoprotein(a) gene is associated with lipoprotein(a) plasma concentrations in Caucasians. J Clin Invest 1995;96:150–157.

38. Amemiya H, Arinami T, Kikuchi S, Yamakawa K, Li L, Fujiwara H, et al. Apolipoprotein(a) and pentanucleotide repeat polymorphisms are associated with the degree of atherosclerosis in coronary heart disease. Atherosclerosis 1996;123:181–191.

39. Suzuki K, Kuriyama M, Saito T, Ichinose A. Plasma lipoprotein(a) levels and expression of the apolipoprotein(a) gene are dependent on the nucleotide polymorphisms in its 5′-flanking region. J Clin Invest 1997;99:1361–1366.

40. Puckey LH, Lawn RM, Knight BL. Polymorphisms in the apolipoprotein(a) gene and their relationship to allele size and plasma lipoprotein(a) concentration. Hum Mol Genet 1997;6:1099–1107.

41. Prins J, Leus FR, Bouma BN, van Rijn HJ. The identification of polymorphisms in the coding region of the apolipoprotein(a) gene-association with earlier identified polymorphic sites and influence on the lipoprotein(a) concentration. Thromb Haemost 1999;82:1709–1717.

42. Kraft HG, Haibach C, Lingenhel A, Brunner C, Trommsdorff M, Kronenberg F, et al. Sequence polymorphism in kringle IV 37 in linkage disequilibrium with the apolipoprotein(a) size polymorphism. Hum Gent 1995;95:275–282.

43. Djurovic S, Berg K. Epidemiology of Lp(a) lipoprotein: its role in atherosclerotic/thrombotic disease. Clin Genet 1997;52:281–292.

44. Borba EF, Santos RD, Bonfa E, Vinagre CG, Pileggi FJC, Cossermelli W, et al. Lipoprotein(a) levels in systemic lupus erythematosus. J Rheumatol 1994;21:220–223.

45. Okawa-Takatsuji M, Aotsuka S, Sumiya M, Ohta H, Kawakami M, Sakurabayashi I. Clinical significance of the serum lipoprotein(a) level in patients with systemic lupus erythematosus: its elevation during disease flare. Clin Exp Rheumatol 1996;14:531–536.

46. Kawai S, Mizushima Y, Kaburaki J. Increased serum lipoprotein(a) levels in systemic lupus erythematosus with myocardial and cerebral infaction. J Rheumatol 1995;22:1210–1211.

47. Rantapää-Dahlqvist S, Wållberg-Jonsson S, Dahlén GH. Lipoprotein(a), lipids, and lipoproteins in patients with rheumatoid arthritis. Ann Rheum Dis 1991;50:366–368.

48. Orem A, Deger O, Memis O, Bahadir S, Ovali E, Cimsit G. Lp(a) lipoprotein levels as a predictor of risk for thrombogenic events in patients with Behçet`s disease. Annals Rheum Dis 1995;54:726–729.

49. Atsumi T, Khamashta MA, Andujar C, Leandro MJ, Amengual O, Ames PRJ, et al. Elevated plasma lipoprotein (a) level and its association with impaired fibrinolysis in patients with antiphospholipid syndrome. J Rheumatol 1998;25:69–73.

50. Yamazaki M, Asakura H, Jokaji H, Saito M, Uotani C, Kumabashiri I, et al. Plasma levels of lipoprotein(a) are elevated in patients with the antiphospholipid antibody syndrome. Thromb Haemost 1994;71:424–427.

51. Eaton DL, Fless GM, Kohr WJ, Mclean JW, Xu QT, Miller CG, et al. Partial amino acid sequence of apolipoprotein(a) shows that it is homologus to plasminogen. Proc Natl Acad Sci USA 1987;84:3224–3228.

52. Grainger DJ, Kemp PR, Metcalfe JC, Liu AC, Lawn RM, Williams NR, et al. The serum concentration of active transforming growth factor-beta severily depressed in advanced atherosclerosis. Nat Med 1995;1:74–79.

53. Etingin OR, Hajjar DP, Hajjar KA, Harpel PC, Nachman RL. Lipoprotein(a) regulates plasminogen activator inhibitor-1 expression in endothelial cells. A potential mechanism in thrombogenesis. J Biol Chem 1991;266:2459–2465.

54. Berge KE, Djurovic S, Muller HJ, Alestrom P, Berg K. Studies on effects of Lp(a) lipoprotein on gene expression in endothelial cells in vitro. Clin Genet 1997;52:314–325.

55. Naruszewicz M, Selinger E, Davignon J. Oxidative modification of lipoprotein (a) and the effect of β-carotene. Metabolism 1992;11:1215–1224.

56. Haberland ME, Fless GM, Scanu AM, Fogelman AM. Malondialdehyde modification of lipoprotein (a) produces avid uptake by human monocyte-macrophages. J Biol Chem 1992;6:4143–4151.

57. Ross R. The pathogenesis of atherosclerosis- an update.

N Engl J Med 1986;314:488–500.

58. Ponn M, Zhang X, Dunsky K, Taubman MB, Harpel PC. Apolipoprotein(a) is a human vascular endothelial cell agonist: studies on the induction in endothelial cells of monocyte chemotactic factor activity. Clin Genet 1997;52:308–313.

59. Parums DV, Brown DL, Mitchinson MJ. Serum antibodies to oxidized low density lipoprotein and ceroid in chronic periaortitis. Arch Pathol Lab Med 1990;114:383–387.

60. Vaarala O, Alfthan G, Jauhiainen M, Leirisalo-Repo M, Aho K, Palosuo T. Crossreaction between antibodies to oxidised low-density lipoprotein and to cardiolipin in systemic lupus erythematosus. Lancet 1993;341:923–925.

61. Romero FI, Amengual O, Atsumi T, Khamashta MA, Tinahones FJ ,Hughes GRV. Arterial disease in lupus and secondary antiphospholid syndrome: association with anti-beta2-glycoprotein I antibodies but not with antibodies against oxidized low-density lipoprotein. Br J Rheumatol 1998;37:883–888.

62. Bellomo G, Maggi E, Poli M, Agosta FG, Bollati P, Finardi G. Autoantibodies against oxidatively modified low-density lipoproteins in NIDDM. Diabetes 1995;44:60–66 .

63. Boullier A, Hamon M, Walters-Laporte E, Martin-Nizart F, Mackereel R, Fruchart JC, et al. Detection of autoantibodies against oxidized low-density lipoproteins and of IgG-bound low density lipoproteins in patients with coronary artery disease. Clinica Chimica Acta 1995;238:1–10.

64. Maggi E, Marchesi E, Ravetta V, Martignoni A, Finardi G, Bellomo G. Presence of autoantibodies against oxidatively modified low-density lipoprotein in essential hypertension: a biochemical signature of an enhanced in vivo low-density lipoprotein oxidation. J Hypertension 1995;13:129–138.

65. Amengual O, Atsumi T, Khamashta MA, Tinaones F, Hughes GRV. Antibodies agaisnt oxidized low-density lipoprotein in antiphospholipid syndrome. Br J Rheumatol 1997;36:964–968.

66. Cuadrado MJ, Tinahones F, Camps MT, de Ramón E, Gómez-Zumaquero JM, Mujic F, et al. Antiphospholipid, anti beta2- glycoprotein-I and anti-oxidized-low-density-lipoprotein antibodies in antiphospholipid syndrome. QJM 1998;91:619–626.

67. Romero FI, Atsumi T, Tinahones FJ, Gómez-Zumaquero JM, Amengual O, Khamashta MA, et al. Autoantibodies against malondialdehyde-modified lipoprotein(a) in the antiphospholipid syndrome. Arthritis Rheum 1999;42:2606–2611.

68. Puurunen M, Mänttäri M, Manninen V, Tenkanen L, Alfthan G, Ehnholm C, et al. Antibody against low-density lipoprotein predicting myocardial infarction. Arch Intern Med 1994;154:2605–2609.

69. Ylä-Herttuala S, Palinski W, Butler SW, Picard S, Steinberg D, Witztum JL. Rabbit and human atherosclerotic lesion contain IgG that recognizes epitopes of oxidized LDL. Arterioscler Thromb, 1994;14:32–40.

70. Palinski W, Hörkkö S, Miller E, Steinbrecher UP, Powell HC, Curtiss LK, et al. Cloning of monoclonal autoantibodies to epitopes of oxidized lipoproteins from apolipoprotein E-deficient mice. J Clin Invest 1996;98:800–814.

71. Mizutani H, Kurata Y, Kosugi S, Shiraga M, Kashiwagi H, Tomiyama Y, et al. Monoclonal anticardiolipin autoantibodies established from the (New Zealand White X BXSB)F1 mouse model of antiphospholipid syndrome cross-react with oxidized low-density lipoprotein. Arthritis Rheum 1995;38:1382–1388.

72. Hörkkö S, Miller E, Dudl E, Reaven P, Curtiss LK, Zvaifler N, et al. Antiphospholipid antibodies are directed against epitopes of oxidized phospholipids. J Clin Invest 1996;98:815–825.

73. George J, Blank M, Hojnik E, Bar-Meir E, Koike T, Matsuura E, et al. Oxidized low-density lipoprotein (Ox-LDL) but not LDL aggravates the manifestations of experimental antiphospholipid syndrome. Clin Exp Immunol 1997;108:227–233.

74. Vaarala O, Puurunen M, Lukka G, Alfthan M, Leirisalo-Repo K, Aho K, et al. Affinity-purified cardiolipin-binding antibodies show heterogeneity in their binding to oxidized low-density lipoprotein. Clin Exp Immunol 1996;104:269–274.

75. Lecerf V, Alhenc-Gelas M, Laurian C, Bruneval P, Aiach M, Cormier JM, et al. Antiphospholid antibodies and atherosclerosis. Am J Med 1992;92:575–576.

76. Lozier J, Takahashi N, Putnan FW. Complete amino acid sequence of human β2-glycoprotein I. Proc Natl Acad Sci USA 1984;81:3640–3644.

77. Matsuura E, Igarashi Y, Fujimoto M, Ichikawa K, Koike T. Anticardiolipin cofactor(s) and differential diagnosis of autoimmune disease. Lancet 1990;336:177–178.

78. McNeil HP, Simpson RJ, Chesterman CN, Krilis SA. Anti-phospholipid antibodies are directed against a complex antigen that induces a lipid-binding inhibitor of coagulation: β2-glycoprotein I (apolipoprotein H). Proc Natl Acad Sci USA 1990;87:4120–4124.

79. Galli M, Comfurius P, Maassen C, Hemker C, DeBaets MH, van Bredavriesman PJC, et al. Anticardiolipin antibodies (ACA) directed not to cardiolipin but to a plasma protein cofactor. Lancet 1990;335:1544–1547.

80. Hunt JE, Krilis S. The fifth domain of β2-glycoprotein I contains a phospholipid binding site (Cys281-Cys288) and a region recognized by anticardiolipin antibodies. J Immunol 1994;152:653–659.

81. Igarashi M, Matsuura E, Igarashi Y, Nagae H, Ichikawa K, Triplett DA, et al. Human β2-glycoprotein I as an anticardiolipin cofactor determined using deleted mutants expressed by a Baculovirus system. Blood 1996;87:3262–3270.

82. Matsuura E, Katahira T, Igarashi Y, Koike T. β2-Glycoprotein I bound to oxidatively modified lipoproteins could be targeted by anticardiolipin antibodies. Lupus 1994;3:314.

83. Roubey RAS. Anticardiolipin antibodies recognize β2-glycoprotein I in the absence of phospholipid: Importance of antigen density and bivalent binding. J Immunol 1995;154:954–960.

84. Schousboe I. β2-glycoprotein I: Plasma inhibitor of contact activation of the intrinsic blood coagulation pathway. Blood 1985;66:1086–1091.

85. Schousboe I, Rasmussen MS. Synchronized inhibition of the phospholipid mediated autoactivation of Factor XII in plasma by β2-glycoprotein I and anti-β2-glycoprotein I. Thromb Haemostas 1995;73:798–804.

86. Shi W, Chong BH, Hogg PJ, Chesterman CN. Anticardiolipin antibodies block the inhibition by β2-glycoprotein I of the factor Xa generating activity of platelets. Thromb Haemost 1993;70:342–345.

87. Nimpf J, Bevers EM, Bomans PHH, Till U, Wurm H, Kostner GM, et al. Prothrombinase activity of human platelets inhibited by β2-glycoprotein I. Biochem Boiphys Acta 1986;884:142–149.

88. Nimpf J, Wurm H ,Kostner M. Interaction of β2-glycoprotein I with human blood platelets: Influences upon the ADP induced aggregation. Thromb Haemostas 1985;54:397–401.

89. Mori T, Takeya H, Nishioka J, Gabazza EC, Suzuki K. β2-glycoprotein I modulates the anticoagulant activity of activated protein C on the phospholipid surface. Thromb Haemost 1996;75:49–55.

90. Blank M, George J, Barak V, Tincani A, Koike T, Shoenfeld Y. Oral tolerance to low dose b2-glycoprotein I: immunomodulation of experimental antiphospholipid syndrome. J Immunol 1998;161:5303–5312.

91. Roubey RAS. Immunology of the antiphospholipid antibody syndrome. Arthritis Rheum 1996;39:1444–1454.

92. George J, Harats D, Gilburd B, Afek A, Levy Y, Schneiderman J, et al. Immunolocalization of b2-glycoprotein I (apolipoprotein H) to human atherosclerotic plaques. potential implications for lesion progression. Circulation 1999;99:2227–2230.

93. Hasunuma Y, Matsuura E, Makita Z, Katahira T, Nishi S, Koike T. Involvement of β2-glycoprotein I and anticardiolipin antibodies in oxidatively modified low-density lipopoprotein uptake by macrophages. Clin Exp Immunol 1997;107:569–573.

94. Amengual O, Atsumi T, Khamashta MA, Koike T, Hughes GRV. Specificity of ELISA for antibody to β2-glycoprotein I in patients with antiphospholipid syndrome. Br J Rheumatol 1996;35:1239–1243.

Atherosclerosis and Autoimmunity
Y. Shoenfeld, D. Harats and G. Wick, editors

"Endotheliology" in Antiphospholipid Antibodies

Tatsuya Atsumi[1], Olga Amengual[2] and Munther A Khamashta[2]

[1]*Department of Medicine II, Hokkaido University School of Medicine, Sapporo, Japan;* [2]*St. Thomas' Hospital, London, UK*

1. INTRODUCTION

Endothelial cells form one of the major organs that covers all of the inner surface of blood vessels and have largely various properties to regulate a number of important physiological and pathological reactions. Antithrombotic properties are the most classical, but also they are involved in inflammatory reactions, immune reactions, blood vessel tonus, angiogenesis and atherosclerosis. The alterations of endothelial functions may lead to vasculitis syndrome, thrombosis, disseminated intravascular coagulation, diabetic retinopathy or many kinds of neovascularising conditions. In those pathological situations, endothelial cells play central roles and they can be considered as a "target organ". Therefore, Maruyama has proposed a new paradigm-shift in medicine, "Endotheliology" [1]. The important points in this area will be 1) multifactoriality, 2) organ specificity, 3) dynamicity (their functions are never static; they are heterogeneously changable) and 4) cross-link between endothelium and blood cells/smooth muscle cells.

In this review, we describe recent topics in the pathophysiology of thrombosis associated with antiphospholipid antibodies (aPL) from a viewpoint of the "Endotheliology", rather than that of the immunological specificity.

2. ANTITHROMBOTIC PROPERTIES OF ENDOTHELIAL CELLS

Endothelial cells play the most important roles to maintain the blood fluidity. At the most basic level, endothelium prevents platelets and plasma coagulation factors from encontering the thrombogenic subendothelial extracellar matrix. Their antithrombotic properties have been widely explored.

Endothelial cells produce nitric oxide (NO; also called as an endothelium derived relaxation factor) and prostacyclin (PGI2). Both mediators are potent vasodilators and inhibitors of thrombocytes' aggregation [2, 3].

Regarding the suppression of coagulation reaction, endothelial cells produce the following molecules; tissue factor pathway inhibitor (TFPI) [4], thrombomodulin [5] and heparin-like proteoglycan [6]. The extrinsic coagulation pathway is modulated by TFPI, a multivalent Kunitz-type plasma proteinase inhibitor [7, 8]. Direct activation of factor X by VIIa-Tissue Factor complex is quickly supressed by TFPI. It has been suggested that TFPI may protect against thrombotic complications following exposure of Tissue Factor (TF) on the surface of intravascular cells. On the other hand, thrombomodulin is a glycoprotein that converts thrombin from a procoagulant protease to an anticoagulant. Thrombin-thrombomodulin complex activate protein C [9–11], leading to inhibiting clotting by proteolytic cleavage of factors Va and VIIIa in the presence of protein S that is synthesised by endothelial cells as a cofactor [12, 13]. Therefore, thrombomodulin is an anticoagulant receptor that plays a crucial role to regulate thrombin generation. Another anticoagulant, heparin-like proteoglycans bind and activate antithrombin that inhibits factor Xa and thrombin immediately [14, 15, 6].

The third antithrombotic player on endothelial cells is tissue type plasminogen activator (t-PA),

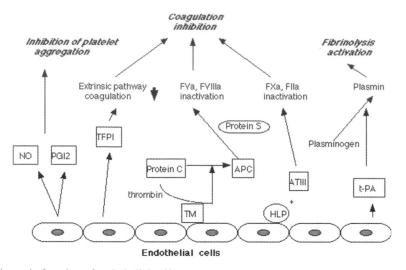

Figure 1. Antithrombogenic function of endothelial cell.
NO: nitric oxide; PGI2: prostacyclin; TFPI: tissue factor patway inhibitor; TM: thrombomodulin; APC: activated protein C; HLP: heparin like proteoglycan; ATIII: antithrombin; t-PA: tissue type plasminogen activator.

which cleaves Arg560-Val561 on plasminogen converting to plasmin [16]. Plasmin breaks down fibrin and interferes with its polymerization. The fibrin degradation products also play a role as a weak anticoagulants.

3. INTERACTION OF ANTIPHOSPHOLIPID ANTIBODIES ON THE ANTITHROMBOTIC ENDOTHELIUM

Although a scenario in which aPL inhibit PGI2 production is one of the most "classic" stories, data presented by some investigators were controversial. Carreras et al. [17] published some data showing inhibited PGI2 production from endothelium by aPL, whereas others have reported no effect, enhanced PGI2 production or mixed results [18–21]. Thus the scenario has failed to arrive a consensus.

On the other hand, many data have supported the suppressed thrombomodulin-protein C system by aPL. The fact that protein C and its cofactor protein S are phospholipid binding plasma proteins has made this system one of the most likely to be involved in the pathophysiology of thrombosis in APS. APL might inhibit phospholipid-dependent reactions of the protein C pathway in different ways. Firstly, they can interfere with the activation of protein C by the thrombin/thrombomodulin complex.

Thrombin formation inhibited by aPL could paradoxically cause a prothrombotic tendency due to insufficient protein C activation [22]. It has also been shown that LA positive IgGs inhibit the activation of purified protein C by thrombin on endothelial cells [23, 18] or by thrombin/purified thrombomodulin [24]. Secondly, the proteolytic effect of APC on factor Va/factor VIIIa can be inhibited by aPL. Marciniak and Romond [25] reported that factor Va degradation was reduced in plasma from patients with lupus anticoagulant (LA). Malia et al. [26] the inhibitory effect of IgGs purified from aPL positive patients on factor Va degradation by activated protein C (APC). Ieko et al. [27] showed that human monoclonal anti-β2glycoprotein I antibodies (anti-β2GPI) inhibit APC function, definitely confirming the autoimmune aPL effect on this system. Finally, the co-factor effect of protein S in the protein C pathway can be affected by aPL [28–30].

Recently, Ieko et al. showed, for the first time, the inhibitory effect of aPL on the t-PA dependent extrinsic fibrinolytic activity [31].

4. PROCOAGULANT PROPERTIES OF ENDOTHELIAL CELLS

Endothelial cells are also prothrombotic, affecting platelets, coagulation proteins, and the fibrinolytic

290

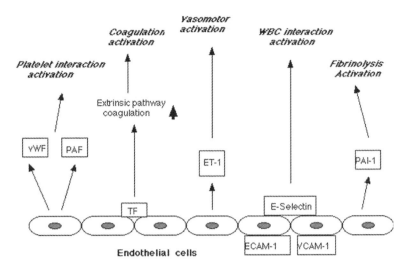

Figure 2. Thrombogenicity of endothelial cells.

vWF: von Willebrand factor; PAF: platelet activator factor; TF: tissue factor; ET-1:endothelin I; PAI-1: plasminogen activator inhibitor; WBC: white blood cells.

system.

Endothelial injury leads to adhesion of platelets to the underlying extracellular matrix, facilitating endothelial production of von Willebrand factor. It functions as an adhesion bridge between subendothelial collagen and the GpIb platelet receptor. Endothelium is one of the pruducers of platelet activating factor (PAF).

Bacterial endotoxin or cytokines (tumor necrosis factor or interleukin 1) induce TF, activating the extrinsic clotting cascade [32, 33]. TF is a single chain transmembrane protein composed of 263 amino acid residues [34]. Of the many factors involved in the activation of the intrinsic and extrinsic pathways of coagulation, TF is the only factor that is fully active in its native form, not dependent on proteolysis, therefore procoagulant activity generation merely requires TF exposure on cell surfaces [35].

Endothelin-1 (ET-1) is the most potent endothelium-derived contracting factor modulating vascular smooth muscle tone [36, 37]. ET-1 is extremely labile, thus the mature peptide is not found within endothelial cells [38]; however, the levels of prepro ET-1 (a precursor of ET-1) mRNA are induced by a range of stimuli, such as thrombin [39] or cytokines. Production and secretion of mature ET-1 peptide occurs within minutes of exposure to these stimuli [40]. Vascular cells are, therefore, able to adjust rapidly ET-1 production as required for the regulation of vasomotor tone [37].

Adhesion receptors are proteins in cell membranes that facilitate the interaction of cells with matrix. Intracellular adhesion molecule-1 (ICAM-1), vascular cell adhesion molecule-1 (VCAM-1) and E-selectin are typical molecules found on activated endothelial cells. Leucocytes stick on endothelial cell via those molecules, further activating endothelium. Some proteases derived from such leukocytes also cause to direct endothelium injury.

Finally, endothelial cells secrete the inhibitor of plasminogen activator-1(PAI-1) to depress fibrinolysis by blocking t-PA activity, when activated.

5. INDUCTION OF PROCOAGULANT TENDENCY ON ENDOTHELIAL CELLS BY ANTIPHOSPHOLIPID ANTIBODIES

Silver et al. [41] reported that aPL enhance PAF production, but it was not confirmed by the others [42]. A few reports showed the increased vWF production by aPL.

In contrast, numerous investigators have focused the upregulation of TF expression by aPL. We [43] and others [44, 45] showed that aPL induce TF activity, antigen or mRNA on endothelial cells as well as on monocytes. As described above, TF does not require activation by other enzymes to function, thus the its expression per se represents hypercoagulation in patients with aPL.

We also showed that markedly increased plasma ET-1 levels were found in APS patients with arterial thrombosis but not those with venous thrombosis [46]. It is so far the only specific marker for arterial thrombosis in APS. Human monoclonal aCL induced prepro ET-1 mRNA levels, confirming aPL's direct effect on endothelium regarding ET-1 production. These data suggest that the production of ET-1 induce by aPL may play an important role in altering arterial tone and probably contributing to arterial occlusion [46].

Cellular interaction of aPL have gained increasing attention. Purified aPL or monoclonal anti-β2GPI induce expression of the adhesion molecules E-selectin, VCAM-1 and ICAM-1. Pierangeli [47] showed an unique *in vivo* model to present the increased leukocyte adhesion by aPL infusion to mice, in which adhered leukocytes are visualised using scrotum under microscope.

Impaired fibrinolysis in APS has been shown in some reports [48–50], but no direct evidence has been reported in the induction of PAI-1 by aPL. Acquired antithrombin deficiency has been hypothesized in APS. In fact, prothrombin fragment 1+2 was markedly elevated in patients with aPL, reflecting the increased thrombin generation, whereas the levels of thrombin-antithrombin complex (TAT) in those patients were not increased [51].

In any case, aPL activate endothelium, leading to its perturbation. The activation may depend on the immune complex formation on cell surface and/or Fcγ receptor stimulation and/or thrombin receptor that delivers a stimularory signal by thrombin [52].

6. APOPTOSIS AND ENDOTHELIAL CELLS

Apoptosis is a regulated mode of cell death characterized by alteration of the overall cell shape and density, cytoplasm blebbing, modification of the chromatin, with digestion of the DNA, and late membrane failures . Death via apoptosis and the ensuing phagocytosis of apoptotic cells by living cells is a common event that is crucial to the homeostasis of organisms [53, 54]. Antigen-presenting cells, such as macrophages are well characterized

scavengers of apoptotic cells [54]. During the early phases of apoptosis, the plasma membrane itself undergoes rearrangements, which include the exposure of anionic phospholipids (PL), confined to the intracellular portion of membrane of viable cells [55, 56]. Phosphatidylserine (PS) recognition, in association with other membrane modifications, triggers the engulfment of apoptotic cells through specific membrane receptors by scavenger phagocytes. This process limits the release of the intracelullar content into the environment [57, 54].

It is widely accepted the concept that autoimmune aPL require PL-binding proteins, most notably β2GPI [58–61]. β2GPI is a plasma protein that binds with high efficiency to membranes of human cells undergoing apoptosis [62]. Apoptotic cells express PS, thus PS-bound β2GPI is selectively bound by human aPL [63–65, 62]. Furthermore aPL-bound apoptotic cells are more efficiently phagocytosed by macrophages, triggering the secretion of soluble factors such as tumor necrosis factor α (TNFα) by scavenger macrophages. TNFα selectively regulates the ability of Fc receptor-positive dendritic cells to further take up antigens at the periphery and possible their terminal differentiation into potent antigen-presenting cells [65]. Thus, the interference with the in vivo clearance and processing of apoptotic cells is a potential pathogenic mechanism of these antibodies [66].

Apoptotic cells contain antigens that can productively activate an immune response [67]. The exposure of PL during the apoptosis may be a driving antigenic stimulus to the production of aPL and PL-protein complexes formed during apoptosis are targeted by pathogenic aPL. The binding and the clearance of apoptotic cells by these antibodies likely enhances the aPL immune response. Therefore, aPL are able of transforming the silent programmed death of single cells in a signal that promotes productive activation of autoactive T cells by dendritic cells [68].

The recognition of β2GPI by the aPL at the surface of the endothelial cell may result in the activation of cultured endothelia [69, 70]. On the other hand, it has been recently reported that antibodies reactive against endothelial cells (AECA) cause apoptosis of endothelial cells [71]. AECA is one of the many factor responsible for the PS reaching the surface of the cell membrane from its intrac-

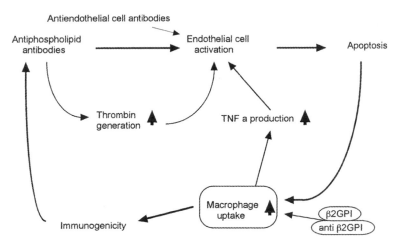

Figure 3. Apoptosis and immunogenicty.

TNF a: tumor necrosis factor alpha; β2GPI: β2 glycoprotein I; antiβ2GPI: antibodies against β2glycoprotein I.
Antiphospholipid antibodies (aPL) and antiendothelial cell antibodies are able to activate endothelial cell leading to apoptosis.
Apoptotic cells are taken up by macrophage scavenger and this phagocytosis is more efficient in the presence of aPL. Macrophage produce a massive amount of TNFα after recognition of aPL-opsonized apoptotic cells. TNFα activate endothelial cell and make them accessible to aPL. Then macrophage uptaking apoptotic cells may provide an antigenic stimulus to the production of aPL.

ellular location, before cells undergo apoptosis. Anionic PL then become available for binding to β2GPI and, subsequently, to aPL. Fig. 3 illustrated the relationship between apoptosis and immunogenicity.

7. CONCLUSION

Too many mechanisms have been reported in the aPL-associated thrombosis in the endotheliology. However, it is not an exaggeration. Antibody mediated thrombosis must be multifactorial and complex. The further clarification should lead to the better management for the affected patients.

REFERENCES

1. Maruyama I. Biology of endothelium. Lupus 1998;7:41–3.
2. Furchgott RF, Zawadzki JV. The obligatory role of endothelial cells in the relaxation of arterial smoth muscle by acetylcholin. Nature 1980;228:373–6.
3. Weksler BB, Marcus AS, Jaffe EA. Synthesis of protaglandin I2 (prostacyclin) by a cultured human and bovine endothelial cells. Proc Natl Acad Sci USA 1977;74:3922–6.
4. Lupu C, Lupu F, Dennehy U, Kakkar VV, Scully MF.

Thrombin induces the redistribution and acute release of tissue factor pathway inhibitor from specific granules within human endothelial cell in culture. Aterioscler Thromb Vasc Biol 1995;15:2055–61.
5. Maruyama I, Bell CE, Majerus PW. Thrombomodulin found on endothelium of arteries, veins, capillaries, and lymphaticas and on syncytiothrophoblast of human placenta. J Cell Biol 1985;101:363–72.
6. Marcum JA, Fritze L, Galli SJ, Karp G, Rosenber RD. Microvascular heparin-like species with anticoagulnt actvity. Am J Physiol 1983;245:725–33.
7. Broze GJJ, Warren LA, Novotny WF, Higuchi DA, Girard JJ, Miletich JP. The lipoprotein associated coagulation inhibitor that inhibits the factor VII-tissue factor complex also inhibits factor Xa: Insight into its possile mechanism of action. Blood 1988;71:335–43.
8. Kazama Y. The importance of the binding of factor Xa to phospholipids in the inhibitory mechanism of tissue factor pathway inhibitor: the transmembrane and cytoplasmic domains of tissue factor are not essential for the inhibitory action of tissue factor pathway inhibitor. Thromb Haemost 1997;77:492–7.
9. Esmon CT, Owen WG. Identification of an endothelial cell cofactor for thrombin-catalysed activation of protein C. Proc Natl Acad Sci USA 1981;78:2249–52.
10. Esmon NL, Owen WG, Esmon CT. Isolation of a membrane-bound cofactor for thrombin-catalyzed activation of protein C. J Biol Chem 1982;257:859–64.
11. Ye J, Esmon NL, Esmon CT, Johnson A. The active

site on thrombin is altered upon binding to thrombomodulin: two distinct structural changes are detected by flourescence, but onlu one correlates with protein C activation. J Biol Chem 1991;266:23016–22.

12. Suzuki K, Stenflo J, Dahlbäck B, Teodorsson B. Inactivation of human coagulation Factor V by activated protein C. J Biol Chem 1983;258:1914–8.

13. Dahlback B. Protein S and C4b-binding protein: Components involved in the regulation of the protein C anticoagulant system. Thromb Haemost 1991;66:49–61.

14. Hatton MWC, Berry LR, Regoeczi E. Inhibition of thrombin by antihrombin III in the presence of certain glycosaminoglycans found in the mammalian aorta. Thromb Res 1978;13:655–70.

15. Marcum JA, Rosenberg RD. Anticoagulantly active heparin-like molecules from vascular tisue. Biochimestry 1984;23:1730–7.

16. Plow EF, Herren T, Redlitz A, Miles LA, Hoover-Plow JL. The cell biology of the plasminogen system. FASEB J 1995;9:939–45.

17. Carreras LO, Defreyn G, Machin SJ, Vermylen J, Deman R, Spitz B et al. Arterial thrombosis, intratuterine death and "lupus" anticoagulanr: Detection of immunoglobulin interfering with prostacyclin formation. lancet 1981;1:244–6.

18. Cariou R, Tobelem G, Bellucci S, Soria J, Soria C, Maclouf J et al. Effect of lupus anticoagulant on antithrombotic properties of endothelial cells - Inhibition of thrombomodulin-dependent protein C activation. Thromb Haemost 1988;60:54–8.

19. Walker TS, Triplett DA, Javed N, Musgrave K. Evaluation of lupus anticoagulants: Antiphospholid antibodies, endothelium associated immunoglobulin, endothelial prostacyclin secretion, and antigenic protein S levels. Thromb Res 1988;51:267–81.

20. Petraioulov W, Bovill E, Hoak J. The lupus anticoagulant stimulates the release of prostacyclin from human endothelial cells. Thromb Res 1988;50:847–55.

21. Hasselaar P, Derksen RHWM, Blokzijil L, de Groot PG. Thrombosis associated with antiphospholipid antibodies cannot be explained by effects on endothelial and platelet prostanoid synthesis. Thromb Res 1988;59:80-.

22. de Groot PG, Derksen RHWM. Protein C pathway, antiphospholipid antibodies and thrombosis. Lupus 1994;3:229–33.

23. Cariou R, Tobelem G, Soria C, Caen J. Inhibition of protein C activation by endothelial cells in the presence of lupus anticoagulant. N Engl J Med 1986;314:1193–4.

24. Taskiris DA, Settas L, Makris PE, Marbet GA. Lupus anticoagulant - antiphospholipid antibodies and thrombophilia. Relation to protein C-protein S-thrombomodulin. J Rheumatol 1990;17:785–9.

25. Marciniak E, Romond EH. Impaired catalytic function

of activated protein C: a new in vitro manifestation of lupus anticoagulant. Blood 1989;71:2426–32.

26. Malia RG, Kitchen S, Greaves M, Preston FE. Inhibition of activated protein C and its cofactor protein S by antiphospholipid antibodies. Br J Haematol 1990;76:101–7.

27. Ieko M, Ichikawa K, Triplett DA, Matsuura E, Atsumi T, Sawada K et al. Beta2-glycoprotein I is necessary to inhibit protein C activity by monoclonal anticardiolipin antibodies. Arthritis Rheum 1999;42:167–74.

28. Oosting JD, Derksen RHWM, Bobbink IWG, Hackeng TM, Bouma BN, Groot PG. Antiphospholipid antibodies directed against a combination of phospholipids with prothrombin, protein C, or protein S: An explanation for their pathogenic mechanism ? Blood 1993;81:2618–25.

29. Atsumi T, Khamashta MA, Ames PRJ, Ichikawa K, Koike T, Hughes GRV. Effect of β2glycoprotein I and human monoclonal anticardiolipin antibody on the protein S / C4b-binding protein system. Lupus 1997;6:358–64.

30. Merrill JT, Zhang HW, Shen C, Butman BT, Jeffries EP, Lahita RG et al. Enhancement of protein S anticoagulant function by beta2-glycoprotein I, a major target antigen of antiphosphoipid antibodies: beta2-glycoprotein I with binding of protein S to its plasma inhibitor, C4b-binding protein. Thromb Haemost 1999;81:748–57.

31. Ieko M, Ichikawa K, Atsumi T, Takeuchi R, Sawada KI, Yasukouchi T et al. Effects of beta2-glycoprotein I and monoclonal anticardiolipin antibodies on extrinsic fibrinolysis. Semin Thromb Hemost 2000;26:85–90.

32. Colucci M, Balconi G, Lorenzet R, Locati PD. Cultured human endothelial cells generate tissue factor in response to endotoxin. J Clin Invest 1983;71:1893–6.

33. Herbert JM, Savi P, Laplaca MC, Lale A. IL-4 inhibits LPS, IL-1 beta and TNF alpha induced expression of tissue factor in endothelial cells and monocytes. FEBS lett 1992;310:31–3.

34. Nemerson Y. Tissue factor and hemostasis. Blood 1988;71:1–8.

35. Petersen LC, Valentin S, Hedner U. Regulation of the extrinsic pathway system in health and disease: The role of fator VIIa and tissue factor pathway inhibitor. Thromb Res 1995;79:1–47.

36. Yanagisawa M, Kurihara H, Kimura S, Tomobe Y, Kobayashi M, Mitsui Y et al. A novel potent vasoconstrictor peptide produced by vascular endothelial cells. Nature 1988;332:411–4.

37. Levin ER. Endothelins. N Engl J Med 1995;333:356–63.

38. Nakamura S, Naruse M, Naruse K, Demura H, Uemura H. Immunocytochemical localization of endothelin in cultured bovine endothelial cells. Histochemistry

1990;94:475–7.

39. Marsen TA, Simonson MS, Dunn MJ. Thrombin induces the preproendothelin-1 gene in endothelial cells by a protein tyrosine kinase-linked mechanism. Circ Res 1995;76:987–95.

40. Inoue A, Yanagisawa M, Takuwa Y, Mitsui Y, Kobayashi M, Masaki T. The human preproendothelin-1 gene. J Biol Chem 1989;264:14954–9.

41. Silver RK, Adler L, Hickman R, Hageman JR. Anticardiolipin antibody-positive serum enhances endothelial cell platelet-activating factor production. Am J Obstet Gynecol 1991;165:1748-.

42. Schorer AE, Duane PG, Woods VL, Niewoehner DE. Some antiphospholipid antibodies inhibit phospholipase A2 activity. J Lab Med 1992;120:67–77.

43. Amengual O, Atsumi T, Khamashta MA, Hughes GRV. The role of the tissue factor pathway in the hypercoagulable state in patients with the antiphospholipid syndrome. Thromb Haemost 1998;79:276–81.

44. Branch DW, Rodgers GM. Induction of endothelial cell tissue factor activity by sera from patients with antiphospholipid syndrome: A possible mechanism of thrombosis. Am J Obstet Gynecol 1993;168:206–10.

45. Kornberg A, Blank M, Kaufman S, Shoenfeld Y. Induction of tissue factor-like activity in monocytes by anticardiolipin antibodics. J Immunol 1994;153:1328–32.

46. Atsumi T, Khamashta MA, Haworth RS, Brooks G, Amengual O, Ichikawa K et al. Arterial disease and thrombosis in the antiphospholipid syndrome. A pathogenic role for endothelin 1. Arthritis Rheum 1998;41:800–7.

47. Pierangelli SS, Colden-Stanfield M, Lie X, Barker JII, Anderson GH, Harris EN. Antiphospholipid antibodies from antiphospholipid patients activate endothelial cells in vivo and in vitro. Circulation 1999;99:1997–2002.

48. Atsumi T, Khamashta MA, Andujar C, Leandro MJ, Amengual O, Hughes GRV. Elevated plasma lipoprotein (a) level and its association with impaired fibrinolysis in patients with antiphospholipid syndrome. J Rheumatol 1998;25:67–73.

49. Yamazaki M, Asakura H, Jokaji H, Saito M, Uotani C, Kumabashiri I et al. Plasma levels of lipoprotein(a) are elevated in patients with the antiphospholipid antibody syndrome. Thromb Haemost 1994;71:424–7.

50. Jurado M, Paramo JA, Gutierrez-Pimentel M, Rocha E. Fibrinolytic potential and antiphospholipid antibodies in systemic lupus erythematosus and other connective tissue disorders. Thromb Haemost 1992;68:516–20.

51. Ames PRJ, Tommasino C, Iannaccone L, Brillante M, Cimino R, Brancaccio V. Coagulation activation and fibrinolytic imbalance in subjects with idopathic antiphospholipid antibodies - a crucial role for acquired free protein S deficiency. Thromb Haemost 1996;76:190–4.

52. Vu T-H, Hung DT, Wheaton VI, Coughlin SR. Molecular cloning of a functional thrombin receptor reveals a novel proteolytic mechanism of receptor activation. Cell 1991;64:1057–68.

53. Kerr JFR, Willie AH, Currie AR. Apoptosis: a basic biological phenomenon with wide-range implications in tissue kinetics. Br J Cancer 1972;26:239–57.

54. Savill J, Fadok V, Henson P, Haslett C. Phagocyte recognition of cells undergoing apoptosis. Immunol Today 1993;14:131–6.

55. Martin SJ, Reutelingsperger CPM, McGrahon AJ, Rader JA, van Schie RCAA, LaFace DM et al. Early redistribution of plasma membrane phosphatidylserine is a general feature of apoptosis regardless of the initiating stimulus: inhibition by overexpression of Bcl-2 and Abl. J Exp Med 1995;182:1545–56.

56. Martin SJ, Finucane DM, Amarantemendes GP, Obrien GA, Green DR. Phosphatidylserine externalization during CD95-induced apoptosis of cells and cytoplasts requires ICE/CED-3 protease activity. J Biol Chem 1996;271:28753–6.

57. Fadok VA, Voelker DR, Kampbel PA, Cohen JJ, Bratton DL, Henson PM. Exposure of phosphatidylserine on the surface of apoptotic lymphocytes triggers specific recognition and removal by macrophages. J Immunol 1992;148:2207–16.

58. McNeil HP, Simpson RJ, Chesterman CN, Krilis SA. Anti-phospholipid antibodies are directed against a complex antigen that induces a lipid-binding inhibitor of coagulation: β2-glycoprotein I (apolipoprotein H). Proc Natl Acad Sci USA 1990;87:4120–4.

59. Matsuura E, Igarashi Y, Fujimoto M, Ichikawa K, Koike T. Anticardiolipin cofactor(s) and differential diagnosis of autoimmune disease. Lancet 1990;336:177–8.

60. Galli M, Comfurius P, Maassen C, Hemker HC, de Baets MH, van Breda-Vriesman PJC et al. Anticardiolipin antibodies (ACA) directed not to cardiolipin but to a plasma protein cofactor. Lancet 1990;335:952–3.

61. Roubey RAS. Immunology of the antiphospholipid antibody syndrome. Arthritis Rheum 1996;39:1444–54.

62. Manfredi AA, Rovere P, Heltai S, Galati G, Nebbia G, Tincani A et al. Apoptotic cell clearance in systemic lupus erythematosus. II. Role of b2-Glycoprotein I. Arthritis Rheum 1998;41:215–23.

63. Price BE, Rauch J, Shia MA, Walsh MT, Lieberthal W, Gilligan HM et al. Anti-phospholipid antibodies bind to apoptotic, but not to viable, thymocytes in a b2-glycoprotein I-dependent manner. J Immunol 1996;157:2201–8.

64. Casciola-Rosen L, Rosen A, Petri M, Shliissel M. Surface blebs on apoptotic cells are sites of enhanced procoagulant activity: implications for coagulations events

and antigenic spread in systemic lupus erythematosus. Proc Natl Acad Sci USA 1996;93:1624–9.

65. Manfredi AA, Rovere P, Galati G, Heltai S, Bozzolo E, Soldini L et al. Apoptotic cell clearance in systemic lupus erythematosus. I. Opsonitazion by antiphospholipid antibodies. Arthritis Rheum 1998;41:205–14.

66. Pittoni V, Ravirajan CT, Donohoe S, Machin SJ, Lydyard PM, Isenberg DA. Human monoclonal anti-phospholipid antibodies selectively bind to membrane phospholipid and beta2-glycoprotein I (beta2-GPI) on apoptotic cells. Clin Exp Immunol, 2000;119:533–43.

67. Vaishnaw AK, McNally JD, Elkon KB. Apoptosis in the rheumatic diseases. Arthritis Rheum 1997;40:1917–27.

68. Rovere P, Sabbadini MG, Vallinot C, Fascio U, Rescigno M, Crosti M et al. Dendritic cell presentation of antigens from apoptotic cells in a proinflammatory context. Arthritis Rheum 1999;42:1412–20.

69. Simantov R, LaSala JM, Lo SK, Gharavi AE, Sammaritano LR, Salmon JE et al. Activation of cultured vascular endothelial cells by antiphospholipid antibodies. J Clin Invest 1995;96:2211–9.

70. Del PaPa N, Guidali L, Sala A, Buccellati C, Khamashta MA, Ichikawa K et al. Endothelial cells as target for antiphospholipid antibodies. Arthritis Rheum 1997;40:551–61.

71. Bordron A, Dueymes M, Levy Y, Leroy JP, Jamin C, Piette JC et al. The binding of some human antiendothelial cell antibodies induce endothelial cell apoptosis. J Clin Invest 1998;101:2029–35.

Atherosclerosis and Autoimmunity
Y. Shoenfeld, D. Harats and G. Wick, editors

Accelerated Atherosclerosis in the Aortic Arch and Cerebral Ischemia in a Patient with Primary Antiphospholipid Syndrome

V Pengo[1], A Zocche[1], R Scognamiglio[1], A Biasiolo[1], T Del Ros[2] and A Ruffatti[2]

[1]Department of Clinical and Experimental Medicine, Thrombosis Center, University of Padova, Italy;
[2]Department of Medical and Surgical Sciences, University of Padova, Italy

1. INTRODUCTION

Antiphospholipid syndrome is characterized by both arterial and venous thromboembolic events in the absence of a precipitating factor. Among arterial thromboses, those in the cerebral circulation are most common [1–2]. Clinical manifestations reflect the duration of cerebral artery occlusion and its recurrence, and range from transient ischemic attacks to dementia sustained by multiple cerebral infarcts. The association between cerebral ischemia and livedo reticularis defines Sneddon syndrome [3].

The source of thrombi in cerebral ischemia (cardiogenic, paradoxical, artery-to-artery) and consequently the type of treatment are important, poorly defined issues in patients with cerebral ischemia and antiphospholipid syndrome [4]. Transesophageal echocardiography (TEE) is an important tool for detecting the cardiac source of embolism in patients with cerebral ischemia of uncertain origin [5]. Using this technique, it is possible to identify intracardiac thrombi and assess and measure a patent foramen ovalis [6], and to determine valve thickness or valvular vegetations, with their size being evaluated by planimetry and expressed in square centimeters [7]. Aortic arch inspection allows detection of atherosclerotic plaques and the assessment of differences in intra-plaque echogenicity [5].

In this paper we describe a patient with antiphospholipid syndrome and cerebral ischemia in whom TEE disclosed two lesions potentially related to cerebral ischemia, i.e., non-thrombotic bacterial endocarditis and accelerated atherosclerosis in the aortic arch.

2. CASE HISTORY

We present a 35 year-old Caucasian female whose clinical history started at the age of 9 years with an episode of purpura associated with thrombocytopenia. The patient was treated with a course of corticosteroids, and subsequently her platelet count never fell below $100,000/mm^3$. At 24 years of age the patient complained of neurological symptoms (facial and right hand paraesthesiae, dysphasia, dysarthria, diplopia and defects in visual field). Laboratory investigations showed a positivity for Lupus Anticoagulant and IgG anticardiolipin antibodies. Cerebral nuclear magnetic resonance revealed several small infarcts in the white matter of the left hemisphere. At the age of 27, after a further episode of transient cerebral ischemia and confirmation of the presence of antiphospholipid antibodies, a treatment with long term oral anticoagulants was initiated. At that time transthoracic echocardiography revealed nodularities on the ventricular side of the mitral valve. Subsequently, at the age of 32 years, the patient had two consecutive episodes of cerebral ischemia (amaurosis fugax) and reported some of the previous neurological complaints with the addition of dizziness. Laboratory tests confirmed high antiphospholipid antibody levels and the presence of anti-β2-glycoprotein I antibodies of the IgG isotype. With the exception of low-titer antinuclear antibodies (fine speckled pattern), no other organ- or non-organ specific autoantibodies were detected. Thus the diagnosis of primary antiphospholipid syndrome was made.

A TEE with a color Doppler imaging system

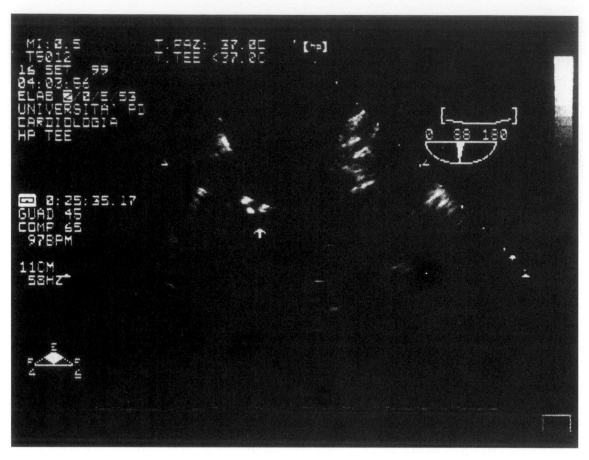

Figure 1. Transesophageal echocardiogram showing rough, nodular, hyperintense thickenings on the mitral valve (arrow).

(Hewlett-Packard 5MHZ transducer) was performed using standard echocardiographic views [8]. This technique revealed rough nodular thickening of mitral valve leaflets (Fig 1). Moreover, a protruding soft plaque in the lateral wall of the aortic arch was also disclosed (Fig 2).

3. DISCUSSION

Transesophageal echocardiography is a valid technical resource superior to transthoracic echocardiography for distinguishing the source of thrombi in unexplained cerebral ischemia. Nevertheless, the presence of multiple lesions at TEE, as reported in the present study, may render it difficult to distinguish between cardiogenic and artery-to-artery embolism.

Mitral and aortic heart valve thickenings repre-

sent the most common echocardiographic feature in patients with antiphospholipid syndrome [9–11]. This feature is considered the result of multiple appositions of thrombi whose organization determines subsequent valve degeneration and incompetence [12–14]. In contrast to the firmly adherent, leukocyte-rich vegetations found on the heart valves of systemic lupus erithematosis (SLE) patients (Libman-Sacks endocarditis), the fresh friable material deposited over the heart valves of antiphospholipid syndrome patients might be easily dislodged. In fact, at 'post mortem' examination of two patients, Fulham and Co-workers [15] found the same material in heart valve vegetations and in cerebral circulation. Although clear vegetations were not seen in the patient described in this study, rough nodular thickenings might well represent a feature of non-bacterial thrombotic endocarditis. When these lesions and the counterpart cerebral ischemic areas are found

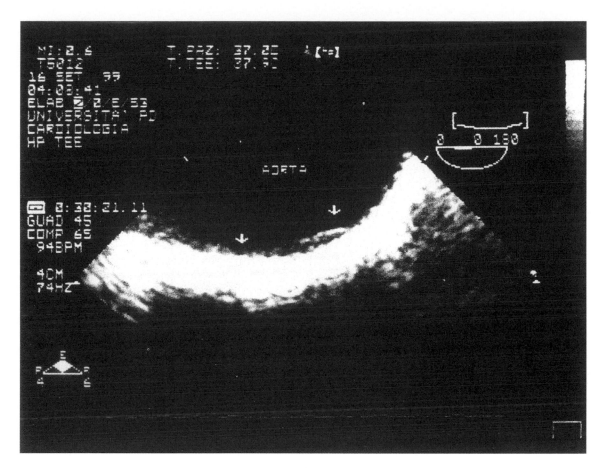

Figure 2. Transesophageal echocardiography showing the aortic arch, whose lateral wall presents a clearly visible atherosclerotic plaque (arrows).

in these patients, the pathogenic link appears obvious. However TEE disclosed a further lesion which is potentially related to cerebral ischemia in this patient. The atherosclerotic plaque present in the aortic arch can be defined as the result of an 'accelerated atherosclerosis', as such plaque formation is uncommon in subjects of the same age. The occurrence of accelerated atheroslerosis was previously reported in young premenopausal females with SLE [16]. This feature is probably the result of autoimmune disease 'per se' independent from classical risk factors [17]. The patient described in this paper had an autoimmune disease characterized by the presence of antiphospholipid antibodies, with cigarette smoking the only classical risk factor present. A relationship between antiphospholipid antibodies and clinical manifestations of atherosclerosis has been postulated but remains to be clarified [18].

Although the pathogenesis of 'accelerated atherosclerosis' is likely to be multifactorial in many instances, the peculiar features of the present case support a major role for antiphospholipid antibodies in the rapid development of atherosclerotic plaques.

REFERENCES

1. Shah NM, Kamashta MA, Atsumi T, Hughes GRV. Outcome of patients with antiphospholipid antibodies: a 10 year follow-up of 52 patients. Lupus 1998;7:3–6.
2. Krnic-Barrie S, O'Connor CR, Looney SW, Pierangeli SS, Harris EN. A retrospective review of 61 patients with antiphospholipid syndrome. Arch Intern Med 1997;157:2101–8.
3. Kalashnikova LA, Nasonov EL, Kushekbaeva AE, Gracheva LA. Anticardiolipin antibodies in Sneddon's syndrome. Neurology 1990;40:464–7.

4. Brey R and Escalante E. Neurological manifestation of antiphospholipid antibody syndrome. Lupus 1998;7(Suppl 2):S67–S74.

5. Pearson AC, Labovitz AJ, Tatineni S, Gomez CR. Superiority of transesophageal echocardiography in detecting cardiac source of embolism in patients with cerebral ischemia of uncertain origin. JACC 1991;17:66–72.

6. Steiner MM, Di-Tullio MR, Rundek T, Gan R, Chen X, Liguori C, Brainin M, Homma S, Sacco RL. Patent foramen ovale size and embolic brain imaging findings among patients with ischemic stroke. Stroke 1998;29:944–8.

7. Roldan CA, Shively BK, Crawford MH. An echocardiographic study of valvular heart disease associated with systemic lupus erythematosus. N Engl J Med 1996;335:1424–30.

8. Seward JB, Khanderia BK, Oh JK, Abel MD, Hughes RWJr, Edwards WD, Nichols BA, Freeman NK, Tajik AJ. Transesophageal echocardiography: technique, anatomic correlations, implementation, and clinical applications. Mayo Clin Proceed 1988;63:649–80.

9. Fulham MJ, Gatenby P, Tuck RR. Focal cerebral ischemia and antiphospholipid antibodies: a case for cardiac embolism. Acta Neurol Scand 1994; 90: 417–23.

10. Barbut D, Borer JS, Wallerson D, Ameisen O, Lockshin M. Anticardiolipin antibody and stroke: possible relation of valvular heart disease and embolic events. Cardiology 1991; 79:99–109.

11. Verro P, Levine SR, Tietjen GE. Cerebrovascular ischemic events with high positive anticardiolipin antibodies. Stroke 1998; 29: 2245–53.

12. Ford SE, Lillicrap D, Brunet D, Ford P. Thrombotic endocarditis and lupus anticoagulant. Arch Pathol Lab Med 1989; 113: 350–3.

13. APASS. Clinical and laboratory findings in patients with antiphospholipid antibodies and cerebral ischemia. Stroke 1990; 21:1268–73.

14. APASS. Clinical, radiological, and patholocical aspects of cerebrovascular disease associated with antiphospholipid antibodies. Stroke 1993;24(Suppl I):I-119–I-123.

15. Fulham MJ, Gatenby P, Tuck RR. Focal cerebral ischemia and antiphospholipid antibodies: a case for cardiac embolism. Acta Neurol Scand 1994;90:417–23.

16. Urowitz MB, Bookman AA, Koehler BE, Gordon DA, Smythe HA, Ogryzlo MA. The bimodal mortality pattern of systhemic lupus erythematosus. Am J Med 1976;60:221–5.

17. Shoenfeld Y, Alarcon-Segovia D, Buskila D, Abu-Shakra M, Lorber M, Sherer Y, Berden J, Meroni PL, Valesini G, Koike T, Alarcon-Riquelme ME. Frontiers of SLE: review of the 5th International Congress of Systemic Lupus Erythematosus, Cancun, Mexico, April 20–25,1998. Semin Arthr Rheum 1999;29:112–130.

18. Schwartz SM, Reidy MA, O'Brien ER. Assessment of factors important in atherosclerosis occlusions and restenosis. Thromb Haemost 1995;74:541–51.

Atherosclerosis and Autoimmunity
Y. Shoenfeld, D. Harats and G. Wick, editors

Rheumatoid Arthritis, Vasculitis and Arteriosclerosis

Paul A. Bacon and G.D. Kitas

Department of Rheumatology, University of Birmingham, Birmingham, United Kingdom

1. INTRODUCTION

1.1. RA Mortality Data – Increased CVS Deaths

Rheumatoid arthritis is a common disease with a world-wide distribution, occurring in 1–2% of the population. The name implies that it is primarily a joint disease. The latter is characterised by persistent inflammation leading to progressive joint destruction and disability. In addition to the morbidity induced by this joint involvement, RA presents aspects of a systemic inflammatory disease with serositis, granulomata, and inflammation in blood vessels. In Europe, as well as most of the western world, this makes a significant contribution to the severity of RA. The frequency of systemic, or extra-articular, disease is debated and probably widely under-estimated. Sub-cutaneous nodules are the most obvious feature and are seen in 30 40% of caucasian patients seen in hospitals in England or USA [1, 2]. Interestingly, the incidence varies with both geography and ethnicity. They are seen at less than half that frequency in Italy and are a rarity in Asia and Africa [3–5]. The incidence of overt internal organ involvement is lower and these are often viewed as rare events of little overall importance. However RA is not a benign disease and carries a definite mortality if this is examined in an actuarial manner. Thus it has been estimated that the prognosis for 5 year survival of patients with RA is worse than either Hodgkins lymphoma or triple vessel coronary disease [6].

The accelerated mortality in RA is more prominent in those with marked locomotor disability [7] – but it is not due to direct effects of arthritis. Indeed detailed follow-up of an inception cohort of RA patients sufficiently severe to attend hospital showed that only a few died from events that could be directly attributed to the arthritis, or even to overt systemic rheumatoid disease [8]. However, mortality may still relate to rheumatoid disease. A survey in one large hospital cohort showed that it was most prominent in males, who suffered a 17 loss of life expectancy [9]. Males tend to have a lower frequency of RA but more severe disease when it does occur, suggesting that mortality does relate to severity of RA. The causes of death in this survey included most of those seen in the population at large but there was a clearcut enhancement of death rates from cardiovascular events. This has been seen in a number of other studies where the rate of CVS mortality has been increased 2–4 fold [10, 11]. The mechanism of this is not immediately clear but it has been suggested that the degree of joint inflammation is predictive of enhanced cardiovascular mortality [12]. The purpose of this chapter is to suggest that the latter relates to accelerated atherosclerosis which itself is a consequence of systemic inflammation and sub-clinical vascular inflammation in active RA.

1.2. CVS Events – Common Problem in Auto-Immune Rheumatic Disease

The proposal that persistent systemic inflammation plus vascular involvement may be a precursor of accelerated atherosclerosis in RA prompts the suggestion that this may be a common mechanism in persistent auto-immune inflammatory rheumatic disease. The best supporting evidence for this suggestion currently comes from studies in Systemic Lupus Erythematosis (SLE). In this disease acute mortality rates have fallen steadily with improved disease control but the longer term mortality is still elevated compared to the general population. Urowitz and colleagues in Canada have observed that there is now a twin peak to mortality in SLE. The early fatalities still relate to complications of active disease. In contrast the late mortality appears due to cardiovascular disease [13]. Studies to examine the prevalence of CVS events in SLE have concentrated on pre-menopausal women, since they have a low risk of such events in the general population but form the largest part of the disease population in SLE. These have revealed that N. American women with SLE have an astonishing increased incidence of CVS events, RR >50 [14]. There is evidence suggesting that this is not due to classical risk factors for CVS disease, but may relate to disease activity [15].

The mechanism of these events has not been established. Although commonly assumed to relate to atherosclerosis, there is no hard evidence at present to ascribe this to fixed changes in the vessel wall, as opposed to the reversible vascular dysfunction suggested by the studies in primary vasculitis (see below). There are well established mechanisms leading to an enhanced thrombotic tendency in SLE, related to the anti-phospholipid syndrome (APS) [16]. This more commonly presents with venous than arterial thrombosis and the incidence of CVS events in primary APS, as opposed to SLE, has not been clearly established. APS is due to the presence of certain specific auto-antibodies directed at lipids relevant to the clotting cascade. SLE is essentially a disease of multiple auto-antibodies, with associated formation of immune complexes, complement consumption, and generation of inflammatory complement breakdown products. Thus the relationship between disease activity and CVS events in SLE may reflect antibody or immune complex mediated endothelial activation and damage rather than thrombotic events. A similar clinical picture of systemic inflammation and vascular events is seen in Behcets syndrome, suggesting it would be reasonable to postulate that any chronic inflammatory autoimmune disease could show a similar increase in CVS events. This challenges the rheumatological community to look beyond the immediate events in a variety of such diseases to establish the longer term prognosis and the causes of death in each

case.

The mechanism that is common to SLE and RA, as well as Behcets, is the frequent presence of vascular inflammation. We have previously put forward the hypothesis that in RA the excess CVS mortality may be a late consequence of earlier vascular inflammation [17], in the same way that vascular inflammation in the arteries of organ grafts promotes accelerated atherosclerosis in both animal models and human disease [18]. Here we examine the new evidence for cardiac dysfunction and ischaemia in RA, and propose the concept of primary systemic vasculitis (1°SNV) as a model to explore the mechanisms involved.

2. CARDIOVASCULAR INVOLVEMENT IN RHEUMATOID DISEASE

2.1. Rheumatoid Arthritis – A Systemic Disease

Rheumatoid Arthritis (RA) is the commonest chronic inflammatory musculoskeletal disease. Its main characteristic is chronic inflammation of synovial joints – but RA is not limited only to joints. Its systemic nature has been recognised for a long time, with acute or chronic inflammatory pathology affecting other tissues as well, including the skin, eye, lung, heart and blood vessels. In this respect, RA should be referred to as Rheumatoid *Disease* rather than Rheumatoid *Arthritis*.

Involvement of the heart in RA was first suggested by Jean Bouillaud in 1836. However, it was Charcot in 1881 who first described endocarditis and pericarditis in the presence of "chronic rheumatism", and attempted to differentiate the cardiac disease of rheumatic fever (rheumatic heart disease) from cardiac disease associated with other forms of rheumatism (rheumatoid heart disease – RHD). In 1941 Baggenstoss and Rosenburg reported on 20 autopsy cases of "infectious" arthritis showing evidence of cardiac lesions typical of rheumatoid heart disease [19]. Since then, many studies have documented that cardiac pathology associated with RA, including pericarditis, endocarditis, myocarditis and vasculitis, is common, occurring in 30–40% of all RA patients during the course of their disease.

Most of the studies documenting cardiac pathology in RA are based on autopsy data. Cardiac complications in RA are rarely clinically apparent. Simple investigations such as the electrocardiogram and chest X ray are useful in certain clinical settings, but grossly non-specific and insensitive at picking up relevant pathology. The most useful investigation is the echocardiogram and Doppler examination, which allows detailed examination of cardiac anatomy and provides information on cardiac function and the haemodynamic effects of the pathological processes observed. In most cases, prevalence of cardiac pathology detected by echocardiography in RA during life, approaches that detected at postmortem. CT scanning, cardiac catheterisation, coronary angiography and endomyocardial biopsy all have specific indications in the clinical setting, but have not been used as research tools in RA, probably due to the associated costs and risks. [67]Gallium scanning has been used successfully to detect cardiac inflammation in a case of rheumatoid coronary arteritis [20], but has not been used as a research tool. Non-invasive investigation of cardiac ischaemia on a population basis in RA may be problematic, as exercise ECG is impractical in patients with considerable physical disability. It may however be achieved using pharmacological stress and either nuclear perfusion imaging or echocardiography. Specifically in RA, pharmacologically-stressed nuclear perfusion imaging may be the most useful investigation for several reasons: it overcomes the difficulties of exercising the disabled patient sufficiently; it provides valuable information into myocardial perfusion abnormalities whether due to epicardial or small vessel disease; the extent of ischaemia can be assessed accurately and is related to prognosis in Ischaemic Heart Disease (IHD), thus it may lead to either the instigation or avoidance of further, more invasive, investigations; it is less operator dependent and more feasible technically than stress echocardiography, due to the difficulties associated with the latter in a predominantly female and commonly obese population.

2.2. Rheumatoid Heart Disease

Pericardial disease is the commonest cardiac complication of RA, found in 30–50% of patients at autopsy [21], and in up to 30% of patients by echocardiography [22–24]. Pericardial disease is however diagnosed clinically in only 2–4% of RA patients and cardiac embarrassment due to tamponade or constriction occurs in less than 0.5% [25–27]. Pericarditis is commoner in male, seropositive patients with active RA and other extra-articular features, but has also been described in sero-negative [27] or quiescent RA [28]. Rarely, it may occur prior to the onset of synovitis [28]. The pathological appearance of rheumatoid pericarditis has been likened to a rheumatoid nodule that has opened into a serous cavity. The pericardium is thickened and fibrotic suggesting a chronic inflammatory process. The pericardial surfaces are fibrinous and the pericardial space may be obliterated. Microscopy of the epithelial surfaces shows palisading epithelial cells and infiltrating polymorphonuclear leukocytes. The deeper parts of the pericardium show perivascular lymphocytic and plasma cell infiltration. Immunofluorescence reveals granular deposits of immunoglobulins in the interstitium and perivascular areas. In contrast to the preponderance of CD4[+] T cells in inflamed synovium, most of the infiltrating T cells in rheumatoid pericarditis are CD8[+], a feature of rheumatoid nodules. This has led to the suggestion that pericarditis may have a different pathogenetic mechanism to synovitis in RA [29]. The inflammatory aetiology of rheumatoid pericarditis is also supported by the nature of the pericardial fluid. This is usually clear, with serosanguinous, haemorrhagic or chylous effusions seen rarely [29, 30]. Biochemical examination reveals a high protein content, typical of an exudate, and a raised LDH with a low glucose. IgE containing immune complexes have been reported, and IgM rheumatoid factor is frequently present [30, 31] On microscopy the cellular content is predominantly neutrophils. Cholesterol crystals have also been reported and are associated with larger effusions and a tendency for reaccumulation [32] – they are believed to be the result of cell debris in chronic inflammation and are not specific for RA, as they are also seen with tuberculous pericarditis.

Endocardial involvement, consisting of non specific changes have been reported in 9–70% of RA patients at autopsy [33–35]. Echocardiographic studies show a high prevalence of valvular thickening, [22, 36] but clinically significant valvular disease is very rare. The valves are affected in an order of preference similar to that of *rheumatic* heart disease, i.e. mitral, aortic, tricuspid, pulmonary, in decreasing order of likelihood. Most cases show non-specific infiltration of the valves with histiocytes, lymphocytes, and other inflammatory cells. Areas of fibrosis and healing suggest a chronic inflammatory process leading to thickening and calcification. This tends to occur in the base of the valve and the valve ring, but rarely causes haemodynamically significant distortion of the valve [33, 35, 37]. The most distinctive rheumatoid valvular lesions are rheumatoid granulomata [35]. They typically appear within the valve leaflets and can progress to deform the leaflet or even cause perforation, leaving the valve incompetent. Most RA patients with valvular involvement are asymptomatic, since the left ventricle can adapt to considerable degrees of mitral and aortic regurgitation without decompensating. It is not only the degree of regurgitation but also the rapidity of onset of the disease which defines its effect on the performance of the left ventricle. In occasional rare but very severe cases, valvular lesions can develop abruptly, with rapid deterioration leading to left ventricular failure.

Myocarditis is found in up to 29% of RA patients on autopsy [34, 35, 38]. It can be diffuse or focal, non-specific or pathognomonic nodular rheumatoid myocarditis [35]. The non-specific form shows sporadic small groups of destroyed myocardial fibres with evidence of scarring. When florid, the process becomes diffuse with widespread necrotising myocarditis. Lymphocytes, plasma cells and eosinophills can be present. Granuloma formation, similar to that found in other cardiac structures, is typical of rheumatoid heart disease [35]. The significance of myocarditis in the clinical setting is unknown. The overwhelming majority of patients are asymptomatic. However, inflammation of the cardiac skeleton can rarely lead to conduction system involvement. The atrio-ventricular node, by nature of its compact anatomy, and its spatial relationship to the aortic root and inter-ventricular septum as it traverses the AV ring, is vulnerable to damage from inflammation of adjacent structures. Complete heart block can be seen in association with rheumatoid arthritis [39]and has also been reported in association with penicillamine induced polymyositis [40].

Coronary arteritis has been reported in up to 20% of

autopsy cases [33–35, 37, 38], but clinically apparent disease is rare. Its relationship to myocardial infarction is controversial [34, 41]. Pathological lesions can be seen in vessels of all sizes in patients with RA. Coronary arteritis mostly affects the medium and small intra-myocardial arteries, although severe arteritis of the epicardial vessels has been reported [34, 41] In most cases involving the epicardial arteries, the arteritis tends to be non occlusive [34] – occlusive large vessel disease leading to myocardial infarction is seen only occasionally [34, 41]. More commonly, smaller vessel involvement leads to patchy areas of myocardial necrosis, possibly due to microinfarction or ischaemia [35]. The inflammation can be non specific, necrotising, or granulomatous and all three can be seen together. Non specific inflammation is characterised by inflammation of the media with extension into the adventitia and intima and disruption of the elastica interna. The inflammatory infiltrate is a mixture of histiocytes, neutrophils, lymphocytes and macrophages. There is often evidence of healing by fibrosis. Fibrinoid necrosis is commonly found, but aneurysm formation is not seen. The granulomatous form of arteritis shows infiltration with macrophages and histiocytes. Occasionally, giant cells can be seen along with lesions resembling rheumatoid nodules.

Studies such as those presented above leave no room for doubt that cardiac structures are commonly affected by rheumatoid inflammation. However, this involvement is largely subclinical. Rheumatoid heart disease as a whole, is clinically apparent in only 2% of RA patients and has direct haemodynamic consequences in less than 0.5%. As such, RHD is unlikely to be the direct explanation for the increased and earlier cardiovascular mortality of RA. However the lesson of subclinical disease becoming apparently more common the harder you look, particularly when sophisticated detection methods are used, is relevant. We suggest that a similar common but sub-clinical incidence of vascular inflammation in RA may be the precursor to accelerated atherosclerotic heart disease, again only appreciated with special testing. Recent studies of this aspect are considered next.

2.3. Cardiac Function in Rheumatoid Disease

Several studies have shown a high prevalence (30–40%) of left ventricular (LV) filling abnormalities in RA compared with age and sex matched controls, even after exclusion of patients with known causes of LV diastolic dysfunction such as hypertension, LV hypertrophy or IHD [42, 43]. Such abnormalities have been detected in other inflammatory conditions as well, including sarcoidosis [44] and SLE [45]. Recent evidence suggests that inflammatory cytokines such as TNFα, IL-1β and IL-6 may play an important role in the pathophysiology of heart failure [46, 47]; indeed, TNFα has become a target for therapeutic intervention in congestive cardiac failure [48]. We have therefore hypothesised that systemic inflammation in RA may be the cause of LV diastolic dysfunction. We have now shown that in RA, LV diastolic filling abnormalities do not associate with hypertension, LV hypertrophy or cardiac ischaemia. Instead, the major predictors of measures of LV diastolic impairment such as E:A ratio or isovolumetric relaxation time are age, levels of C-reactive protein and IL-6 [49]. Levels of von Willebrand Factor (vWF), considered a surrogate serological marker of endothelial damage or dysfunction, and endothelium-dependent vasodilatation measured *in vivo* using high resolution vascular ultrasound of the brachial artery, also associated inversely with LV diastolic function. Endothelial dysfunction leading to altered vascular responses may result in increased afterload, increased end diastolic pressures and thus the development of LV filling abnormalities. These findings suggests a close association of the systemic inflammatory response and endothelial dysfunction with impaired LV filling in RA.

The long term sequelae of this remain undetermined. Impairment of LV filling however, is believed to represent the earliest detectable evidence of LV impairment, has been recognised as a cause of congestive heart failure in the absence of systolic dysfunction, has been identified as an early sign of the cardiomyopathy associated with other conditions such as diabetes and hypertension and has been associated with increased mortality. In this respect, impaired myocardial function in RA may be important in the increased cardiovascular mortality seen in this disease. Frank congestive heart failure in RA is well described but rare and may be the result of several processes operating alone or in tandem. In addition to the above, restrictive cardiac involvement due to amyloid, can lead to predominant diastolic heart failure. This is seen rarely, since although cardiac amyloid has been reported in 10–20% of rheumatoid hearts in pathological series in the past [39] – amyloidosis in RA is now considered a rarity, probably due to improved therapeutic control of the inflammatory response. Rheumatoid pancarditis and small vessel vasculitis *without* evidence of myocarditis can both lead to systolic pump failure [28, 50]. Other system involvement, for example pulmonary fibrosis, may lead to right ventricular failure. RA patients suddenly developing overt heart failure should be actively investigated for many possible causes, including coronary vasculitis, hypertensive heart disease, valvular disease, subacute bacterial endocarditis, cor-pulmonale due to pulmonary fibrosis, or constrictive pericarditis. However, as in the general population, atherosclerotic ischaemic heart disease is still the most likely cause.

2.4. Myocardial Perfusion in RD

The commonest cause of premature death in the general population is coronary artery disease leading to IHD. This, together with the rarity of significant haemodynamic compromise due to RHD, suggests that IHD is also the major cause of cardiovascular death in RA. Despite this, IHD has been ignored as a significant comorbid condition or cardiovascular complication of RA. Post-mortem studies have reported a similar or slightly increased prevalence of coronary artery disease in RA compared with age and sex-matched controls [51]. These findings can only be viewed with caution, as age matched controls for a population such as RA, characterised by increased mortality and reduced life expectancy, must also have died earlier. There are no published studies addressing the prevalence, clinical expression and causes of IHD in a *living* population of RA patients. We have recently completed a study assessing the prevalence of IHD in RA compared with matched non-inflammatory osteoarthritis controls, using stress myocardial perfusion imaging with SPECT [52]. The two populations were matched for all classical cardiovascular risk factors, including age, sex, hypertension, smoking, family history, diabetes, cholesterol, body mass index (including body fat/lean percentage), menopausal status and their total composite 10 year cardiovascular event risk (based on the Framingham data) [53]. They were also matched for the use of non-steroidal anti-inflammatory drugs, which may have significant antiplatelet, aspirin-like effects. IHD was almost twice as prevalent in RA (49%) as in the controls (27%), both in males and females. More than half (52%) of RA patients with IHD had clinically silent ischaemia as opposed to only 20% of controls. The systemic inflammatory response (erythrocyte sedimentation rate, C-reactive protein) and fibrinogen were significantly higher in RA than controls; although there were trends, there were no significant differences in these parameters between RA patients with and without IHD. RA patients with IHD were more likely to be older, male, obese, hypertensive, hypertriglyceraemic and had a significantly higher composite 10 year cardiovascular event risk than those without IHD. This suggests that the fingerprint of classical cardiovascular risk factors operates in RA as it does in the general population, but having RA (like having diabetes) confers extra, additive risk. Indeed, logistic regression analysis showed that age, sex, RA and body mass index operate as independent predictors for IHD; hypertension was collinear with age and triglycerides collinear with body mass index.

There are several mechanisms through which the systemic inflammation of RA may be linked to accelerated atherosclerosis and earlier development of IHD. We have previously suggested that clinical or subclinical vascular inflammation (vasculitis) involving cardiac vessels of all sizes in RA may be one of the most important. Addressing this hypothesis accurately *in vivo* is very difficult without the availability of tissue from endomyocardial biopsies. Such an invasive and potentially risky approach is difficult to justify ethically, particularly in the absence of clinical symptoms. Recent technical developments have allowed the investigation of patients with primary systemic necrotising vasculitis as an *in vivo* model to address some aspects of this hypothesis.

3. 1°SNV – A MODEL FOR CVS EVENTS IN RA?

3.1. EDVD in 1°SNV and Ways to Investigate It

Primary systemic vasculitides (1°SNV) are a group of diseases characterised by inflammation in blood vessels. They are largely of unknown aetiology and can present in a bewildering variety of ways to many specialities. However, there are well defined patterns of organ involvement underlying the various syndromes which have been incorporated into the Chapel Hill consensus criteria [54], widely accepted as a basis for classification of these diseases. There is extensive evidence for immune mechanisms in the pathogenesis of these disorders, particularly for the subgroup known as the ANCA-associated vasculitides (AASNV). The latter include Wegeners syndrome, Churg-Strauss, and microscopic poly-angiitis (MPA) which all present clinically with disease primarily involving small blood vessels, particularly those in the kidneys and lungs. This contrasts with classic polyarteritis nodosa (PAN) which is a disease of muscular arteries and does not involve the smaller arterioles. In AASNV vascular inflammation may at times extend into medium-sized vessels but unlike PAN they are characterised by antibodies to antigens present in neutrophil cytoplasmic granules (ANCA). Much research has shown that such antibodies can mediate inflammation with the potential to directly injure endothelial cells in vivo in a similar fashion to that established in vitro (Ref. [55]). The immuno-pathogenic mechanisms underlying PAN are less well defined, although intriguingly some may be initiated by infection, but there is again a picture of inflammation at the endothelial level. Thus these diseases appear good candidates to study the outcome of acute endothelial injury and the mechanisms involved in the development of persistent endothelial dysfunction.

The outcome of 1°SNV has markedly improved with modern therapy, with a greater than 80% 2 year survival now [56]. However this is unfortunately not providing cure of disease. Rather it appears that therapy has transformed acute life-threatening vasculitis into chronic disease with a high level of ongoing morbidity and a significant tendency to relapse. We have derived and validated improved methods to quantitate this disease burden in terms of activity of the inflammatory vascular process and of damage related to disease scars [57, 58]. The importance of the latter has only recently become apparent. Our studies have established that damage occurs surprisingly early in disease and that it contributes directly to disease severity [64–66]. We therefore postulated that damage would involve the endothelial cells themselves, which would contribute both to the progression of organ dysfunction and to the tendency to relapse. We set out to investigate this directly, using the non-invasive methods developed recently by cardiologists. The intention was to examine vessels not involved in the primary pattern of clinical disease, since relapse can often involve new organs.

The investigation of blood vessel status by non-invasive methods has progressed rapidly in the past decade [59]. There are two broad approaches, aimed either at detection of structural changes in the vessel wall or at estimation of vascular reactivity. The former, such as carotid wall thickness measurement by ultra-sound, provide an alternative to invasive procedures like angiography in detecting established atheromatous deposits. The latter, such as flow mediated endothelial responses by brachial artery ultra-sound, actually assess the ability to respond to important physiological stimuli in disease situations. Both are used as surrogate markers of atherosclerosis in clinical research and practice, since they can detect pre-clinical abnormalities. However, endothelial dysfunction is one of the earliest changes. It thus seemed to provide us with the tool needed to directly measure endothelial function in an artery not clinically involved in the patients with 1°SNV. Basically the test of endothelial dependant vasodilatation (EDV) measures the NO dependant response to altered blood flow induced by the release of a cuff that had temporarily occluded fore-arm blood flow. The control, essential to show that the target artery is capable of reactivity, is the response to a small dose of glyceryl trinitrate which acts directly on vascular smooth muscle. We therefore applied this test to 1°SNV, starting with classic PAN which, although it affects muscular arteries (both small and medium-sized), does not commonly involve the brachial artery. These results were then compared to those obtained in cases of AASNV, which primarily affects small blood vessels.

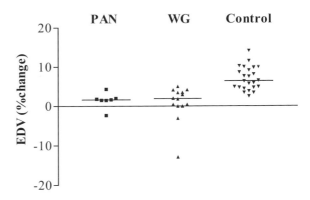

Figure 1. Cross-sectional study of endothelium dependent vasodilatation. Individual values and medians (horizontal bars) are shown. 7 polyarteritis nodosa (PAN) patients, 14 Wegener's granulomatosis (WG) patients, 24 controls.

3.2. Endothelial Dysfunction in 1°SNV

Our preliminary study in 1°SNV involved 24 unselected patients from the vasculitis clinic [60]. These patients showed a marked depression of endothelial dependent vasodilatation (EDV), The group as a whole was significantly impaired compared to matched controls (median EDV 1.7 [0–3.4] v 6.4[4.7–9.5]; p<0.0001). However there was no significant difference between the two groups for the control responses to GTN (11.7 [9.2–17.0] vs 16.6 [10.8–19.1]). These heterogenous patients also showed no significant differences between those with active disease, as classified by either a clinical activity score (BVAS) [57] or by CRP. This established for the first time that endothelial function in vivo, assessed in a clinically uninvolved vessel, was abnormal in patients with 1°SNV.

The next question was whether this represented aberrations due to systemic or local inflammation. We used subgroups of 1°SNV to address this, comparing the 7 cases of classic PAN with 14 cases of Wegeners and found no obvious differences between them (Fig. 1). PAN is a disease of muscular arteries, so here the explanation could be local vessel inflammation, although the brachial artery was not clinically involved in these patients. However identical changes were seen in the patients with Wegeners (WG), which is primarily a small vessel disease. In this latter case a systemic response to distant inflammation appears far more likely. The mecha-

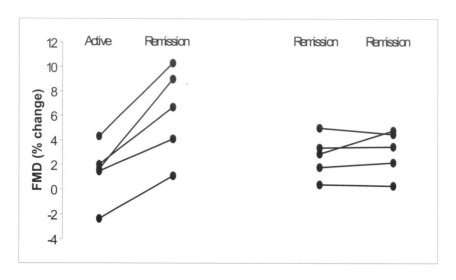

Figure 2. Longitudinal study of endothelial responses. In acute flares versus chronic stable disease.

nism for such change occurring at a site distant from the specific inflammation of 1°SNV is not clear but it may be an example of the "endothelial stunning" described by Vallance and colleagues. This has been shown to occur experimentally after exposure to both bacterial lipopolysaccharide and to inflammatory mediators such as TNFα [61] and has been suggested as a link between infection and atherosclerosis [62].

The second question was whether this endothelial dysfunction was another aspect of the accumulating damage, representing scars of disease, that is so common in vasculitis [63]. Endothelial dysfunction was also documented in the follow-up clinic in 1°SNV patients with apparently well controlled disease, suggesting it can indeed be an aspect of the organ damage following flares of vasculitis. This may predispose to atheroma in an analogous manner to the accelerated disease seen in transplanted organ grafts. The probable mechanisms for this are simple to understand where there has been direct inflammation in a vessel wall involved in active vasculitis, with cell infiltrates closely similar to those seen in the vessels wall in organ graft rejection. There are also potential mechanisms whereby endothelial stunning could predispose to chronic atherosclerosis, as discussed below, so it appeared important to investigate further the relationship to disease activity and whether there was an element of reversibility. The correlation of endothelial dysfunction with

the activity or damage occurring in vasculitis was examined further in serial studies of disease flares before and after the active therapy, including pulses of cyclophosphamide plus steroid as well as daily interval steroids. The results in the first 5 PAN patients studied showed enhanced responses in all, coincident with suppression of disease activity as documented by either clinical score or CRP. The responses post therapy were not significantly different from the range seen in normal controls. Similar improvement has also been seen in Wegeners patients. These improvements contrast to the lack of change seen in a further group of patients in clinical remission whose repeat scans showed no change after a similar interval – but in this case on stable therapy (Fig. 2).

A larger cross-sectional study is currently underway in patients with small or large vessel disease to address a number of other issues. The first was whether the same dysfunction would be seen in those with a variety of syndromes within 1°SNV, irrespective of size of vessel involved in the disease. The second was whether it would occur in localised versions of disease as well as systemic cases. This was examined both within a single syndrome (eg. local versus systemic forms of Wegeners) and by comparing intrinsically organ-limited disease, such as vasculitis of the eye, to systemic syndromes. These studies, which are still ongoing, show that the endothelial dysfunction detected in the preliminary study is a surprisingly common factor in systemic vasculitis. So far we have detected it to occur in at least the majority of all cases of systemic small or medium vessel vasculitis examined, although not in the few cases of large vessel giant cell arteritis examined to date. This finding of frequent and severe endothelial dysfunction in patients with vasculitis of several types suggests that they may be prone to an increased incidence of diffuse atheroma, probably occurring at an earlier age. The improvement seen in active disease treated with aggressive immuno-suppression is an important lesson for 1°SNV and may also have messages for the therapy of primary atherosclerosis in view of the postulated link with endothelial stunning. The possible mechanisms for this need to be examined further.

3.3. Mechanisms and Consequences of Endothelial Stunning (ECS)

Both direct endothelial injury in vasculitis and endothelial stunning resulting from distant inflammation may initiate chronic changes of atherosclerosis. The former allows entry of acute and chronic inflammatory cells as well as plasma. As the acute changes resolve the macrophages ingest the debris, including serum proteins and lipids and so resemble the foamy cells seen atheroma. Indeed there are many pointers to support the concept of primary atherosclerosis as an inflammatory immune process [64], although it occurs in a more patchy, localised fashion. This model provides convincing explanations for the atheroma seen in transplanted organs, which may be accelerated as a result of the more diffuse and extensive nature of the rejection process occurring within the graft. A closely related process would be predicted to occur in local vessels directly affected by the primary disease process in 1°SNV. This would not initially appear to provide an explanation for chronic changes occurring systemically in vasculitis after ECS. In fact the mechanisms may have many similarities, based on the role of the endothelial cell as a central player in both processes.

Endothelial cells (EC), once seen as passive victims of inflammation in vasculitis, are now viewed as key players, attracting and localising circulating cells to a site of inflammation. The main function of resting endothelial cells may be maintenance of the blood/tissue barriers. However, activated cells express a number of cell surface receptors, such as adhesion and selectin molecules, that slow, retain, and guide circulating cells to leave the blood stream and enter local tissues under the influence of a number of cytokines and chemokines. Key cytokines involved in EC activation include TNFα and Il-1. These activate EC, causing them to both upregulate surface expression of selectins such as E-selectin; adhesion molecules such as ICAM-1; and secrete cytokines such as Il-1 which may continue the process into a chronic stage. These molecules first slow the progress of circulating inflammatory cells such as neutrophils and monocytes, then cause them to adhere to the endothelium before migrating into the local tissues. This is a normal patho-physiological response but the unusual, and unexplained, aspect of vasculitis is that these cells are retained in the vessel wall rather than migrating straight through into the tissues. At the site of local inflammation driven by antigen deposition from infection or other causes, this chain of events has clear host advantage. Thus in most respects the inflammation in the vessel wall in sites directly involved in 1°SNV is essentially similar to other types of immune inflammation. What is less clear is the sequence of events occurring in the vascular bed which is not directly involved in the local inflammation.

Endothelial stunning was described as acute endothelial dysfunction induced by the same key cytokines involved in EC activation, namely TNFα and Il-1, together with bacterial products such as lipopolysaccharide. A relatively brief exposure could induce changes that lasted over a week [65]. Thus the changes of up-regulation of certain factors such as adhesion molecules discussed above was combined with down-regulation of normal NO related responses. The effects of chronic exposure of EC to such cytokines has not been studied and it is not clear that the chronic release of TNFα etc driving distant endothelial stunning has a physiological role. In the acute stages of infection it may have survival advantages in increasing circulation of cells with a surveillance role through the tissues but in the chronic phase the persistence of this mechanism may be seen as a disadvantage. Persistence of local organ inflammation is a common factor in vasculitis, as it is in the synovial inflammation of RA, and both illustrate the common observation that chronic inflammation changes from a protective to an injurious response. The chronic release of cytokines like TNFα may have very different effects from its acute actions. In T lymphocytes, for example, the acute and chronic effects of exposure to TNFα on receptor signalling appear to be very different. Our preliminary experiments suggest the same holds true in EC. Thus chronic activation of EC could potentially lead to both continuing attraction of circulating inflammatory cells together with a down-regulation of the process that normally leads to their rapid transmigration through into the local tissues. The retention of chronic inflammatory monocytic cells in the vessel wall, under the endothelium, is a characteristic feature of the lesions of atherosclerosis.

The detailed mechanisms whereby endothelial stunning can lead to the chronic vessel wall changes seen in atheroma clearly require further study. However the importance of at least two effects appear well established. The relevance of upregulation of adhesion molecules has been well studied in knock out mice models [66, 67]. This has shown that the enhanced atheroma formation following lipid feeding is greatly diminished when one or several adhesion molecules are absent. The relevance of the chronicity is stressed by the demonstration that the relative risk for cardiovascular death in RA increases with the duration as well as the severity of the arthritis [6]. The relevance of attracting T-cells into the vessel wall has been investigated by examining the effects of blockading CD40L, the receptor involved in T-cell/endothelial cell interactions [68]. Such blockade in hyperlididaemic mice lacking the receptor for low-density lipoproteins limited atherosclerosis after high cholesterol diet. Doubtless there are other important factors still to be defined. The important point is that distant inflammation, particularly when it is chronic, can lead to endothelial cell injury not confined to the organs directly involved in the vascular inflammatory process in 1°SNV. Such endothelial injury or dysfunction is seen as the primary starting point in the response to injury hypothesis of atherosclerosis [64]. It can promote systemic atherosclerosis which once initiated is influenced by all the classical risk factors for CVS disease (see diagram). In this aspect, 1°SNV provides a model for the enhanced risk of CVS events occurring in the more common rheumatic diseases. This model is open to therapeutic modulation with the potential

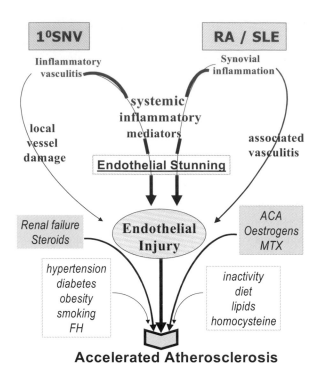

Figure 3. 1°SNV as a model for CVS events in RA.

to provide new insights into treatments for primary atheroma.

4. DISCUSSION

The studies in 1°SNV have a number of implications requiring further study. The finding of endothelial dysfunction in several main syndromes within 1°SNV, with no difference between muscular artery disease like PAN and small vessel disease, indicates that this is not a direct effect of inflammation vasculitis in the local vessel wall. The implication is that it is an effect of the systemic inflammation seen in these diseases. The prediction from this is that it may be a precursor of accelerated atherosclerosis in 1°SNV and epidemiologic studies are needed to examine this concept.

The evidence so far supports the hypothesis that 1°SNV forms a useful model for the development of atherosclerosis in systemic rheumatic diseases such as RA and SLE. We already have evidence to show that similar endothelial dysfunction is seen in both these conditions. We now need to examine the speed of development of such dysfunction, the relationship to disease activity and duration, and the response to therapy. The most important aspect of the 1°SNV model may be that it allows the study of the development of endothelial responses from the onset of disease, the factors influencing severity and progression to chronic changes, the responses to therapy and whether they influence the long term outcome. The therapies used in all these diseases are similar, although the extent to which they are applied varies according to concepts of disease severity. Interestingly the recent studies of TNFα blockade in RA has illustrated the improvement in clinical response that can occur with effective therapy in RA. Since similiar aberations of TNFα are also seen in 1°SNV, this is now seen as a promising therapy to apply here also. Thus there may be even more confluence of therapies and greater opportunities to treat or prevent endothelial dysfunction in rheumatic diseases in future.

REFERENCES

1. Wollhcim FA. Rheumatoid Arthritis – the clinical picture. In: Oxford Textbook of Rheumatology. Maddison PJ, Isenberg DA, Wood P, Glass DN, eds. 1993;2:639–661.
2. Moots R, Bacon PA. Extra-articular manifestations of Rheumatoid Arthritis. In: Arthritis and Allied Conditions 13th Edition. Koopman WJ, ed. 1997;1:1071–1088.
3. Salvarani C, Macchioni P, Mantovani W, Rossi F, Veneeiani M, Bioardi L, Lodi L, Portoli I. Extra-articular manifestations of RA and HLA antigens in Northern Italy. J Rheum 1992;1(2):242–246.
4. Sattar MA, Sughayer AA. A clinical profile of rheumatoid arthritis in Kuwait. Med Assoc 1986;20:21–28.
5. Moolenburgh JD, Valkenburg HA, Fourie PB. A population study on rheumatoid arthritis in Lesotho, Southern Africa. Ann Rheum Dis 1986;45:691–695.
6. Wolfe FA, DM Mitchell, JT Sibley, JF fries, DA Bloch, CA Williams, PW Spitz, M Haga, SM Kleinheksel, M.A.Cathey. The mortality of Rheumatoid arthritis. Arthritis Rheum 1994;37:481–494.
7. Pincus T, Callahan LF, Sale WG, Brooks AL, Payne LE, Vaughn WK: Severe functional declines, work disability, and increased mortality in seventy-five Rheumatoid arthritis patients studied over nine years. Arthritis Rheum 1984;27:864–872.
8. Rasker JJ, Cosh JA. Cause and Age of Death in a Prospective Study of 100 patients with Rheumatoid. Ann Rheum Dis 1981;40:115–20.
9. Prior P, Symmonds DPM. Cause of Death in Rheumatoid Arthritis. Brit J Rheumatol 1984;23:92–99.
10. Grabriel SE, Crowson CS, O'Fallon Wn. Mortality in rheumatoid arthritis: have we made an impact in four decades. J Rheumatol 1999;26:2529–33.
11. Myllykangas-Luosujärvi R, Aho K, Kautiainen H, Isomäki H. Cardiovascular Mortality in Women with Rheumatoid Arthritis. J Rheumatol 1995;22:1065–1067.
12. Wallberg-Jonsson S, Johansson H, Ohman ML, Rantapaa-Dahlqvist S. Extent of inflammation predicts cardiovascular disease and overall mortality in seropositive Rheumatoid arthritis: a retrospective cohort study from disease onset. J Rheumatol 1999;26:2562–71.
13. Urowitz MB, Bookman AA, Koehler BE, Gordon DA, Symthe HA, Ogryzlo MA. The bimodal mortality pattern of systemic lupus erythematosus. Arthritis Rheum 1999;42:338–46.
14. Manzi S, Meilahn En, Rairie JE, Conte CG, Medsger TA Jr, Jansen McWilliams L, et al. Age-specific incidence rates of myocardial infarction and angina in women with systemic lupus erythematosus: comparison with the Framingham Study. Am J Epidemiol 1997;145:408–15.
15. Esdaile JM, Abrahamowicz M. Grodzicky T, Senecal JL, Panaritis T, Li Y, et al. Myocardial infarction and stroke in SLE: markedly increased incidence after controlling for risk factors. Arthritis Rheum 1998;41(suppl 9):A639.
16. Cuadrado MJ, Khamashta MA. The antiphospholipid antibody syndrome (Hughes Syndrome): therapeutic aspects. Baillieres Clin Rheum 2000;14:1,151–163.
17. Bacon PA, Kitas GD. The significance of vascular inflammation in Rheumatoid arthritis. Ann Rheum Dis 1994;53:621–623.
18. Gao SZ, Schroeder JS, Hunt S, Strinson EB. Retransplantation for severe accelerated coronary disease in heart transplant recipients. Am J Cardiol 1988;62:867.
19. Bahgenstoss AH, Rosenburg EF. Viceral Lesions Associated with Chronic infectious (Rheumatoid) arthritis. Arch Path 1943;199:855–7.
20. Khan AH, Spodick DH. Rheumatoid Heart Disease. Sem Arth Rheum 1972;1:327–37.
21. Cathcart ES, Spodick DH. Rheumatoid Heart Disease. N Eng J Med 1962;266:959–64.
22. Bacon PA, Gibson DG. Cardiac Involvement in Rheumatoid Arthritis. Acta Morph Hum 1992;40:149–86.
23. Macdonald WJ, Crawford MH. Echocardiographic assessment of cardiac structure and function in patients with RA. Am J Med 1977;63:890–6.
24. Mody GM, Stevens JE. The heart in rheumatoid arthritis – a clinical and echocardiographic study. Q J Med 1987;65(247):921–8.

25. Kirk J, Cosh J. Rheumatoid heart disease. Ann Rheum Dis 1969;28(6):680–1.
26. Prakash R, Atassi A, Poske R. Prevalence of Pericardial Effusion in Rheumatoid Arthritis. NEJM 1973;289:597–600.
27. Escalante A, Kaufman R. Cardiac compression in Rheumatoid arthritis. Semin Arthritis Rheum 1990;20:148–63.
28. Sigal LH, Friedman HD. Rheumatoid Pancarditis in a patient with well controlled arthritis. J Rheumatol 1988;16:373–86.
29. TravaglioA, Anaya J-M. Rheumatoid Periarditis: New immunopathological aspects. Clin Exp Rheum 1994;12:313–6.
30. Stables RH, Campbell S. Haemopericardium in pericarditis. Int J Cardiol 1989;23:268–70.
31. Ball GV, Schrohenloher R. Gammaglobulin complexes in Rheumatoid pericardial fluid. Am J Med 1975;58:123–8.
32. Van Offel JF, De Clerk LS. Cholesterol Crystals and IgE containing complexes in rheumatoid pericarditis. Clin Rheumatol 1991;10:78–80.
33. Liebowitz WB. The Heart in Rheumatoid Arthritis. Ann Int med 1963;58:102–110.
34. Karten I. Arteritis, Myocardial Infarction and Rheumatoid Arthritis. JAMA 1969;210:1717–20.
35. Bely M, Apathy A. Cardiac Changes in Rheumatoid Arthritis. Acta Morph Hum 1992;40:149–86.
36. Corrao S, Armone S. Echodoppler left vetricular filling abnormalities in patients with rheumatoid arthritis without clinically evident cardiovascular disease. Europ J Clin Invest 1996;26:293–297.
37. Sokolof L. The Heart in Rheumatoid Arthritis. Am Heart J 1953;45:635–43.
38. Cruikshank B. Heart Lesions in Rheumatoid Arthritis. J Path Bacteriol 1958;76:223–40.
39. Ahern M, Lever JV. Complete Heart Block in Rheumatoid Arthritis. Ann Rheum Dis 1983;42:389–95.
40. Christensen PD, Sorensen Ke. Pencillamine Induced Polymyositis with Complete Heart Block. Euro Heart J 1989;10:1041–4.
41. Sweezy R. Myocardial Infarction due to Rheumatoid Arthritis. JAMA 1967;199:855–7.
42. Kitas GD, Banks M, Bacon PA. Accelerated atherosclerosis as a cause of cardiovascular death in RA. Pathogenesis 1998;1(2):78–83.
43. Corrao S, Salli L, Arnone S, Scaglione L, Pinto A, Licata G. Echodoppler abnormalities in patients with rheumatoid arthritis without clinically evident cardiovascular disease. Euro J Clin Inv 1996;26:293–297.
44. Fahy J, Marnick T, Mcreevy C, Quigley J, Maurer B. Doppler echocardiographic detection of left ventricular diastolic dysfunction in patients with pulmonary sar-

coidosis. Chest 1996;109:62–66.
45. Leung WG, Wong KL, Wong CK, Lan CP, Cheng CH, Tai YT. Doppler echocardiographic evaluation of left ventricular diastolic dysfunction in patients with systemic lupus erythematosis. Am Heart J 1987;113:966–71.
46. Ungureanu-Longrois D, Balligand JL, Kell RA, Smith TW. Myocardial contractile dysfunction in the systemic inflammatory response syndrome: role of cytokines-inducible nitric oxide synthase. J Molecular and Cellular Cardiology 1995;27:155–67.
47. Price S, Anning PB, Mitchell JA, Evans TW. Myocardial dysfunction in sepsis: mechanisms and therapeutic implications. Eur Heart J 1999;20:715–24.
48. Deswal A, Bozkurt B, Seta Y, Parilti-Eiswirth S, Hayes FA, Blosch C, Mann DL. Safe and efficacy of a P75 tumour necrosis factor receptor (Enbrel, etanercept) in patients with advanced heart failure. 1999;99:3224–6.
49. Banks MJ, Bacon PA, Flint EJ, Forsey PR, Kitas GD. Left Ventricular Diastolic Filling Abnormalities Associate With Systemic Inflammation In Rheumatoid Arthritis. Brit J Rheumatol 2000 (in press).
50. Monson R, Hall P. Mortality Amongst Arthritics. J Chronic Dis 1976;29:459–67.
51. Suzuki A, Ohosone Y. Cause of death in 81 patients with rheumatoid arthritis. J Rheumatol 1994;21:33–60.
52. Banks MJ, Kitas GD, Foresey PR et al. Ischaemic heart disease in rheumatoid arthritis: a silent killer? (submitted).
53. Banks MJ, Flint EJ, Foresey PR, Bacon PA, Kitas GD. Risk factors for ischaemic heart disease (IHD) in rheumatoid arthritis (RA). Rheumatol 39(suppl.1):40.
54. Jeannette JC, Falk RJ, Andrassy K, Bacon PA, Churg J, Gross WL, Hagen EC, Hoffman GS, Hunder GG et al. Nomenclature of systemic vasculitides: the proposal of an international consensus conference. Arthritis Rheum 1994;37:187–192.
55. Kallenberg CG, Tervaert JW. What is new with antineutrophil cytoplasmic antibodies: diagnostic, pathogenetic and therapeutic implications. Curr Opin Nephrol Hypertens 1999;8:307–15.
56. Carruthers CD, Bacon PA. Combination therapy in vasculitis. Springer Seminars in Immunopathology 2000 (in press).
57. Luqmani RA, Bacon PA, Moots RJ, Janssen BA, Pall A, Emery P, Savage C, Adu D. Birmingham Vasculitis Activity Score (BVAS) in systemic necrotizing vasculitis. QJM 1994;87:671–8.
58. Exley AR, Bacon PA, Luqmani RA, Kitas GD, Gordon C, Savage CO, Adu D. Development and initial validation of the Vasculitis Damage Index for the standardized clinical assessment of damage in the systemic vasculitides. Arthritis Rheum 1997;40:371–80.

59. Adams MR, Celermajer DS. Detection of presymptomatic atherosclerosis: a current perspective. Clin Sci 1999;97:615–624.

60. Raza K, Thambyrajah J, Townend JN, Exley AR, Hortas C, Filer A, Carruthers DM, Bacon PA Suppression of inflammation in primary systemic vasculitis restores vascular endothelial function – lessons for atherosclerotic disease? Circulation 2000 (in press).

61. Bhagat K, Moss R, Collier J, Vallance P. Endothelial "stunning" following a brief exposure to endotoxin: a mechanism to link infection and infarction? Cardiovasc Res 1996;32:822–9.

62. Vallance P, Collier J, Bhagat K. Infection, inflammation, and infarction: does acute endothelial dysfunction provide a link? Lancet 1997;349:1391–2.

63. Exley AR, Bacon PA, Luqmani RA, Kitas GD, Carruthers DM, Moots R. Examination of disease severity in systemic vasculitis from the novel perspective of damage using the vasculitis damage index (VDI). Br J Rheumatol. 1998;37:57–63.

64. Ross R. Atherosclereosis – an inflammatory disease. N Engl J Med 1999;340:115–26.

65. Bhagat K, Vallance P. Inflammatory cytokines impair endothelium-dependent dilatation in human veins in vivo. Circulation 1997;96:3042–7.

66. Nakashima Y, Raines EW, Plump AS, Breslow JL, Ross R. Upregulation of VCAM-1 and ICAM-1 at atherosclerosis-prone sites on the endotherlium in the ApoE-deficioent mouse. Arterioscler Thromb Vasculitis Biol 1998;18:842–51.

67. Hynes RO, Wagner DD. Genetic manipulation of vascular adhesion molecules in mice. J Clin Invest 1996 15;98:2193–5.

68. Mach F, Schönbeck, Sukhova GK, Libby P. Reduction of atherosclerosis in mine by inhibition of CD40 signalling. Nature 1998;394:200–203.

Atherosclerosis and Autoimmunity
Y. Shoenfeld, D. Harats and G. Wick, editors

Vasculitis of the Coronary Arteries and Atherosclerosis: Random Coincidence or Causative Relationship?

Viera Štvrtinová[1], Lubica Rauová[2], Alena Tuchyňová[2] and Jozef Rovenský[2]

[1]Medical Faculty, Comenius University, Bratislava, Slovak Republic; [2]Research Institute of Rheumatic Diseases, Piešt'any, Slovak Republic

1. INTRODUCTION

Myocardial ischemia and its extreme consequence, acute myocardial infarction are generally accepted to be a result of transient or prolonged discrepancy between real myocardial needs for oxygen and the actual blood flow through the coronary arteries into the cardiac muscle. There may be a variety of reasons for insufficient blood supply into the coronary arteries [1]. In industrialized countries, coronary heart disease (CHD) is caused by atherosclerosis in more than 90% of the cases; it should be borne in mind however that there is a wide range of other pathological processes that eventually may result in myocardial infarction [2] (Table 1).

Inflammatory affection of the coronary arteries may present a life-threatening condition and the underlying reason for CHD in all age groups. Since the epicardial coronary arteries are not easily accessible to biopsy, as well as the pathogenesis and classification of various forms of vasculitis are rather confusing, diseases involving the coronary arteries are rarely diagnosed correctly during the lifetime of the patients. However, a correct and timely diagnosis has become vitally important not only for the necessity to aggressively manage some "malignant" forms of vasculitis by immunosuppressive therapy, but also because of the needless administration of such therapy may lead to serious complications and adverse effects [3]. It is therefore rather crucial to make an early distinction between vasculitis, i.e. inflammatory condition of the coronary artery, and atherosclerotic alterations since the management of the two conditions would be approached differently.

On the other hand, underlying vasculitis may enhance atherogenesis and the development of atherothrombosis. Smoking, hyperlipidemia, hypertension and diabetes mellitus as the major risk factors for the development and progression of atherosclerosis can not explain atherosclerosis in many patients [4]. A number of additional risk factors, which might be affected by systemic or local inflammation, have been identified during recent years – including elevated levels of homocysteine, lipoprotein (a), oxidative or enzymatic modifications of lipoproteins, estrogen deficiency, hypercoagulability and last but not least infection [5]. Increasing evidence suggests that atherosclerosis is a chronic inflammatory disease developing in response to certain specific injury of vascular wall. Vascular wall inflammation plays a significant role in both the evolvement of atherosclerosis and during the later stages when inflammation is considered to be the reason for the instability of the atherosclerotic plaque [6]. Macrophages, endothelial cells, smooth muscle cells and activated lymphocytes are the principal constituents of the atherosclerotic plaque. Similar to an inflammatory process there is an interaction between effector cells of the immune response and the production of soluble mediators (cytokines, chemokines and soluble adhesion molecules) [7]. Markers of systemic inflammation such as C-reactive protein or serum amyloid A appear to predict cardiovascular events in healthy men and aspirin seems to significantly reduce the risk of myocardial

Table 1. Causes of myocardial ischemia (adjusted according to Cheitlin and Virmani [2])

1. Coronary atherosclerosis

2. Other diseases involving coronary arteries
    - arteritis (occurring in the framework of primary and secondary vasculitis)
    - metabolic disease (mucopolysaccharidoses, homocysteinuria, Fabry's disease, amyloidosis, pseudoxanthoma elasticum etc.)
    - compression of the coronary artery from the outside (e.g. by tumor)

3. Coronary artery aneurysms

4. Coronary artery thrombosis

5. Coronary artery spasms

6. Coronary artery embolism

7. Congenital abnormalities of coronary arteries

8. Injuries and dissections

9. Disproportion between oxygen needs and supply (aortic stenosis, aortic insufficiency, thyreotoxicosis, pheochromocytoma, etc.)

10. Syndrome X (small vessel disease)

infarction in individuals with high CRP levels only [8]. Statins in addition to blood lipid levels reduction modify endothelial function, inflammatory responses, plaque stability, and thrombus formation and thus reduces the risk of cardiovascular complications [9].

For the human vasculitides as well as atherosclerosis both autoimmune and infectious causes have been proposed. The primary symptoms of many vasculitides resemble those of infectious diseases and moreover, vasculitis is a well-documented manifestation of infection by some known microbial agent. In addition, in chronic or "extinguished" syphilitic arteritis, alterations of the intima resemble atherosclerotic changes, and atherosclerotic lesions may frequently be layered onto old syphilitic lesions [10]. The organism implicated (*Chlamydia pneumoniae, Helicobacter pylori* as well as herpes viruses (mainly cytomegalovirus) are ubiquitous and this has raised question whether they may in some patients enhance inflammation in atherosclerosis whereas in others, e.g. in patients with altered immune function, lead to systemic vasculitis [11]. It however remains unclear whether infectious agents act in the development of atherosclerotic lesions as a cause or as a cofactor or whether they are present just as an innocent commensal [12]. The indirect evidence for

their causative role in induction of atherosclerosis is provided by the potentially reducing effects of tetracycline or quinolone antibiotics on the risk of acute myocardial infarction [13].

The aim of the present work is to point to the possible association between atherosclerosis and coronary vasculitis in the clinical picture of the various types of the primary vasculitis. Coronary vasculitis is associated with Takayasu's arteritis, polyarteritis nodosa as well as diffuse connective tissue diseases-associated vasculitis, less frequently with giant cell arteritis, Wegener's granulomatosis, Churg-Strauss syndrome, Winiwarter-Buerger's disease and secondary infectious vasculitis. Isolated coronary vasculitis as a limited variant of various vasculitides is very rare, however sudden cardial death was reported in Churg-Strauss syndrome [14, 15], polyarteritis nodosa [16, 17], Takayasu's arteritis [18] and inactive SLE [19]

2. TAKAYASU'S ARTERITIS

2.1. Background

Takayasu's arteritis (TA) is a non-specific chronic inflammatory arteritis, mainly involving the aorta and its main branches as well as the coronary and pulmonary arteries developing in two clinical stages. The first, initial inflammatory stage develops suddenly, mostly between the age from 10 to 20 and presents by non-specific symptoms such as fever, lack of appetite, weight loss, nocturnal sweating, weakness, nausea, muscular and articular pain. Symptoms of the second, chronic occlusive stage appear after several months up to years. This chronic occlusive stage is characterized by ischemia of the tissues and organs involved, in particular upper extremities, central nervous system and eyes. Arterial renovascular hypertension occurs in about 50% of the cases [20]. The majority of cases are diagnosed but at the chronic occlusive stage. Epidemiologically, it affects mostly female patients and is most prevalent in Asian and Latin Americans countries.

2.2. Coronary Involvement and Atherosclerosis in Takayasu's Arteritis

The most frequent clinical manifestation of cardiac involvement is cardiac failure due to hypertension. Coronary arteries are involved in about 15–25% of the cases of TA [3] with the narrowing of the coronary arteries usually due to the inflammatory process spreading from the aorta to the coronary arteries [21]. The typical lesion is stenosis or occlusion of coronary ostia found in 73% cases [22], followed by stenosis of the proximal segments of the coronary arteries with the distal parts of the coronary arteries remaining usually intact. Diffuse or focal coronary arteritis, which may extend diffusely to all epicardial branches or may involve focal segments and coronary aneurysm seem to be very rare in TA [23]. Angina pectoris may be the very first sign of TA, however frequently no subjective symptoms are present and the first sign of coronary involvement are myocardial infarction or heart failure. Coronary bypass is effective therapy for this disease [21], even excessively thickness of ascending aorta may sometimes cause technical problems during the surgery and inflammation of the aortic wall may contribute to the late occlusion of the origin of the bypass grafts. The surgery should be performed during the inactive phase of the disease, however, if clinical or histological signs of active disease are identified during the surgery, steroids have to be administered

postoperatively until erythrocyte sedimentation rates reduce and C-reactive protein values normalize. In 63 undergoing coronary artery surgery for TA between 1961 and 1989 revascularization was performed in 49 patients and endarterectomy in the remaining 14 patients. Operative mortality was 7.9%, and late deaths were reported in three patients. [22]. The success rates of bypass surgery point to the importance of early recognition of coronary involvement in TA to prevent myocardial infarction.

Among the 8 patients with TA followed at our Institute of Rheumatic Diseases during the recent 5 years (Table 2), the only male patient developed pressure pain behind the sternum at the age of 43, after six years of the disease, with resting ECG showing no signs of ischemia. However, coronarographic investigation showed 25% reduction of the left coronary artery lumen with smooth walls, the ramus interventricularis anterior showed marginal atherosclerotic irregularities of the vessel wall and the right coronary artery was obliterated shortly after ostium. In this patient, the process of atherosclerosis could be enhanced by smoking and rise of cholesterol and triglyccride levels induced by the steroid therapy. The acceleration of atherosclerosis in TA is also due to arterial hypertension related to the involvement of renal arteries. This could be observed in one of our female patient in whom the disease was manifested at the age of 31 as subclavian steal phenomenon due to the narrowing of the a. subclavia. The patient underwent a successful surgery and was only temporarily (about 1 year) on steroid therapy. To manage hypertension she received calcium blockers. A marked irregularity of the abdominal aorta lumen with extensive calcifications in the wall along with a stenosis of the right-sided renal artery were identified upon angiographic investigation at the age of 47 years. Spiral CT identified diffuse thickening of the aortic wall with diffuse calcifications. These findings suggest a combination of inflammatory and atherosclerotic alterations. Apparently, TA patients may develop "secondary atherosclerosis" of the thickened intima [24], similarly as secondary atherosclerosis developing in experimental animals at the site of arterial wall injury [25]. However, some individuals may have some segments of their arteries altered by inflammation and the others altered due to atherosclerosis. A male patient was reported with severe form of

Table 2. The group of our patients with Takayasu's arteritis

Patient	Gender	Year of birth	Age at onset	First symptons
1	female	1974	19 years	arterial hypertension
2	female	1966	27 years	pressure difference between upper extremities
3	female	1949	31 years	pressure difference between upper extremities
4	female	1956	39 years	arterial hypertension
5	male	1955	38 years	acute stroke
6	female	1983	14 years	lack of radial and ulnar artery pulsations
7	female	1980	17 years	arterial hypertension
8	female	1971	15 years	headaches and collapse

angina pectoris aggravated with activity of arteritis despite administration of prednisolone. Post-mortem examination revealed severe atherosclerosis of the aorta, with the large arteries arising from the aorta showing signs of the fibrotic stage of TA, and the atherosclerotic coronary arteries without signs of arteritis [26]

3. GIANT CELL ARTERITIS

3.1. Background

Giant cell arteritis (GCA) is an inflammatory vasculitis that affects the medium and large arteries. Temporal arteritis represents the most frequently occurring type of GCA [27]. Clinically, temporal arteritis was first described by Hutchinson in 1890, the histopathological picture in relation to the clinical syndrome was provided by Horton in 1932, but it only was Jenning in 1938 who recognized the association with blindness as a serious complication [3]. Shortly thereafter, GCA was found to involve also extracranial arteries, including coronary arteries.

Unlike Takayasu's arteritis, this is a disease affecting older patients, mostly occurring after the age of 50. Typically, it involves branches of the carotic artery (temporal artery), but it is actually a systemic granulomatous panarteritis that may involve any medium or large artery. The clinical picture includes headaches as well as painful swelling over the temporal artery, claudication pain in jaw mus-

cles, chronic pain in the throat, pressure sensitivity, redness and loss of hair over the temporal artery. The most feared complication of GCA is blindness that may occur suddenly, with both eyes being involved within a short interval of time [28]. Polymyalgia rheumatica occurs in about half of the patients with temporal arteritis, and vice versa, about 50% of the patients with symptoms of polymyalgia show positive findings upon temporal biopsy [29]. Involvement of the aorta and its branches is observed in approximately 10–15% of the patients suffering from GCA, with the symptoms suggesting the involvement of large arteries such as intermittent claudication of an extremity, paresthesias, and Raynaud's phenomenon [30]. The alteration of the aorta may be life threatening due to the development of dissecting aneurysm or aortic rupture [3].

The diagnosis is based on the typical finding of panarteritis identified upon the biopsy of the temporal artery. Since the vessels are involved segmentally, the biopsy need not catch the site involved. Therefore, the biopsy of a 5–8 cm long segment of the temporal artery is recommended [31]. Histology shows a typical infiltration of the vessel wall by lymphocytes and macrophages, disruption or loss of the lamina elastica interna, and – typically – also the presence of multinuclear giant cells.

Table 3. The group of our patients with giant cell arteritis

Patient	Gender	Year of birth	Age at the onset	Histology	Stroke	IM	PMR	
1	male	1926	74	+	0	0	0	
2	female	1919	76	+	0	0	0	
3	female	1931	66	+	0	+	0	
4	female	1925	73	+	0	0	0	
5	male	1941	51	+	0	0	0	
6	female	1921	75	+	0	0	0	
7	female	1924	72	+	0	0	0	
8	female	1939	54	+	0	0	0	
9	male	1926	70	+	0	0	0	
10	female	1917	81	+	0	0	0	
11	female	1919	55	+	0	0	0	IDLE
12	female	1924	73	+	0	+	0	
13	female	1914	84	+	0	0	0	
14	male	1926	64	not done	+	0	1	
15	male	1923	77	+	+	+	0	
16	female	1936	56	not done	0	0	1	
17	female	1912	61	+	0	++	1	
18	female	1926	58	+	0	0	1	
19	female	1920	55	+	0	0	1	
20	female	1912	64	+	0	0	1	
21	male	1919	67	+	0	0	1	
22	male	1903	72	+	0	0	1	
23	male	1903	75	+	0	0	1	

IM: myocardial infarction; PMR: polymyalgia rheumatica; IDLE: ischemic disease of the lower extremities

3.2. Coronary Involvement and Atherosclerosis in GCA

The involvement of the coronary arteries is rarely recognized, though deaths have been reported due to acute myocardial infarction [28, 32, 33]. Freddo and co-workers [34] suggest that myocardial infarction may be a more common early complication of temporal arteritis than appreciated and can occur despite administration of high-dose corticosteroid therapy.

In our group of 23 patients (15 females and 8 males) with the diagnosis of GCA (Table 3) four patients developed myocardial infarction, 2 patients suffered stroke and 1 patient both myocardial infarction and stroke. One female patient developed ischemic disease of the lower extremities.

With regard to the high age of patients with GCA their coronary heart disease may be assumed to atherosclerotic alterations of the coronary arteries. However, vasculitis can set in the vascular wall already damaged by the atherosclerotic process and

319

the inflammatory response can be triggered by so far unknown mechanism. Moreover, when healed up, temporal arteritis may only hardly be distinguished from atherosclerosis, and some pathologists claim that atherosclerosis and temporal arteritis may be based on a common pathological process [35]. This could explain why GCA develops mainly in elderly patients. A multicentric prospective study involving 400 patients with the diagnosis of GCA or polymyalgia rheumatica identified smoking and previous arterial disease as a risk factor for the development of the GCA in women [36]. Interestingly, patients with GCA had lower cholesterol levels at the time of the diagnosis compared to a control group of healthy volunteers; the cholesterol levels may however have been influenced by the inflammatory process [37].

4. POLYARTERITIS NODOSA

4.1. Background

Polyarteritis nodosa (PAN) represents necrotizing vasculitis of small and medium sized muscular arteries. The etiology of the condition is unknown, however deposition of immune complexes into the arterial walls is considered as an important pathophysiological mechanism. Currently, two forms of PAN are recognized. *Classical* PAN is defined as necrotizing inflammation involving small and medium sized arteries without vasculitis affecting arterioles, capillaries or venules, and without glomerulonephritis. *Microscopic* polyarteritis and/or microscopic polyangiitis is necrotizing vasculitis with minimum or no deposits of immune complexes, affecting small vessels, i.e. capillaries, venules or arterioles with or without affecting small and medium sized arteries [38].

4.2. Coronary Involvement and Atherosclerosis in PAN

Coronary artery vasculitis is a well-recognized complication of PAN and both the large epicardial and small intramural coronary arteries may be affected [3]. It can be found in as many as 80% cases during autopsy, however, the clinical diagnosis is much less frequent [31]. Heart failure is the cause of death in as many as 44% of the patients, resulting from dif-

fuse damage to the heart muscle secondary to arteritis of the coronary arteries or secondary hypertension in renal arteritis [29]. Pericarditis is rather frequent finding, and involvement of the myocardial conducting system has been reported as well [10].

Coronary vasculitis should be considered particularly in young patients with multisystem involvement, because of the different therapy as compared with coronary heart disease determined atherosclerosis. Combined steroid and cyclophosphamide therapy has improved the 5-year survival rate to 75–80% compared to 12% survival of untreated patients [3]. Such an immunosuppressive therapy however has a number of adverse effects including an extremely rapid progression of atherosclerotic alterations. It remains unclear whether steroids are directly atherogenic or whether they enhance atherosclerosis indirectly inducing other risk factors such as dyslipoproteinemia [39] or hyperglycemia, which may result in hypertension and obesity.

5. CHURG-STRAUSS SYNDROME

Churg-Strauss syndrome (CSS) or allergic angiitis and granulomatosis was described by Churg and Strauss in 1951. It is a rare condition characterized by granulomatous vasculitis of multiple organ systems with frequent involvement of the lungs. Its incidence is slightly higher in males, with an average age at the onset of around 44 years. The syndrome occurs in patients with bronchial asthma or another atopic disease in their history, and eosinophilia is a typical feature [29]. The cause of the disease remains unknown. Serum IgE levels are elevated at the vasculitis phase and elevated IgE-immune complex values in the serum have been reported. It belongs to the ANCA-associated vasculitides with the presence of perinuclear type (p-ANCA) namely autoantibodies against myeloperoxidase. All ANCA-associated vasculitides share a number of common pathologic features, ie, focal distribution, necrosis, and neutrophil infiltration. [40]. The clinical features of CSS and PAN are similar, with a higher incidence of pulmonary symptoms in Churg-Strauss syndrome. The disease develops in three clinical stages. There is an allergic condition during the prodromal stage, most frequently asthma or allergic rhinitis. Eosinophilic tissue infiltrations and eosinophilia in the blood are typical of the second stage, and systemic vasculitis appears during the third stage [10]. The heart is one of the most frequently involved organs, with symptoms of granulomatous vasculitis of the coronary arteries or granulomatous myocarditis [15]. Half of the patients die of myocardial infarction or congestive heart failure [10].

6. WEGENER´S GRANULOMATOSIS

6.1. Background

Wegener's granulomatosis (WG) is a necrotizing granulomatous vasculitis involving the respiratory system associated with focal segmental glomerulonephritis and a variable extent of disseminated vasculitis of small vessels. Autoantibodies directed against cytoplasmic antigens of neutrophils (ANCA), especially those with specificity for proteinase 3 (PR-3), are valuable markers for differential diagnosis and monitoring of disease activity in WG [41]. The initial stage of WG is often marked by symptoms of infection and it has been postulated that a bacterial infection could be the etiologic factor of this disease. Due to the infection, neutrophils are locally activated and lysosomal enzymes get released. These may directly damage the vascular wall and/or induce the production of autoantibodies. The presence of c-ANCA may further prime neutrophils resulting in their enhanced activation and further release of oxygen radicals and lysosomal enzymes [42]. If the therapy is successful, c-ANCA titers drop [43].

6.2. Coronary Artery Involvement and Atherosclerosis in WG

The heart is involved in almost one third of the patients with Wegener's granulomatosis. Necrotizing vasculitis of small intramural coronary arteries is present in about 25% of the cases, occasionally also involvement of epicardial coronary arteries has been reported. Moreover, myocarditis occurs, and patients with dysrhythmias have been reported, resulting from granulomatous lesions of the conducting system of the heart muscle, as well as patients with symptoms of myocarditis [10].

7. THROMBOANGIITIS OBLITERANS

7.1. Background

Felix von Winiwarter first described the pathologic-anatomical signs of thromboangiitis in 1879 in the amputated leg of a 57-year old male. In the same year, Leo Buerger, who summarized both the clinical and the histological symptoms of the disease in 1908 and used the term thromboangiitis obliterans for the first time, was born in Vienna [44]. Buerger described the obliterating disease, typically involving medium-sized arteries and veins (both superficial and deep) in the extremities, developing in three stages [45]. The disease mainly involves lower extremity vessels and only occasionally cerebral or coronary arteries.

Buerger's disease affects young individuals presenting frequently as superficial migrating phlebitis along with claudication in palms and soles. Cyanosis and necroses of the digits may be present at the onset of the disease since the claudication pain in the calves and thighs appears but during the later stages of the disease.

7.2. Coronary Involvement and Atherosclerosis in Buerger's Disease

The coronary arteries are involved rarely. Ohno and co-workers [46] reported acute myocardial infarction in a 32-year old male in whom the diagnosis of Buerger's disease was established both clinically and angiographically but not histologically. We reported myocardial infarction in a 19-year old patient with the clinical diagnosis of obliterating thromboangiitis confirmed angiographically [47]. As compared to a previous investigation (Fig. 1), the ECG recording showed a substantial alteration, with the pathological Q wave in leads II, III and VF (Fig. 2). Furthermore, myocardial infarction has been reported in a patient with aorto-coronary bypass using vena saphena for the bypass [10].

Smoking as one of the risk factors for development atherosclerosis is the only known and generally accepted risk factor for obliterating thromboangiitis so far. Moreover, the only way to halt the progression of the disease is to give up smoking [48]. The disease mostly affects young males [49], but has shown increasing incidences in females

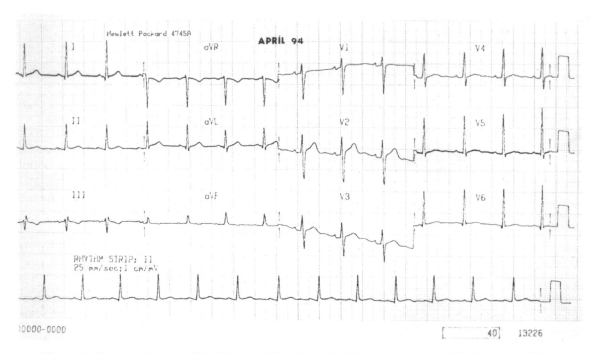

Figure 1. Electrocardiogram of the 19-years old patient with obliterating thrombangiitis from April 1994.

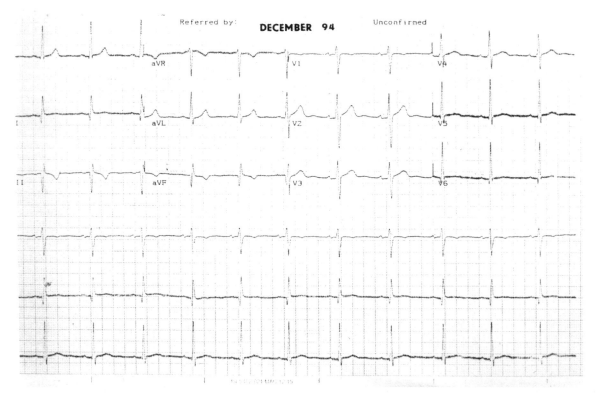

Figure 2. Electrocardiogram of the 19-years old patient with obliterating thrombangiitis from December 1994 showing substantial alteration with pathological Q wave in leads II, III and aVF.

in recent times, probably reflecting the increasing prevalence of smoking among women [50]. Nevertheless, with the progression of the disease only some patients develop atherosclerotic vascular alterations. Probably, the enhancement of the atherosclerotic alterations is determined by the occurrence of other risk factors of atherosclerosis. We observed the development of gangrene of the right toe in one of our female patient 16 years after the onset of obliterating thromboangiitis, after the patient developed high glycemia levels. Since the underlying disease itself had been in inactive phase for 10 years, the development of the gangrene could be explained by associated diabetic microangiopathy. Higher homocysteine levels [51] and lipoprotein (a) [52] were observed in some patients with obliterating thromboangiitis. Hyperhomocystinemia is considered a significant independent risk factor of arterial wall damage for its unfavorable action on endothelial cells, assisting atherogenic processes [53]. Nevertheless, it remains unclear why identical risk factors determine inflammatory alterations of the vascular wall in some individuals, while inducing atherosclerotic changes in others. Inflammatory and atherosclerotic alterations may both represent an "extreme" reflexion of vascular wall damage.

8. INFECTIOUS ANGIITIS

Infectious angiitis may have a variety of consequences – from minimal damage with minute structural alterations to extensive fibrosis with calcifications and luminal stenoses, thrombosis and rupture of blood vessels with resulting hemorrhages, dilation of vessels and formation of mycotic aneurysms [3]. The clinically important infectious angiitis are associated with spirochaetes, mycobacteria, pyogenic bacteria, rickettsiae, viruses or protozoa.

8.1. Syphilis

All the 3 stages of syphilis bear some features of arteritis. Probably, syphilitic aneurysms were first described as early as in 1554, and syphilitic aortitis is mentioned in the book by Joseph Hodgson *Treatise on Diseases of Arteries and Veins* published in London in 1815, i.e. 180 years ago [54]. Syphilitic aortitis is the most significant vascular lesion during the third, last stage of syphilis, and frequently causes stenosis of the coronary artery at its arisal from the aorta; however, coronary arteritis in syphilis may be independent of the aortic involvement. In a study of 223 cases of syphilitic aortitis, coronary artery involvement was observed in 17% of the patients [55]. In chronic or "extinguished" syphilitic arteritis, alterations of the intima resemble atherosclerotic changes, and atherosclerotic lesions may frequently be layered onto old syphilitic lesions [10]. In these cases the diagnosis can be confirmed by positive results of serological testing for syphilis.

8.2. Lyme Diseases

Nowadays, in the antibiotic era, syphilitic arteritis is rare; however, another disease induced by spirochaetes and described in 1977 has come to the foreground: Lyme disease caused by *Borrelia burgdorferi*. With the course in 3 stages, multisystemic involvement as well as by imitating other diseases very much resembles syphilis. In both conditions, spirochaetes may persist in the body for several years and, after the latency period, cause slowly progression particularly to the central nervous system. The underlying mechanism damaging host tissues by spirochaetes remains unclear [56]. In various vessels, a certain degree of vascular damage, including vasculitis up to occlusion has been observed, but no reports of any damage to coronary arteries have appeared so far in the available literature.

8.3. Tuberculosis

About 140 cases of tuberculosis-associated aortitis have been reported so far, but coronary arteritis is extremely rare even in countries with high incidences of tuberculosis [3]. Mycobacterium-induced coronaritis has been described in one heart transplant recipient [10].

Viruses may induce vasculitis either by direct invasion or through immunopathological mechanisms. Examples of viral vasculitis in humans include antigenemia associated with hepatitis B in PAN, association of Herpes zoster virus infection and granulomatous angiitis, or association of visceral vasculitis and cytomegalovirus infection.

9. VASCULITIS IN DIFFUSE DISEASES OF CONNECTIVE TISSUE

9.1. Systemic Lupus Erythematosus

Coronary artery disease has emerged as an important cause of death in young patients with SLE both secondary to premature atherosclerosis and, rarely, coronary arteritis. Women with SLE in the 35- to 44-year age group were over 50 times more likely to have a myocardial infarction than were women of similar age in the Framingham Offspring Study [57]. Prevalence of severely narrowed coronary arteries is 80% in SLE comparing to 30% in age matched healthy controls [58]. The subclinical coronary artery disease is reported to be about 40% [59]. Although vasculitis is a common feature of SLE, necropsies have failed to provide evidence of active coronary arteritis, carditis, or valvular heart disease as a common cause of death [60], however, necrotizing coronaritis may result in fatal thrombosis particularly in young patients [31].

On the other hand, atherosclerotic processes is pronouncedly enhanced in patients with SLE [61]. The risk factors of atherosclerosis development in SLE patients seem similar to those for the general population – dyslipoproteinemia, arterial hypertension, smoking, obesity, diabetes mellitus, sedentary lifestyle. The important additional risk factors are steroid therapy, renal disease with resulting hypertension, and the presence of antiphospholipid antibodies. However, having SLE appears to be an independent risk factor for development of early atherosclerosis [62]. In addition to unspecific inflammatory process, immune dysregulation typical for SLE may also play a significant role in atherogenesis. Dysfunction of endothelial cells secondary to a number of harmful factors such as superoxide and other reactive oxygen intermediates, immune complexes and autoantibodies has been implicated in development and progression of atherosclerosis. [63]. Endothelial damage results in enhanced permeability and adhesiveness, procoagulation characteristics and expression of vasoactive molecules [64]. Injury of the arterial endothelium is the initial event leading to the atherosclerosis according to "response to injury" hypothesis and generation of modified LDL mediates further its progression. Important mechanism of endothelial cell activation

in SLE might be mediated by CD40 molecule, constitutively expressed on endothelial cells. Patients with SLE express excessive amounts of CD40L on both T and B cells, resulting in the production of pathological autoantibodies [65, 66]. Interaction of CD40 on endothelial cells and CD40L on activated T and B cells and platelets then activates endothelial cells and enhances expression of E selectin, ICAM-1, VCAM-1 [67]. Moreover, soluble CD40L released from the membrane of activated cells enhances production of chemoattractant peptide-1 from mononuclear cells further promoting accumulation of immune cells in the atherosclerotic lesion. Soluble as well as membrane bound CD40L are also potent inducers and activators of MMPs in vascular smooth muscle cells and macrophages. enhanced CD40L-CD40 interaction may promote thrombotic activity by enhancing tissue-factor expression in macrophages and through the direct regulation of endothelium-procoagulant activity. Thus CD40-CD40L interaction induced may lead to procoagulant responses and MMP activation which, in patients with an preexisting atherosclerotic lesion, ultimately may lead to plaque rupture and the development of an acute coronary syndrome [68].

Among wide spectrum of autoantibodies presented in SLE, antiphospholipid antibodies are associated not only with venous and arterial thromboembolism, stroke, or recurrent abortions in primary and secondary antiphospholipid syndrome [69], but also with myocardial infarction in patients who do not suffer from lupus [70]. Some anticardiolipin antibodies may cross-react with oxLDL due to cross-reactivity between oxidized lipids. Indeed, it was shown recently, that antibodies to oxLDL were raised in the sera of lupus patients and cross-reacted with cardiolipin and with beta2GPI. Moreover, oxLDL containing immune-complexes of the IgG and IgM isotypes were both elevated in the SLE patients as compared with healthy controls [61].

9.2. Rheumatoid Arthritis

Histologically confirmed coronary arteritis occurs in as many as 20% of patients with rheumatoid arthritis [71]. In RA coronary arteritis-coronary arteriolitis can be isolated or part of generalized vasculitis. Moreover, vasculitis can be early preceding articular complaints. Small intramural arteries are mainly involved. Multifocal microinfarction of the myocardium due to vasculitis of the intramural arterioles and small arteries may lead to the progressive cardiac insufficiency, the direct cause of death [72]. Necrotizing arteritis of epicardial arteries is less frequent but usually causes myocardial infarction [10]. Aortitis can be also a feature of severe rheumatoid arthritis and is often associated with rheumatoid vasculitis, however the diagnosis is extremely rarely made until autopsy [73]. Occasional reports of the involvement of coronary arteries during rheumatic fever may be found in older literature [3]. Interestingly, currently most widely used MTX therapy may promote atherosclerosis in patients who have already signs of atherosclerotic vascular disease probably due to increase concentrations of homocysteine [74]

10. CONCLUSION

It is evident, that the classical risk factors of atherosclerosis per se cannot be the reason for the enhanced atherosclerotic process observed in young patients with vasculitis. Inflammation plays an important role, although the exact mechanism through which acute or chronic inflammation results in acceleration of atherosclerosis remains unknown. Crucial is to timely seek for the various risk factors and attempt to eliminate or at least attenuate them. It seems rather important to instruct the patient correctly and to achieve a change in his/her unfavorable lifestyle. Namely, it has been recognized that atherosclerosis in general develops as a result of a combination of several risk factors. In the case of vasculitis, traditional risk factors get combined with inflammatory process, which is responsible for the acceleration of atherosclerotic alterations in young individuals. The clarification of the relationship between inflammation, vasculitis and atherosclerosis therefore represents a challenge to both the basic and the clinical research.

REFERENCES

1. Cheitlin MD, McAllister HA and de Castro CM. Myocardial infarction without atherosclerosis. JAMA 1975;231:951–9.

2. Cheitlin MD and Virmani R. Myocardial infarction in the absence of coronary atherosclerotic disease. In: R. Virmani and M.B. Forman, editors. Nonatherosclerotic ischemic heart disease. New York: Raven Press, 1989;1–30.

3. Lie JT. Coronary vasculitis. A review in the current scheme of classification of vasculitis. Arch Pathol Lab Med 1987;111:224–33.

4. Mehta JL, Saldeen TG and Rand K. Interactive role of infection, inflammation and traditional risk factors in atherosclerosis and coronary artery disease [see comments]. J Am Coll Cardiol 1998;31:1217–25.

5. Braunwald E. Shattuck lecture – cardiovascular medicine at the turn of the millennium: triumphs, concerns, and opportunities. N Engl J Med 1997;337:1360–9.

6. Pasterkamp G, Schoneveld AH, van der Wal AC et al. Inflammation of the atherosclerotic cap and shoulder of the plaque is a common and locally observed feature in unruptured plaques of femoral and coronary arteries. Arterioscler Thromb Vasc Biol 1999;19:54–8.

7. George J, Harats D and Shoenfeld Y. Inflammatory and immune aspects of atherosclerosis. Isr Med Assoc J 1999;1: 112–6.

8. Ridker PM, Cushman M, Stampfer MJ, Tracy RP and Hennekens CH. Inflammation, aspirin, and the risk of cardiovascular disease in apparently healthy men. N Engl J Med 1997;336:973–9.

9. Rosenson RS and Tangney CC. Antiatherothrombotic properties of statins: implications for cardiovascular event reduction [see comments]. JAMA 1998;279:1643–50.

10. Darcy TP and Virmani R, Coronary vasculitis. In: R. Virmani and M.B. Forman, editors. Nonatherosclerotic ischemic heart disease. New York.: Raven Press, 1989;237–275.

11. Dal Canto AJ and Virgin HWt. Animal models of infection-mediated vasculitis. Curr Opin Rheumatol 1999;11:17–23.

12. Quaschning T and Wanner C. The role of Chlamydia in coronary heart disease-fact or fiction? [editorial]. Nephrol Dial Transplant 1999;14:2800–3.

13. Meier CR, Derby LE, Jick SS, Vasilakis C and Jick H. Antibiotics and risk of subsequent first-time acute myocardial infarction. JAMA 1999;281:427–31.

14. Hunsaker JCd, O'Connor WN and Lie JT. Spontaneous coronary arterial dissection and isolated eosinophilic coronary arteritis: sudden cardiac death in a patient with a limited variant of Churg-Strauss syndrome. Mayo Clin Proc 1992;67:761–6.

15. Lie JT and Bayardo RJ. Isolated eosinophilic coronary arteritis and eosinophilic myocarditis. A limited form of Churg-Strauss syndrome. Arch Pathol Lab Med 1989;113:199–201.

16. Paul RA, Helle MJ and Tarssanen LT. Sudden death as sole symptom of coronary arteritis. Ann Med 1990;22:161–2.

17. Swalwell CI, Reddy SK and Rao VJ. Sudden death due to unsuspected coronary vasculitis. Am J Forensic Med Pathol 1991;12:306–12.

18. Tanaka A, Fukayama M, Funata N, Koike M and Saito K. Coronary arteritis and aortoarteritis in the elderly males. A report of two autopsy cases with review of the literature. Virchows Arch A Pathol Anat Histopathol 1988;414:9–14.

19. Korbet SM, Schwartz MM and Lewis EJ. Immune complex deposition and coronary vasculitis in systemic lupus erythematosus. Report of two cases. Am J Med 1984;77:141–6.

20. Fauci AS, Haynes B and Katz P. The spectrum of vasculitis: clinical, pathologic, immunologic and therapeutic considerations. Ann Intern Med 1978;89:660–76.

21. Cipriano PR, Silverman JF, Perlroth MG, Griepp RB and Wexler L. Coronary arterial narrowing in Takayasu's aortitis. Am J Cardiol 1977;39:744–50.

22. Amano J and Suzuki A. Coronary artery involvement in Takayasu's arteritis. Collective review and guideline for surgical treatment. J Thorac Cardiovasc Surg 1991;102:554–60.

23. Matsubara O, Kuwata T, Nemoto T, Kasuga T and Numano F. Coronary artery lesions in Takayasu arteritis: pathological considerations. Heart Vessels Suppl 1992;7: 26–31.

24. Lande A. Abdominal Takayasu's aortitis, the middle aortic syndrome and atherosclerosis. A critical review [editorial]. Int Angiol 1998;17:1–9.

25. Titus JL and Kim HS, Blood vessels and lymphatics. In: J.M.Kissane, Editor. Anderson´s pathology, St.Louis: Mosby, 1990;752–803.

26. Okada H, Suzuki H, Murakami M et al. Takayasu's arteritis with heart failure due to atherosclerosis. Jpn J Med 1990;29:309–12.

27. Huston KA, Hunder GG, Lie JT, Kennedy RH and Elveback LR. Temporal arteritis: a 25-year epidemiologic, clinical, and pathologic study. Ann Intern Med 1978;88:162–7.

28. Lie JT, Failoni DD and Davis DC, Jr. Temporal arteritis with giant cell aortitis, coronary arteritis, and myocardial infarction. Arch Pathol Lab Med 1986;110:857–60.

29. Cupps TR, Cardiac and vascular diseases. In: D.P.Stites and A.I.Terr, editors. Basic and Clinical Immunology, Appleton a Lange, 1991, 492–505.

30. Klein RG, Hunder GG, Stanson AW and Sheps SG. Large artery involvement in giant cell (temporal) arteritis. Ann Intern Med 1975;83:806–12.

31. Joyce JW. Arteritis. In: H.H.G.Eastcott, editor. Arterial Surgery, Madrid, Melbourne, New York and Tokyo:

Churchill Livingstone, 1992;211–222.

32. Martin JF, Kittas C and Triger DR. Giant cell arteritis of coronary arteries causing myocardial infarction. Br Heart J 1980;43:487–9.

33. Save Soderbergh J, Malmvall BE, Andersson R and Bengtsson BA. Giant cell arteritis as a cause of death. Report of nine cases. JAMA 1986;255:493–6.

34. Freddo T, Price M, Kase C and Goldstein MP. Myocardial infarction and coronary artery involvement in giant cell arteritis. Optom Vis Sci 1999;76:14–8.

35. O'Brien JP. A new risk factor in vascular disease. Excessive solar and other actinic radiation in giant-cell arteritis and atherosclerosis. Int J Dermatol 1987;26:345–8.

36. Duhaut P, Pinede L, Demolombe Rague S et al. Giant cell arteritis and cardiovascular risk factors: a multicenter, prospective case-control study. Groupe de Recherche sur l'Arterite a Cellules Geantes. Arthritis Rheum 1998;41:1960–5.

37. Ettinger WH, Jr., Harris T, Verdery RB, Tracy R and Kouba E. Evidence for inflammation as a cause of hypocholesterolemia in older people [see comments]. J Am Geriatr Soc 1995;43:264–6.

38. Jennette JC, Falk RJ, Andrassy K et al. Nomenclature of systemic vasculitides. Proposal of an international consensus conference. Arthritis Rheum 1994;37:187–92.

39. Ettinger WH, Goldberg AP, Applebaum Bowden D and Hazzard WR. Dyslipoproteinemia in systemic lupus erythematosus. Effect of corticosteroids. Am J Med 1987;83:503–8.

40. Jennette JC. Antineutrophil cytoplasmic autoantibody-associated diseases: a pathologist's perspective. Am J Kidney Dis 1991;18:164–70.

41. van der Woude FJ, Rasmussen N, Lobatto S et al. Autoantibodies against neutrophils and monocytes: tool for diagnosis and marker of disease activity in Wegener's granulomatosis. Lancet 1985;1: 425–9.

42. Falk RJ, Terrell RS, Charles LJ and Jennette JC. Anti-Neutrophil Cytoplasmic Autoantibodies Induce Neutrophils to Degranulate and Produce Oxygen Radicals in vitro. Proc. Natl. Acad. Sci. USA. 1990;87:4115–4119.

43. Stegeman CA, Tervaert JW, Sluiter WJ, Manson WL, de Jong PE and Kallenberg CG. Association of chronic nasal carriage of Staphylococcus aureus and higher relapse rates in Wegener granulomatosis. Ann Intern Med 1994;120:12–7.

44. Shionoya S and Eastcott HHG. Buerger´s disease. In: H.H.G.Eastcott, editor. Arterial Surgery. Madrid, Melbourne, New York and Tokyo: Churchill Livingstone, 1992;153–173.

45. Horowitz SA. Case records of the Massachusetts general hospital, Case 16. N. Engl. J. Med. 1989;320:1068–1076.

46. Ohno H, Matsuda Y, Takashiba K, Hamada Y, Ebihara H

and Hyakuna E. Acute myocardial infarction in Buerger's disease. Am J Cardiol 1986;57:690–1.

47. Stvrtinova V. Vasculitides of the coronary arteries. Bratisl Lek Listy 1995;96:544–51.In Slovak

48. Shigematsu H and Shigematsu K. Factors affecting the long-term outcome of Buerger's disease (thromboangiitis obliterans). Int Angiol 1999;18:58–64.

49. Williams G. Recent views on Buerger's disease. J Clin Pathol 1969;22:573–8.

50. Stvrtinova V, Ambrozy E, Stvrtina S and Lesny P. 90 years of Buerger's disease--what has changed? Bratisl Lek Listy 1999;100:123–8.

51. Caramaschi P, Biasi D, Carletto A et al. Three cases of Buerger's disease associated with hyperhomocysteinemia. Clin Exp Rheumatol 2000;18:264–5.

52. Biasi D, Caramaschi P, Carletto A, Pasqualini R and Bambara LM. A case of Buerger's disease associated with high levels of lipoprotein(a). Clin Rheumatol 1999;18:59–60.

53. Rodgers GM and Conn MT. Homocysteine, an atherogenic stimulus, reduces protein C activation by arterial and venous endothelial cells. Blood 1990;75:895–901.

54. Lie JT. The Canadian Rheumatism Association, 1991 Dunlop-Dottridge Lecture. Vasculitis, 1815 to 1991: classification and diagnostic specificity. J Rheumatol 1992;19:83–9.

55. Scharfman W, B., Wallach JB and Angrist A. Myocardial infarction due to syphilitic coronary ostial stenosis. Amer Heart J 1950;40:603–613.

56. Steere AC, Lyme Disease. In: M.Schaechter, G.Medoff, and B.I.Eisenstein, editors. Mechanisms of microbial disease., Baltimore-London-Philadelphia-Tokyo: Williams and Wilkins, 1993;343–349.

57. Manzi S, Meilahn EN, Rairie JE et al. Age-specific incidence rates of myocardial infarction and angina in women with systemic lupus erythematosus: comparison with the Framingham Study. Am J Epidemiol 1997;145:408–15.

58. Haider YS and Roberts WC. Coronary arterial disease in systemic lupus erythematosus; quantification of degrees of narrowing in 22 necropsy patients (21 women) aged 16 to 37 years. Am J Med 1981;70:775–81.

59. Ilowite NT. Premature atherosclerosis in systemic lupus erythematosus. J Rheumatol 2000; Suppl 58:15–9.

60. Manzi S. Systemic lupus erythematosus: a model for atherogenesis? Rheumatology (Oxford) 2000;39:353–9.

61. George J, Harats D, Gilburd B, Levy Y, Langevitz P and Shoenfeld Y. Atherosclerosis-related markers in systemic lupus erythematosus patients: the role of humoral immunity in enhanced atherogenesis. Lupus 1999;8: 220–6.

62. Shoenfeld Y, Alarcon Segovia D, Buskila D et al. Frontiers of SLE: review of the 5th International Congress of Systemic Lupus Erythematosus, Cancun, Mexico, April 20–25, 1998. Semin Arthritis Rheum 1999;29:112–30.

63. Stvrtinova V, Ferencik M, Hulin I and Jahnova E. Vascular endothelium as a factor in information transfer between the cardiovascular and immune systems. Bratisl Lek Listy 1998;99:5–19. In Slovak

64. Ross R. Atherosclerosis is an inflammatory disease. Am Heart J 1999;138: S419–20.

65. Desai Mehta A, Lu L, Ramsey Goldman R and Datta SK. Hyperexpression of CD40 ligand by B and T cells in human lupus and its role in pathogenic autoantibody production. J Clin Invest 1996;97:2063–73.

66. Koshy M, Berger D and Crow MK. Increased expression of CD40 ligand on systemic lupus erythematosus lymphocytes. J Clin Invest 1996;98:826–37.

67. Hollenbaugh D, Mischel Petty N, Edwards CP et al. Expression of functional CD40 by vascular endothelial cells. J Exp Med 1995;182:33–40.

68. Aukrust P, Muller F, Ueland T et al. Enhanced levels of soluble and membrane-bound CD40 ligand in patients with unstable angina. Possible reflection of T lymphocyte and platelet involvement in the pathogenesis of acute coronary syndromes. Circulation 1999;100:614–20.

69. Gharavi AE and Wilson WA. The syndrome of thrombosis, thrombocytopenia, and recurrent spontaneous abortions associated with antiphospholipid antibodies: Hughes syndrome. Lupus 1996;5: 343–4.

70. Vaarala O, Manttari M, Manninen V et al. Anti-cardiolipin antibodies and risk of myocardial infarction in a prospective cohort of middle-aged men. Circulation 1995;91:23–7.

71. Morris PB, Imber MJ, Heinsimer JA, Hlatky MA and Reimer KA. Rheumatoid arthritis and coronary arteritis. Am J Cardiol 1986;57:689–90.

72. Bely M, Apathy A and Beke Martos E. Cardiac changes in rheumatoid arthritis. Acta Morphol Hung 1992;40:149–86.

73. Gravallese EM, Corson JM, Coblyn JS, Pinkus GS and Weinblatt ME. Rheumatoid aortitis: a rarely recognized but clinically significant entity. Medicine Baltimore 1989;68:95–106.

74. Landewe RB, van den Borne BE, Breedveld FC and Dijkmans BA. Methotrexate effects in patients with rheumatoid arthritis with cardiovascular comorbidity [letter]. Lancet 2000;355:1616–7.

Dyslipoproteinemia and Premature Atherosclerosis in the Pediatric Rheumatic Diseases

Diana Milojevic and Norman T. Ilowite

Division of Pediatric Rheumatology, Schneider Children's Hospital, Long Island Jewish Medical Center, Albert Einstein College of Medicine, New Hyde Park, NY 11040, USA

1. INTRODUCTION

Premature atherosclerosis and its sequelae, myocardial infarction (MI) and cerebrovascular accident (CVA), are recognized complications of systemic lupus erythematosus (SLE) [1–5]. Prevalence of severely narrowed coronary arteries has been demonstrated to be approximately 80% vs 30% in otherwise healthy age matched controls [4, 5]. Proposed etiologies include dyslipoproteinemia (DL), vasculitis, hypertension and increased tendency for thrombosis associated with the presence of antiphospholipid antibodies. With advances in medical therapy of the underlying chronic rheumatic disease, life expectancy has been improved, and complications of premature atherosclerosis have become significant causes of morbidity and mortality. Most investigators agree that the atherosclerosis process begins in childhood. Thus interventions directed toward prevention of premature atherosclerosis should also begin in childhood. This review will concentrate on recent developments in the understanding of DL in childhood rheumatic disorders.

2. THE SCOPE OF THE PROBLEM

Numerous case reports and series have documented the occurrence of complications of premature atherosclerosis in young adults and children with SLE [1–5]. The frequency of clinically recognizable coronary artery disease (CAD) in adults has been reported to be about 9%. Subclinical CAD is considerably higher in adults, approaching 40%. Autopsy studies show the incidence to be 45%. In a study of 40 children and adolescents with SLE and no cardiac symptoms, myocardial perfusion and function were assessed by thallium myocardial perfusion scans, radionuclide angiography with multiple gated acquisition and resting M-mode, and 2-dimensional echocardiography [6]. Perfusion abnormalities were found in 16%, including a large fixed defect in one patient. Low ejection fractions were found in 19% although exercise responses were normal [6]. In the group with abnormal thallium scans, three of five patients had antiphospholipid antibodies detected, and two of four had an abnormal plasma lipid profiles.

3. SERUM LIPOPROTEIN CONCENTRATIONS

DL is common in rheumatic disease patients. Ettinger found elevated plasma triglyceride, cholesterol and low-density lipoprotein cholesterol (LDL-C) to be elevated in 46 female SLE patients as compared to normal controls [7]. In this study, SLE patients who were being treated with corticosteroids had higher triglycerides and LDL-C than those who were not taking corticosteroids. The authors concluded that prednisone plays an important role in the lipoprotein abnormalities. In contrast, in prospective studies of children and adolescents with SLE before ever receiving corticosteroids and after corticosteroid treatment, two distinct patterns of DL were demonstrated: one related to the underlying disease, and another caused by administration of

329

systemic corticosteroids [8]. The DL secondary to the disease itself is characterized by depressed high density lipoprotein cholesterol (HDL-C), with elevated very low density lipoprotein cholesterol (VLDL-C) and triglycerides (TG) (the DL of active disease); whereas DL related to corticosteroid therapy consists of increased total cholesterol (TC), VLDL-C and TG (the DL of steroid therapy). Both of these patterns are atherogenic.

This pattern of active disease was confirmed, and shown to correlate with SLEDAI scores and presence of vasculitis in adults [9].

A similar pattern of DL consisting of low total cholesterol, low HDL-C and LDL-C with high VLDL-C and triglycerides has been demonstrated in patients with juvenile rheumatoid arthritis (JRA) [10]. Abnormalites in serum lipoprotein concentrations were most pronounced in patients with active arthritis and in systemic onset disease patients. These results were confirmed in another study showing correlation of ESR and CRP levels with dyslipoproteinemia in patients with JRA [11]. Patients with active JRA exhibit low levels of HDL2 and HDL3 and are deficient in plasma platelet-activating factor acetylhydrolase activity, suggesting the loss of anti-inflammatory activity of plasma ApoB- and ApoA-I-containing lipoproteins [12].

Lipoprotein (a) (Lp(a)), a cholesterol-rich plasma lipoprotein and a newly emerging risk factor for coronary artery disease and stroke, has been found to be elevated in adult SLE, but has not been systematically studied in children [13, 14].

4. MECHANISMS OF DYSLIPOPROTEINEMIA OF ACTIVE DISEASE

One potential mechanism for the low HDL levels found in untreated SLE patients is removal of antibodies complexed with Apo A1, the major apolipoprotein of HDL. To investigate the immunoreactivity of SLE sera with Apo A1, a mouse complementary DNA lambda phage expression library was screened by Merrill et al [15]. Using serum from an SLE patient who had had a cerebrovascular accident, 650,000 plaques were screened. Eighteen positive clones were identified, and 12 sequenced. One clone (MA1) had 82% DNA sequence homology

to human Apo A1. The protein produce of the MA1 clone reacted with Apo A1 antiserum but not normal mouse or human serum. Apo A1 competitively inhibited binding of ApoA1 antiserum to MA1. The authors conclude that MA1 may have both structural homology and immunologic relatedness to human Apo A1 and could represent a mouse homolog of this protein. Additionally, human Apo A1 could be an antigenic target in SLE patients.

One biochemical mechanism which may explain the lipoprotein abnormalities in untreated SLE patients is decreased lipoprotein lipase activity. This membrane bound enzyme is responsible for liberation of fatty acids from VLDL, resulting in the formation of LDL. LPL activity can be suppressed by tumor necrosis factor, interleukin-1, and gamma interferon. Magilavy et al postulated that deficiency of <u>hepatic</u> lipase may also play a role in the lipoprotein abnormalities in chronic inflammatory states such as JRA or SLE [16]. Hepatic lipase activity in MRL/lpr mice was 29.5% of that in age-matched control MRL/++ mice (p<.005). Polyinosinic-polycutidylic acid complex treatment (inducing reticuloendothelial activation) of control mice resulted in decreased hepatic lipase activity. Northern blot analysis of liver poly (A)+RNA showed no difference in hepatic lipase mRNA abundance in the two strains. The authors concluded, therefore, that the deficience in the MRL/lpr mice was at the translational or post-translational level.

In another study, chylomicron metabolism was found to be markedly abnormal; chylomicron removal dysfunction may also partially be responsible for this dyslipoproteinemic pattern [17].

The relationships between antiphospholipid antibodies and dyslipoproteinemia has been examined extensively in adults, and is reviewed elsewhere in this monograph.

5. HOMOCYSTEINE

Homocysteine is a nonessential amino acid produced by transamination of amino acids. Premature atherosclerosis has been identified in patients with familial homocysteinemia, prompting examination of the relationship of this amino acid to atherosclerosis. Several studies identified an association between hyperhomocysteinemia and occlusive vascular disease. Potential causal mechanisms include direct toxic effects on endothelium, as well as indirect effects including induction of vascular endothelial cell activator, promotion of smooth muscle proliferation, and inhibition of endothelial growth. Folic acid supplementation has been shown to lower plasma homocysteine concentrations. In a prospective study, Petri et al, followed 337 patients with SLE for 1619 person-years for occurrence of stroke and arterial or venous thrombotic events, as well as time of entry fasting plasma homocysteine levels [18]. Elevated homocysteine concentrations were found in 15% of the SLE patients, correlated with low serum folate levels, and were significantly associated with stroke and arterial thrombotic events (odds ratios 2.24 and 3.74, respectively).

6. MANAGEMENT

In the NZB/NZW murine SLE model, DL consisting of hypertriglyceridemia (similar to DL of active disease), responded to a menhaden oil diet which has high levels of omega-3 fatty acids [19]. In another murine SLE model, the MRL/lpr mouse was treated with estrogen to determine the effects on serum lipoprotein profiles [20]. A significant shift of cholesterol from HDL to LDL resulted in an increase in the amount of cholesterol on LDL particles after 1 week of treatment, and was significantly more pronounced than that seen in Balb/c or MRL/++ mice. The authors interpreted these results to mean that pharmacologic doses of estrogen may contribute to cardiovascular disease in this murine model. In another study, the effects of cholesterol loading on the MRL/lpr mouse were studied [21]. Mice getting a high cholesterol diet showed a rise in serum cholesterol 2.5 times that in mice on control diets, however the triglycerides, HDL-C and lipid peroxides significantly decreased. Aortic cholesterol content was significantly higher in mice fed the high cholesterol diet. The authors concluded that this murine SLE model is susceptible to diet-induced hypercholesterolemia and aortic cholesterol deposition. The mouse, while being a good model of SLE, may be a poor model in which to study DL and atherosclerosis, because of sharp differences in lipoprotein metabolism as compared to humans.

Studies of dietary intervention and fish oil sup-

plementation in children and adolescents with SLE were performed [22]. Twenty-four consecutive adolescents fulfilling SLE classification criteria were screened with fasting lipid profiles. Patients were identified as having DL of active disease or of corticosteroid therapy. Patients were treated for 6 weeks with dietary modification and if DL did not normalize, with another six weeks of dietary modification and fish oil supplementation. Seventeen patients (71%) had DL; 10 of active disease; 4 of steroid therapy; 3 with a combined pattern. Eleven patients underwent dietary modification including counseling on the Expert Panel on Blood Cholesterol Levels in Children and Adolescents NCEP step one Diet. This diet consists of no more than 30% of calories from fat, and less than 10% total calories from saturated fat, less than 300 mg/day of dietary cholesterol, and adequate energy intake to promote growth. There was a significant decrease in serum triglyceride concentrations (p<.05). Total cholesterol, LDL cholesterol and HDL cholesterol did not significantly change. A further significant decline in serum triglycerides was achieved with fish oil supplementation consisting of 1800 mg eicosapentaenoic and 620 mg of docosahexaenoic acids (p<.05). Five of the 11 patients who underwent treatment continued to have DL. The authors concluded that DL is common in pediatric SLE; dietary modification and fish oil supplementation appear to be effective in improving serum lipid profiles, and blinded studies are warranted. A significant number of patients may require pharmacologic therapy for persistent DL to prevent complications of premature atherosclerosis, which is similar to recommendations made for adults [23].

Lower cholesterol, LDL-C, triglyceride and Apo CIII levels were seen in adults with RA and SLE who were being treated with hydroxychloroquine, as compared to those not so treated [24–26]. Hydroxychloroquine treatment may be useful in improving lipoprotein levels in children as well.

Supplementation with antioxidant vitamins C and E has been found to improve arterial dilatation in children with familial hypercholesterolemia or combined hyperlipoproteinemia. [27]. Although the role of low dose aspirin in active young children is not known, there is good evidence that antithrombotic therapy is effective in prevention of complications of atherosclerosis, specifically myocardial infarctions.

Our current atherosclerosis preventive management in childhood SLE includes: discontinuation of smoking, control of hypertension, encouragement of regular aerobic activity and weight loss if obese, supplemental folate, vitamin E, vitamin C, and in older adolescents or children with antiphospholipid antibodies, consideration of low dose aspirin, as well as consideration of supplemental estrogen in patients who have ovarian failure secondary to cyclophosphamide therapy. We assess fasting lipoproteins. If dyslipoproteinemia is present we prescribe an NCEP step I diet, and reassess. If dyslipoproteinemia persists we supplement with fish oil. If DL of active disease persists (high TG, low HDL-C), we consider treatment with nicotinic acid or fibric acids. If DL of corticosteroid therapy is found (increased TC, VLDL-C, LDL-C, and TG), we consider treatment with HMG-CoA reductase inhibitors.

7. SUMMARY

DL is common in the pediatric rheumatic diseases, and may play a significant role in development of premature atherosclerosis. Both chronic inflammatory disease and its treatment with corticosteroids contribute to DL, however, differential patterns of DL are evident. Antiphospholipid antibody presence which increases the risk of thrombosis, may also be associated with DL, further increasing the atherosclerosis risk. Prevention of premature atherosclerosis with treatment of DL should begin in the pediatric age group. Initial treatment with dietary modification and physical activity is indicated. In select patients, fish oil supplementation or pharmacologic intervention with lipid lowering agents may be indicated.

REFERENCES

1. Meller J, Conde CA, Deppisch LM, et al. Myocardial infarction due to coronary atherosclerosis in three young adults with systemic lupus erythematosus. Am J Cardiol 1975;35:309–314.
2. Spiera H, Rothenberg RR. Myocardial infarction in four young patients with systemic lupus erythematosus. J Rheumatol 1983;10:464–466.
3. Homey CJ, Liberthson RR, Fallon JT, et al. Ischemic heart disease in systemic lupus erythematosus in the young patient: report of six cases. Am J Cardiol 1982;49:478–484.
4. Haider VS, Roberts WC. Coronary arterial disease in systemic lupus erythematosus: qualification of degrees of narrowing in 22 necropsy patients (21 women) aged 16–37 years. Am J Med 1981;70:775–781.
5. Bulkley BH, Roberts WC. The heart in systemic lupus erythematosus and the changes induced in it by corticosteroid therapy. A study of 36 necropsy patients. Am J Med 1975;58:243–264.
6. Gazarian M, Feldman BM, Benson LN et al. Assessment of myocardial perfusion and function in childhood systemic lupus erythematosus. J Pediatr 1998;132:109–16.
7. Ettinger W, Appelbaum-Bouden D, Wylez F, et al. Dyslipoproteinemia in systemic lupus erythematosus. Arthritis Rheum 1985;28:S46.
8. Ilowite N, Samuel P, Ginzler E, and Jacobson MS. Dyslipoproteinemia in pediatric systemic lupus erythematosus. Arthritis Rheum 1988;31:859–63.
9. Borba EF, Bonfa E. Dyslipoproteinemias in systemic lupus erythematosus: influence of disease, activity, and anti-cardiolipin antibodies. Lupus 1997;6:533–9.
10. Ilowite N, Samuel P, Beseler L, and Jacobson MS. Dyslipoproteinemia in juvenile rheumatoid arthritis. J Pediatr 1989;114:823–826.
11. Bakkaloglu A, Kirel B, Ozen S et al. Plasma lipids and lipoproteins in juvenile chronic arthritis. Clin Rheumatol 1996;15:341–5.
12. Tselepis AD, Elisaf M, Besis S et al. Association of the inflammatory state in active juvenile rheumatoid arthritis with hypo-high-density lipoproteinemia and reduced lipoprotein-associated platelet-activating factor acetylhydrolase activity. Arthritis Rheum 1999;42:373–83.
13. Borba EF, Santos RD, Bonfa E, Vinagre CG, Pileggi FJ, Cossermelli W, Maranhao RC. Lipoprotein(a) levels in systemic lupus erythematosus. J Rheumatol 1994;21:220–223.
14. Kawai S, Mizushima Y, Kaburaki J. Increased serum lipoprotein(a) levels in systemic lupus erythematosus with myocardial and cerebral infarctions. J Rheumatol 1995;22:1210–1211.
15. Merrill JT, Rivkin E, Shen C, Lahita RG. Selection of a gene for apolipoprotein A1 using autoantibodies from a patient with systemic lupus erythematosus. Arthritis Rheum 1995;38:1655–1659.
16. Magilavy DB, Zhan R, Black DD. Modulation of murine hepatic lipase activity by exogenous and endogenous Kupffer-cell activation. Biochem J 1993;292:255.
17. Borba EF, Bonfa E, Vanagre CG et al. Chylomicron

metabolism is markedly altered in systemic lupus erythematosus. Arthritis Rheum 2000;43:1033–40.

18. Petri M, Roubenoff R, Dullal G et al. Plasma homocyteine as a risk factor for atherosclerotic events in systemic lupus erythematosus. J Rheumatol 1995;22:450–4.

19. Jacobson MS, Tractman H, Feldman J, Samuel P, Ilowite NT. Dyslipoproteinemia in murine systemic lupus erythematosus. Atherosclerosis, 1989;79:205–211.

20. Zuckerman SH, Bryan-Poole N. Estrogen-induced alterations in lipoprotein metabolism in autoimmune MRL/lpr mice. Arterioscler Thromb Vasc Biol 1995;15:1556–1562.

21. Yamaguchi Y, Kitagawa S, Imaizumi N, Kunitomo M, Fujiwara M. Effects of cholesterol loading on autoimmune MRL-lpr/lpr mice: susceptibility to hypercholesterolemia and aortic cholesterol deposition. Jpn J Pharmacol 1993;61:291–298.

22. Ilowite NT, Copperman N, Leicht T, Kwong T, Jacobson MS. Effects of dietary modification and fish oil supplementation on dyslipoproteinemia in pediatric systemic lupus erythematosus. J Rheumatol 1995;22:1347–1351.

23. Hearth-Holmes M, Baethge BA, Broadwell L, Wolf RE. Dietary treatment of hyperlipidemia in patients with systemic lupus erythematosus. J Rheumatol 1995;22:450–454.

24. Wallace DJ, Metzger AL, Stechler VJ, Turnbull BA, Kern PA. Cholesterol lowering effect of hydroxychloroquine in patients with rheumatic disease: reversal of deleterious effects of steroids on lipids. Am J Med 1987;89:322–326.

25. Hodis HN, Quismorio FP, Wickham E, Blankenhorn DH. The lipid, lipoprotein, and apolipoprotein effects of hydroxychloroquine in patients with systemic lupus erythematosus. J Rheumaol 1993;20:661–5.

26. Petri M, Lakatta C, Magder L, Goldman D. Effect of prednisone and hydroxychloroquine on coronary artery disease risk factors in systemic lupus erythematosus: a longitudinal data analysis. Am J Med 1994;96:254–259.

27. Mietus-Snyder M, Malloy MJ. Endothelial dysfunction occurs in children with two genetic hyperlipidemias: improvement with antioxidant vitamin therapy. J Pediatr 1998;133:35–40.

Atherosclerosis and Autoimmunity
Y. Shoenfeld, D. Harats and G. Wick, editors

Atherosclerosis and Familial Mediterranean Fever

Pnina Langevitz[1], Avi Livneh[1], Lily Neumann[2], Dan Buskila[2], Joshua Shemer[1] and Mordechai Pras[1]

[1]*The Heller Institute of Medical Research, Sheba Medical Center, Tel-Hashomer and Sackler Faculty of Medicine, Tel Aviv University, Tel Aviv, Israel;* [2]*Rheumatic Disease Unit and Epidemiology Department, Soroka Medical Center, Faculty of Health Sciences, Ben Gurion University of the Negev, Beer Sheva, Israel*

Familial Mediterranean fever (FMF) is an autosomal recessive disease, found more commonly among Sephardi and North African Jews, Armenians, Arabs, Druze and Turks, and characterized by recurrent, self limited febrile attacks of serosal inflammation, involving the peritoneum, pleura and synovium [1]. The attacks may also involve the pericardium, skin, muscles and testes [1–3]. In a large proportion of untreated patients, amyloidosis may develop [1]. FMF patients are treated with colchicine in a dose of 1–2 mg/day continuously. This drug prevents the febrile attacks in most patients and amyloidosis in practically all [4, 5]. The attacks of FMF are associated with various markers of inflammation, reflected clinically by fever and pain in the affected sites; histologically by an invasion of polymorphonuclear leukocytes to the serosal membranes. During the febrile attacks, an acute-phase response develops, manifested by marked increase in erythrocyte sedimentation rate (ESR), white blood cell (WBC) count, fibrinogen, serum amyloid A (SAA), phospholipase A$_2$ (PLA$_2$), and C-reactive protein (CRP) [6–8]. Inflammatory mediators like IL-6 and soluble receptors of TNF were recently found to be also increased during the FMF attacks [7].

The FMF gene, which is mapped to chromosome 16p, was recently cloned and found to encode a previously unknown protein thought to be a transcription factor [9–11]. Although the role of the FMF gene in the development of FMF attacks is yet to be determined, its malfunction results eventually in inflammation with local and systemic consequences.

Systemic inflammation is an important factor in the initiation and development of atherosclerosis [12–15]. A recent study showed that in normal men, serum levels of CRP may predict future myocardial infarction and ischemic stroke. The increased risk of elevated CRP was independent of lipid-related and non-lipid related cardiovascular risk factors and was reduced by treatment with aspirin, causing a fall in the base-line CRP levels [16]. With respect to the inflammatory background of atherosclerosis, one may expect an increased morbidity of IHD in patients with FMF. To examine this hypothesis, we performed a study looking for the prevalence of IHD in patients with FMF. However, we did not find an increased prevalence of IHD in FMF patients compared to that in the Israeli population (16%) of similar age and sex, but it was significantly lower than in patients with other inflammatory conditions [17].

Inflammation has a role in both the precipitation of acute ischemic events and the chronic development of atherosclerosis underlying IHD. This notion is supported by several lines of evidence: elevated serum levels of CRP are predictive of future myocardial infarction and ischemic stroke, and administration of aspirin decreases this risk in direct correlation to the reduction in CRP values. Elevated levels of CRP were found in patients with unstable angina [18] and are associated with a risk of fatal coronary disease among smokers [19]. In addition, inflammatory cell infiltrates and evidence for immunologic activation of these cells may be found in atheromatous plaques in both acute and chronic ischemic syndromes [13–15]. IL-6 was found to be

335

associated with the recruitment of macrophages and monocytes into atherosclerotic plaques [20]. And finally, patients who develop a significant increase of their serum amyloid A in the first 24 hours after percutaneous coronary angioplasty (PTCA) had a high relative risk for developing restenosis in the first year after PTCA [21].

Since inflammation is a risk factor for ischemic events and is a sine qua non of FMF attacks, and since colchicine completely prevents attacks in only 60% of FMF patients, 30% experience significant improvement but still suffer from some inflammatory FMF attacks, and the rest, 10%, of the patients remain unaffected, we expected an increased frequency of IHD in FMF patients, a hypothesis that allegedly was not confirmed in our study [17]. Failure to display higher than normal rates of IHD in FMF may still be attributed to the continuous life-long therapy with colchicine, started in most FMF patients before age 20 [4, 5]. This treatment probably reduces the expected increased frequency of IHD in FMF patients. The fact that less FMF patients are obese could also be related to colchicine therapy, which may cause a decrease in appetite, nausea and diarrhea [4], or simply to more careful eating employed by patients as a means of protection from abdominal attacks.

FMF is very common among the ethnically predisposed population. The frequency of the gene in carriers was computed to be 1:7–1:20 in North African Jews [22]. Such frequency favors a protecting role for the gene. However, in order to be widely scattered among the population, a protective gene should offer its benefits prior to or during the childbearing age. Protection against IHD, which is a disease of the elderly, does not carry any evolutionary advantage and therefore it is unlikely to be related to the FMF gene. Possible benefits of the FMF gene should be explored elsewhere. Similar conclusion, that the FMF gene does not provide protection against IHD was obtained in another study [23]. Our study supported a probable role for colchicine in the protection against inflammation induced by atherosclerosis [17].

In conclusion, colchicine treated FMF patients, despite being subjected continuously to inflammation, a novel risk factor for IHD, sustain IHD with a frequency comparable to the general population, probably due to the favorable effect of colchicine.

REFERENCES

1. Sohar E, Gafni J, Pras M, Heller H. Familial Mediterranean fever. A survey of 470 cases and review of the literature. Am J Med 1967;43:227–53.
2. Kees S, Langevitz P, Zemer D, Padeh S, Pras M, Livneh A. Attacks of pericarditis as a manifestation of familial Mediterranean fever. Q J Med 1997;90:643–7.
3. Livneh A, Langevitz P, Zemer D, Migdal A, Sohar E, Pras M. The changing face of familial Mediterranean fever. Semin Arthritis Rheum 1996;26:612–27.
4. Zemer D, Revach M, Pras M, Modan B, Schor S, Sohar E, Gafni J. A controlled trial of colchicine in preventing attacks of familial Mediterranean fever. N Engl J Med 1974;291:932–4.
5. Zemer D, Pras M, Sohar E, Modan M, Cabili S, Gafni J. Colchicine in the prevention and treatment of the amyloidosis of familial Mediterranean fever. N Engl J Med 1986;314:1001–5.
6. Knecht A, de Beer FC, Pras M. Serum amyloid A protein in familial Mediterranean fever. Ann Int Med 1985;102:71–72.
7. Gang N, Drenth YPH, Livneh A, Langevitz P, Zemer D, Brezniak N, Pras M, van der Meer YWM. Activation of the cytokine network in familial Mediterranean fever. In: Familial Mediterranean Fever, Sohar E, Gafni J, Pras M. (eds.) Freund Publishing House Ltd. 1997;193–6.
8. Cang J, Musser JH, McGregor H. Phospholipase A$_2$: Function and pharmacological regulation. Biochem Pharmacol 1987;36:2429–36.
9. Pras E, Aksentijevich I, Gruberg L, Prosen L, Dean M, Pras M, Kastner DL. Mapping of a gene causing familial Mediterranean fever to the short arm of chromosome 16. N Engl J Med 1992;326:1509–13.
10. The International FMF Consortium. Ancient missense mutations in a new member of the RoRet gene family are likely to cause familial Mediterranean fever. Cell 1997;90:797–807.
11. The French FMF Consortium. A candidate gene for familial Mediterranean fever. Nature Genetics 1997;17:25–31.
12. Munro JM, Cotran RS. The pathogenesis of atherosclerosis: atherogenesis and inflammation. Lab Invest 1988;58:249–61.
13. Fuster V, Badimon L, Badimon JJ, Chesebro YM. The pathogenesis of coronary artery disease and of the acute coronary symptoms. N Engl J Med 1992;326:242–50.
14. Ross R. The pathogenesis of artherosclerosis: a prospective for the 1990's. Nature 1993;362:801–9.
15. Alexander RW. Inflammation and coronary artery disease. N Engl J Med 1994;331:468–9.
16. Ridker PM, Cushman M, Stampfer MJ, Tracy RP, Hennekens CH. Inflammation, aspirin and the risk of car-

diovascular disease in apparently healthy men. N Engl J Med 1997;336:973–9.

17. Langevitz P, Livneh A, Neumann L, Buskila D, Pras M. The prevalence of ischemic heart disease in patients with familial Mediterranean fever. IMAJ (accepted for publication).

18. Liuzzo G, Biasucci LM, Gallimore JR, Grillo RL, Rebuzzi AG, Pepys MB, Maseri A. The prognostic value of C-reactive protein and serum anyloid A protein in severe unstable angina. N Engl J Med 1994, 331:417–24.

19. Kuller LH, Tracy RP, Shaten J, Meilahn EN. Relation of C-reactive protein and coronary artery disease in the MRFIT nested case-control study. Am J Epidermiol 1996, 14:537–47

20. Biasucci LM, Viterlli A, Liuzzo G, Almatura S, Cali-giuri G, Monaco C, Rebuzzi AG, Gilibero G, Maseri A. Elevated levels of interleukin-6 in unstable angina. Circulation 1996;94:874–7.

21. Blum A, Vardinon N, Kaplan G, Laniado S, Yust I, Burk M, Miller H. Autoimmune and inflammatory responses may have an additive effect in postpercutaneous transluminal coronary angioplasty restenosis. Am J Cardiol 1988, 81:339–41.

22. Daniels M, Shohat T, Brenner-Ullman A. Familial Mediterranean fever. High gene frequency among the non-Ashkenazic and Ashkenazic Jewish population in Israel. Am J Med Genet 1995;55:311–4.

23. Brenner-Ullman A, Melzer-Ofir H, Daniels M, Shohat M. Possible protection against asthma in heterozygotes for familial Mediterranean fever. Am J Med Genet 1994;53:172–75.

GENETIC OF THROMBOSIS

Atherosclerosis and Autoimmunity
Y. Shoenfeld, D. Harats and G. Wick, editors

Genetics of Arterial Thrombosis: Contribution to Atherosclerosis

Eduardo C. Lau

Specialty Laboratories, Inc., Santa Monica, CA 90404, USA

1. INTRODUCTION

Arterial thrombosis (AT) is a pivotal event in the natural history of coronary heart disease (CHD), stroke (cerebrovascular ischemic disease), and peripheral vascular disease. CHD represents a continuum of myocardial ischemia ranging from unstable angina to coronary artery disease (CAD), and to myocardial infarction (MI). Although a family history of CAD is a risk factor for cardiovascular ischemic episodes, the overall impact of family history is modest [1]. Common forms of AT segregate in a non-Mendelian inheritance pattern. Over 95% of early CHD cases are not caused by monogenic defects such as familial hypercholesterolemia (FH), but rather by multiple genetic and environmental determinants. The pathogenesis of AT is probably different from that of venous thrombosis (VT). Most forms of AT are multifactorial disorders resulted from many different combinations of genetic prothrombotic polymorphisms and environmental atherogenic factors, even though some by themselves may not be sufficient to cause disease [2]. Environmental risk factors for AT include high fat diets, cigarette smoking, increased salt consumption, and decreased intake of folate.

Intravascular thrombogenesis is influenced by a complex display of procoagulant, anticoagulant, and fibrinolytic factors. The elucidation of genes responsible for CHD or stroke is difficult, because the relative importance of genetic factors is often affected by environmental factors. Traits governed by a small number of genes are reflected in discontinuous distributions, whereas very complex genetic traits determined by the additive action of a large number of genes yield a Gaussian distribution for continuously variable susceptibility. Thus, polygenic inheritance traits of AT can be represented by a Gaussian distribution, in which a threshold for susceptibility is postulated [3]. When affected individuals inherit a combination of susceptibility genes that raise the susceptibility beyond the threshold, thrombotic events occur.

2. GENETIC DETERMINANTS FOR SUSCEPTIBILITY TO ARTERIAL THROMBOSIS

Common forms of atherosclerosis and AT result from the interaction of many different combinations of genetic and environmental factors. In the presence of unfavorable environmental factors, genetic factors are the primary determinants of AT. Linkage and association studies have identified a number of candidate genes, polymorphic DNA markers, and nongenetic risk factors for atherosclerosis and AT [4]. Potential polymorphic genetic markers for predisposition to CHD include lipid- and lipoprotein-related risk factors, thrombotic and fibrinolytic variables, platelet-related factors, inflammatory markers, homocysteine levels, and von Willebrand factors [5, 6].

Although a wide variety of candidate genes are available for the study of genotype-AT phenotype association, it is not easy to demonstrate associations between genetic risk factors and AT. Initial studies of these genetic risk factors for AT are commonly conducted in small numbers of individuals. Subsequent confirmation of these candidate genetic markers for AT, which necessitate large population studies, is hampered by the poor definition and/or the high complexity of the diseases. In addition, the clinical significance of many of these polymorphic genetic markers is often disputed by prospective studies. Because AT is determined by both genetic and environmental factors, it may not be possible to extrapolate those genetic markers established for the US Caucasians to subjects of other countries with different ethnic populations and environmental background.

3. ATHEROSCLEROSIS: PREDISPOSITION TO ARTERIAL THROMBOSIS

3.1. Atherosclerotic Coronary Artery Diseases

Atherosclerotic vascular thrombosis is a multifactorial disease caused by the interaction of genetic and acquired risk factors [7]. Atherosclerosis denotes a heterogeneous disease, under which etiologically distinct diseases are subsumed. Traditional risk factors for premature CHD (under the age of 60) include gender, hyperlipidemia, diabetes mellitus, hypertension, cigarette smoking, and obesity [2, 8, 9]. The most common form of CHD is atherosclerotic coronary artery disease (CAD) resulted from genetic factors for atherosclerosis. By considering atherosclerosis as a chronic inflammatory process predisposing an individual to AT, ischemic CHD and stroke are linked with a common mechanism [10].

3.1.1. Risk profiles for atherosclerosis

Early atherogenesis: Prospective studies of atherosclerosis show that the risk profile of early atherogenesis includes traditional vascular risk factors such as hypertension, hyperlipidemia and cigarette smoking [2], as well as several less well-established risk factors including iron overload, hypothyroidism, microalbuminuria, and high alcohol consumption [11]. Iron overload might contribute to gender-related difference in the manifestation of AT phenotype [11]. Although cigarette smoking increases the risk of early carotid atherogenesis, this correlation is confined to smokers with high circulating bacterial endotoxin [11].

Advanced atherogenesis: The majority of patients experiencing acute MI (AMI) have advanced atherosclerotic CAD and occlusive AT. With increasing severity of atherosclerosis, the risk profile undergoes substantial changes and most traditional risk factors lose their predictive significance [11]. The risk profile for advanced atherosclerosis includes markers for enhanced prothrombotic activity, attenuated fibrinolysis, as well as clinical conditions that promote coagulation such as high fibrinogen, low antithrombin, factor V (*FV*) gene Leiden mutation, high lipoprotein(a) [Lp(a)], high platelet count, cigarette smoking, and diabetes mellitus [2, 11]. These findings suggest that atherothrombosis is a key mechanism in the development of advanced stenotic atherosclerosis, while hyperlipidemia and hypertension are of only minor relevance for advanced atherogenesis. Cigarette smoking initiates a variety of dose-dependent prothrombotic conditions at both platelet and coagulation levels, and thus is a prominent risk factor for advanced stenotic atherogenesis [11].

Gene-environment interactions are important for the expression of familial combined hyperlipidemia, which is characterized by increased plasma concentrations of cholesterol, triglyceride, apolipoprotein B (apoB), and/or low-density lipoprotein (LDL). Elevated levels of D-dimer indicate the presence of a chronic hypercoagulable state (thrombophilia); whereas, low levels of apoA-I (the major protein constituent of HDL), and high levels of apoB indicate lipid transport disorder that contributes to enhanced deposition of lipids in atherosclerotic plaques. Combined with elevated levels of D-dimer, low apoA-I and high apoB levels enhance thrombogenic activity, that contributes to recurrent coronary events [12].

Whereas atherosclerosis predisposes an individual to the risk of AT, the development of thrombosis over atherosclerotic plaques is due to either superficial or deep intimal injury [13]. Platelets participate in the formation of thrombotic plugs on injured arterial wall, notably the atherosclerotic arterial wall. A high platelet count confers an increased risk of advanced atherogenesis [11]. The progression of atherosclerosis to thrombotic occlusion involves complex biochemical processes [10, 14], including synthesis and secretion of various mediators of coagulation, such as ADP, thromboxane A_2, and von-Willebrand factor (vWF) [15]. Activated platelets expose the cell surface receptor (GP) IIb/IIIa, which binds fibrinogen (Fg), vWF, and fibronectin. Fg is a bivalent protein, which is responsible for cross-linking platelets and causing platelet to aggregate. vWF is responsible for the adhesion of platelets to abnormal endothelium at sites of damage. Collagens and other prothrombic molecules also bind to specific platelet receptors. Eventually, platelet aggregation leads to the formation of thrombus on the diseased vessel wall, and occlusive AT [10].

3.1.2. Initiation and progression of atherogenesis

Initiation of atherosclerotic plaques: In the initial stage, atherosclerotic plaques are generated, but there are no clinical symptoms. Platelets and fibrinogen participate in the formation of arterial thrombi. Within the vessel, fibrinogen derived from the infiltration of plasma appears to directly enhance atherogenesis by converting to fibrin, which binds LDL and stimulates proliferation of vascular smooth muscle cells (SMC).

Progression of atherosclerotic plaques: In the later stage, advanced atherosclerotic plaques cause symptomatic diseases, in which thrombosis plays a major role in precipitating acute clinical symptoms, such as ischemic MI caused by sudden arterial occlusion. The density of atherosclerotic plaques present in the coronary and cerebral arteries is a determinant for the risk of disease progression. Plaques with high lipid and macrophage content, in which the number of smooth muscle cells is low, are at the greatest risk of disruption.

3.2. Non-atherosclerotic Coronary Artery Diseases

Although atherosclerotic AT is the most common pathophysiologic mechanism underlying CHD, AMI also occurs in the absence of significant coronary obstruction in 5–10% of cases [9, 16]. These non-atherosclerotic AMI cases, which lack traditional risk factors, can be either congenital or acquired CAD, or a hereditary connective tissue disorder with coronary artery involvement [9]. Sometimes in AMI, cocaine-induced vasospasm and coronary obstruction need to be considered.

4. LIPID- AND LIPOPROTEIN-RELATED GENETIC MARKERS OF PREDISPOSITION TO ATHEROSCLEROTIC ARTERIAL THROMBOSIS

Lipids and lipoproteins play an important role in the pathogenesis of CHD. Polymorphic genes, whose products are involved in the metabolism of lipids and lipoproteins, e.g. apolipoproteins (apo), LDL-receptors (LDL-R), lipoprotein lipase (LPL), and cholesteryl ester transfer protein (CETP), are potential determinants for susceptibility to CHD. Hyperlipidemia plays a crucial role in early atherogenesis, and is a traditional risk factor for CHD. Hypertension, cigarette smoking, and diabetes mellitus are primary risk factors for hyperlipidemia. Hypertension plays an important role in early atherogenesis [11]. The incidence of CHD is directly related to plasma levels of LDL and apoB, and is inversely related to plasma levels of HDL and apoA-I [5]. Total cholesterol, LDL-C, apolipoprotein B (apoB), low high-density lipoprotein cholesterol (HDL-C), and total cholesterol/HDL-C ratio, are all risk predictors of atherogenesis [11]. Genes involved in fatty acid and lipoprotein metabolism, such as genes encoding LDL-R, LPL, PAI-1, stromelysin, apolipoproteins (apo) A-I, and apo C-III are also candidates for CHD involvement. Polymorphisms in the promoter region of many of these genes substantially alter gene transcription.

4.1. Apolipoprotein Genes

Apolipoprotein(a) gene [Apo(a)]: Apo(a) encodes a lipoprotein composed of a serine protease domain, a kringle V-like domain, and 15–40 tandem repeats resembling the kringle IV domain of plasminogen [17, 18]. Variability in the number of kringle IV repeats, together with polymorphism in the promoter region of *Apo(a)* gene, accounts for most of the genetic variability. The *Apo(a)* gene determines greater than 90% of variation in plasma levels of Lp(a) in a given population [19]. Plasma concentrations of lipoprotein(a) [Lp(a)] are inversely correlated with the size of apo(a) molecules.

Lp(a), a cholesterol-carrying lipoprotein, shows an independent dose-response relation with the risk of early atherogenesis [11]. Polymorphisms in the

Apo(a) gene that increase the plasma level of Lp(a) are associated with increased risk of AT [20, 21]. A high plasma level of Lp(a) might be a monogenic risk factor which accounts for a major portion of familial predisposition to CHD [22]. Because plasma Lp(a) concentrations are inversely correlated with the size of apo(a) molecules, low molecular weight isoforms of apo(a) are more frequently found in patients with CHD [21].

Lp(a) localized in the intima, subintima, and plaque shoulder adhere to fibrin monolayers. Lp(a) competes with plasminogen for binding to fibrinogen and fibrin, and attenuates lysis of fibrin clots [23]. An elevated plasma level of Lp(a) is an indicator of rapid progression of atherosclerosis, and a strong risk factor for stenosis [11]. In addition, Lp(a) induces the expression and secretion of plasminogen activator inhibitor (PAI), which reduces vascular fibrinolytic capacity and thromboresistance. A prospective study, however, did not support the association of Lp(a) level with MI [24].

Although measurement of plasma Lp(a) is not recommended as a general screening test for assessing cardiovascular risk, this assay should be considered for patients with premature CHD who have relatively normal lipid levels, and for patients who have a family history of premature CHD or stroke.

Apolipoprotein B (apoB) gene: apoB is a glycoprotein existing in two isoforms, apoB-100 and apoB-48. The apoB-100 isoform, a polypeptide of apparent 550 kDa synthesized primarily in the liver, constitutes the protein component of LDL, and is essential for the assembly of very low-density lipoproteins (VLDL) in the liver. apoB-100 serves as a ligand for LDL-receptors (LDL-R) involved in the recognition and catabolism of plasma LDL. The apoB-48 isoform, a truncated form of apoB-100 synthesized primarily in the small intestine, is a structural protein which is crucial for the formation of chylomicrons in the intestine.

Genetic variations in the *ApoB* gene influence the plasma levels of apoB-containing lipoproteins [21, 25]. Elevated serum levels of apoB are associated with increased risk of premature atherosclerosis [26]. An insertion-deletion (*I/D*) polymorphism in the signal peptide of apoB modulates the effect of *ApoE2* genotype on plasma levels of cholesterol, LDL-cholesterol (LDL-C) [27], and very low-density lipoprotein-triglyceride (VLDL-TG) [28, 29]. In addition, an interaction between a common *ApoB X2* allele and the *ApoE E4* allele(s) increases the risk of cerebrovascular atherosclerosis [30].

Apolipoprotein E (ApoE) gene: apoE, an arginine-rich glycoprotein (34 kDa) composed of 299 amino acid residues, is an integral component of lipoproteins. The apoE molecule has a receptor-binding domain between codons 140 and 160, and acts as a ligand for LDL-receptors (LDL-R) on liver cells to direct lipoprotein metabolism. Two common polymorphisms in the *ApoE* gene, C112R and C158R, yield three alleles, *E2*, *E3* and *E4*, which code for apoE2 (112C, 158C), apoE3 (112C, 158R), and apoE4 (112R, 158R) isoforms, respectively [31]. These different apoE isoforms have different affinity for liver LDL-R, and subsequent up-regulation of LDL-R.

Plasma concentrations of apoE and cholesterol are partially determined by the *ApoE* genotype. *ApoE3* is the most frequent allele in the US population. The *ApoE2* allele is associated with lower plasma cholesterol and higher apoE concentrations. The ApoE4 allele present in approximately 25% of the general population is associated with higher plasma cholesterol and lower apoE concentrations [32]. Both the *E2* and *E4* alleles of *ApoE* are associated with hypertriglyceridemia, which is a common metabolic disorder occurring in greater than 5% of Western populations. The *ApoE4* allele promotes atherosclerosis and is associated with increased risk for both ischemic CHD [33] and stroke [34, 35]; whereas, the *ApoE2* allele is either pro- or anti-atherogenic, depending on the influence of environmental and other genetic factors [36]. The prevalence of *MTHFR* C677T homozygosity is significantly higher among premature MI patients [2].

The combination of *ApoE4* genotype and prothrombic factors such as smoking increases the risk of AMI [2]. The current concept is that the *ApoE* gene is a susceptibility locus, and the *ApoE4* genotype predisposes an individual to CAD, but the utility of *ApoE* genotyping in assessing the risk for CAD is not fully defined.

4.2. Lipoprotein-modifying Genes

Lipoprotein lipase (LPL) gene: LPL, a glycoprotein particularly abundant in muscle, adipose tissue and macrophages is bound to glycosaminoglycans of the capillary endothelium. Because LPL regulates the rate of hydrolysis and removal of core triglyceride in chylomicrons, as well as very-low-density lipoprotein (VLDL) triglycerides from the circulation, it affects plasma lipid levels and plays a central role in lipoprotein metabolism [37]. Plasma triglyceride levels are simultaneously modulated by polymorphisms at the *LPL* and *ApoE* genes [38]. The *LPL* gene is a candidate for predisposition to dyslipidemia and risk of atherosclerosis.

A *Hind* III polymorphism in intron 8 of the *LPL* gene influences plasma levels of triglyceride and HDL-C [39, 40]. The *H*-allele of *Hind* III polymorphism, which occurs at an allelic frequency of approximately 30%, is associated with reduced plasma triglyceride (TG) levels, and lower risk for coronary atherosclerosis and premature MI [41].

Common variations, D9N, N291S and S447X (X indicates a stop codon), within the coding region of the *LPL* gene affect plasma lipid levels [31]. Heterozygosity for the D9N or N291S mutation in *LPL* gene, which occurs at frequencies of up to approximately 5% in the general population, predisposes an individual to elevated levels of plasma triglyceride (TG), as well as reduced levels of HDL-C. These genetic variations, which results in decrease in amount or catalytic activity of LPL, as well as reduced HDL-C levels, are correlated with increased progression of coronary atherosclerosis, and enhanced susceptibility to premature CAD [42, 43]. The relative frequency of LPL N291S mutation increases in patients with lower HDL-C levels, hypoalphalipoproteinemia.

The nonsense S447X mutation of *LPL* gene causes premature translational termination and truncates the LPL polypeptide by two amino acids. This S447X polymorphism, which is in very strong allelic association with the *H*-allele of *Hind* III polymorphism in intron 8 of the *LPL* gene, occurs at carrier frequency of approximately 20% in the general population, and is associated with lower plasma levels of triglycerides (TG), as well as lower risk of coronary atherosclerosis and premature MI [41].

Cholesteryl ester transfer protein (CETP) gene: CETP is an extremely hydrophobic, heat stable glycoprotein synthesized in the liver, small intestine, spleen, and adrenal glands. CETP-mediated plasma lipid transfer processes play a central role in the metabolism of HDL-C, and may alter the susceptibility to atherosclerosis [44]. An increased plasma activity of CETP results in atherogenic change in lipoprotein metabolism in obese children [45].

Among men with established CAD, the CETP Taq IB polymorphism in intron 1 is associated with higher plasma CETP concentrations and progression of coronary atherosclerosis [46]. *B1* and *B2* alleles denote the presence and absence of the *Taq* I restriction site, respectively. Pravastatin therapy slows the progression of coronary atherosclerosis in patients with *B1/B1* genotype, but not with *B2/B2* genotype [46]. Besides the *Taq* IB polymorphism, *Msp* I (intron 8) and *Rsa* I (intron 14) polymorphisms of the *CETP* gene also influence plasma levels of CETP and HDL-C [47].

Paraoxonase (PON) genes: Paraoxonase (PON), a 44-kDa glycoprotein, is a HDL-associated enzyme that hydrolyzes lipid peroxides. The paraoxonase gene family contains at least three members, *PON1*, *PON2* and *PON3,* clustered at the q21.3–22.1 region of chromosome 7 [48]. They may have arisen from tandem duplication of a common evolutionary precursor. The *PON1* gene is expressed mainly in the liver. Its gene product, PON1, plays an important role in lipoprotein metabolism and might be associated with risk of atherosclerotic CHD. The activity of plasma PON1 influences the oxidation of lipids and phospholipids in LDL and HDL. Some oxidized LDL (oxLDL) and PL, which participate in atherogenesis, are also substrates for paraoxonase.

Common polymorphisms, Q192R and M55L, in the *PON1* gene determine the variation in plasma PON activity among individuals, as well as the antioxidant capacity of HDL to protect LDL against oxidative modification. Individuals with the 192Q-allele of *PON1* show lower plasma activity of PON than those with the 192R-allele [49]. Polymorphisms in the *PON1* gene modulate the plasma levels of most lipoproteins including LDL-C and HDL-C, and thus the resistance to atherogenesis and CHD [50–54].

4.3. Genes Related to Cellular Lipid Metabolism

Low-density lipoprotein receptor (LDL-R) gene: LDL, a hydrophilic complex of lipid and apoB-100, is one of the major cholesterol-carrier lipoproteins in plasma. Elevated plasma levels of LDL are an important risk factor for atherogenesis. The *LDL-R* gene encodes a mature membrane glycoprotein of 839 amino acid residues. Approximately 35% of patients with familial hypercholesterolemia (FH) have mutations in the *LDL-R* gene. More than 150 small mutations and extensive structural rearrangements have been detected in the *LDL-R* gene, that alter its receptor function in different ways [21]. Homozygosity in the *Pvu* II-polymorphism of *LDL-R* gene results in lower plasma levels of cholesterol in carriers of the *ApoE2* allele, but higher cholesterol levels in carriers of the *ApoE4* allele [55].

5. HEMOSTASIS- AND THROMBOSIS-RELATED GENETIC MARKERS OF PREDISPOSITION TO ARTERIAL THROMBOSIS

Under physiologic conditions, procoagulant and anticoagulant mechanisms ensure that the production and inhibition of thrombin are in equilibrium. There are two major anticoagulant mechanisms involved in the suppression of excessive thrombin generation: (i) The antithrombin pathway: Antithrombin forms an inactive complex with thrombin, which is then rapidly removed from the circulation; (ii) The protein C pathway: Activated protein C (APC), together with its cofactor protein S, suppress the major positive feedback mechanism in coagulation by inactivating FVa and FVIIIa [56]. Low antithrombin levels and factor V gene (*FV*) Leiden mutation are significant risk factors for advanced atherogenesis [11]. APC resistance (APC-R) caused by "acquired" antibodies against APC is a potential cause for severe AT and VT [57]. Acquired APC-R, which is independent of *FV* gene mutation, can also be derived from protein C deficiency or the presence of lupus anticoagulant (LAC), and is a prominent risk predictor for advanced atherosclerosis and CAD [58].

Elevated plasma levels of thrombotic and fibrino-lytic markers, such as fibrinogen, plasminogen activator inhibitor-1 (PAI-1), coagulation factors FVII and FVIII, are all important risk factors for AT [9]. These hemostatic markers may be useful in understanding the pathophysiology underlying AT, and in identifying subjects at high risk for recurrent CHD and stroke.

Factor V (FV) gene: The G1691A (Leiden) mutation in the coagulation *FV* gene, which replaces arginine 506 in the APC cleavage site of FV with glutamine, is responsible for poor response or *resistance to activated protein C* (APC-R) in more than 90% of thrombotic cases [59]. Factor V Leiden (*FVL*; R506Q) mutation or APC-R is an anticoagulant defect that is correlated with VT. In addition, *FVL* mutation or APC-R also increases the risk for AT among patients with a history of CHD or primary hypertension (PH) [60–62]. Heterozygosity for the *FVL* mutation is associated with 5–10 fold increase in risk of thrombosis [59]. Some other studies did not identify association of *FVL* mutation or APC-R with CHD [58, 63–72].

An interaction between *FVL* mutation and "environmental" risk factors leads to AT and VT [73–75]. Nongenetic determinants of APC-R include behavioral, hormonal, and environmental factors, some of which are potentially modifiable. Among current smokers, *FVL* mutation increases the risk for MI, as well as early complications after AMI [73, 76]. The *FVL* mutation is also correlated with risk of ischemic stroke; this association is even greater in women, possibly due to an interaction of the *FVL* genotype with female hormones [77].

Despite the absence of *FVL* mutation, "acquired" APC-R has been observed during pregnancy, in patients on oral contraceptives, in patients with ischemic stroke, and in the presence of aPL antibodies [78–83]. Although estrogen replacement therapy (ERT) may reduce the risk of AT for individuals with normal ("wildtype") *FV* genotype, exogenous estrogens can result in acquired APC-R that promotes atherosclerotic AT, VT, unstable angina, CHD, ischemic stroke, and osteonecrosis in heterozygous carriers of *FVL* mutation [84, 85].

Prothrombin (PT) gene: The G20210A transition in the 3'-noncoding region of prothrombin (*PT*) gene, which is a regulatory site for gene expression, results in increased risk for CHD [86–89]. This genetic variation is correlated with elevated plasma levels of PT (also known as coagulation factor II), excessive thrombin generation, and increased risk for MI in carriers [89].

Some studies did not confirm an association of the *PT* G20210A mutation alone with CHD, but detected increased risks for MI in individuals with additional major cardiovascular risk factor(s), such as smoking, hypertension, diabetes mellitus, obesity, high plasma Lp(a) levels, or high apoA-I/apoB ratios [2, 86, 90, 91]. Some other studies did not detect any association between the *PT* G20210A mutation and AT [92–94].

Factor VII (FVII) gene: Coagulation FVII, a glycoprotein synthesized principally in the liver, is a serine protease and a vitamin K-dependent coagulation factor. Coagulation defects resulted from elevated levels of plasma FVII are associated with increased risk of MI [95–98]. High plasma levels of FVII provide a link between hypertriglyceridemia and vascular risk [99]. Other studies did not support the association of *FVII* gene polymorphisms with AT [100].

A genetic variant R353Q (G353A) in exon 8 of the *FVII* gene is correlated with plasma FVII levels. Homozygous 353R allele of the *FVII* gene is associated with higher levels of FVII, which are not a causal determinant of AT [101, 102]. A 10-bp insertion/deletion (I/D) polymorphism in the promoter (–323) region of *FVII* gene, which is in linkage disequilibrium with the R353Q polymorphism [103], is associated with reduced transcription activity and lower plasma FVII levels [104], which are also not a causal determinant for AT [102]. Thus, the predictive value of FVII testing for AT remains uncertain.

Plasminogen activator inhibitor-1 (PAI-1) gene: PAI-1 is a 50-kDa glycoprotein that belongs to the superfamily of serine protease inhibitors. Elevated levels of PAI-1 are found in individuals with CAD and type II diabetes mellitus [105]. Elevated PAI-1 activity is associated with reduced plasma fibrinolytic activity, that increases the risk of CHD [106]. The plasma level of PAI-1, which is related to the extend of atherosclerosis in the vessel wall, is a reliable predictor of coronary events in patients with angina pectoris.

A common 4/5-guanine (4G/5G) polymorphism in the promoter (–675) region of the *PAI-1* gene, which influences its transcriptional activity and plasma PAI-1 activity, is associated with risk of premature MI and stroke [107]. The promoter 4G-allele specifically increases the basal transcription of *PAI-1* due to a differential binding of transcription factors to the polymorphic site, that results in elevated plasma PAI-1 activity [107]. Increase in plasma PAI-1 activity results in impaired endogenous fibrinolytic function that predisposes to CAD. Homozygous 4G/4G genotype of the *PAI-1* promoter is a risk factor for the development of CAD in type II diabetes mellitus [105].

Homozygous 4G/4G genotype of the *PAI-1* promoter is also associated with a family history of MI [108]. Homozygous 4G/4G genotype of *PAI-1* increases the risk for AT in individuals with inherited protein S (PS) deficiency, but is not associated with thrombosis in individuals without PS deficiency [109]. Other studies did not identify the 4G-polymorphism of *PAI-1* as a risk factor for AT [71, 110].

b-fibrinogen (β-Fg) gene: Fibrinogen (Fg) is a glycoprotein comprising pairs of three non-identical polypeptides: α, β and γ chains. The genes encoding these Fg polypeptides lie within a 50-kb region, and the direction of transcription of the β-*Fg* gene is opposite to that of the other two genes. High plasma levels of Fg result in a hypercoagulable state, that is strongly associated with advanced stenotic atherosclerosis and increased risk for MI or stroke [11, 111]. Both genetic and environmental factors contribute to plasma Fg levels, which increase with age, menopause, hypertension, and obesity. Plasma Fg concentrations are also positively correlated with total cholesterol and LDL-C levels, but are inversely correlated with HDL-C levels, exercise, and the use of hormone replacement therapy (HRT). G(-455)A polymorphism in the promoter region of β-*Fg* gene is associated with high plasma Fg levels, progression of coronary atherosclerosis, and increased risk of CHD [112, 113], and ischemic stroke [35]. In addition, G448A polymorphism in the β-*Fg* gene is correlated with fibrinogen levels in males [114].

Thrombomodulin (TM) gene: Thrombomodulin

(TM), a transmembrane glycoprotein expressed mainly on the endothelial surface of blood vessels, functions as a receptor for thrombin. Thrombin, the key enzyme in blood coagulation, promotes clot formation, activation of platelets, activation of FV and FVIII, that are involved in atherogenesis and arterial thrombus formation. The thrombin-TM complex is much more efficient in the activation of protein C than thrombin alone. Thus, TM functions as a natural anticoagulant by greatly accelerating the activation of protein C. Activated protein C (APC), together with its cofactor protein S, cleaves and inactivates FVa and FVIIIa, and results in inhibition of thrombin generation [115]. On binding to TM, thrombin undergoes conformational change and loses most of its procoagulant properties, such as its ability to cleave Fg and activate platelets [116].

G127A mutation in the *TM* gene leading to A25T substitution is a potential risk factor for AT and VT [86]. Besides this, G(-33)A mutation in the promoter region of *TM* gene is associated with increased risk for AT [117]. In addition, a frameshift insertion mutation (1589insT) in the TM gene was detected in a kindred with premature MI. This mutant TM has normal sequences for its extracellular and transmembrane domains, but an elongated intracellular carboxyl terminus [118]. This *TM* 1589insT mutation reduces the expression level of mutant TM on coronary endothelial cell surface, and decreases the plasma level of TM, that may promote thrombus formation at the site of plaque injury and the development of AT [118].

Stromelysin-1 gene: Stromelysin-1, previously known as matrix metalloproteinase 3, is a member of the metalloproteinase family, and is able to degrade many of the constituents of the extracellular matrix such as types III, IV, V and IX collagens, proteoglycans, laminin, fibronectins, gelatin, and elastin. Stromelysin-1 is extensively expressed by foam cells of macrophage origin and smooth muscle cells (SMC) in atherosclerotic plaques. Stromelysin-1 may play an important role in connective tissue remodeling by degrading fibrinogen and cross-linked fibrin clots during atherogenesis, plaque rupture, wound healing, and other pathophysiological processes [119].

The stromelysin-1 gene is regulated primarily at the transcription level. The 5/6-adenosine (5A/6A) polymorphism in the promoter (-1171) region of stromelysin-1 gene regulates its expression. Homozygosity for the 6A-allele (6A/6A) is correlated with reduced stromelysin-1 expression, lower enzyme activity, increased vessel wall thickness, and vessel dilation of the common carotid artery, as well as more rapid progression of atherosclerosis and CHD [120, 121].

6. ANGIOTENSIN-RELATED GENETIC MARKERS OF PREDISPOSITION TO ARTERIAL THROMBOSIS

AMI is thought to result from the rupture of a susceptible atherosclerotic plaque rich in tissue factor (TF), which is a cell surface receptor mediating cellular initiation of the coagulation serine protease cascades [122]. TF plays a pivotal role with certain other cellular receptors in the initiation and regulation of coagulation, hemostasis, thrombogenesis, and some thrombohemorrhagic diseases [123, 124]. Susceptible plaques, which are weakened by internal proteolysis of the fibrous cap, are rendered more susceptible to rupture by hypertensive flow and pressure. Essential hypertension is clinically associated with increased risk of CHD.

Angiotensin-converting enzyme (ACE) gene: In the renin-angiotensin system (RAS), ACE is the enzyme that converts angiotensin I into angiotensin II. ACE is predominantly located on capillary endothelial cells of vascular beds, and is involved in vasoconstriction. ACE inhibitors reduce the morbidity and mortality of MI and the risk of heart failure. An *I/D polymorphism in the ACE gene* refers to the presence and absence of a 287-bp *Alu* sequence in intron 16, respectively. Homozygous *D* (*D/D*) genotype of *ACE* is associated with high levels of *ACE* expression, which increases the risks for CHD, cardiomyopathy, left ventricular hypertrophy, and stroke [125–130]. The *ACE D/D* genotype is also associated with parental history of CHD [131, 132]. Some other studies did not identify the association of the *ACE D/D* genotype with CHD [133, 134]. It seems that the *ACE D/D* genotype is associated with CHD in European and Japanese populations, but not in the US and Korean populations [21].

Angiotensinogen (AGT) gene: AGT is the precursor of angiotensin II. T704C transition in exon 2 of the *AGT* gene, resulting in M235T substitution, is correlated with coronary atherosclerosis and CHD [135, 136]. Some other studies did not confirm the correlation between M235T variant and MI [136].

7. PLATELET-RELATED AND OTHER GENETIC MARKERS OF PREDISPOSITION TO ARTERIAL THROMBOSIS

Platelet glycoprotein IIIa (GPIIIa) gene: Platelet glycoprotein (GP) IIb/IIIa, a membrane receptor for fibrinogen and von Willebrand factor, is involved in the pathogenesis of premature AMI. A common polymorphism, T1565C (*Pl^{A1/A2}* genotype), in exon 2 of the platelet *GPIIIa* gene results in proline for leucine substitution at amino acid residue 33. This *T1565C variant of GPIIIa*, also known as the *Pl^{A2}* or *HPA-1b* allele, is a prothrombotic predisposition factor for those who have family history of premature MI (with onset age before 60 years), but with no obvious conventional risk factors for premature CAD [137, 138]. In Caucasians, approximately 2% of the population have homozygous *Pl^{A2/A2}* genotype, and approximately 16% are heterozygous carriers with the *GPIIIa Pl^{A1/A2}* genotype who may also develop acute CAD [137, 139]. The clinical expression of this genetic predisposition seems to interact with cholesterol levels [138], and is enhanced by cigarette smoking [2, 140]. Some other studies did not confirm the association between *GPIIIa Pl^{A2}* allele and increased risks of CAD, stroke, or VT [141–143].

5,10-Methylenetetrahydrofolate reductase (MTHFR) gene: MTHFR catalyzes the reduction of 5,10-methylenetetrahydrofolate to 5-methyltetrahydrofolate, which is a cofactor required for the methylation of homocysteine to methionine. A common C677T variant in the *MTHFR* gene yields an A223V substitution which results in thermolabile MTHFR phenotype, reduced enzymatic activity, and mild elevation in homocysteine levels [144]. The prevalence of homozygous *MTHFR* C677T missense mutation is approximately 10% in the general population. Homozygous *MTHFR* C677T genotype is associ-

ated with increased risks for MI in young males, especially in the presence of atherogenic factors such as hypertension, hypercholesterolemia, and diabetes mellitus.

Although homozygosity for the C677T mutation in *MTHFR* gene is associated with high plasma homocysteine level and low plasma folate level, the role of this mutation as a predisposing factor for CHD is disputed [145–150]. Recent data suggest the association of homozygous *MTHFR* C677T genotype with a family history of MI [151]. In addition, the prevalence of MTHFR C677T homozygosity is significantly higher among premature MI patients [2].

Selectin genes: Selectins, one class of cell adhesion proteins (CAM) expressed on the vascular endothelial cell surface, are designated according to the cell type on which originally identified: E-selectin for endothelium, P-selectin for platelets, and L-selectin for lymphocytes.

Selectins are involved in thrombus formation through the coagulation pathway with leukocyte integrins, as well as in platelet adhesion and aggregation with β_1– and β_3–integrins. E- and P-selectins bind to common carbohydrates sites such as sialylated Lewis x (sLe^x)-related structures, sulfated polysaccharides, phosphated monosaccharides and polysaccharides [152]. E-selectin participates in the adhesion of neutrophils, monocytes, and a subpopulation of memory T lymphocytes to endothelial cells that have been activated by cytokines or bacterial endotoxin. The S128R variant of E-selectin is correlated to CHD [134]. Other studies, however, did not identify the association of selectins in atherosclerosis and CHD [153, 154]. Although the plasma concentration of E-selectin is elevated in the presence of clinically relevant atherosclerosis, it is not a reliable indicator of a complicated atherosclerotic plaque [155].

Interleukin-6 (IL-6) gene: Infection is a risk factor for early atherogenesis, and inflammation may play a role in the development of CHD [11]. IL-6 is a circulating proinflammatory cytokine expressed and secreted by activated macrophages, lymphocytes, macrophage foam cells, and smooth muscle cells (SMC) in atherosclerotic plaques. Inflammatory cells release a wide range of cytokines, such as IL-1,

IL-6, and tumor necrosis factor-α (*TNF-α*), which are involved in inflammatory processes in atherosclerotic plaques and in acute CAD [156]. Plasma TNF-α increases with acute coronary ischemia [157]. IL-1 and TNF-α induce SMC in atherosclerotic plaques to express and secrete IL-6, that further contributes to vascular damage [158]. Among post-MI patients, elevated plasma levels of TNF-α are correlated with inflammatory instability and increased risk for recurrent CAD [159].

G(-174)C polymorphism in the promoter region of the *IL-6* gene may modulate the effect of environmental insults on acute phase activation, and thereby on cardiovascular risk [160]. Individuals homozygous for the *IL-6* promoter (-174)C allele have significantly lower circulating concentrations of IL-6 than those with the G allele, and might be protected from CHD [160]. IL-6 activates monocytes in vessel walls and contributes to deposition of fibrinogen. In addition, IL-6 also decreases plasma LPL levels and activity.

8. ARTERIAL THROMBOSIS IN ANTIPHOSPHOLIPID SYNDROME

Antiphospholipid syndrome (APS): APS, one of the most common "acquired" thrombophilia, is manifest as AT, VT, stroke, intrauterine fetal loss and/or thrombocytopenia in the presence of antiphospholipid (aPL) antibodies. The PL target is located on the platelet inner membrane. aPL play a major role in coagulation defects, thrombosis, MI, and ischemic stroke [161–163]. aPL cause thrombosis by inducing platelet activation and aggregation. AT and VT are the complications most likely to affect morbidity and mortality in patients with APS [162]. In patients with APS, hypertension and hyperlipidemia are significantly associated with AT [164].

APS-associated aPL are a heterogeneous family of autoantibodies with diverse cross-reactivity, including anticardiolipin (aCL) and lupus anticoagulant (LAC) autoantibodies, which are detected in a variety of autoimmune diseases such as systemic lupus erythematosus (SLE). Although Phospholipids (PL) do not elicit autoantibodies per se, complexes of PL and PL-binding proteins stimulate the production of aPL autoantibodies. The resulting antibodies can bind to PL moieties. Cardiolipin (CL) requires a plasma protein, apoH, previously known as β$_2$-glycoprotein I (β$_2$GPI), as cofactor to elicit aCL production. The presence of prothrombin (PT) and apoH are required for LAC production. LAC can react with prothrombin, PL-bound prothrombin, or PL alone. In patients with primary APS or SLE, aPL are markers for increased risk of AT and VT.

The risk of CHD is 9-fold greater in SLE patients than the normal population [165]. aPL are present in more than 30% of patients with SLE, and only a proportion of patients with aPL develop thrombosis. Because the risk for thrombosis is variable among patients with aPL, discovery of additional risk factors for thrombophilia are expected.

The aCL and LAC subgroups of aPL antibodies have distinct specificities and functional properties. In patients with APS, the presence of persistent LAC or high aCL titers is associated with higher risk of pregnancy loss, as well as VT during pregnancy and the postpartum period [166]. LAC are involved in atherogenesis, AT, VT, fetal loss and thrombocytopenia, and seem to be a specific marker for APS. Anti-PT autoantibodies occur frequently in patients with a history of thrombosis (AT or VT), either with or without aPL [167].

Endothelin 1 (ET-1) is the most potent endothelium-derived contracting protein that modulates vascular smooth muscle tone. APS may involve vasomotor disorder. In APS patients, an elevation in plasma ET-1 levels is a risk marker for AT, especially arterial stroke [168]. Thrombin, cytokines, hypoxia, shear stress, and aPL induce the transcriptional levels of prepro-ET-1 (a precursor of ET-1) mRNA in endothelial cells, that might contribute to AT [168].

Apolipoprotein H (APOH) gene: The *APOH* gene encodes apoH, which is previously known as β$_2$-glycoprotein I (β$_2$GPI), and is a glycoprotein of approximately 50 kDa with 326 amino acid residues. In patients with autoimmune diseases such as SLE, apoH is PL-binding plasma protein which provides target antigen for aPL. Predominant aPL found in many patients with primary APS or SLE recognize apoH as a target antigen [169–171].

Polymorphism in the *APOH* gene is a significant determinant of interindividual variations in plasma apoH concentration, that may affect the generation of anti-apoH or aPL in SLE patients [173, 173].

Two common polymorphisms, C306G and W316S, in the *APOH* gene alter the amino acid sequence in the fifth domain of apoH, that prevents its binding to PL [174–176], and precludes these individuals from production of apoH-dependent aPL antibodies [173–176].

Patients with anti-apoH may have increased risk of clinical complications of the APS [177, 178], as well as higher risk of recurrent thrombotic events and pregnancy loss [166, 179–181]. The presence of anti-apoH is significantly associated with VT, but not AT [177]. Patients with high aCL and LAC titers have increased risk for AT, whereas those without LAC do not develop AT [182].

Oxidized low-density lipoprotein (OxLDL) antibodies in APS: Oxidation of LDL plays a role in the initiation and progression of atherosclerosis [183]. OxLDL is present in atherosclerotic lesions [184], chronic periaortitis [185], progressive carotid atherosclerosis [186, 187], and SLE, but not in normal arteries. OxLDL is more immunogenic than its native counterpart in eliciting anti-OxLDL antibodies. Because LDL contains both PL and apoB, anti-OxLDL might be considered as aPL and represent a distinct subset of autoantibodies [188]. In SLE, there is cross-reaction between anti-OxLDL and some but not all aCL [184, 188].

Anti-OxLDL induce progression of atherosclerosis and increase the risk for CAD and MI [166, 188–190]. Patients with anti-OxLDL have higher risk for AT, but lower risk for thrombocytopenia [165]. Because the anti-OxLDL titers are elevated in APS patients with a history of AT, anti-OxLDL may be a potential marker for AT in APS [188].

Oxidized low-density lipoprotein receptor-1 (LOX-1) gene: The *LOX-1* gene is expressed in luminal endothelial cells in early atherogenesis, as well as in macrophages and smooth muscle cells (SMC) in the intima of carotid atherosclerotic plaques [191]. Changes in the expression level of *LOX-1* gene may affect atherogenesis and the development of hypertension [192–193]. LOX-1 binds OxLDL, PL, and apoptotic or aged cells. In atherosclerotic lesions, LOX-1 may participate in the uptake of OxLDL by activated macrophages and SMC, and subsequent transformation of these endothelial cells into foam cells and fatty streaks that accumulate in the athero-sclerotic intima [191].

9. MEDICAL IMPACT OF GENETIC SUSCEPTIBILITY TESTING FOR ARTERIAL THROMBOSIS

AT disorders, predominantly ischemic AMI and stroke, are the leading cause of morbidity and mortality in the US. The inheritance of gene(s) for susceptibility to AT is neither necessary nor sufficient for induction of CAD, but rather predisposes an individual to AT and makes it more likely that one will develop AT disorders. Because common forms of AT are adult-onset disorders, the most effective intervention may be at early asymptomatic stage of atherogenesis that prevents the development of clinical phenotypes. Beyond the traditional risk factors, less well-established risk factors for atherogenesis and AT are now being evaluated in clinical practice for disease prevention [11].

Nucleic acid-based testing will contribute to our understanding of the genetic basis of AT, our ability to assess risks for AT, and have a major impact on the health care. Even though common ATs are multifactorial disorders that involve both genetic and environmental risk factors, it may be possible to use polymorphic genetic markers to classify different kinds of AT disorders according to genetic defects, and then to assess the risks for subsets of vascular disorders. If genetic tests are readily available for assessing the state of balance between intravascular thrombosis and anticoagulation, more customized and efficient therapy will be developed for the management of CHD. By developing effective genetic susceptibility testing for risk assessment, it may be possible to implement efficient screening procedures, effective preventive measures, and pharmacological intervention by altering one or more of the pathological causes.

REFERENCES

1. Nora JJ, Lortscher RH, Spangler RD, Nora AH, Kimberling WJ. Genetic epidemiologic study of early onset ischemic heart disease. Circulation 1980;61:503–8.
2. Inbal A, Freimark D, Modan B, Chetrit A, Matetzky S, Rosenberg N, Dardik R, Baron Z, Seligsohn U. Syn-

ergistic effects of prothrombotic polymorphisms and atherogenic factors on the risk of myocardial infarction in young males. Blood 1999;93:2186–90.

3. Falconer DS. Introduction to quantitative genetics, 2nd edn., London: Longman, 1991.

4. Di Minno G, Grandone E, Margaglione H. Clinical relevance of polymorphic markers of arterial thrombosis. Thromb Haemost 1997;78:462–6.

5. Hegele RA. Dyslipidaemia and coronary heart disease: nature vs nurture. Br J Hosp Med 1995;54:142–6.

6. Ridker PM. Fibrinolytic and inflammatory markers for arterial occlusion: the evolving epidemiology of thrombosis and hemostasis. Thromb Haemost 1997a;78:53–9.

7. Siscovick D, Schwartz S, Rosendaal F, Psaty B. Thrombosis in the young: effect of atherosclerotic risk factors on the risk of myocardial infarction associated with prothrombotic factors. Thromb Haemost 1997;78:7–12.

8. Humphries S, Panahloo A, Montgomery H, Green F, Yudkin J. Gene-environment interaction in the determination of levels of haemostatic variables involved in thrombosis and fibrinolysis. Thromb Haemost 1997;78:457–61.

9. Ridker PM, Antman EM. Pathogenesis and pathology of coronary heart disease syndromes. J thrombosis Thrombolysis 1999;8:167–89.

10. Gonzalez ER, Kannewurf BS. Atherosclerosis: a unifying disorder with diverse manifestations. Am J Health-Syst Pharm 1998;55 (Suppl. 1) S4–7.

11. Willeit J, Kiechl S, Oberhollenzer F, Rungger G, Egger G, Bonora E, Mitterer M, Muggeo M. Distinct risk profiles of early and advanced atherosclerosis: prospective results from the Bruneck study. Arterioscler Thromb Vasc Biol 2000;20:529–37.

12. Moss AJ, Goldstein RE, Marder VJ, Sparks CE, Oakes D, Greeberg H, et al. Thrombogenic factors and recurrent coronary events. Circulation 1999;99:2517–22.

13. Davies MJ. Pathology of arterial thrombosis. Brit Med Bulletin 1994;50:789–802.

14. Wu KK. Platelet activation mechanisms and markers in arterial thrombosis. J Intern Med 1996;239:17–34.

15. Becker RC. Thrombosis and the role of the platelet. Am J Cardiol 1999;83:3E-6E.

16. Roberts WC, Buja LM. The frequency and significance of coronary arterial thrombi and other observations in fatal acute myocardial infarction: a study of 107 necropsy patients. Am J Med 1972;52:425–43.

17. McLean JW, Tomlinson JE, Kuang WJ, Eaton DL, Chen EY, Fless GM, et al. cDNA sequence of human apolipoprotein (a) is homologous to plasminogen. Nature 1987;330:132–7.

18. Kratzin H, Armstrong VW, Niehaus M, Hilschmann N, Seidel D. Structural relationship of an apolipoprotein (a) phenotype (570 kDa) to plasminogen: homologous kringle domains are linked by carbohydrate-rich regions. Hoppe-Seylers Z. Biol Chem 1987;368:1533–44.

19. Boerwinkle E, Leffet CC, Lin J, Lackner C, Chiesa G, Hobbs HH. Apolipoprotein (a) gene accounts for greater than 90% of the variation in plasma lipoprotein (a) concentrations. J Clin Invest 1992;90:52–60.

20. Kim JQ, Song JH, Lee MM, Park YB, Chung HK, Tchai BS, Kim SI. Evaluation of Lp(a) as a risk factor of coronary artery disease in the Korean population. Ann Clin Biochem 1992;29:226–8.

21. Kim JQ, Song JH, Park YB, Hong SH. Molecular bases of coronary heart disease in Koreans. J Korean Med Sci 1998;13:1–15.

22. Wang KL, Tam C, McCredie RM, Wilken DEL. Determinants of severity of coronary heart disease in Australian men and women. Circulation 1994;89:1974–81.

23. Miles LA, Fless GM, Levin EG, Scanu AM, Plow EF. A potential basis for the thrombotic risks associated with lipoprotein(a). Nature 1989;339:301–3.

24. Ridker PM, Hennekens CH, Stampfer MJ. A prospective study of lipoprotein(a) and the risk of myocardial infarction. JAMA 1993;270:2195–9.

25. Schonfeld G. Genetic variation of apolipoprotein B can produce both low and high levels of apoB-containing lipoproteins in plasma. Can J Cardiol 1995;11 (Suppl G):86G-92G.

26. Brunzell JD, Sniderman Ad, Albers JJ, Kwiterowich PQ Jr. Apoprotein B and A-I and coronary artery disease in humans. Arteriosclerosis 1984;4:79–83.

27. Visvikis S, Cambou JP, Arveiler D, Evans AE, Parra HJ, Aguillon D, et al. Apolipoprotein B signal peptide polymorphism in patients with myocardial infarction and controls. Hum Genet 1993;90:561–5.

28. Renges HH, Wile DB, McKeigue PM, Marmot MG, Humphries SE. Apolipoprotein B gene polymorphisms are associated with lipid levels in men of South Asian descent. Atherosclerosis 1991;91:267–75.

29. Hong SH, Lee CC, Kim JQ. Genetic variation of the apolipoprotein B gene in Korean patients with coronary artery disease. Mol Cells 1997;7:521–5.

30. Aalto-Setala K, Palomaki H, Miettinen H, Vuorio A, Kuusi T, et al. Genetic risk factors and ischaemic cerebrovascular disease: role of common variation of the genes encoding apolipoproteins and angiotensin-converting enzyme. Ann Med 1998;30:224–33.

31. Emi M, Wu LL, Robertson MA, Myers RL, Hegele RA, Williams RR, White R, Lalouel JM. Genotyping and sequence analysis of apolipoprotein E isoforms. Genomics 1988;3:373–9.

32. Siest G, Pillot T, Regis-Bailly A, Leininger-Muller B, Steinmetz J, Galteau M, Visvikis S. Apolipoprotein E: an important gene and protein to follow in laboratory

medicine. Clin Chem 1995;41:1068–86.

33. Wilson PWF, Schaefer EJ, Larson MG, Ordovas JM. Apolipoprotein E alleles and risk of coronary disease: a meta-analysis. Arterioscler Thromb Vasc Biol 1996;16:1250–55.

34. Margaglione M, Seripa D, Gravina C, Grandone E, et al. Prevalence of apolipoprotein E alleles in healthy subjects and survivors of ischemic stroke: an Italian case-control study. Stroke 1998;29:399–403.

35. Kessler C, Spitzer C, Stauske D, Mende S, Stadlmuller J, Walther R, Rettig R. The apolipprotein E and β-fibrinogen G/A–455 gene polymorphisms are associated with ischemic stroke involving large-vessel disease. Arterioscler Thromb Vasc Biol 1997;17:2880–4.

36. Davignon J, Cohn JS, Mabile L, Bernier L. Apolipoprotein E and atherosclerosis: insight from animal and human studies. Clin Chim Acta 1999,286:115–43.

37. Fisher RM, Humphries SE, Talmud PJ. Common variation in the lipoprotein lipase gene: effects on plasma lipids and risk of atherosclerosis. Atherosclerosis 1997;135:145–59.

38. Salah D, Bohnet K, Gueguen R, Siest G, Visvikis S. Combined effects of lipoprotein lipase and apolipoprotein E polymorphisms on lipid and lipoprotein levels in the Stanislas cohort. J Lipid Res 1997;38:904–12.

39. Mitchell RJ, Earl L, Bray P, Fripp YJ, Williams J. DNA polymorphisms at the lipoprotein lipase gene and their association with quantitative variation in plasma high-density lipoproteins and triacylglycerides. Hum Biol 1994;66:383–97.

40. Chen L, Patsch W, Boerwinkle E. Hind III DNA polymorphism in the lipoprotein lipase gene and plasma lipid phenotypes and carotid artery atherosclerosis. Hum Genet 1996;98:551–6.

41. Humphries SE, Nicaud V, Margalef J, Tiret L, Talmud PJ. Lipoprotein lipase gene variation is associated with a paternal history of premature coronary artery disease and fasting and postprandial plasma triglycerides: The European Atherosclerosis Research Study. Arterioscler Thromb Vasc Biol 1998;18:526–34.

42. Jukema JW, van Boven AJ, Groenemeijer B, Zwinderman AH, Reiber JHC, Bruschke AVG, Henneman JA, et al. The Asp_9 Asn mutation in the lipoprotein lipase gene is associated with increased progression of coronary atherosclerosis. Circulation 1996;94:1913–8.

43. Gerdes C, Fisher RM, Nicaud V, Boer J, Humphries SE, et al. Lipoprotein lipase variants D9N and N291S are associated with increased plasma triglyceride and lower high-density lipoprotein cholesterol concentrations. Studies in the fasting and postprandial states: the European Atherosclerosis Research Studies. Circulation 1997;96:733–40.

44. Tall AR. Plasma cholesteryl ester transfer protein and their high-density lipoproteins: new insights from molecular genetic studies. J Intern Med 1995;237:5–12.

45. Hayashibe H, Asayama K, Nakane T, Uchida N, Kawada Y, Nakazawa S. Increased plasma cholesteryl ester transfer activity in obese children. Atherosclerosis 1997;129:53–8.

46. Kuivenhoven JA, Jukema JW, Zwinderman AH, de Knijff P, McPherson R, et al. The role of a common variant of the cholesteryl ester transfer protein gene in the progression of coronary atherosclerosis. New Engl J Med 1998;338:86–93.

47. Kuivenhoven JA, Knijff P, Boer JMA, Samlheer HA, Botma GJ, Seidell JC, Kastelein JJP, Pritchard PH. Heterogeneity at the CETP gene locus: influence on plasma CETP concentration and HDL cholesterol levels. Arterioscler Thromb Vasc Biol 1997;17:506–8.

48. Hegele RA. Paraoxonase genes and disease. Ann Med 1999;31:217–24.

49. Humbert R, Adler DA, Disteche CM, Hassett C, Omiecinski CJ, Furlong CE. The molecular basis of the human serum paraoxonase activity polymorphism. Nat Genet 1993;3:73–6.

50. Ruiz J, Blanche H, James RW, Blatter-Garin M-C, Vaise C, Charpentier G. Gln-Arg 192 polymorphism of paraoxonase and coronary heart disease in type 2 diabetes. Lancet 1995;346:869–72.

51. Serrato M, Marian AJ. A variant of human paraoxonase/arylesterase (HUMPONA) gene is a risk factor for coronary artery disease. J Clin Invest 1995;96:3005–8.

52. Blatter-Garin M-C, James RW, Dussoix P, Blanche H, Passa P, Froguel P, et al. Paraoxonase polymorphism Met-Leu 54 is associated with modified serum concentrations of the enzyme. J Clin Invest 1997;99:62–6.

53. Sanghera DK, Saha N, Aston Ce, Kamboh MI. Genetic polymorphism of paraoxonase and the risk of coronary heart disease. Arterioscler Thromb Vasc Biol 1997c;17:1067–73.

54. Mackness MI, Mackness B, Durrington PN, Fogelman AM, Berliner J, et al. Paraoxonase and coronary heart disease. Curr Opin Lipidol 1998;9:319–24.

55. Pedersen JC, Berg K. Interaction between low-density lipoprotein receptor (LDLR) and apolipoprotein E (apoE) alleles contribute to normal variation in lipid level. Clin Genet 1989;35:331–7.

56. Esmon CT. The regulation of natural anticoagulant pathways. Science 1987;235:1348–52.

57. Zivelin A, Gitel S, Griffin JH, Xu X, Fernandez JA, Martinowitz U, et al. Extensive venous and arterial thrombosis associated with an inhibitor to activated protein C. Blood 1999;94:895–901.

58. Kiechl S, Muigg A, Santer P, Mitterer M, Egger G, Oberhollenzer M, et al. Poor response to activated protein C as a prominent risk predictor of advanced atherosclero-

sis and arterial disease. Circulation 1999;99:614–9.

59. Bertina RM, Koeleman BPC, Koster T, Rosendaal FR, Dirvey RJ, et al. Mutation in blood coagulation factor V associated with resistance to activated protein C. Nature 1994;369:64–7.

60. Marz W, Seydewitz H, Winkelmann B, Chen M, Nauck M. Mutation in coagulation factor V associated with resistance to activated protein C in patients with coronary artery disease. Lancet 1995;345:526–7.

61. Holm J, Zoller B, Berntorp E, Erhardt L, Dahlback B. Prevalence of factor V gene mutation amongst myocardial infarction patients and healthy controls is higher in Sweden than in other countries. J Intern Med 1996;239:221–6.

62. Makris TK, Krespi PG, Hatzizacharias AN, Gialeraki AE, Anastasiadis G, et al. Resistance to activated protein C and FV Leiden mutation in patients with a history of acute myocardial infarction or primary hypertension. Am J Hypertens 2000;13:61–5.

63. Emmerich J, Poirier O, Evans A, Marques-Vichal O, Arveiler D, Luc G. Myocardial infarction: Arg506 to Gln factor V mutation, and protein C resistance. Lancet 1995;345:321.

64. Ridker PM, Hennekens CH, Lindpaintner K, Stampfer MJ, et al. Mutation in the gene coding for coagulation factor V and the risk of yocardial infarction, stroke, and venous thrombosis in apparently healthy men. N Engl J Med 1995;332:912–7.

65. Kontula K, Ylikorkala A, Miettinen H, Vuorio A, Kauppinen-Makelin R, et al. Arg506Gln factor V mutation (factor V Leiden) in patients with ischemic cerebrovascular disease and survivors of myocardial infarction. Thromb Haemost 1995;73:558–601.

66. Prohaska W, Mannebach H, Schmidt M, Gleichmann U, Kleesiek K. Evidence against heterozygous coagulation factor 1691 G to A mutation with resistance to activated protein C being a risk factor for coronary artery disease and myocardial infarction. J Mol Med 1995;73:521–4.

67. Emmerich J, Alhenc-Gelas M, Aiach M, Fiessinger JN. Resistance to activated protein C: role in venous and arterial thrombosis. Biomed Pharmacother 1996;50:254–60.

68. Fang JC, Miletich JP, Ridker PM. Prevalence of factor V Leiden in accelerated forms of coronary artery disease. Thromb Haemost 1997;78:1161–2.

69. Cushman M, Rosendaal FR, Psaty BM, Cook EF, Valliere J, Kuller LH, Tracy RP. Factor V Leiden is not a risk factor for arterial vascular disease in the elderly: results from the Cardiovascular Health Study. Thromb Haemost 1998;79:912–5.

70. Dunn ST, Roberts CR, Schechter E, Moore WE, Lee ET, Eichner JE. Role of factor V Leiden mutation in patients with angiographically demonstrated coronary artery disease. Thromb Res 1998;91:91–9.

71. Junker R, Heinrich, J, Schulte H, Tataru M, Kohler E, Schonfeld R, et al. Plasminogen activator inhibitor-1 4G/5G-polymorphisms and factor V Q506 mutation are not associated with myocardial infarction in young men. Blood Coag Fibrinol 1998;9:597–602.

72. Amowitz LL, Komaroff AL, Miletich JP, Ridker PM. Factor V Leiden is not a risk factor for myocardial infarction among young women. Blood 1999;93:1432–3.

73. Rosendaal FR, Siscovick DS, Schwartz SM, Beverly RK, Psaty BM, Longstreth WT, et al. Factor V Leiden increases the risk of myocardial infarction in young women. Blood 1997a;89:2817–21.

74. Hallak M, Senderowisz J, Cassel A, Shapira C, Aghai E, Auslender R, Abramovili H. Activated protein C resistance (factor V Leiden) associated with thrombosis in pregnancy. Am J Obstet Gynecol 1997;176:889–93.

75. Eskandari MK, Bontempo FA, Hassett AC, Faruki H, Makaroun MS. Arterial thromboembolic events in women with the factor V Leiden mutation. Am J Surg 1998;176:122–5.

76. Holm J, Hillarp A, Zoller B, Erhardt L, Berntorp E, Dahlback B. Factor V Q506 (resistance to activated protein C) and prognosis after acute coronary syndrome. Thromb Haemost 1999;81:857–60.

77. Margaglione M, D'Andrea G, Giuliani N, Brancaccio V, De Lucia D, Grandone E, De Stefano V, Tonali PA, Di Minno G. Inherited prothrombotic conditions and premature ischemic stroke: sex difference in the association with factor V Leiden. Arterioscler Thromb Vasc Biol 1999;19:1751–6.

78. Amer L, Kisiel W, Searles RP, Williams RC. Impairment of the protein C anticoagulant pathway in a patient with systemic lupus erythematosus, anticardiolipin antibodies and thrombosis. Thromb Res 1990;57:247–58.

79. Cumming AM, Tait RC, Fildes A, Yoong A, Keeney S, Hay CRM. Development of resistance to activated protein C during pregnancy. Br J Haematol 1995;90:725–727.

80. Henkens CMA, Bom VJJ, Seinen AJ, van der Meer J. Sensitivity to activated protein C: influence of oral contraceptives and sex. Thromb Haemost 1995;73:402–4.

81. Ehrenforth S, Radtke KP, Scharrer I. Acquired activated protein C-resistance in patients with lupus anticoagulant. Thromb Haemost 1995;74:797–8.

82. Fisher M, Fernandez JA, Ameriso SF, Dangci X, Gruber A, Paganini-Hill A, Griffin JH. Activated protein C resistance in ischemic stroke not due to factor V arginine[506] → glutamine mutation. Stroke 1996;27:1163–6.

83. Van der Bom JG, Bots ML, Haverkate F, Slagboom E, Meijer P, de Jong PTVM, Hofman A, et al. Reduced response to activated protein C is associated with

increased risk for cerebrovascular disease. Ann Intern Med 1996;125:265–9.

84. Glueck CJ, McMahon RE, Bouquot J, Triplett D, Gruppo R, Wang P. Heterozygosity for the Leiden mutation of the factor V gene, a common pathoetiology for osteonecrosis of the jaw, with thrombophilia augmented by exogenous estrogens. J Lab Clin Med 1997;130:540–3.

85. Glueck CJ, Wang P, Fontaine RN, Tracy T, Sieve-Smith L, Lang JE. Effect of exogenous estrogen on atherothrombotic vascular disease risk related to the presence or absence of the factor V Leiden mutation (resistance to activated protein C). Am J Cardiol 1999;84:549–54.

86. Doggen CJM, Cats VM, Bertina RM, Rosendaal FR. Interaction of coagulation defects and cardiovascular risk factors: increased risk of myocardial infarction associated with factor V Leiden or prothrombin 20210A. Circulation 1998;97:1037–41.

87. Watzke HH, Schuttrumpf J, Graf S, Huber K, Panzer S. Increased prevalence of a polymorphism in the gene coding for human prothrombin in patients with coronary heart disease. Thromb Res 1997;87:521–6.

88. Arruda VR, Siquiera LH, Chiaparini LC, Coelho OR, Mansur AP, et al. Prevalence of the prothrombin gene variant 20210 G→A among patients with myocardial infarction. Cardiovasc Res 1998;37:42–5.

89. Franco RF, Trip MD, Ten Cate H, van den Ende A, Prins MH, Kastelein JJP, Reitsma PH. The 20210 G→A mutation in the 3'-untranslated region of the prothrombin gene and the risk for arterial thrombotic disease. Br J Haematol 1999;104:50–4.

90. Rosendaal FR, Siscovick DS, Schwartz SM, Psaty BM, Raghunathan TE, Vos HL. A common prothrombin variant (20210 G to A) increases the risk of myocardial infarction in young women. Blood 1997;90:1747–50.

91. Gardemann A, Arsic T, Katz N, Tillmanns H, Hehrlein FW, Haberbosch W. The factor II G20210A and factor V G1691A gene transitions and coronary heart disease. Thromb Haemost 1999;81:208–13.

92. Corral A, Gonzalez-Conejero R, Lozano ML, Rivera J, Heras I, Vicente V. The venous thrombosis risk factor 20210 A allele of the prothrombin gene is not a major risk factor for arterial thrombotic disease. Br J Haematol 1997;99:304–7.

93. Ferraresi P, Marchetti G, Legnani C, Cavallari E, Castoldi E, Mascoli F, et al. The heterozygous 20210 G/A prothrombin genotype is associated with early venous thrombosis in inherited thrombophilias and is not increased in frequency in artery disease. Arterioscler Thromb Vasc Biol 1997;17:2418–22.

94. Ridker PM, Hennekens CH, Miletich JP. G20210A mutation in prothrombin gene and risk of myocardial infarction, stroke, and venous thrombosis in a large cohort of US men. Circulation 1999;99:999–1004.

95. Ruddock V, Meade TW. Factor VII activity and ischaemic heart disease: fatal and non-fatal events. QJM 1994;87:403–6.

96. Wang XL, Wang J, McCredie RM, Wilcken DEL. Polymorphisms of factor V, factor VII, and fibrinogen gene: relevance to severity of coronary artery disease. Arterioscler Thromb Vasc Biol 1997;17:246–51.

97. de Maat MPM, Green F, de Knijff P, et al. Factor VII polymorphisms in populations with different risk of cardiovascular disease. Arterioscler Thromb Vasc Biol 1997;17:1918–23.

98. Iacoviello L, Castelnuovo AD, de Knijff P, D'Orazio A, Amore C, et al. Polymorphism in the coagulation factor VII gene and the risk of myocardial infarction. N Engl J Med 1998;338:79–85.

99. Di Castelnuovo A, D'Orazio A, Amore C, Falanga A, Donati MB, Iacoviello L. The decanucleotide insertion/deletion polymorphism in the promoter region of the coagulation factor VII gene and the risk of familial myocardial infarction. Thrombosis Res 2000;98:9–17.

100. Feng YJ, Draghi A, Linfert DR, Wu AHB, Tsongalis GJ. Polymorphisms in the genes for coagulation factors II, V, and VII in patients with ischemic heart disease. Arch Pathol Lab Med 1999;123:1230–5.

101. Doggen CJM, Cats VM, Bertina RM, Reitsma PH, Vandenbroucke JP, Rosendaal FR. A genetic propensity to high factor VII is not associated with the risk of myocardial infarction in men. Thromb Haemost 1998;80:281–5.

102. Corral J, Gonzalez-Conejero R, Lozano ML, Rivera J, Vicente V. Genetic polymorphisms of factor VII are not associated with arterial thrombosis. Blood Coag Fibrinol 1998;9:267–72.

103. Marcheti G, Patracchini P, Papacchini M, Ferrati M, Bernardi F. A polymorphism in the 5' region of coagulation factor VII gene (F7) caused by an increased decanucleotide. Hum Genet 1993;90:575–6.

104. Sacchi E, Tagliabue L, Scoglio R, Baroncini C, Coppola R, Bernardi F, et al. Plasma factor VII levels are influenced by a polymorphism in the promoter region of the FVII gene. Blood Coag Fibrinolysis 1996;7:114–7.

105. Mansfield MW, Stickland MH, Grant PJ. Plasminogen activator inhibitor-1 (PAI-1) promoter polymorphism and coronary artery disease in non-insulin-dependent diabetes. Thromb Haemostasis 1995;74:1032–4.

106. Wilman B. Plasminogen activator inhibitor 1 (PAI-1) in plasma: its role in thrombotic disease. Thromb Haemost 1995;74:71–6.

107. Eriksson P, Kallin B, van 't Hooft FM, Bavenholm P, Hamsten A. Allele-specific increase in basal transcription of the plasminogen-activator 1 gene is associated with myocardial infarction. Proc Natl Acad Sci

1995;92:1851–5.

108. Margaglione M, Cappucci G, Colaizzo D, Giuliani N, Vecchione G, Grandone, E, et al. The PAI-1 gene locus 4G/5G polymorphism is associated with a family history of coronary artery disease. Arterioscler Thromb Vasc Biol 1998;18:152–6.

109. Zoller B, de Frutos PG, Dahlback B. A common 4G allele in the promoter of the plasminogen activator inhibitor-1 (PAI-1) gene as a risk factor for pulmonary embolism and arterial thrombosis in hereditary protein S deficiency. Thromb Haemost 1998;79:802–7.

110. Ridker PM, Hennekens CH, Kindpaintner K, Stampfer MJ, Miletich JP. Arterial and venous thrombosis is not associated with the 4G/5G polymorphism in the promoter of the plasminogen activator inhibitor gene in a large cohort of US men. Circulation 1997;95:59–62.

111. Ma J, Hennekens CH, Ridker PM, Stampfer MJ. A prospective study of fibrinogen and risk of myocardial infarction in the physicians' health study. J Am Coll Cardiol 1999;33:1347–52.

112. Carter AM, Mansfield MW, Stickland MH, Grant PJ. β-fibrinogen gene –455 G/A polymorphism and fibrinogen levels: risk factors for coronary artery disease in subjects with NIDDM. Diabetes Care 1996;19:1265–8.

113. de Maat MPM, Kastelein JJP, Jukema JW, Zwinderman AH, Jansen H, Groenemeier B, et al. –455G/A polymorphism of the β-fibrinogen gene is associated with the progression of coronary atherosclerosis in symptomatic men. Arterioscler Thromb Vasc Biol 1998;18:265–71.

114. Carter AM, Catto AJ, Bamford JM, Grant PJ. Gender-specific association of the fibrinogen Bβ 448 polymorphism, fibrinogen levels, and acute cerebrovascular disease. Arterioscler Thromb Vasc Biol 1997;17:589–94.

115. Esmon CT, Esmon NL, Harris KW. Complex formation between thrombin and thrombomodulin inhibits both thrombin-catalyzed fibrin formation and factor V activation. J Biol Chem 1982;257:7944–7.

116. Esmon NL, Carroll RC, Esmon CT. Thrombomodulin blocks the ability of thrombin to activate platelets. J Biol Chem 1983;258:12238–42.

117. Ireland H, Kunz G, Kyriakoulis K, Stubbs PJ, Lane DA. Thrombomodulin gene mutations associated with myocardial infarction. Circulation 1997;96:15–18.

118. Kunz G, Ireland HA, Stubbs PJ, Kahan M, Coulton GC, Lane DA. Identification and characterization of a thrombomodulin gene mutation coding for an elongated protein with reduced expression in a kindred with myocardial infarction. Blood 2000;95:569–576.

119. Bini A, Itoh Y, Kudryk BJ, Nagase H. Degradation of cross-linked fibrin by matrix metalloproteinase 3 (stromelysin 1): hydrolysis of the γ Gly 404-Ala 405 peptide bond. Biochemistry 1996;35:13056–63.

120. Ye S, Eriksson P, Hamsten A, Kurkinen M, Humphries SE, Henny AM. Progression of coronary atherosclerosis is associated with a common genetic variant of the human stromelysin-1 promoter which results in reduced gene expression. J Biol Chem 1996;271:13055–60.

121. Gnasso A, Motti C, Irace C, Carallo C, Liberatoscioli L, Bernardini S, Massound R, et al. Genetic variation in human stromelysin gene promoter and common carotid geometry in healthy male subjects. Arterioscler Thromb Vasc Biol 2000;20:1600–5.

122. Edgington TS. Association between the molecular pathobiology of essential hypertension and thrombotic diseases. Amer J Pathol 2000;157:5–6.

123. Nemerson Y. Tissue factor and hemostasis. Blood 1988;71:1–8.

124. Bach RR. Initiation of coagulation by tissue factor. CRC Crit Rev Biochem 1988;23:339–68.

125. Cambien F, Poirier O, Lecerf L, Evans A, Cambou JP, Arveiler D, Lue G, et al. Deletion polymorphism at the angiotensin-converting enzyme gene is a potent risk factor for myocardial infarction. Nature 1992;359:641–4.

126. Raynolds MV, Bristow MR, Bush E, Abraham WT, Lowes BD, Zisman LS, et al. Angiotensin-converting enzyme DD genotype in patients with ischaemic or idiopathic dilated cardiomyopathy. Lancet 1993;342:1073–5.

127. Schunkert H, Hense HW, Holmer SR, Stender M, Perz S, Keli U, et al. Association between a deletion polymorphism of the angiotensin-converting enzyme gene and left ventricular hypertrophy. N Engl J Med 1994;330:1634–8.

128. Ruiz J, Blanche H, Cohen N, Velho G, Cambien F, Cohen D, et al. Insertion/deletion polymorphism of the angiotensin-converting enzyme is strongly associated with coronary heart disease in non-insulin dependent diabetes mellitus. Proc Natl Acad Sci USA 1994;91:3662–5.

129. Nakai K, Itoh C, Miura Y, Hotta K, Mush T, Itoh T, Miyakawa R, et al. Deletion polymorphism of the angiotensin I-converting enzyme is associated with serum ACE concentration and increased risk for CAD in the Japanese. Circulation 1994;90:2199–202.

130. Mattu RK, Needham EWA, Galton DJ, Frangos E, Clark AJL, Caulfield M. A DNA variant at the angiotensin-converting enzyme gene locus associates with coronary artery disease in the Caerphilly Heart Study. Circulation 1995;91:270–4.

131. Tiret L, Kee F, Poirer O, Nicaud V, Lecerf L, Evans A, Cambou JP, et al. Deletion polymorphism in the angiotensin-converting enzyme gene associated with parental history of myocardial infarction. Lancet 1993;341:991–2.

132. Badenhop RF, Wang XL, Wilken DEL. Angiotensin-converting enzyme genotype in children and coronary events

in their grandparents. Circulation 1995;91:1655–8.

133. Lindpaintner K, Pfeffer MA, Kreutz R, Stampfer MJ, Grodstein F, et al. A prospective evaluation of an angiotensin-converting-enzyme gene polymorphism and the risk of ischemic heart disease. N Engl J Med 1995;332:706–11.

134. Wenzel K, Blackburn A, Ernst M, Affeldt M, Hanke R, Baumann G, et al. Relationship of polymorphisms in the renin-angiotensin system and in E-selectin of patients with early severe coronary heart disease. J Mol Med 1997;75:57–61.

135. Ishigami T, Umemura S, Iwamoto T, Tamura K, Hibi K, et al. Molecular variant of angiotensinogen gene is associated with coronary atherosclerosis. Circulation 1995;91:951–4.

136. Tiret L, Ricard S, Poirier O, Arveiler D, Cambou JP, Luc G, et al. Genetic variation at the angiotensinogen locus in relation to high blood pressure and myocardial infarction: the ECTIM dtudy. J Hypertension 1995;13:311–7.

137. Weiss EJ, Bray PF, Tayback M, Schulman SP, Kickler TS, Becker LC, et al. A polymorphism of a platelet glycoprotein receptor as an inherited risk factor for coronary thrombosis. New Engl J Med 1996;334:1090–4.

138. Carter AM, Ossei-Gerning N, Wilson IJ, Grant PJ. Association of the platelet Pl^A polymorphism of glycoprotein IIb/IIIa and the fibrinogen Bβ 448 polymorphism with myocardial infarction and extent of coronary artery disease. Circulation 1997;96:1424–31.

139. Goldschmidt-Clermont, PJ, Shear WS, Schwartzberg J, Varga CF. Bray PF. Clues to the death of an Olympic champion. Lancet 1996;347:1833.

140. Ardissino D, Mannucci PM, Merlini PA, Duca F, Fetiveau R, Tagliabue L, Tubaro M, et al. Prothrombotic genetic risk factors in young survivors of myocardial infarction. Blood 1999;94:46–51.

141. Corral J, Gonzalez-Conejero R, Rivera J, Iniesta JA, Lozano ML, Vicentc V. HPA-1 genotype in arterial thrombosis – role of HPA-1b polymorphism in platelet function. Blood Coag Fibrinol 1997b;8:284–90.

142. Ridker PM. Hennekens CH, Schmitz C, Stampfer MJ, Lindpaintner K. Pl$^{A1/A2}$ polymorphism of platelet glycoprotein IIIa and risks of myocardial infarction, stroke, and venous thrombosis. Lancet 1997;349:385–8.

143. Cenarro A, Casao E, Civeira F, Jensen HK, Faergeman O, Pocovi M. PlA1/A2 polymorphisms of platelet glycoprotein IIIa and the risk of acute coronary syndromes in heterozygous familial hypercholesterolemia. Atherosclerosis 1999;143:99–104.

144. Kluijtmans LA, van den Heuvel LP, Boers GH, Frosst P, Stevens EM, van Oost BA, den Heijer M, et al. Molecular genetic analysis in mild hyperhomocysteinemia: a common mutation in the methylenetetrahydrofolate

reductase gene is a genetic risk factor for cardiovascular disease. Am J Hum Genet 1996;58:35–41.

145. Schwartz SM, Siscovick DS, Malinow R, Rosendaal FR, Beverly K, Hess DL, et al. Myocardial infarction in young women in relation to plasma total homocysteine, folate, and a common variant in the methylenetetrahydrofolate reductase gene. Circulation 1997;96:412–7.

146. Morita H, Taguchi J, Kurihara H, Kitaoka M, Kaneda H, Kurihara Y, et al. Genetic polymorphism of 5,10-methylenetetrahydrofolate reductase (NTHFR) as risk factor for coronary artery disease. Circulation 1997;95:2032–6.

147. Malinow MR, Nieto FJ, Kruger WD, Duell PB, Hess DL, et al. The effects of folic acid supplementation on plasma total homocysteine are modulated by mulivitamin use and methylenetetrahydrofolate reductase genotypes. Arterioscler Thromb Vasc Biol 1997;17:1157–62.

148. Ma J, Stampfer MJ, Hennekens CH, Frosst P, Selhub J, Horsford J, et al. Methylenetetrahydrofolate reductase polymorphism, plasma folate, homocysteine, and risk of myocardial infarction in US physicians. Circulation 1996;94:2410–6.

149. Christensen B, Frosst P, Lussier-Cacan S, Selhub J, Goyette O, et al. Correlation of a common mutation in the methylenetetrahydrofolate reductase gene with plasma homocysteine in patients with premature coronary artery disease. Arterioscler Thromb Vasc Biol 1997;17:569–73.

150. Anderson JL, King GJ, Thomson MJ, Todd M, Bair TL, Muhlestein JB, Carlquist JF. A mutation in the methylenetetrahydrofolate reductase gene is not associated with increased risk for coronary artery disease or myocardial infarction. JACC 1997;30:1206–11.

151. Margaglione M, Colaizzo D, Cappucci G, del Popolo A, Vecchione G, Grandone E, Di Minno G. Genetic polymorphism of 5,10-MTHFR reductase gene in offspring of patients with myocardial infarction. Thromb Haemost 1999a;82:19–23.

152. Jang Y, Lincoff M, Plow EF, Topol EJ. Cell adhesion molecules in coronary artery disease. J Am Coll Cardiol 1994;24:1591–601.

153. Hollander JE, Muttreja MR, Dalesandro MR, Shofer FS. Risk stratification of emergency department patients with acute coronary syndromes using P-selectin. J Amer Coll Cardiol 1999;34:95–105.

154. Paiker JE, Raal FJ, Veller M, von Arb M, Chetty N, Naran NH. Cell adhesion molecules – can they be used to predict coronary artery disease in patients with familial hypercholesterolemia. Clin Chim Acta 2000;293:105–13.

155. Galvani M, Ferrini D, Ottani F, Nanni C, Ramberti A, et al. Soluble E-selectin is not a maker of unstable coronary plaque in serum of patients with ischemic heart disease. J Thrombosis Thrombolysis 2000;9:53–60.

156. Yudkin JS, Kumari M, Humphries SE, Mohamed-Ali V. Inflammation, obesity, stress and coronary heart disease: is interleukin-6 the link? Atherosclerosis 2000;148:209–14.

157. Basaran Y, Basaran MM, Babacan KF, Ener B, Okay T, Gok H, Ozdemir M. Serum tumor necrosis factor levels in acute myocardial infarction and unstable angina pectoris. Angiology 1993;44:332–7.

158. Pang G, Couch L, Batey R, Clancy R, Cripps A. GM-CSF, IL-1α, IL-Iβ, IL-6, IL-8, IL-10, ICAM-1 and VCAM-1 gene expression and cytokine production in human duodenal fibroblasts stimulated with lipopolysaccharide, IL-1αand TNF-α. Clin Exp Immunol 1994;96:437–43.

159. Ridker PM, Rifai N, Pfeffer M, Sacks F, Lepage S, Braunwald E. Elevation of tumor necrosis factor-α and increased risk of recurrent coronary events after myocardial infarction. Circulation 2000;101:2149–53.

160. Fishman D, Faulds G, Jeffery R, et al. Novel polymorphisms in the interleukin-6 gene: their effect on IL-6 transcription, plasma IL-6 levels and an association with systemic-onset juvenile chronic arthritis. J Clin Invest 1998;102:1369–76.

161. Vaarala O. Antiphospholipid antibodies and myocardial infarction. Lupus 1998;7 (Suppl 2):S132–4.

162. Tanne D, D'Olhaberriague L, Schultz LR, Salowich-Palm L, Sawaya KL, Levine SR. Anticardiolipin antibodies and their associations with cerebrovascular risk factors. Neurology 1999;52:1368–73.

163. Kenet G, Sadetzki S, Murad H, Martinowitz U, Rosenberg N, Gitel S, Rechavi G, Inbal A. Factor V Leiden and antiphospholipd antibodies are significant risk factors for ischemic stroke in children. Stroke 2000;31:1283–8.

164. Krnic-Barrie S, O'Connor CR, Looney SW, Pierangeli SS, Harris EN. A retrospective review of 61 patients with antiphospholipid syndrome: analysis of factors influencing recurrent thrombosis. Arch Intern Med 1997;157:2101–8.

165. Johnsson H, Nived O, Sturfelt G. Outcome in systemic lupus erythromatosus: a prospective study of patients from a defined population. Medicine 1989;68:141–50.

166. Cuadrado MJ, Tinahones F, Camps MT, De Ramon E, Gomez-Zumaquero JM, Mujic F, et al. Antiphospholipid, anti-β₂-glycoprotein-1 and anti-oxidized-low-density-lipoprotein antibodies in antiphospholipid syndrome. Q J Med 1998;91:619–26.

167. Forastiero R, Martinuzzo M, Adamczuk Y, Carreras LO. Occurrence of anti-prothrombin and anti-β₂-glycoprotein antibodies in patient with history of thrombosis. J Lab Clin Med 1999;134:610–5.

168. Atsumi T, Khamashta MA, Haworth RS, Brooks G, Amengual O, et al. Arterial disease and thrombosis in the antiphospholipid syndrome. Arthritis Rheumatism 1998;41:800–7.

169. Arvieux J, Roussel B, Ponard D, Columb MG. IgG2 subclass restriction of anti-β2 glycoprotein I antibodies in autoimmune patients. Clin Exp Immunol 1994;95:310–5.

170. Cabiedes J, Cabral, AR, Alarcon-Segovia D. Clinical manifestations of the antiphospholipid syndrome in patients with systemic lupus erythematosus associate more strongly with anti-β₂-glycoprotein-I than with antiphospholipid antibodies. J Rheumatol 1995;22:1899–1906.

171. Cabral AR, Cabiedes J, Alarcon-Segovia D. Antibodies to phospholipid-free β₂-glycoprotein-I in patients with primary antiphospholipid syndrome. J Rheumatol 1995;22:1894–8.

172. Mehdi H, Aston CE, Sanghera DK, Hamman RF, Kamboh MI. Genetic variation in the apolipoprotein H (β₂-glycoprotein I) gene affects plasma apolipoprotein H concentrations. Hum Genet 1999;105:63–71.

173. Kamboh MI, Manzi S, Mehdi H, Fitzgerald S, Sanghera DK, Kuller LH, Atson CE. Genetic variation in apolipoprotein H (β₂-glycoprotein I) affects the occurrence of antiphospholipid antibodies and apolipoprotein H concentrations in systemic lupus erythematosus. Lupus 1999;8:742–50.

174. Sanghera DK, Kristensen T, Hamman RF, Kamboh MI. Molecular basis of the apolipoprotein H (β₂-glycoprotein I) protein polymorphism. Hum Genet 1997;100:57–62.

175. Sanghera DK, Wagenknecht DR, McIntyre JA, Kamboh MI. Identification of structural mutations in the fifth domain of apolipoprotein H (β₂-glycoprotein I) which affect phospholipid binding. Hum Molec Genet 1997;6:311–6.

176. Kamboh MI, Mehdi H. Genetics of apolipoprotein H (β₂-glycoprotein I) and anionic phospholipid binding. Lupus 1998;7 (Suppl 2):S10–13.

177. Forastiero RR, Martinuzzo ME, Cerrato GS, Kordich LC, Carreras LO. Relationship of anti-β₂-glycoprotein I and anti-prothrombin antibodies to thrombosis and pregnancy loss in patients with antiphospholipid antibodies. Thromb Haemost 1997;78:1008–14.

178. Romero FI, Amengual O, Atsumi T, Khamashta MA, Tinahones FJ, Hughes GRV. Arterial disease in lupus and secondary antiphospholipid syndrome: association with anti-β₂-glycoprotein I antibodies but not with antibodies against oxidized low-density lipoprotein. Br J Rheumatol 1998;37:883–8.

179. Martinuzzo ME, Forastiero RR, Carreras LO. Anti β₂-glycoprotein I antibodies: detection and association with thrombosis. Br J Haematol 1995;89:397–402.

180. Teixido M, Font J, Reverter JC, et al. Anti β₂-glycoprotein I antibodies: a useful marker for the antiphospholipid

syndrome. Br J Rheumatol 1997;36:113–6.

181. McNally T, Mackie IJ, Machin SJ, Isenberg DA. Increased levels of β_2-glycoprotein I antigen and β_2-glycoprotein I binding antibodies are associated with a history of thromboembolic complications in patients with SLE and primary antiphospholipid syndrome. Br J Rheumatol 1995;34:1031–6.

182. Noijima J, Suehisa E, Akita N, toku M, Fushimi R, Tada H, et al. Risk of arterial thrombosis in patients with anticardiolipin antibodies and lupus anticoagulant. Br J Haematol 1997;96:447–50.

183. Steinberg D. Low density lipoprotein oxidation and its pathobiological significance. J Biol Chem 1997;272:20963–6.

184. Vaarala O, Alfthan G, Jauhiainen M, Leirisalo-Repo M, Aho K, Palosuo T. Cross-reaction between antibodies to oxidised low-density lipoprotein and to cardiolipin in systemic lupus erythematosus. Lancet 1993;341:923–5.

185. Parums DV, Brown DL, Mitchinson MJ. Serum antibodies to oxidized low-density lipoprotein and ceroid in chronic periaortitis. Arch Pathol Lab Med 1990;114:383–7.

186. Witztum JL, Steinberg D. Role of oxidized low density lipoprotein in atherogenesis. J Clin Invest 1991;88:1785–92.

187. Yla-Herttuala S. Macrophages and oxidized low density lipoproteins in the pathogenesis of atherosclerosis. Ann Med 1991;23:561–7.

188. Amengual O, Atsumi T, Khamashta MA, Tinahones F, Hughes GRV. Autoantibodies against oxidized low-density lipoprotein in antiphospholipid syndrome. Br J Rheumatol 1997;36:964–8.

189. Maggi E, Finardi G, Poli M, Bollati P, Filipponi M, Stefano PL. et al. Specificity of autoantibodies against oxidized LDL as an additional marker for atherosclerotic risk. Coron Artery Dis 1993;4:1119–22.

190. Puurunen M, Manttari M, Manninen V, et al. Antibody against oxidized low-density lipoprotein predicting myocardial infarction. Arch Intern Med 1994;154:2605–9.

191. Kataoka H, Kume N, Miyamoto S, Minami M, Moriwaki H, Murase T, et al. Expression of lectinlike oxidized low-density lipoprotein receptor-1 in human atherosclerotic lesions. Circulation 1999;99:3110–7.

192. Sawamura T, Kume N, Aoyama T, Moriwaki H, Aiba Y, Tanaka t, Miwa S, et al. A novel receptor for oxidized low-density lipoprotein. Nature 1997;386:73–7.

193. Aoyama T, Sawamura T, Furutani Y, Matsuoka R, Yoshida MC, Fujiwara H, Masaki T. Structure and chromosomal assignment of the human lectin-like oxidized low-density-lipoprotein receptor-1 (LOX-1) gene. Biochem J 1999;339:177–84.

Subject Index

Apolipoprotein E3 Leiden mice 44
Apolipoprotein E4 alleles 345
Apolipoprotein H 140, 256
    gene 350, 351
Apoptosis 44, 51, 55, 58, 59, 61, 64, 65, 81, 133, 206, 207, 292
    cells 42, 156
ARA criterion 229
Arachidonate cascade 90
Arachidonic acid 92
Arginines 81
Arterial thrombosis 270, 341, 342, 344, 346, 351
Arteriosclerosis 6
Arthritis 255
Aspirin 252
Asthma 62
Atherogenesis 5, 32, 34, 132, 143
    autoimmune 6
Atheroma 41, 267, 310
Atherosclerosis 6
    autoimmune 17
Atherosclerotic plaques 29, 49, 214, 343, 348, 350
Atherothrombosis 342
Azithromycin 130, 133

B cells 7, 18, 162
Bacterial endotoxin 342
BALB/c mice 101
Basic transcriptional element binding protein-2 145
Bcl2 59, 60, 62
Bcl-xL 60
Behçet's disease 213–215, 280, 302
Bimodal pattern of mortality 255, 258
Borage oil 102
Borderline hypertension 163, 213
Bovine serum albumin 175
Bovine serum proteins 215
Bradykinin 93
DL-Buthionine-[S,R]-sulfoximine 55
Buerger's disease 321

c-Jun 11
C-reactive protein 1, 11, 81, 96, 115, 116, 119, 121, 123, 133, 161, 256, 260, 267, 305–308, 315–317, 330, 335
C1q 228, 233, 237
C3 229
C3a 233
C3b 233, 236
    receptors, 7
C3b1 receptors 7
C57BL/6 mice 18, 20, 21, 139, 233
C57BL/6J mice 10, 64, 130, 162
C5a 233, 236

Calcification 304
Carbon monoxide 51
Cardiac sudden death 257
Cardiolipin 151–153, 155, 270
Cardiovascular disease 310
Carnitine 96
Carotid atherosclerosis 11, 174
Carotid duplex 251
Caspases 59, 60, 62, 65
Catastrophic antiphospholipid syndrome 234
CCR2 receptor 20, 35
CCR2/apoE-double deficient mice 35
CD1 receptors 165
CD11b 101
CD11b/CD18 235
CD14 36
CD25 192, 193
CD3+ 7
CD36 30, 41–44, 145, 146
    null strain, 44 45
CD4 62, 268, 282
    lymphocytes 141
CD4+ 7, 21, 122, 162
    T cells 9, 192, 303
    Th1 cells, 13
CD40 21, 145, 237, 324
    ligand 145
    CD40L 233, 237
CD40L 21, 237, 310, 324
CD45RO 7
CD58 100
CD68 35, 41
    macrosialin, 30
CD8 62, 267
CD8+ 21, 122, 303
    T cells, 18
Cell adhesion molecules 151
Cell adhesion proteins 349
Cellscan 191, 192
Cellular lipid metabolism 346
Central nervous system 216, 229
Ceramide 58, 61, 62, 64, 65, 94
    pathways 55
    sphingomyelin 56
Ceramide-activated protein 57
Cerebral endothelial cells 215, 216
Cerebral ischemia 297
Cerebrospinal fluid 133
Cerebrovascular accident 329
Cerebrovascular disease 255, 273
Cerebrovascular ischemic disease 341
Chemokine monocyte chemotactic protein-1 133
Chemokines 5, 49, 115, 241